STEP-UP to

EMERGENCY MEDICINE

EDITORS

Martin Huecker, MD, FAAEM
Assistant Professor
Department of Emergency Medicine
University of Louisville
Louisville, Kentucky

Scott H. Plantz, MD, FAAEM
Associate Professor
Department of Emergency Medicine
University of Louisville
Louisville, Kentucky

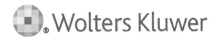

Philadelphia • Baltimore • New York • London
Buenos Aires • Hong Kong • Sydney • Tokyo

Acquisitions Editor: Shannon W. Magee
Product Development Editor: Greg Nicholl
Marketing Manager: Michael McMahon
Production Project Manager: Joan Sinclair
Design Coordinator: Holly McLaughlin
Manufacturing Coordinator: Margie Orzech
Prepress Vendor: Absolute Service, Inc.

9 8 7 6 5

Printed in the United States of America

Library of Congress Cataloging-in-Publication Data available on request from the Publisher.

ISBN: 978-1-4511-9514-9

LWW.com

DEDICATION

We would like to dedicate this book to Daniel Danzl, MD; Royce Coleman, MD; and Salvator Vicario, MD; who have respectively served as Chairman, Medical Director, and Residency Director of the Department of Emergency Medicine, University of Louisville. Over their long academic careers, these individuals have given their support, guidance, and experience to generations of emergency physicians as well as making substantial contributions to the field of emergency medicine.

CONTRIBUTING AUTHORS AND EDITORS

WILLIAM B. ADAMS, MD
Associate Professor
Department of Dermatology
University of Louisville
Louisville, Kentucky

YAMAN ADDAS
Medical Student
MISR University for Science and Technology
6th of October City, Egypt

JOSEPH BALES, MD
Resident
Department of Emergency Medicine
University of Louisville
Louisville, Kentucky

NATHAN BERGER, MD, FAAEM
Faculty
Department of Emergency Medicine
University of Louisville
Louisville, Kentucky

GEORGE BOSSE, MD, FACEP, FAAEM
Professor
Department of Emergency Medicine
University of Louisville
Louisville, Kentucky

ROYCE COLEMAN, MD, FAAEM
Associate Professor
Department of Emergency Medicine
University of Louisville
Louisville, Kentucky

THOMAS CUNNINGHAM, MD
Chief Resident
Department of Emergency Medicine
University of Louisville
Louisville, Kentucky

JESSICA DENNISON, MD, FAAEM
Faculty
Department of Emergency Medicine
University of Louisville
Louisville, Kentucky

CHELSEA GARRISON, MD
Resident
Department of Emergency Medicine
University of Louisville
Louisville, Kentucky

WILLIAM GOSSMAN, MD, FAAEM
Professor
Department of Emergency Medicine
Creighton University
Omaha, Nebraska

SANDRA HERR, MD, FACEP
Professor of Pediatrics
Emergency Department Medical Director
Kosair Children's Hospital and Kosair
    Children's Medical Center
Louisville, Kentucky

AMANDA KORZEP
Medical Student
University of Louisville
Louisville, Kentucky

KRISTINE J. KRUEGER, MD
Professor
Assistant Dean
Chief of Academic and Clinical Affairs
Division of Gastroenterology, Hepatology
    and Nutrition
University of Louisville
Louisville, Kentucky

PETER LATINO, MD, FAAEM
Faculty
Department of Emergency Medicine
University of Louisville
Louisville, Kentucky

DANIEL O'BRIEN, MD, FACEP
Associate Professor
Department of Emergency Medicine
University of Louisville
Louisville, Kentucky

**RAYMOND ORTHOBER, MD, FACEP,
    NREMT-P**
Assistant Professor
Department of Emergency Medicine
University of Louisville
Louisville, Kentucky

STEVE PAHNER, MD, FACEP
Faculty
Department of Emergency Medicine
University of Louisville
Louisville, Kentucky

MELISSA PLATT, MD, FACEP
Associate Professor
Department of Emergency Medicine
University of Louisville
Louisville, Kentucky

TIMOTHY G. PRICE, MD, FAAEM
Associate Professor
Department of Emergency Medicine
University of Louisville
Louisville, Kentucky

JAY SCHUHMANN, MD, FAAEM
Faculty
Department of Emergency Medicine
University of Louisville
Louisville, Kentucky

HUGH W. SHOFF, MD, MS
Assistant Professor
Department of Emergency Medicine
University of Louisville
Louisville, Kentucky

PETER VAN LIGTEN, MD, JD, FACEP
Chief, Emergency Medicine Service
Robley Rex VA Medical Center
Louisville, Kentucky

SALVATOR VICARIO, MD
Associate Professor
Department of Emergency Medicine
University of Louisville
Louisville, Kentucky

ERIC YAZEL, MD, FAAEM
Faculty
Department of Emergency Medicine
University of Louisville
Louisville, Kentucky

PREFACE ● ● ●

Emergency medicine is one of the most comprehensive and difficult specialties; ready knowledge of all aspects of medical training is essential. The typical 1-month student rotation in emergency medicine is often challenging because students are expected to quickly acquire a knowledge base and procedural skills to face an ever-changing array of patient problems.

In keeping with the purpose of the Step-Up series, this textbook has been written to provide residents, medical students, physician assistants, and nurse practitioners with a basic introduction to the core content of emergency medicine in a format that can be quickly assimilated for practical use in the evaluation and treatment of patients in the emergency department and quickly prepare for the NBME® Emergency Medicine Advanced Clinical (Shelf) Exam. The narrative outline allows the concise presentation of large amounts of material. Clinical features, differential diagnoses, patient evaluation, therapy, and patient disposition are discussed for most disorders. Study questions that mimic those found in the NBME® Emergency Medicine Advanced Clinical (Shelf) Examination are included with the e-book, and are accompanied by complete explanations.

The authors and editors hope that you will find the book practical and the subject matter exciting.

CONTENTS ● ◆ ●

Contributing Authors and Editors iv
Preface vi

1 RESUSCITATION

Discussion *1*
Approach to the Patient *2*
Airway *3*
Breathing (Ventilation) *9*
Circulation *11*
Specific Resuscitation Situations *16*

2 CARDIOVASCULAR EMERGENCIES

Chest Pain *25*
Myocardial Ischemic Disease *28*
Congestive Heart Failure and Pulmonary Edema *38*
Rhythm Disturbances *42*
Hypertension *49*
Syncope *52*
Valvular Disease *55*
Pericardial Disease *61*
Primary Myocardial Diseases *66*
Infectious Endocarditis *71*
Vascular Disease *74*

3 PULMONARY EMERGENCIES

Acute Respiratory Failure *84*
Asthma *86*
Chronic Obstructive Pulmonary Disease *88*
Noncardiogenic Pulmonary Edema *90*
Hemoptysis *91*
Pulmonary Embolism *93*
Pleural Effusion *97*
Pneumonia *99*
Mycobacterial Pulmonary Disease *102*
Pneumothorax *104*

4 GASTROINTESTINAL EMERGENCIES

Abdominal Pain *107*
Esophageal Disorders *111*
Gastrointestinal Foreign Bodies *115*
Peptic Ulcer Disease *116*
Gastroenteritis of Infectious Origin *118*
Intestinal Disorders *120*
Anorectal Disorders *125*
Hepatitis, Pancreatitis, Cholecystitis, and Appendicitis *127*
Hernia *132*
Vascular Disorders *134*

5 UROGENITAL EMERGENCIES

Urinary Tract Infections (UTIs) *136*
Nephrolithiasis *138*
Urinary Retention *140*
Renal Failure *141*
Genital Lesions *143*
Male Urogenital Problems *146*

6 INFECTIOUS DISEASE EMERGENCIES

Sepsis *153*
AIDS *156*
Central Nervous System Infections *161*
Sexually Transmitted Diseases (Other than AIDS) *166*
Upper Respiratory Tract Infections *169*
Skin and Soft Tissue Infections *174*
Bone Infections (Osteomyelitis) *177*
Other Infections *178*

7 METABOLIC EMERGENCIES

Sodium Imbalance *184*
Potassium Imbalance *186*
Calcium Imbalance *189*
Magnesium Imbalance *191*
Acid–Base Imbalance *192*

8 ENDOCRINE EMERGENCIES

Hypoglycemia *196*
Diabetic Ketoacidosis *197*
Nonketotic Hyperosmolar Coma *198*
Alcoholic Ketoacidosis *199*
Lactic Acidosis *200*
Thyroid Disorders *201*
Adrenal Insufficiency and Adrenal Crisis *204*

9 NEUROLOGIC EMERGENCIES

Altered Mental Status and Coma *206*
Headache *211*
Cerebrovascular Accident *216*
Vertigo *221*
Seizures *222*
Peripheral Neuropathies *225*
Muscle Disorders *226*
Neuroleptic Malignant Syndrome *228*

10 RHEUMATOLOGIC AND ALLERGIC EMERGENCIES

Anaphylaxis 230
Urticaria and Angioedema 233
Neck Pain 236
Thoracic and Lumbar Back Pain 240
Monarticular Arthritis 244
Polyarticular Arthritis 249

11 DERMATOLOGIC EMERGENCIES

Approach to the Patient with Dermatologic Lesions 254
Disorders Characterized by Vesicular Lesions 255
Disorders Characterized by Vesiculobullous Lesions 256
Disorders Characterized by Papulosquamous Eruptions 259
Dermatitis 261
Erythema Nodosum 262
Fungal Skin Infections 263
Parasitic Skin Infections 265
Viral Exanthems 266
Bacterial Skin Infections 268
Life-Threatening Dermatoses 270

12 EYE, EAR, NOSE, THROAT, AND DENTAL EMERGENCIES

Eye 272
Ear 288
Nose 292
Throat 297
Teeth, Maxilla, and Mandible 300

13 PSYCHIATRIC EMERGENCIES

Organic Brain Disorders and Psychosis 306
Anorexia Nervosa and Bulimia Nervosa 307
Anxiety Disorders and Panic Attacks 308
Conversion Reactions 309
Depression and Suicide 310

14 OBSTETRIC AND GYNECOLOGIC EMERGENCIES

Pelvic Pain 312
Ectopic Pregnancy 314
Vaginal Bleeding during Pregnancy 317
Hypertension in Pregnancy 321
Complications of Parturition 323
Vaginitis, Cervicitis, and Pelvic Inflammatory Disease 326
Abnormal Vaginal Bleeding in Nonpregnant Patients 329

15 PEDIATRIC EMERGENCIES

Approach to the Ill Pediatric Patient *331*
Pain *335*
Sudden Infant Death Syndrome *337*
Foreign Bodies *339*
Respiratory Tract Infections *342*
Otitis Media *352*
Congenital Heart Disease *354*
Kawasaki Disease *357*
Bacteremia, Meningitis, and Sepsis *359*
Gastrointestinal Disorders *361*
Seizures *373*
Child Abuse *376*

16 HEMATOLOGIC AND ONCOLOGIC EMERGENCIES

Approach to the Bleeding Patient *379*
Hematologic Emergencies *383*
Oncologic Emergencies *396*

17 TRAUMATIC EMERGENCIES

Introduction *401*
General Approach to the Trauma Patient *401*
Traumatic Shock *401*
Head Injuries *402*
Spinal Injuries *404*
Penetrating and Blunt Neck Trauma *405*
Thoracic Trauma *406*
Abdominal Trauma *408*
Pelvic Trauma *409*
Genitourinary Trauma *410*
Pediatric Trauma *413*
Trauma in Pregnancy *414*
Burns *416*

18 ORTHOPEDIC EMERGENCIES

Introduction *419*
Hand and Wrist Injuries *425*
Forearm, Elbow, Upper Arm, and Shoulder Injuries *429*
Pelvis, Hip, and Femur Injuries *431*
Knee Injuries *431*
Lower Leg, Ankle, and Foot Injuries *432*
Complications of Orthopedic Injuries *433*

19 WOUND EMERGENCIES

Stages of Wound Healing *434*
Evaluation of Wounds in the Emergency Department *434*
Wound Care *435*
Wound Closure *439*
Care of Specific Wound Types *441*
Follow-up Care *442*

20 TOXICOLOGIC EMERGENCIES

Approach to the Patient *444*
Over-the-counter Drugs *447*
Prescription Drugs *451*
Drugs of Abuse *459*
Alcohols *462*
Carbon Monoxide *465*
Anticholinergics *466*
Industrial Chemicals *467*

21 ENVIRONMENTAL EMERGENCIES

Introduction *470*
Cold-Related Illness and Injury *470*
Heat-Related Illness *478*
Inhalation Injuries *482*
Venomous Snakebites *484*
Insect and Arachnid Bites and Stings *486*

22 MEDICOLEGAL CONSIDERATIONS

Introduction *491*
Informed Consent *491*
Patient Confidentiality and Reportable Conditions *493*
Involuntary Holds *493*
Patient Transfer Laws *495*

Index 497

RESUSCITATION

Timothy G. Price

I. DISCUSSION

- **A. Definitions**
  1. **Cardiopulmonary arrest.** The sudden cessation of cardiac and respiratory function
  2. **Resuscitation.** The revival of a patient from potential or apparent death. Clinically, death is defined by the loss of heartbeat, respirations, and cerebral function. The goal in resuscitation is to perfuse the brain and myocardium with oxygenated blood while trying to correct the cause of the arrest.
  3. **ABCs (*airway patency*, *breathing*, and *circulation*).** Successful resuscitation restores ventilatory and circulatory function while maintaining cerebral viability. The overall hierarchy of management during resuscitation is directed toward restoring or preventing loss of the physiologic systems most immediately responsible for supporting cerebral function. Some scenarios are best approached C-A-B, others A-B-C.
     a. **Airway.** A patent airway is necessary for gas exchange.
     b. **Breathing.** Airway patency alone does not ensure adequate ventilation. Breathing involves oxygenation of the blood and elimination of carbon dioxide (see Clinical Pearl 1-1).
     c. **Hypoventilation** may occur if any aspect of normal ventilatory control is disrupted. The chemoreceptors, brain stem, and effector neurons are sensitive to prolonged hypoxia and acidosis. The spinal column, chest wall, and lung parenchyma may all be affected by ischemia, acidosis, or traumatic injury.
     d. **Circulation.** Circulatory function is necessary to distribute oxygen to, and remove carbon dioxide from, distal end organs. Circulatory failure represents either inadequate blood volume or inadequate pump function.

- **B. Prognosis.** The general outcome of cardiac arrest is poor. Factors influencing outcome include the time between arrest and the institution of therapy, the type of cardiac arrest, and the underlying cause.
  1. **Predictors of outcome.** Studies of comatose survivors of cardiac arrest suggest that a definitive prognosis of poor outcome can be made on the basis of the neurologic examination 72 hours after the hypoxic–ischemic event. The lack of motor response to pain is the best predictor of poor outcome at 72 hours.
  2. **Termination of resuscitation attempts.** Resuscitation attempts may be terminated following adequate trial of advanced cardiac life support (ACLS) protocols if no reversible causes of arrest are identified and arrest persists despite resuscitative efforts. The duration of the attempt depends on numerous variables including the likely etiology of the arrest, age of the patient, comorbid diseases, initial cardiac rhythm, and time from collapse until cardiopulmonary resuscitation (CPR).
  3. **Do not resuscitate (DNR) situations.** CPR and ACLS protocols should be withheld under the following circumstances:
     a. A valid DNR order has been established prior to arrest.
     b. The resuscitation is deemed "futile" given the patient's underlying medical condition.

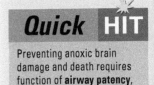

Quick HIT

Preventing anoxic brain damage and death requires function of **airway patency**, **breathing**, and **circulation**.

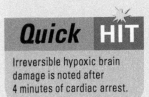

Quick HIT

Irreversible hypoxic brain damage is noted after 4 minutes of cardiac arrest.

Resuscitation

CLINICAL PEARL 1-1

Normal ventilatory control is mediated by the:
- **Central** and **peripheral chemoreceptors,** which detect changes in the pH and arterial oxygen tension (PO_2), respectively
- **Respiratory control center** (brain stem–integrating and motor neurons)
- **Respiration effectors**
  - **Neuromuscular** (spinal cord, nerves, muscles)
  - **Ventilatory** (chest wall, pleura, airways, lung parenchyma)

II. APPROACH TO THE PATIENT

A. **Primary survey.** A rapid (10-second) assessment of the ABCs
  1. **Circulation** is assessed by palpating either a carotid or femoral pulse. If no pulse is palpable, chest compressions should be performed to promote blood flow until a defibrillator is available. Cardiac rhythm should be assessed immediately with the defibrillator paddles to identify ventricular fibrillation (VF) or another rhythm responsive to cardioversion (see Clinical Pearl 1-2).
  2. **Airway** and **breathing** are assessed by visualizing spontaneous respirations while hearing or feeling expired air from the patient's airway. Head tilt and chin lift procedures may be performed for patients without risk of cervical spine injury. If spontaneous respirations are not present, ventilation should be assisted by mouth-to-mask or bag-valve-mask breathing.
  3. **Secondary survey.** More definitive management of the **ABCs** and **investigating the underlying cause**
     a. **Airway.** The decision to perform **endotracheal intubation** or use **other airway adjuncts** to maintain and protect the airway must be made.
     b. **Breathing.** The **administration of oxygen** and **assessment of need for ventilatory support** with positive pressure
     c. **Circulation**
        i. **Intravenous access** should be obtained for the delivery of fluids and medications required for resuscitation. Standard intravenous access for resuscitation is two 14- or 16-gauge peripheral intravenous catheters. Intraosseous or central venous access may be obtained.
        ii. **Electrocardiographic monitoring** should be instituted, and the cardiac rhythm identified and treated using ACLS guidelines. The underlying cause of the arrest should be identified and treated if possible.
     d. **Other interventions**
        i. **Laboratory studies** including hemoglobin, electrolytes, and serum and urine toxicology should be considered.
        ii. **Bladder catheterization** with a Foley catheter should be considered to assist in fluid management.
        iii. **Nasogastric tube placement** should be considered for patients who are being mechanically ventilated (to decrease aspiration risk). Nasogastric tube placement should also be considered for patients suspected of drug overdose (to allow administration of decontamination agents).
  4. **Reassessment.** The patient should be reassessed frequently using both the primary and secondary surveys until stabilized.

CLINICAL PEARL 1-2

Early defibrillation (direct current [DC] cardioversion) is the most important intervention for successful resuscitation during known VF cardiac arrest and should take precedence over intravenous line placement and intubation. In a witnessed arrest, the initial therapy should be application of an automated external defibrillator as soon as one is available.

III. AIRWAY

A. **Assessment:** Airway management includes assessing immediate airway patency as well as determining future risk of airway compromise.

1. **Airway patency**
   a. The airway should be assessed for patency first by **looking, listening**, and **feeling for air exchange.** The patient without spontaneous respirations requires an attempt at ventilation to assess airway patency.
   b. The most common cause of airway obstruction is prolapse of the tongue into the posterior oropharynx. Physical examination may also reveal foreign body or facial, mandibular, or tracheal–laryngeal fractures resulting in airway obstruction.

2. **Airway protection**
   a. Testing the **gag reflex** is one way to assess airway protection. This method predominantly assesses the sensory afferent component of cranial nerves IX and X.
   b. A superior alternative is to assess the posterior oropharynx for pooled secretions and, time permitting, to observe the patient for the **ability to swallow.** Swallowing is the natural means of protecting the airway and clearing secretions; a patient with pooled oral secretions requires definitive airway management. Intact swallowing requires coordinated function of the sensory and motor components of cranial nerves V_2, V_3, IX, and X.

B. **Interventions**

1. **General guidelines**
   a. **Protection of the cervical spine.** All trauma victims should be placed in a **protective cervical spine collar** (this step is often performed in the prehospital setting). However, intubation is best performed with the collar off and experienced hands maintaining spinal immobilization.
   b. **Prevention of aspiration.** Vomiting and aspiration are common in resuscitation. Immediate suctioning of the lower pharynx and oropharynx is mandatory for proper airway management. A vomiting patient should be rolled to the left lateral decubitus position and the entire spine properly protected so the airway can be cleared.

2. **Simple maneuvers and airway adjunct devices**
   a. **Head tilt/chin lift.** This maneuver is performed by simultaneously lifting the chin forward while applying pressure to the forehead and is contraindicated if neck trauma is suspected.
   b. **Jaw thrust.** Applying pressure behind the angles of the mandible to thrust the entire mandible forward simultaneously lifts the tongue and epiglottis forward. The jaw thrust maneuver is the preferred method for patients with possible cervical spine injury.
   c. **Oropharyngeal airway (OPA).** Curved, hollow plastic device that is placed over the top of the tongue. Its curved shape allows the distal portion of the device to fit behind the base of the tongue, lifting it forward and preventing obstruction.
      i. **Indications.** Obstructed airway in an obtunded individual. Conscious patients will not tolerate an OPA.
      ii. **Sizing.** Compare its length to the distance between the corner of the mouth and the angle of the mandible externally.
   d. **Nasopharyngeal airway (nasal trumpet).** Soft rubber tube, 15 to 20 cm long, which is lubricated and passed through an open nasal passage so the distal tip lies behind the tongue.
      i. **Indications.** Conscious and semiconscious patients can tolerate a nasopharyngeal airway. Use when oral trauma precludes OPA usage or when an OPA may not be tolerated by a semiconscious or conscious patient requiring limited airway management.
      ii. **Complications.** Nasal trauma (sustained during placement) and laryngospasm and vomiting in a conscious patient with a sensitive oropharynx
   e. **Laryngeal mask airway (LMA).** Composed of a mask with an inflatable rim attached to a 15- to 20-cm long tube. The mask fits over the larynx the

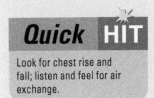

Look for chest rise and fall; listen and feel for air exchange.

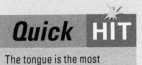

The tongue is the most common cause of airway obstruction.

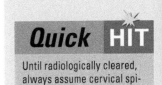

Until radiologically cleared, always assume cervical spinal trauma.

Resuscitation

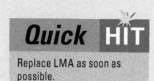

Quick HIT

Replace LMA as soon as possible.

Quick HIT

Intubation is the treatment of choice to maintain a patent airway.

Quick HIT

In children, the diameter of the tube is calculated by adding 16 to the patient's age and dividing by 4.

Quick HIT

Maintain cervical immobilization when spinal instability is of concern (e.g., in trauma victims).

same way a face mask fits over the nose and mouth. The tube communicates with the mask allowing for direct ventilation of the larynx or trachea.

  i. **Indications.** The LMA is very easy to place, even in the neutral position, and is indicated when the airway cannot be secured by endotracheal intubation in an unconscious patient. This device does not protect the airway from aspiration and should be replaced as soon as possible with an endotracheal tube.

  ii. Although the LMA is used frequently in the operating room, this adjunct is not commonly used in the emergency department.

3. **Intubation.** A more secure airway than simple interventions. The treatment of choice for any patient who is unable to safely maintain a patent airway or who cannot sustain adequate ventilation

  a. **Orotracheal intubation.** See Table 1-1.

  b. **Nasotracheal intubation.** Easiest if the patient is awake and spontaneously breathing. Use of a tube with directional tip control (e.g., a "ringed" or Endotrol tube [Covidien, Dublin, Ireland]) may facilitate the procedure. Guidelines for nasotracheal intubation are given in Table 1-2.

  c. **Rapid sequence intubation (RSI).** A series of steps to maximize success and minimize complications. RSI incorporates muscle paralysis in association with sedatives. Sedative agents are not as effective as paralytic agents in decreasing muscle tone, and they do not facilitate intubation to the degree provided by paralytics.

    i. **Overview**

      a) **Indications and contraindications**

        1) **Relative indications** for RSI include the inability to cooperate with intubation while awake, combative behavior, a depressed level of consciousness, active seizure activity, clenched oral musculature, severe trauma, and risk of complications resulting from intubation in the setting of head injury, stroke, or aortic dissection (e.g., increased intracranial pressure [ICP] or increased systolic blood pressure).

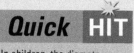

TABLE **1-1** Guidelines for Performing Orotracheal Intubation
1. **Determine tube size.** Usual endotracheal tube sizes are 6.5–8.0 mm for women and 7.0–8.5 mm for men.
2. **Assemble all equipment.** Suction device, supplemental oxygen, bag-valve-mask device, endotracheal tubes, cricothyroidotomy or needle-jet equipment, carbon dioxide indicator, laryngoscope, pulse oximeter
3. **Prepare medications.** Medications necessary for rapid sequence induction should also be assembled.^a
4. **Position the patient's head.** "Sniffing" position: with the neck flexed on a pillow and the head extended.
5. **Preoxygenate the patient.** 100% oxygen for 5 minutes. Avoid unnecessary gastric filling by minimizing assisted bag-valve-mask ventilation. The patient should be oxygenated to an oxygen saturation of 100%.
6. **Position the laryngoscope.** Handle in the left hand, inserting the laryngoscope along the right side of the mouth to the base of the tongue and pushing the tongue to the left. If using a curved blade, advance the laryngoscope to the vallecula (superior to epiglottis) and lift anteriorly. If using a straight blade, place the laryngoscope beneath the epiglottis and lift anteriorly.
7. **Intubate the patient.** Stop just after the cuff disappears behind the vocal cords. If the intubation attempt is unsuccessful after 30 seconds or the oxygen saturation goes below 90%, stop and resume bag-valve-mask ventilation before reattempting intubation.
8. **Secure the tube.** Use a syringe to inflate the cuff and attach the tube to bag valve or ventilator.
9. **Confirm placement.** Check for equal bilateral breath sounds and the absence of gastric air sounds while bagging. Carbon dioxide monitoring or a chest radiograph may also be useful for checking tube location. If any question remains regarding the placement of the endotracheal tube, repeat laryngoscopy with the tube in place to be sure it is endotracheal.
10. **Secure the tube.** Use tape or tracheostomy ties and note the centimeter mark at the mouth. Suction the patient's oropharynx and trachea.

^aIf sedation or paralysis is employed, the patient is at risk for vomiting and aspiration.

TABLE 1-2	Guidelines for Nasotracheal Intubation

1. Determine tube size. Common tube sizes are 6–7 mm for women and 7–8 mm for men.

2. Administer medications.

  a. Spray the nasal passage with a **vasoconstrictor spray** such as cocaine 4% (4 mL) or phenylephrine 0.25% (2 mL), unless contraindicated.

  b. Apply a **topical anesthetic** (e.g., lidocaine gel or a topical spray).

  c. If **sedation** is required, administer fentanyl (1 μg/kg) or midazolam (0.05 to 0.1 mg/kg) and titrate to effect.

3. Position the patient. Nasotracheal intubation may be performed with the patient sitting up.

4. Intubate the patient. Place the tube in the nasal passage and guide it into the nasopharynx. Monitor progress by listening for air movement and observing fogging of the tube. As the tube enters the oropharynx, gradually guide the tube downward. If using a tube with a directional tip control, pull on the ring to direct the tube anteriorly. If the sounds stop, withdraw the tube approximately 1 to 2 cm until breath sounds can be heard again. Reposition the tube, extending the patient's head if necessary. Successful intubation occurs when the tube passes through the cords; the patient may cough and breath sounds will reach maximum intensity if the tube is correctly positioned.

5. Confirm the placement of the tube. Check for equal bilateral breath sounds and the absence of gastric air sounds while bagging. Carbon dioxide monitoring, a syringe test, or a chest radiograph may also be useful for checking tube location. If any question remains regarding the placement of the endotracheal tube, repeat laryngoscopy with the tube in place to be sure it is endotracheal.

2) **Relative contraindications** include airway distortion (which could interfere with the ability to intubate once the patient is paralyzed) and the presence of viable alternatives to RSI.

b) **Goals.** The goals of RSI are to:
1) Preoxygenate the patient
2) Avoid positive-pressure ventilation
3) Induce unawareness
4) Prevent complications, including aspiration
5) Atraumatically intubate the patient

c) **Guidelines** for performing RSI are summarized in Table 1-3.

ii. **Pharmacologic adjuncts**

a) **Atropine** (0.01 mg/kg). Prevents muscarinic bradycardia, which can be associated with the administration of succinylcholine (especially in children). Atropine should be strongly considered for children younger than 6 years who require RSI.

b) **Lidocaine** (1.5 mg/kg administered intravenously approximately 3 minutes before intubation). May blunt the increases in ICP, systolic blood pressure, and pulse that are usually associated with intubation, and it may have other direct benefits in patients with injured brain tissue. Although the efficacy of lidocaine administration is controversial, the administration of lidocaine may be helpful and is unlikely to be harmful, and lidocaine is readily available and inexpensive. Fentanyl appears to have some role in these patients as well, with the effect of blunting the catecholamine surge during laryngoscopy.

iii. **Induction of unawareness. Sedative–induction agents** are used to decrease consciousness during intubation. Properties of these agents are summarized in Tables 1-4 and 1-5.

a) **Thiopental**
1) **Effects.** Lowers the ICP by reducing cerebral blood flow. Rapid redistribution of thiopental out of the brain results in a short duration of action and light anesthesia. Thiopental, a myocardial depressant, decreases systolic and mean arterial pressure.

TABLE 1-3   Guidelines for Performing Rapid Sequence Induction

1. Decide whether to use a depolarizing or nondepolarizing agent.

2. Decide whether a priming dose of a nondepolarizing agent is indicated.

3. Assemble and check all equipment, including a pulse oximeter, a cricothyroidotomy tray, a Yankauer suction, laryngoscope blades, and a carbon dioxide detector. Include equipment necessary for an alternative plan if the intubation attempt is unsuccessful (e.g., cricothyroidotomy, bag-valve-mask ventilation, transtracheal needle-jet insufflation).

4. Reassure the patient and describe the procedure.

5. Preoxygenate the patient with 100% oxygen. Avoid gastric filling by avoiding unnecessary respiratory assistance.

6. Premedicate the patient to block increases in intracranial pressure and blood pressure as indicated by the patient's condition. Consider lidocaine for patients in whom increased intracranial pressure and blood pressure are a concern, and fentanyl for patients in whom increased blood pressure is a concern.

7. Administer a priming dose of the nondepolarizing agent if the decision is made to prime.

8. Sedate the patient using the agent of choice.

9. Paralyze the patient using the agent of choice.

10. Intubate the patient.

11. Confirm placement of the tube by checking for equal bilateral breath sounds and the absence of gastric air sounds while bagging. Carbon dioxide monitoring or a chest radiograph may be useful for checking tube location. If any question remains regarding placement of the endotracheal tube, repeat laryngoscopy with the tube in place to be sure it is endotracheal.

12. Continue sedation, analgesia, and paralysis as appropriate for the patient's condition.

TABLE 1-4   Sedative–Induction Agents

Agent	Class	Onset	Duration	Induction Dose
Thiopental	Barbiturate	30–60 seconds	5–10 minutes	3.0–5.0 mg/kg intravenous push in adults and children (approximately 300 mg), may be titrated
Methohexital	Barbiturate	30–60 seconds	5–10 minutes	5–12 mL of 1% solution at 1 mL/5 sec (1–2 mg/kg)
Fentanyl	Opiate	2–4 minutes	45 minutes	3–5 μg/kg (approximately 200–300 μg) for adults; 2–3 μg for children 2–11 years
Midazolam	Benzodiazepine	1–5 minutes	30 minutes	0.1 mg/kg (approximately 5 mg) for adults; 0.05–0.1 mg/kg for children[a]
Etomidate	Benzodiazepine derivative (imidazole)	30–60 seconds	4–6 minutes	0.3 mg/kg (approximately 20 mg); not recommended for children younger than 10 years
Propofol	Diisopropylphenol	30 seconds	5–10 minutes	1.5–3.0 mg/kg (approximately 140 mg)
Ketamine	Arylcyclohexylamine	1 minute	10–20 minutes	1–2 mg/kg

[a]Midazolam may also be administered rectally, intranasally, or orally. Lower doses can be used to assist in sedation.

TABLE 1-5	**Hemodynamic and Intracranial Effects of Sedative–Induction Agents**		

Agent	Effect on MAP	Effect on Pulse	Effect on ICP
Thiopental	↓	↑	↓↓
Methohexital	↓	↑↑	↓↓
Fentanyl	No effect or ↓	No effect or ↓	No effect
Midazolam	No effect or ↓	↓↑	↓
Etomidate	No effect	No effect	↓↓
Propofol	↓↓	↓	↓
Ketamine	↑↑	↑↑	↑

ICP = intracranial pressure; MAP = mean arterial pressure; ↑ = increase, ↓ = decrease.

2) **Adverse effects.** Airway hyperactivity and laryngospasm following mechanical stimulation of the airway during instrumentation. Hypotension may also occur.
3) **Contraindications.** Hemodynamic instability
b) **Methohexital.** Lowers the ICP and has the same adverse effects as thiopental
c) **Fentanyl.** Rarely used as a sole inducing agent
1) **Effects.** Fentanyl appears to blunt increases in blood pressure and pulse associated with intubation and thus may be useful for patients in whom such increases could be catastrophic.
2) **Adverse effects.** Fentanyl can cause bradycardia and hypotension secondary to parasympathetic stimulation and blunting of catecholinergic activity.
d) **Midazolam.** Minimal cardiovascular effects and may blunt the increase in ICP associated with intubation. Additionally, it is a drug familiar to most emergency physicians.
e) **Etomidate.** Minimal cardiovascular effects (as compared with thiopental). Often used for induction of trauma patients. It has a rapid onset and short duration of action.
1) **Adverse effects.** Etomidate can suppress cortisol production, even with a single dose.
2) **Contraindications.** Etomidate is contraindicated in children younger than 10 years and in pregnant or lactating women.
f) **Propofol.** Lowers ICP and causes as much or greater hypotension when compared with thiopental. It has a rapid onset of action as well as rapid resolution of sedation.
g) **Ketamine**
1) **Effects.** Chemically related to phencyclidine and causes a dissociative, cataleptic state. Ketamine also has analgesic properties. Ketamine relaxes bronchial smooth muscle and rarely causes respiratory depression. These characteristics make ketamine a particularly appropriate induction agent for patients with isolated respiratory failure, especially asthmatics.
2) **Adverse effects.** Dreams or hallucinations occur in 30% to 50% of adults and 5% to 10% of prepubescent children. These may be recalled as being dysphoric. Benzodiazepine medications are given to minimize this side effect. Ketamine increases skeletal muscle tone and is associated with nonpurposeful movements.

It increases the mean arterial pressure, the pulse rate, and possibly the ICP.

3) **Contraindications.** Patients with elevated ICP and those in whom an increase in mean arterial pressure could be harmful.

iv. **Neuromuscular blockade.** To relax musculature to facilitate intubation. Neuromuscular transmission is mediated by acetylcholine (ACh), which is created from acetyl coenzyme A and choline. ACh is stored in synaptic vesicles in axon terminals and, after it is released, is hydrolyzed by acetylcholinesterase in the synaptic cleft or by pseudocholinesterase in the plasma.

a) **Depolarizing blockade.** Achieved with **succinylcholine** which binds to end-plate ACh sites and causes depolarization in the same manner as ACh. Succinylcholine results in a brief period of repetitive muscle contractions manifested by fasciculations, followed by block of neuromuscular transmission.

1) **Dose.** Intravenously (1.5 mg/kg for adults and children older than 10 to 12 years); 100 mg is the average adult dose. Dosing is increased to 2 mg/kg for children younger than 10 to 12 years of age.

2) **Onset and duration of action.** Succinylcholine is the fastest acting paralytic agent—satisfactory relaxation occurs within 30 to 60 seconds. Succinylcholine is hydrolyzed rapidly by pseudocholinesterase and as a result has the shortest duration of action of the paralytic agents (3 to 5 minutes, occasionally as long as 10 minutes).

3) **Adverse effects. Increased intragastric and intraocular pressures.** It is unclear whether succinylcholine alone causes increased ICP. Succinylcholine has also been associated with **malignant hyperthermia** and **arrhythmias** (especially bradycardia in children). Succinylcholine is associated with **risk for prolonged paralysis in patients with abnormal pseudocholinesterase levels** (e.g., some pregnant women, patients with severe hepatic dysfunction, patients with renal failure, and patients with bronchogenic carcinoma). Due to release of potassium from muscle tissue during depolarization, succinylcholine can lead to lethal arrhythmias.

4) **Contraindications.** Penetrating ocular trauma or glaucoma, patients with unstable fractures (which may be worsened by fasciculations), patients with neuromuscular diseases, and burn patients more than 24 hours after injury

b) **Nondepolarizing blockade.** Competitive inhibition of postsynaptic ACh receptors. Nondepolarizing agents cause more prolonged paralysis than succinylcholine (Table 1-6).

1) **Vecuronium.** Lacks any histamine-releasing or ganglion-blocking activity. Advantages include no fasciculations and no increase in ICP, intragastric pressure, or intraocular pressure. Vecuronium has a long duration of action; therefore, it must be used with caution because if the attempt at intubation fails, the patient will require prolonged ventilatory support using bag-valve-mask ventilation until another attempt can be made.

2) **Pancuronium.** May increase the pulse and blood pressure, although the increase is not usually clinically significant.

3) **Rocuronium.** Newer nondepolarizing agent—created in an attempt to achieve the rapid onset and short duration of action of succinylcholine. Rocuronium has the fastest onset of the nondepolarizing agents (see Table 1-6).

c) **"Priming."** Administration of a less-than-paralytic dose of a nondepolarizing agent (e.g., vecuronium, 0.01 mg/kg) to bind postsynaptic ACh receptor sites prior to the administration of a second dose of a depolarizing paralytic agent. Evidence is controversial. Priming blocks succinylcholine-induced fasciculations and their sequelae,

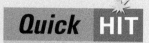

Quick HIT

Succinylcholine is associated with increased intragastric and intraocular pressures and possibly ICP.

Quick HIT

Succinylcholine is contraindicated in patients with ocular trauma, glaucoma, unstable fractures, neuromuscular disease, and burn patients.

TABLE 1-6 Neuromuscular Blocking (Paralytic) Agents			
Agent	**Onset**	**Duration**	**Induction Dose**
Depolarizing Agents			
Succinylcholine	30–60 seconds	3–5 minutes; occasionally as long as 10 minutes	1.5 mg/kg for adults and children older than 10–12 years (approximately 100 mg for adults); 2.0 mg/kg for children younger than 10–12 years
Nondepolarizing Agents			
D-Tubocurarine	1–5 minutes	40–60 minutes; longer in infants	0.03 mg/kg for children younger than 1 week; 0.06 mg/kg for children older than 6 weeks
Vecuronium	2–3 minutes	20–40 minutes	0.1 mg/kg (approximately 7 mg for adults)
Pancuronium	2–3 minutes	40–80 minutes	0.1 mg/kg (approximately 7 mg for adults)
Rocuronium	1.5 minutes	30 minutes	0.6 mg/kg

and likely decreases the onset time and duration of action when followed by an appropriate dose of a nondepolarizing agent. However, there is little evidence that priming affects the ICP or provides significant benefit when succinylcholine is used for paralysis.

IV. BREATHING (VENTILATION)

A. **Assessment.** Spontaneous ventilation requires function of the nervous system, lungs, chest wall, and diaphragm. Each component should be examined and evaluated rapidly.
   1. **Physical examination.** This component of assessing the patient's ability to ventilate can be combined with the initial assessment of airway patency.
      a. **Observation.** One should observe and palpate the chest wall, searching for spontaneous respirations and evidence of crepitus or trauma. It is also

---

CLINICAL PEARL 1-3

Techniques for Managing the Difficult Airway

A. **Cricothyrotomy.** A vertical skin incision is made over the cricothyroid membrane and extended through the membrane. The hole is dilated and maintained with a dilator, or a hook and tracheostomy tube are inserted into the trachea.

B. **Transtracheal jet insufflation.** Needle cricothyrotomy is performed by inserting a large-caliber (12- to 14-gauge) plastic cannula into the trachea, again through the cricothyroid membrane. The cannula is attached to a high-pressure oxygen source; oxygen is delivered with manually controlled intermittent insufflation.

C. **Fiberoptic intubation.** Fiberoptic laryngoscopy precedes intubation, and the endotracheal tube is advanced over fiberoptic cable into the trachea.

D. **Lighted stylet intubation.** A stylet with a bright light source at the tip is used in a darkened room to help identify the trachea. An endotracheal tube is advanced over the stylet into the airway.

E. **Video-assisted laryngoscopy.** A modified laryngoscope is used to improve visualization of the oropharynx and pass the endotracheal tube into the trachea.

F. **Retrograde wire intubation.** A needle and subsequently a long wire are passed from the cricothyroid membrane up the pharynx and out the nose or mouth, which is then used to guide the endotracheal tube into position.

necessary to feel and listen for oral air exchange (it may be difficult to hear in the setting of a noisy emergency department).

i. Patients may present with **agonal gasps** at varied rates.

ii. In the nonarrest patient, **tachypnea** is an indication that additional airway management is necessary.

b. **Auscultation.** Provides clues to possible causes of respiratory arrest or distress, including pneumothorax, congestive heart failure (CHF), pulmonary edema, pneumonia, asthma, or pleural effusions.

2. **Monitoring. Pulse oximetry** monitoring should be instituted for all resuscitation patients. In pulse oximetry, oxygen saturation is estimated based on spectrophotometric analysis of light absorption by oxyhemoglobin and deoxyhemoglobin using red and infrared light.

3. **Diagnostics.** A portable chest radiograph may aid in diagnosis of pneumothorax, CHF, or pericardial tamponade. However, acute intervention based on clinical grounds supersedes radiologic investigation.

B. **Interventions**

1. **Supplemental oxygen.** Mandatory for all resuscitation patients. Oxygen should initially be provided at a concentration as close to 100% as possible. Concentrations may be decreased once the patient has been stabilized. Oxygen may be delivered by the following methods:

a. **Nasal cannula.** Delivers oxygen at concentrations of 25% to 45% at a flow rate of 1 to 6 L/min. This device is not optimal for resuscitation due to the low concentration of oxygen delivered and the fact that delivery of oxygen requires spontaneous respirations and the actual inspired oxygen concentration depends on the respiration depth.

b. **Simple (standard) face mask.** Plastic mask with side holes that allow inhalation and exhalation of room air and supplemental oxygen. An oxygen flow rate of greater than 5 L/min is necessary to fill the mask reservoir; the recommended flow rate is 8 to 10 L/min for delivery of oxygen at a concentration of 40% to 60%. The limitations of a simple face mask in an arrest setting are the same as those of the nasal cannula.

c. **Venturi mask.** Similar to a simple face mask but modified to allow more precise delivery of oxygen. The Venturi mask is appropriate for **conscious patients with chronic obstructive pulmonary disease in whom tight control of the oxygen concentration is required.** The limitations of the Venturi mask in an arrest setting are the same as those of the nasal cannula and the simple face mask.

d. **Nonrebreather mask.** A one-way exhalation valve prevents mixing of room air and expired air with the reservoir bag of 100% oxygen. In order to be effective, the patient must have spontaneous respirations, the mask must fit tightly, and the reservoir bag must be completely filled (necessitating an oxygen flow rate of 10 to 15 L/min).

2. **Assisted ventilation.** The decision to institute prolonged mechanical ventilation may be guided by continuous oxygen saturation trends and arterial blood gas determinations to assess acid-base status and ventilation effectiveness. The recommended tidal volume for resuscitation is 10 to 15 mL/kg.

a. **Rescue breathing.** Direct mouth-to-mouth; mouth-to-mask breathing is considered optional by the American Heart Association.

i. Concern from bystander rescuers about infection transmission may limit the use of rescue breathing; however, the estimated rate of infectious disease transmission is very low.

ii. Exhaled gas contains 16.6% to 17.1% oxygen and 3.5% to 4.1% carbon dioxide.

b. **Bag-valve-mask ventilation ("bagging the patient").** Manually controlled delivery of tidal volumes—the standard of ventilation for **apneic, nonintubated patients.** Bag-valve-mask ventilation allows the operator to estimate lung compliance through the amount of force required to ventilate the patient.

i. **Components.** Clear mask with an air-cushion rim to provide a tight face seal, a true nonrebreathing valve, a no-pressure release valve, and

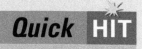

Quick HIT

Oxygen saturations of 100%, 90%, 60%, and 50% correlate with approximate arterial oxygen tensions of 90 mm Hg, 60 mm Hg, 30 mm Hg, and 27 mm Hg, respectively.

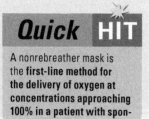

Quick HIT

A nonrebreather mask is the **first-line method** for the delivery of oxygen at concentrations approaching 100% in a patient with spontaneous respirations.

an attached bag and reservoir that may accept oxygen flow at a rate of 12 to 15 L/min for a delivered oxygen concentration of almost 100%.

    ii. **Disadvantages**

        a) Inexperienced operators may find it difficult to maintain the mask seal while coordinating bag ventilation. The use of two operators is superior for optimal usage.

        b) Large tidal volumes may inadvertently cause gastric distention, increasing the risk of aspiration and limiting effective tidal volume. Large tidal volumes also increase the risk of pneumothorax.

  c. **Endotracheal intubation.** Allows for delivery of 100% oxygen directly to the trachea and for direct monitoring of expired carbon dioxide, which may be helpful in optimizing chest compressions during CPR (see V.B.1.a.iii.c). Endotracheal intubation affords increased protection against aspiration.

  d. **Mechanical positive-pressure ventilation.** Allows maximal control of the tidal volume and airway pressures, decreasing the risk of barotrauma, and is the optimal method of ventilating unconscious patients. However, this method of ventilation may be difficult to initiate during the immediate resuscitation phase.

C. **Failure to oxygenate or ventilate** may occur for multiple reasons.

  1. **Mechanical failure.** The ventilatory circuit should be systematically evaluated.

    a. Check for monitor malfunction/accuracy.

    b. Ensure all interventional equipment is properly positioned. (Is the endotracheal tube in the esophagus? Is the mask seal tight?)

    c. Ensure the oxygen supply is adequate.

  2. **Organic source.** Development of tension pneumothorax or the existence of preexisting conditions (e.g., pleural effusions, acquired respiratory distress syndrome, pulmonary edema, CHF) can lead to inadequate oxygenation or ventilation. Any specific cause that can be identified should be treated appropriately (e.g., chest tube thoracostomy, furosemide, thoracocentesis).

V. CIRCULATION

A. **Assessment**

  1. **Physical examination**

    a. The physical examination may provide clues to the cause of arrest (e.g., shock, pericardial tamponade, dysrhythmia, tension pneumothorax).

    b. The pulses, neck veins, skin color, and quality of the heart sounds should be rapidly assessed (see Clinical Pearl 1-4).

  2. **Monitoring**

    a. **Defibrillator paddles or pads** to identify VF or ventricular tachycardia (VT) is one of the most important steps in treating cardiac arrest.

    b. **Continuous electrocardiographic rhythm monitoring** and **noninvasive blood pressure monitoring** (updated every 2 minutes) should also be instituted, regardless of the cause of arrest.

  3. **Diagnostics**

    a. A **12-lead electrocardiogram (ECG)** and a **stat potassium level.** For patients with nonshockable rhythms (as identified during the quick look)

    b. **Immediate bedside ultrasound.** Useful in observing for cardiac activity and in diagnosing pericardial tamponade–induced pulseless electrical activity (PEA)

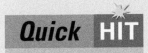

Quick HIT

Endotracheal intubation is the optimal means of ventilating the **unconscious patient** or the **patient with severe respiratory compromise.**

Resuscitation

CLINICAL PEARL 1-4

Pulses may correlate roughly with the systolic blood pressure, although these findings are not very reliable: a palpable radial pulse = a systolic blood pressure greater than 80 mm Hg, a palpable femoral pulse = a systolic blood pressure greater than 70 mm Hg, and a palpable carotid pulse = a systolic blood pressure greater than 60 mm Hg.

B. Interventions
  1. Maintaining cerebral and cardiac perfusion
      a. **Noninvasive (closed chest) compression.** Provides only 25% to 30% of normal cardiac output. Successful CPR is dependent on the **return of spontaneous circulation (ROSC).** ROSC is directly related to the ability to supply myocardial blood flow (i.e., the **coronary perfusion pressure**). Coronary perfusion pressure (CPP) is the gradient across the coronary vasculature and is equal to the difference between the aortic diastolic pressure and the right atrial pressure. During CPR, the maximal CPP occurs between chest compressions. Standard CPR provides a CPP of only 1 to 8 mm Hg, and the estimated CPP required for ROSC is 15 to 30 mm Hg. Epinephrine, which increases systemic vascular resistance and the aortic diastolic pressure, thereby increasing the CPP, is a useful adjunct in CPR.
          i. **Standard technique.** Place the heel of one hand two fingerbreadths above the xiphoid on the sternum, with the other hand covering the first. Force is transmitted downward with the elbows locked so that the patient's chest is compressed (1.5 to 2 inches for adults; 1 to 1.5 inches for children) at a rate of 100 compressions per minute. The individual performing compressions should also be comfortably positioned above the patient, with the aid of a footstool if necessary, to minimize rescuer fatigue.
          ii. **Mechanism of action.** Unknown. The two leading theories are:
              a) **Cardiac pump theory.** Suggests that the heart is squeezed between the sternum and spine, leading to the forward flow of blood. Backflow is prevented by the cardiac valves, and the heart passively fills between compressions. Criticisms of this theory are that the arteriovenous pressure gradient may be equalized during arrest and the mitral or semilunar valves may be incompetent.
              b) **Thoracic pump theory.** Suggests that the intrathoracic veins collapse with chest compression and blood is forced forward through the aorta. Backflow of blood in the venous circulation is prevented by valves located in the large veins at the thoracic inlet. Between compressions, the central venous circulation fills and the cycle is repeated.
          iii. **Monitoring the effectiveness of chest compressions.** Not currently the accepted standard, although compressions are often not optimally applied during resuscitation. Techniques include:
              a) **Invasive blood pressure monitoring.** Allows direct calculation of CPP
              b) **Assessment of central venous oxygen saturation.** May be predictive of ROSC: a central venous oxygen saturation of 72% is associated with 100% ROSC, whereas a central venous oxygen saturation of 30% is associated with 0% ROSC
              c) **Capnometry.** Measurement of the end-tidal carbon dioxide concentration correlates directly with cardiac output when the minute ventilation is constant. The monitoring device is attached to the endotracheal tube or ventilator system. Calorimetric capnometry may provide an inexpensive and readily available means of gauging CPR effectiveness. Capnography can assist in determining when resuscitation is futile, with CO_2 level below 10 after 30 minutes of CPR predicting zero chance of neurologic recovery.
          iv. **Complications.** Usually result from inappropriately placed or excessive force
              a) **Rib fractures (30%)**
              b) **Sternal fractures (20%)**
              c) **Pneumothorax, cardiac contusion, pericardial hemorrhage, cardiac laceration, gastroesophageal tears,** and **liver or splenic lacerations**
          v. **Variations or augmentations to the standard closed chest compression technique**
              a) **Impedance threshold device.** Applied between the endotracheal tube or supraglottic airway and the ventilation bag. It contains a pressure triggered valve that prevents air from passively entering

the thorax via the trachea during the decompression phase. This results in maximal negative intrathoracic pressure, recruits increased venous return, and increases cardiac output, cerebral perfusion pressure, and CPP.

    b) **Circumferential chest compression.** Use of a pneumatic vest, which inflates to compress the chest circumferentially. Circumferential chest compression generates greater fluctuations in intrathoracic pressure and increases intrathoracic airway collapse, resulting in air-trapping. Air-trapping increases the intrathoracic pressure by increasing the intrathoracic volume, potentiating the external compressive force. Use of a pneumatic vest has been shown in early studies to increase short-term survival in humans, but disadvantages include cost and availability.

    c) **Active compression–decompression.** Thought to increase the net negative intrathoracic pressure during the relaxation/decompression phase (following the thoracic pump model). Active decompression of the chest during the relaxation phase of chest compression is provided through a handheld suction cup device. A possible advantage is the simultaneous ventilation of the patient provided through chest wall compression–decompression.

b. **Open cardiac massage.** Provides up to 55% of the baseline cardiac output, as compared with the 25% to 30% output generated by closed chest compression

    i. **Standard technique.** Performed after thoracotomy by positioning the heart between both hands, with the palms at the base. Massage is conducted by compressing the heart from the palms at the apex toward the fingertips at the base. Defibrillation may be carried out with internal paddles at 0.5 joule/kg.

    ii. **Indications**

        a) Cardiac arrest in the setting of penetrating chest trauma

        b) In patients with chest deformities that preclude effective closed chest compressions

        c) In some patients with pulmonary embolism, hypothermia, pericardial tamponade, or abdominal hemorrhage

c. **Cardiopulmonary bypass.** Access is obtained via the femoral artery and vein. Disadvantages include the need for a skilled operator and for special equipment.

2. **Restoring rhythm. Defibrillation (countershock):** the passing of energy through the chest in an attempt to produce momentary asystole, allowing the natural pacemaker and electrical conduction tracts of the heart to reestablish normal function. Success is inversely proportional to the time between arrest and countershock. **Early defibrillation is the only intervention consistently proven to improve outcome in cardiac arrest.**

a. **Automatic external defibrillator (AED).** Portable device that analyzes the cardiac rhythm and automatically delivers DC countershocks if a shockable rhythm is detected. The strength of the energy (in Joules) and the waveform morphology used for countershock varies depending on manufacturer and model. Some AED devices (semiautomatic AEDs) read the rhythm but require an operator to initiate countershock delivery. The goal of the AED is to provide early defibrillation without expert training.

b. **Manual defibrillator**

    i. **Synchronized versus unsynchronized countershock**

        a) **Synchronized mode.** Defibrillator delivers the countershock within milliseconds of the ECG R wave to prevent administration of the shock during the absolute refractory period of the ECG cycle. Most defibrillators require the three-lead or four-lead monitoring cables be attached to the patient to deliver a synchronized shock (or to provide pacing).

b) **Unsynchronized mode.** Defibrillator delivers countershock on demand, irrespective of the point in the ECG cycle. The unsynchronized mode should be used initially for patients with VF or pulseless VT. It may also be used for patients with unstable VT with a pulse if an undue delay in synchronization occurs.

ii. **Considerations. Implantable cardioverter-defibrillator.** Implanted in survivors of non-myocardial infarction (MI)–related VF or VT arrest, or in patients with recurrent VT that is not responsive to pharmacotherapy. When externally defibrillating a patient with an implantable cardioverter-defibrillator or other pacemaker, the paddles should be positioned 5 inches away from the device to prevent damage to the implanted device.

iii. **Pharmacologic adjuncts to defibrillation.** The administration of epinephrine, lidocaine, amiodarone, procainamide, or magnesium sulfate may be indicated. Anti-arrhythmics have not been proven to improve survival from cardiac arrest; however, they may raise the fibrillation threshold and prevent recurrent fibrillation following successful countershock.

3. **Electrical pacing.** Maintains cardiac rhythm when contractions initiated by the natural pacemaker are inadequate to maintain sufficient blood pressure
   a. **Indications**
      i. **Refractory tachycardia**
      ii. **Polymorphic VT (torsades de pointes)**
      iii. **Bradycardia with unstable presentation** (i.e., a systolic blood pressure of less than 80 mm Hg, a change in mental status, MI, or pulmonary edema)
   b. **Settings.** In general, output is increased until effective capture is achieved, then decreased by 5 joules. The target rate should be 80 to 100 beats/min. The mode should be asynchronous in the setting of emergency pacing for arrest.
   c. **Methods**
      i. **Transcutaneous pacing.** The fastest and least invasive technique; pacing leads are applied directly to the chest wall. The ability to capture is related to the energy of pacing and transthoracic resistance. Higher energy may be required in obese, barrel-chested individuals, and in the setting of a large pericardial effusion.
      ii. **Transvenous pacing.** Requires placement of temporary pacing wires through a central vein so the catheter tip lies against the apex of the right ventricle. Transvenous pacing may be instituted after successful transcutaneous pacing.

4. **Establishing intravenous access.** Required for administration of drugs and fluids during resuscitation. The type of intravenous catheter and the placement site vary according to the situation. The standard recommendation is two 14- to 16-gauge catheters inserted peripherally in the upper extremity. Intraosseous access may also be used in emergency settings.
   a. **Complications.** Hematoma formation, cellulitis, thrombosis, phlebitis, sepsis, pulmonary thromboembolism, catheter-fragment embolism, and air embolism.
   b. **Flow rate.** Directly proportional to the radius of the catheter raised to the fourth power and inversely proportional to the catheter length. Therefore, flow rate is limited by the catheter diameter and length, not the size of the vein cannulated. The fastest flow rate has been observed in large-bore (9 French), short-length (5.5-inch) introducer catheters, which may be placed at any central access point (Table 1-7).
   c. **Circulation time.** Increased in patients with cardiac/circulatory arrest.
      i. Drugs administered centrally achieve the most rapid onset of action.
      ii. Drugs administered via upper extremity peripheral intravenous sites require 1 to 2 minutes to reach the central circulation. Delivery of medications administered by a peripheral intravenous may be

TABLE **1-7**	Flow Rates Through Standard Resuscitation Catheters	
Catheter Type	**Location**	**Tap Water Flow Rates by Gravity (mL/min)**
USCI 9-French introducer, 5½"	Central	247
USCI 8-French introducer, 5½"	Central	243
Deseret Angiocath (gauge 16, 5½")	Central	91
Deseret subclavian jugular catheter (gauge 16, 12")	Central	54
Deseret Angiocath (gauge 14, 2")	Peripheral	173
Deseret Angiocath (gauge 16, 2")	Peripheral	108

Modified with permission from Mateer JR, Thompson BM, Aprahamian C, et al. Rapid fluid resuscitation with central venous catheters. *Ann Emerg Med* 1983;12:149–152.

accelerated by following it immediately with a 20-mL bolus of intravenous fluid and elevation of the extremity.

   iii. Use of a femoral or lower extremity vein for drug administration during cardiac arrest is not recommended due to prolonged circulation time and altered blood flow with chest compressions.

  d. **Access site.** Limited by the success of line placement, the potential for interference with other resuscitative measures (e.g., chest compressions, intubation), and preexisting injuries (e.g., cervical trauma).

    i. **Peripheral sites**

     a) **Basilic** or **median veins** in the antecubital fossa. The first choices for intravenous access due to ease of cannulation, lack of interference with chest compressions, acceptable circulation time of infused drugs, and minimal complications. Access may be more difficult to obtain in hypovolemic patients, intravenous drug abusers, and morbidly obese individuals.

     b) **External jugular vein.** A peripheral vein that may be easily cannulated and provides rapid access to the central circulation. Disadvantages include difficult placement in hypovolemic patients, interference with airway management measures, easy dislodgement, and variable function with head movement (e.g., turning of the head may cause the catheter to kink).

    ii. **Central venous cannulation.** Indicated if peripheral access attempts fail, if central pressure monitoring or pulmonary artery catheterization is required, or if administration of hypertonic or irritating fluids (pressor agents) is required.

     a) **Right internal jugular vein.** Preferred over the left because it is directly aligned with the right atrium, the dome of the diaphragm and pleura are lower on the right side, and there is no thoracic duct on the right side. Intravenous access is usually obtained using the Seldinger (catheter over a guidewire) technique (Table 1-8).

      1) **Advantages.** Rapid circulation time, easier access during chest compressions, easy compression in the event of a hematoma, and decreased risk of pneumothorax (as compared with a subclavian approach).

      2) **Disadvantages.** Interference with airway management and increased rate of carotid artery puncture (2% to 10%), pneumothorax, and hemothorax

     b) **Subclavian vein.** Easily cannulated and allows for rapid central administration of drugs. Left subclavian vein catheterization is the

TABLE 1-8 Guidelines for Right Internal Jugular Catheterization (Central Approach)

1. Prepare a percutaneous central venous access kit.
2. Position the patient in the Trendelenburg position (10 to 15 degrees), with the head turned to the left if possible.
3. Identify landmarks. The insertion site is the cephalad apex of the triangle formed by the two heads of the sternocleidomastoid muscle and the clavicle. Use ultrasound to identify and guide placement, if necessary.
4. Sterile preparation and drape of the area.
5. In conscious patients, infiltrate the skin overlying the area of puncture with 1% lidocaine.
6. With the finder needle attached to a 5-mL syringe, puncture the skin at a 45-degree angle at the apex of the triangle and advance the needle toward the ipsilateral nipple while gently drawing back on the syringe plunger. Ultrasound guidance, where available, is superior to use of a finder needle in venipuncture.
7. Entry into the internal jugular vein is marked by the return of nonpulsatile venous blood into the syringe. Typically, the internal jugular vein should be entered no more than 5 cm from the skin surface. Return of pulsatile arterial blood indicates puncture of the carotid artery. If this occurs, remove the needle and apply direct pressure for 5 to 10 minutes.
8. Following successful cannulation of the internal jugular vein, advance the larger needle along the tract of, or right over, the finder needle. Some operators skip the step of using the finder needle.
9. Holding the needle firmly in place, remove the syringe and insert the guidewire through the needle. Note that whenever the needle hub is open to air, there is a threat of air embolism. **Always cover the open hub to prevent air entry.** The wire should advance smoothly. Do not let go of the guidewire.
10. While controlling one end of the wire, remove the needle. Puncture the skin at the site of wire entry with a scalpel. Some kits have the catheter over a dilator; some require a separate step of advancing a dilator over the wire before advancing the catheter over the wire. Remove the wire.
11. Attach a syringe to the line and demonstrate easy draw of blood. Flush the line and suture in place.
12. Obtain a portable chest radiograph to rule out pneumothorax and confirm line placement.

preferred route for placement of transcutaneous pacing wires. The infraclavicular approach to obtaining intravenous access via the subclavian vein is summarized in Table 1-9.

1) **Advantages.** Low infection rate and superior patient comfort
2) **Disadvantages.** Risk of pneumothorax (1% to 2%), subclavian artery puncture (1%), and interference with chest compressions

c) **Femoral vein.** Easily cannulated (the success rate is 90%). Guidelines for femoral vein catheterization are given in Table 1-10 (see Figure 1-1).

1) **Advantages.** No interference with airway management or chest compressions and no risk of pneumothorax
2) **Disadvantages.** Highest rate of infection of all central lines if left in for days, increased risk of thrombosis (10%) and femoral artery puncture (5%), and prolonged circulation time in arrest situation if the catheter does not reach above the diaphragm

VI. SPECIFIC RESUSCITATION SITUATIONS

A. **Dysrhythmias.** The American Heart Association prepared the first **ACLS guidelines** in 1974 to provide an organized algorithmic approach to victims of cardiac arrest based on presenting cardiac rhythm. In addition, **all patients with arrest caused by a dysrhythmia should receive standard resuscitation measures** (i.e., ABCs, **establishment of intravenous access, administration of supplemental oxygen**, and **monitoring**).

1. **VF.** Possibly the most common arrest rhythm. Occurs commonly in the setting of coronary artery disease (CAD). VF has the best outcome of all arrest

TABLE **1-9**	Guidelines for Subclavian Vein Catheterization (Infraclavicular Approach)

1. Prepare a percutaneous central venous access kit. Attach the needle to a syringe.

2. Position the patient in the Trendelenburg position if possible.

3. Identify landmarks. The insertion site is 1 cm inferior to the clavicle at approximately the distal third of the clavicle length. This point is also identified as the superior inflection point of the clavicle and is just lateral to the insertion of the sternocleidomastoid muscle on the clavicle.

4. Sterile preparation and drape.

5. Infiltrate the skin at the insertion point with 1% lidocaine. Direct the needle down to the clavicle and infiltrate the periosteum with 1% lidocaine.

6. Insert and advance the needle parallel to the skin along a horizontal line between the shoulders toward the sternal notch. Apply gentle back pressure on the syringe plunger while advancing the needle. The needle should just skirt the clavicle (on the underside) while being advanced toward the sternal notch.

7. Entry into the subclavian vein is marked by the return of nonpulsatile venous blood. Sudden aspiration of air is a marker of entry into the pleural space and indicates induction of a pneumothorax. In the event of pneumothorax, remove the needle, obtain a stat chest radiograph, and prepare to perform tube thoracostomy.

8. Following successful cannulation of the subclavian vein, advance the needle several millimeters so that the tip is in the lumen of the vein.

9. Holding the needle firmly in place, remove the syringe and insert the guidewire through the needle. Note that whenever the needle hub is open to air, there is a threat of air embolism. **Always cover the open hub to prevent air entry.** The wire should advance smoothly. Do not let go of the guidewire.

10. While controlling one end of the wire, remove the needle. Puncture the skin with a scalpel at the site of wire entry. Some kits have the catheter over a dilator; some require a separate step of advancing a dilator over the wire before advancing the catheter over the wire. Remove the wire.

11. Attach a syringe to the line and demonstrate easy draw of blood. Flush the line with heparin solution or initiate fluid flow through the line and suture in place.

12. Obtain a portable chest radiograph to rule out pneumothorax and confirm line placement.

rhythms because of its responsiveness to DC countershock; the survival rate associated with VF arrest is estimated at 15%.

  a. **Clinical evaluation**

    i. **Patient history.** VF is often seen in the setting of CAD accompanied by angina, with or without MI.

    ii. **Physical examination.** No palpable pulse

  b. **Differential diagnoses.** Asystole and motion artifact from the ECG leads.

  c. **Therapy:** The ACLS algorithm for VF is shown in Figure 1-2.

2. **PEA.** Electrical activity without significant contraction of the heart muscle. PEA is the most common arrest rhythm, next to VF, and often occurs after prolonged VF. Reversible causes include hypovolemia (most commonly the result of hemorrhage), hypoxia, cardiac tamponade, tension pneumothorax, hypothermia, massive pulmonary embolism, drug overdose, hyperkalemia, and acidosis.

  a. **Clinical features.** No palpable pulse. However, lack of a palpable pulse does not imply absolute absence of cardiac activity; invasive monitoring detects arterial pulse waveforms in 40% to 50% of patients.

  b. **Evaluation**

    i. **Diagnostic studies.** ECG shows cardiac rhythm. Inefficient ventricular wall motion corresponding to the ECG cycle is noted in up to 80% of arrest victims using ultrasound. Invasive arterial monitoring may show a low-amplitude pulse waveform.

    ii. **Laboratory evaluation.** Serum electrolyte profile (especially the potassium level) and arterial blood gas should be obtained.

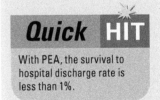

***Quick* HIT**

With PEA, the survival to hospital discharge rate is less than 1%.

TABLE 1-10	Guidelines for Femoral Vein Catheterization

1. Prepare a percutaneous central access kit. The catheter may be the large introducer type (e.g., an 8.5-gauge French catheter) for rapid volume administration, or a 16–20-cm 16-gauge catheter.

2. Identify landmarks. If the femoral artery is palpable just below the inguinal ligament, then the femoral vein lies 1–2 cm medial to the palpable pulse. If no palpable pulse is present, then the insertion point is blind. Imagine a line between the superior iliac crest and the pubic tubercle. Divide the line into three intervals. The femoral artery lies at the junction of the medial and middle intervals. The femoral vein lies 1–2 cm medial to this junction. Remember the NAVEL mnemonic (*nerve, artery, vein, empty space, lymphatics*) to help visualize the anatomy.

3. Sterile preparation and drape

4. Guard the femoral artery pulse with one hand and insert the needle attached to a 5-mL syringe 1–2 cm medially with the other hand. Advance the needle cephalad at a 30-degree angle to the skin.

5. Entry into the femoral vein is marked by the return of nonpulsatile venous blood. If pulsatile arterial flow is noted, withdraw the needle and compress the site for 5–10 minutes.

6. Following successful cannulation of the femoral vein, advance the larger needle along the tract of, or right over, the finder needle. Some operators skip this step if using the small finder needle.

7. Holding the needle firmly in place, remove the syringe and insert the guidewire through the needle. Note that whenever the needle hub is open to air, there is a threat of air embolism. **Always cover the open hub to prevent air entry.** The wire should advance smoothly. Do not let go of the guidewire.

8. While controlling one end of the wire, remove the needle. Puncture the skin at the site of wire entry with a scalpel. Some kits have the catheter over a dilator; some require a separate step of advancing a dilator over the wire before advancing the catheter over the wire. Remove the wire.

9. Attach a syringe to the line and demonstrate easy draw of blood. Flush the line with heparin solution or initiate fluid flow through the line and suture in place.

Quick HIT

Less than 1% of patients with asystolic out-of-hospital cardiac arrest survive to hospital discharge.

    c. **Therapy.** Reversible causes must be addressed. For acute therapy, the ACLS PEA algorithm is followed (see Figure 1-2).

3. **Asystole.** Can result from profound myocardial injury (e.g., as a result of infarction, hypoxia, hyperkalemia, hypokalemia, acidosis, drug overdose, hypothermia, or trauma) and is responsible for 25% to 56% of arrests
    a. **Clinical features.** Physical examination reveals no pulse or heartbeat.
    b. **Evaluation.** No detectable cardiac activity on the ECG monitor. **Must be confirmed in two leads**
    c. **Therapy.** The ACLS asystole algorithm is shown in Figure 1-2.

4. **Atrial fibrillation.** The most common serious arrhythmia, frequently seen in elderly patients. Causes include CAD, CHF, cardiomyopathy, thyrotoxicosis, rheumatic heart disease, hypertension, alcohol ingestion, and pulmonary embolism. In atrial fibrillation, multiple atrial ectopic foci stimulate an irregular ventricular response. The enlarged and poorly contracting left atrium predisposes the patient to thrombus formation, emboli, and stroke.
    a. **Clinical features**
       i. **Patient history.** May be chronic (and asymptomatic) in patients with longstanding arteriosclerotic heart disease. In paroxysmal situations, palpitations may be accompanied by weakness and near-syncope.
       ii. **Physical examination.** Irregularly irregular rhythm (approximately 80 to 180 beats/min). The heart rate in patients with chronic atrial fibrillation is usually 80 to 120 beats/min. A "pulse deficit" is not uncommon (i.e., electrical depolarization is seen on the monitor at a frequency greater than that of the palpable pulses).
    b. **Differential diagnoses.** Multifocal atrial tachycardia, paroxysmal supraventricular tachycardia, and atrial flutter
    c. **Evaluation.** ECG shows a small, irregular baseline rhythm without discernible P waves. The QRS complex is narrow but can be wide if aberrant conduction is present.

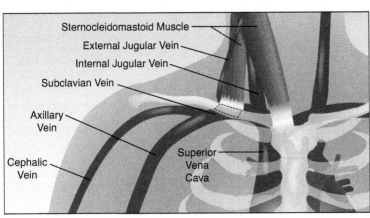

A

B

FIGURE
1-1 Schematics of anatomy and landmarks for placement of internal jugular and subclavian (A) and femoral (B) lines.

    d. Therapy. Treated according to the ACLS algorithm shown in Figure 1-3. A slow response rhythm (less than 120 beats/min) usually requires no immediate therapy.

      i. Anticoagulation therapy. Considered for patients who have been in atrial fibrillation for longer than 48 hours.

      ii. Diltiazem. Preferred agent for ventricular rate control in stable patient. It is a negative inotrope and can cause hypotension.

      iii. Sedation and **cardioversion** beginning at 100 joules is indicated for unstable patients (i.e., those with chest pain, dyspnea, hypotension, CHF, or cardiac ischemia).

    e. Disposition: Patients should be admitted to a telemetry unit or a cardiac care unit (CCU).

  5. Atrial flutter. Result of an ectopic focus originating in a small area of the atrium. Causes include CAD, chronic obstructive pulmonary disease, and rheumatic heart disease

    a. Clinical features

      i. Patient history. Often a history of heart palpitations, with or without symptoms.

      ii. Physical examination. Pulse is approximately 150 beats/min (with a 2:1 block) and is usually regular. Rates of 75 beats/min occur with a 4:1 block. Rate and rhythm may be irregular, alternating between a 2:1 and 4:1 block.

    b. Evaluation. The ECG shows characteristic "sawtooth" flutter waves with an atrial rate between 250 and 350 per minute (see Figure 1-5B). AV block is usually present.

    c. Therapy. The ACLS tachycardia algorithm is followed (see Figure 1-3).

      i. Calcium channel blockers, as described for atrial fibrillation.

      ii. Cardioversion. Starting at 25 to 50 joules of synchronized energy for unstable patients

    d. Disposition. Patients should be admitted to a telemetry unit or the CCU.

  6. Paroxysmal supraventricular tachycardia. Sudden increase in heart rate resulting from a reentrant signal that travels in a circular fashion through the AV node and an accessory pathway, resulting in sustained tachycardia. Causes include congenital conditions (e.g., mitral valve prolapse),

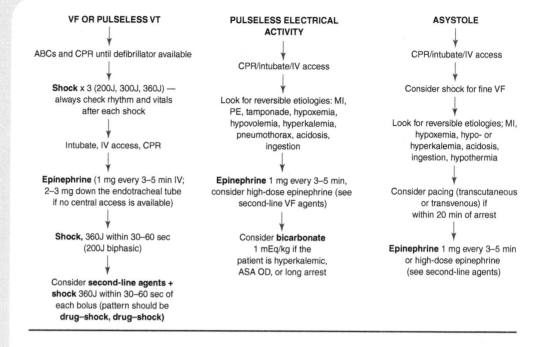

VF OR PULSELESS VT	PULSELESS ELECTRICAL ACTIVITY	ASYSTOLE
ABCs and CPR until defibrillator available	CPR/intubate/IV access	CPR/intubate/IV access
Shock x 3 (200J, 300J, 360J) — always check rhythm and vitals after each shock	Look for reversible etiologies: MI, PE, tamponade, hypoxemia, hypovolemia, hyperkalemia, pneumothorax, acidosis, ingestion	Consider shock for fine VF
Intubate, IV access, CPR	Epinephrine 1 mg every 3–5 min, consider high-dose epinephrine (see second-line VF agents)	Look for reversible etiologies; MI, hypoxemia, hypo- or hyperkalemia, acidosis, ingestion, hypothermia
Epinephrine (1 mg every 3–5 min IV; 2–3 mg down the endotracheal tube if no central access is available)	Consider bicarbonate 1 mEq/kg if the patient is hyperkalemic, ASA OD, or long arrest	Consider pacing (transcutaneous or transvenous) if within 20 min of arrest
Shock, 360J within 30–60 sec (200J biphasic)		Epinephrine 1 mg every 3–5 min or high-dose epinephrine (see second-line agents)
Consider second-line agents + shock 360J within 30–60 sec of each bolus (pattern should be drug–shock, drug–shock)		

Second-line agents

Amiodarone: 300 mg IV, repeat doses 150 mg

Lidocaine: 1.5 mg/kg (avg dose 100 mg) IVB, repeat in 3–5 min to max 3 mg/kg load

Magnesium sulfate: 1–2 g IV, especially consider if patient is in torsades de pointes, known hypomagnesemia, or refractory VF

Procainamide: infuse 30 mg/min to max 17 mg/kg load (avg dose 1–1.2 g)

Bicarbonate: 1 mEq/kb, consider for nephrine hyperkalemic patients, TCA OD, ? long arrest

Epinephrine: 1 mg 3–5 min apart

FIGURE
1-2 **Advanced cardiac life support (ACLS) algorithms for the treatment of pulseless dysrhythmias.**
ABCs, airway, breathing, circulation; ASA, acetylsalicylic acid; CPR, cardiopulmonary resuscitation; IV, intravenous; MI, myocardial infarction; OD, overdose; PE, pulmonary embolism; TCA, tricyclic antidepressant; VF, ventricular fibrillation; VT, ventricular tachycardia. Reprinted with permission from the *Massachusetts General Hospital Medical Housestaff Manual 1996–1997.*

Wolff-Parkinson-White syndrome, hyperthyroidism, and arteriosclerotic heart disease.

    a. **Clinical features**
        i. **Patient history.** Heart palpitations, which may be accompanied by near-syncope
        ii. **Physical examination.** Pulse rate is 120 to 280 beats/min (typically 160 to 200 beats/min) and regular. The patient may present with angina, signs of CHF, or hypotension.
    b. **Differential diagnoses.** Digitalis toxicity (i.e., paroxysmal supraventricular tachycardia with block), paroxysmal atrial fibrillation, VT, and atrial flutter
    c. **Evaluation.** The ECG usually shows a narrow QRS complex with flattened or notched P waves. In patients with Wolff-Parkinson-White syndrome, a "delta" wave may be noted. P waves are seldom identified at heart rates greater than 200 beats/min.
    d. **Therapy.** The ACLS tachycardia algorithm is followed (see Figure 1-3).
        i. **Vagal maneuvers** (e.g., the **Valsalva maneuver, carotid massage**): Occasionally effective. Carotid massage is contraindicated in patients with a history of vascular disease or carotid bruits.
        ii. **Adenosine** (for narrow QRS complexes) or **amiodarone** (for wide complexes)
        iii. **Cardioversion:** Beginning at 50 joules, for unstable patients
  7. **VT.** Three or more consecutive premature ventricular contractions from an ectopic focus in the ventricle at a rate greater than 100 beats/min. Causes

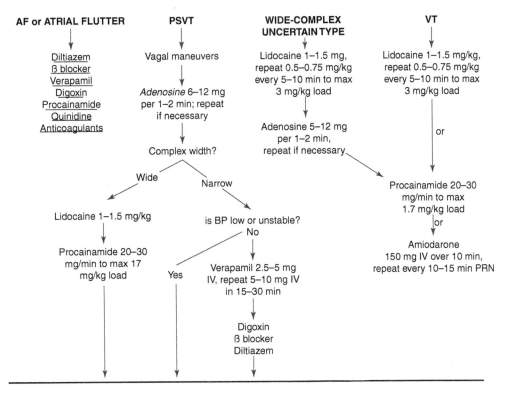

ABCs, oxygen 12-lead ECG, IV access, review history
if unstable →SYNCHRONOUS CARDIOVERSION (see below);
cardioversion seldom needed for HR <150 beats/min

AF or ATRIAL FLUTTER

Diltiazem
ß blocker
Verapamil
Digoxin
Procainamide
Quinidine
Anticoagulants

PSVT

Vagal maneuvers

Adenosine 6–12 mg
per 1–2 min; repeat
if necessary

Complex width?

Wide → Lidocaine 1–1.5 mg/kg → Procainamide 20–30 mg/min to max 17 mg/kg load

Narrow → is BP low or unstable?
No → Verapamil 2.5–5 mg IV, repeat 5–10 mg IV in 15–30 min → Digoxin / ß blocker / Diltiazem
Yes

WIDE-COMPLEX UNCERTAIN TYPE

Lidocaine 1–1.5 mg,
repeat 0.5–0.75 mg/kg
every 5–10 min to max
3 mg/kg load

Adenosine 5–12 mg
per 1–2 min,
repeat if necessary

VT

Lidocaine 1–1.5 mg/kg,
repeat 0.5–0.75 mg/kg
every 5–10 min to max
3 mg/kg load

or

Procainamide 20–30
mg/min to max
1.7 mg/kg load

or

Amiodarone
150 mg IV over 10 min,
repeat every 10–15 min PRN

SYNCHRONOUS CARDIOVERSION
Have suction and intubation kit ready
If awake, sedate with diazepam, midazolam, barbiturates
with or without morphine/fentanyl
VT/AF: 100J, 200J, 300J, 360J
PSVT/atrial flutter: 50J, 100J, 200J, 300J, 360J
Polymorphic VT: treat as VF 200J, 300J, 360J

FIGURE 1-3 **Advanced cardiac life support (ACLS) algorithms for the treatment of tachycardias.**
AF, atrial fibrillation; ABCs, airway, breathing, circulation; BP, blood pressure; ECG, electrocardiogram; HR, heart rate; IV, intravenous; PSVT, paroxysmal supraventricular tachycardia; VF, ventricular fibrillation; VT, ventricular tachycardia. Reprinted with permission from the *Massachusetts General Hospital Medical Housestaff Manual 1996–1997*.

include MI, hypertrophic cardiomyopathy, drug toxicity, hypoxia, alkalosis, and electrolyte abnormalities.

    a. **Clinical evaluation**
       i. **Patient history.** Usually in the setting of ischemic heart disease or MI
      ii. **Symptoms.** May be asymptomatic. Unstable VT may present with angina, hypotension, signs of CHF, or a decreased level of consciousness.
     iii. **Physical examination.** The pulse is regular with a rate of 150 to 200 beats/min, or absent.
    b. **Differential diagnoses.** Any atrial tachycardia with aberrant conduction
    c. **Evaluation.** The ECG shows wide QRS complexes in a sustained pattern or in short bursts. Stat electrolytes and arterial blood gas may be useful.
    d. **Therapy.** The ACLS tachycardia algorithm is followed (see Figure 1-3). Pulseless VT should be treated in a manner similar to that of VF.
  8. **Polymorphic VT (torsades de pointes).** ECG demonstrates alteration in the amplitude and direction of electrical activity around the baseline. Polymorphic VT is usually related to prolonged QT intervals and may be congenital (long QT syndrome), drug-induced (e.g., by procainamide, quinidine, cyclic antidepressants), or caused by an electrolyte imbalance.
    a. **Clinical features.** Irregular pulse greater than 150 beats/min. The patient may present with palpitations, near-syncope, or syncope.

    b. **Evaluation.** The ECG shows an irregular rhythm with a wide QRS complex and independent or no P waves. The QRS complexes appear to gradually increase and decrease in amplitude. Stat electrolyte and drug levels should be considered.

    c. **Therapy** (see Figure 1-3)

    d. **Disposition.** Patients should be admitted to the CCU.

  9. **Bradyarrhythmias**

    a. **Clinical features.** Heart rate is less than 60 beats/min and may be regular or irregular.

      i. Many athletes and other individuals have normal resting heart rates that are less than 60 beats/min and are asymptomatic. Treatment of bradycardia should be based on clinical symptoms.

      ii. Symptomatic bradycardia may be clinically manifested as a decreased level of consciousness, hypotension, chest pain, shortness of breath, pulmonary congestion, CHF, or acute MI.

    b. **Evaluation.** The ECG may show narrow-QRS sinus bradycardia, junctional rhythm, second-degree AV block, or third-degree AV block. Wide-QRS AV block bradycardia can also occur.

    c. **Therapy.** Described in the ACLS bradycardia algorithm (Figure 1-4)

      i. **Atropine** (0.5 to 1.0 mg for adults; 0.01 to 0.02 mg/kg for pediatric patients). Intravenously every 3 to 5 minutes to a total dose of 3 mg for adults and 0.04 mg/kg for children

      ii. **Transcutaneous pacing**

      iii. **Epinephrine** (2 to 10 μg/min for adults; 0.05 to 2 μg/kg/min for pediatric patients)

    d. **Disposition.** The patient should be admitted to a telemetry unit or the CCU.

B. Acute MI is discussed in Chapter 2.II.B.

C. Stroke is discussed in Chapter 9.III.A.

D. Electrocution

  1. Victims of electrocution may present with **cardiac arrest** due to depolarization of the myocardium by the external energy source. VF is common with alternating current electricity and asystole is common with lightning. **Respiratory arrest** may occur secondary to direct damage to the midbrain respiratory center or as a result of tetanic contraction of the respiratory musculature. **Associated conditions** that can complicate the resuscitation effort include fractures, myoglobinuria, head injury, and nerve injury.

  2. The **extent of injury** is determined by:

    a. The **type of current**

    b. The **duration of exposure**

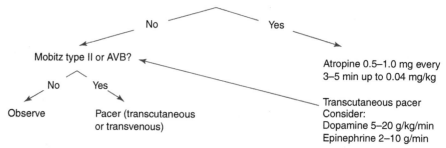

FIGURE 1-4 Advanced cardiac life support (ACLS) algorithm for bradycardia.

ABCs, airway, breathing, circulation; AVB, atrioventricular block; CHF, congestive heart failure; ECG, electrocardiogram; IV, intravenous. Reprinted with permission from the *Massachusetts General Hospital Medical Housestaff Manual 1996–1997*.

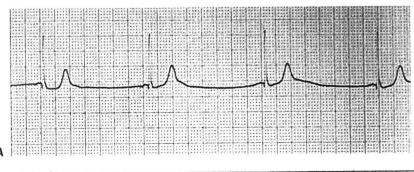

A

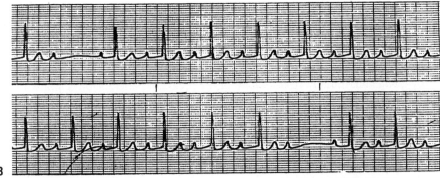

B

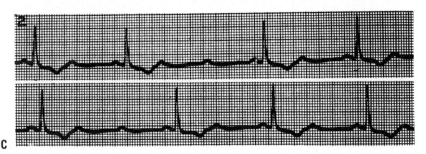

C

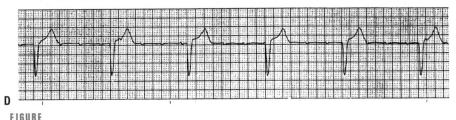

D

FIGURE 1-5 Figure of the above arrhythmias in rhythm strips.

    c. The **pathway of the current** (the hand-to-hand transthoracic path is associated with a higher mortality rate than the hand-to-foot path)

  3. The **mortality rate** ranges from 15% to 30%.

E. **Near-drowning or submersion incident.** Applied to patients who recover after a significant submersion injury

  1. Adverse consequences causing arrest are **hypoxemia, acidosis,** and **pulmonary edema** caused by alveolar damage.

  2. Resuscitation as usual with particular **emphasis on airway management.** Over-aggressive suctioning (to remove fluid from the airway) may cause aspiration and prolong definitive airway management. An orogastric tube may be placed after intubation to decrease the risk of further aspiration.

F. **Hypothermia.** Decrease in the core body temperature to below 35°C. Severe hypothermia is defined as a decrease in the core body temperature to below 30°C.

  1. Patients may have **severe depression of cerebral and cardiac function,** appearing clinically dead. Resuscitation from this state is possible and all appropriate efforts must be made to warm the patient and restore vital signs

before declaring death (thus the phrase, "You are not dead until you are warm and dead").

    a. Symptoms of moderate hypothermia include lack of shivering, decreased respiratory rate, depressed mental status, muscular rigidity, bradyarrhythmias, and decreased reflexes.

    b. Symptoms of severe hypothermia may include hypotension, apnea, severe bradycardia, VF, and asystole.

2. Resuscitation efforts follow the standard format. Warm, humidified oxygen should be provided. **Rapid core rewarming** is the key to resuscitation. Rewarming alternatives include warmed intravenous fluids provided centrally, peritoneal lavage with warm, potassium-free fluid, pleural lavage via a chest tube thoracostomy, and cardiopulmonary bypass. Selection of rewarming modality depends on the patient's condition and available alternatives.

G. **Pregnancy.** Cardiac arrest is rare during pregnancy. Causes include pulmonary embolism, trauma, CHF, MI, amniotic fluid embolism, and peripartum hemorrhage or hypovolemia. Initially, resuscitation of the pregnant patient should follow the same guidelines as if there were no pregnancy. **Special considerations** include the following:

1. Hemodynamic changes of pregnancy include an increase in maternal blood volume and cardiac output of up to 50%. Uterine blood flow accounts for 20% of cardiac output at term. Systemic peripheral vascular resistance is decreased.

2. Pulmonary changes include a decrease in the functional residual capacity and decreased pulmonary vascular resistance.

3. The enlarged uterus compresses the inferior vena cava and impedes venous return in the supine position.

4. In the setting of cardiac arrest unresponsive to standard therapy after 5 minutes, perimortem cesarean section should be performed immediately if the fetus is past the age of viability (if possible, ultrasound is used to assess fetal size and cardiac activity). Perimortem cesarean section may be lifesaving for both the fetus and the mother.

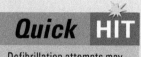

Quick HIT

Defibrillation attempts may be ineffective until the core temperature is greater than 30°C.

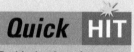

Quick HIT

Positioning the patient on her left side and displacing the uterus from the inferior vena cava may resolve hypotension and hasten stabilization.

CARDIOVASCULAR EMERGENCIES

Thomas Cunningham • Raymond Orthober

I. CHEST PAIN

A. **Discussion**

1. **Visceral pain.** Visceral afferent fibers are present in the sympathetic and parasympathetic nerves of the chest. These nonmyelinated fibers provide sensation from the heart, pericardium, lungs, and all visceral structures embryologically derived from the foregut.

2. **Somatic pain.** Somatic innervation gives rise to sensation from the mesodermal structures (e.g., the parietal pleura and peritoneum and muscular, skeletal, and dermal structures).

3. **Referred pain.** Both visceral and somatic afferent fibers share synaptic projections in the spinal cord and brain stem, which can cause visceral pain signals to be perceived in somatic structures. An example is the classic radiation of cardiac pain to the arms, neck, teeth, or jaw.

4. **"Atypical" chest pain** is a term often used to refer to chest pain that does not clearly fit in any category. The use of this term as shorthand for "nonsignificant chest pain" should be avoided because many serious diseases present atypically.

B. **Clinical features**

1. **History.** The history is the most important tool in determining the cause of a patient's pain.

   a. **Description of pain.** A description of the pain with regard to its onset, location, quality, duration, and radiation must be obtained.

      i. The patient should be questioned regarding exacerbating and relieving factors, such as activity, position, exertion, swallowing (solids versus liquids), meals, respiration, and medications (especially analgesic and antacid use).

      ii. The distinction between visceral and somatic pain is clinically useful but not well defined. Deep skeletal structures such as joint capsules and vertebrae are innervated by poorly localized nonmyelinated fibers. Conversely, disease processes in visceral organs can irritate adjacent somatically innervated structures; for example, myocardial infarction (MI) can cause pericardial irritation, leading to the typical sharp pain of pericarditis.

   b. **Description of previous episodes.** A history of previous episodes of chest pain or trauma should be sought.

   c. **Determination of risk factors.** Many significant causes of chest pain have identifiable risk factors; therefore, the patient's family history, medical history, and social history (especially concerning the use of tobacco, cocaine, or alcohol) may reveal clues pertinent to the current episode.

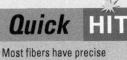

Quick HIT

Most fibers have precise somatotropic and dermatomal organization, giving rise to **pain perceived as well localized** and **"sharp."**

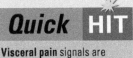

Quick HIT

Visceral pain signals are **poorly localized** and **perceived as "dull"** or **"aching."**

2. Symptoms
   a. **Symptoms of acute, critical illness.** Recognition of the following symptoms mandates immediate intervention according to the ABC principle (airway, breathing, and circulation; see Chapter 1) prior to further evaluation or work-up.
      i. **Inability to speak**
      ii. **Difficulty breathing**
      iii. **Thready pulse**
      iv. **Rapid or very slow heart rate**
      v. **Systolic blood pressure less than 100 mm Hg**
      vi. **Diaphoresis**
      vii. **Confusion**
   b. **Autonomic symptoms** (e.g., nausea, vomiting, diaphoresis, tachypnea, eructation) are often associated with visceral chest pain as a result of neural connections in the brain stem and in autonomic ganglia.
   c. **Palpitations, dizziness, fever, coughing,** or **weakness** may be seen, depending on the underlying cause of the chest pain.

C. **Differential diagnoses**
   1. **Life-threatening causes of chest pain**
      a. **Myocardial ischemia.** The signs and symptoms of MI and stable and unstable angina are discussed in section II.
      b. **Pulmonary embolism** causes a spectrum of symptoms ranging from no chest pain at all to sharp, pleuritic, or dull chest pain (see Chapter 3.VI). The dogma that pulmonary embolism always causes pleuritic chest pain is based on studies of hospitalized patients, and even in this group, pleuritic chest pain is described only 75% of the time.
      c. **Aortic dissection** is discussed in XII.A.
      d. **Cardiac tamponade** is discussed in IX.C.
      e. **Tension pneumothorax.** Patients usually present with dyspnea accompanied by the signs or symptoms of shock. In most cases, the complaint of pain occurs in the context of a known history of trauma. Tension pneumothorax evolving from spontaneous pneumothorax is a consideration in a patient with respiratory distress and chest pain.
      f. **Acute esophageal perforation** (Boerhaave syndrome) can cause sharp pleuritic, poorly localized, midline pain anywhere from the base of the neck to the epigastrium. Pain is not invariably present initially, but with the development of mediastinitis over the following days, pain becomes more diffuse, constant, and severe and is associated with systemic signs of infection.
   2. **Serious but not immediately life-threatening causes of chest pain**
      a. **Stable angina** is discussed in II.A.
      b. **Pneumothorax** (see also Chapter 3.X) can be traumatic or spontaneous (i.e., atraumatic). The former usually presents little diagnostic difficulty. Spontaneous pneumothorax is often associated with minimal symptoms and mild chest discomfort without significant dyspnea. In view of these nonspecific clinical findings, the emergency physician should have a low threshold for obtaining chest radiographs in patients with atypical chest discomfort.
      c. **Pneumonia** is suggested by cough and fever with or without chest pain. The pain is classically sharp, localized, and pleuritic in nature.
      d. **Abdominal processes.** Diseases of the stomach, liver, gallbladder, spleen, and kidneys can cause chest pain by one of several mechanisms.
         i. **Referred pain.** Pain fibers from the gallbladder can lead to the perception of pain in the right scapular region, and pain fibers from the spleen can lead to the perception of pain in the left scapular area. Painful processes affecting the central diaphragm can be referred to the third and fourth cervical dermatomes.
         ii. **Pain originating from structures in direct proximity to the diaphragm** can be perceived as originating in the chest. Sources of this type of pain include **subdiaphragmatic abscesses** and **perforated peptic ulcers.**

iii. **Extension of abdominal disease processes** into the chest can lead to chest pain. Examples include diaphragmatic herniation of abdominal viscera and the development of pleural effusions or empyema secondary to a hepatic or subdiaphragmatic abscess.

3. **Chronic or benign causes of chest pain**

a. **Pericarditis** is discussed in IX.A.

b. **Mitral valve prolapse** is discussed in VIII.B.3.

c. **Esophageal diseases** usually cause a poorly defined, burning, midsternal chest pain that can often be reproduced by asking the patient to swallow cold fluids or food. Pain of esophageal origin is referred in the same pattern as that of the heart, making for diagnostic difficulties.

d. **Musculoskeletal disorders.** Patients describe well-localized pain that can be reproduced by palpation or specific movements. Causes include muscle strain, costosternal and costochondral inflammation, osteoarthritis of the spine, and bursitis, arthritis, or tendinitis of the shoulder girdle. Such conditions can coexist with serious causes of chest pain.

e. **Pulmonary** and **abdominal processes** of a less life-threatening nature include viral pneumonitis, pleurisy, nonperforating peptic ulcer, biliary disease, chronic pancreatitis, and most forms of hepatitis.

D. **Evaluation.** Most patients with chest pain should be placed on supplemental oxygen and monitored using a pulse oximeter, cardiac monitor, and blood pressure monitor until it is determined that they are not at risk for acute decompensation and do not require emergent intervention.

1. **Physical examination**

a. As a part of the initial assessment of the ABCs, the vital signs should be noted prior to obtaining the history.

b. Initial attention to the cardiopulmonary examination should be followed by a comprehensive examination in all stable patients.

2. **Diagnostic tests**

a. **Electrocardiography.** The electrocardiogram (ECG) gives direct and indirect information about many of the causes of chest pain. ECG should be obtained in all patients in whom the history and physical examination have not definitively ruled out a cardiopulmonary etiology. A normal ECG does not exclude any cause of chest pain.

b. **Radiography.** A chest radiograph, like electrocardiography, is a rapid, noninvasive, and inexpensive way of ruling out or identifying many of the diseases in the differential diagnosis (e.g., pneumothorax, pneumonia, congestive heart failure [CHF], and, indirectly, pulmonary embolus and aortic dissection). A chest radiograph should be obtained unless the patient clearly has a disorder for which it is noncontributory.

c. **Arterial blood gas (ABG).** An ABG is rarely diagnostic but can be used as a measure of severity of illness or to assess acid–base status.

d. **Pulse oximetry** provides instant information about a patient's oxygenation status.

e. **Serum markers of myocardial injury**

i. **Cardiac troponins.** The troponin complex is the main protein of the thin filament of the myofibrils that regulate the calcium-dependent adenosine triphosphate hydrolysis of actomyosin. Levels are reliably elevated in myocardial ischemia in all patients at 6 hours, peak at 12 hours, and remain elevated for 7 to 10 days.

ii. **Creatine kinase (CK), CK-MB subunit, and myoglobin.** CK is an intracellular enzyme involved in the transfer of high-energy phosphate groups from adenosine triphosphate to creatine. CK-MB from cardiac muscle becomes elevated within 4 to 8 hours after coronary artery occlusion, peaks between 12 to 24 hours, and returns to normal between 3 and 4 days (Table 2-1).

f. **Bedside echocardiography** is diagnostic of cardiac tamponade and can provide information about cardiac wall motion and valvular function.

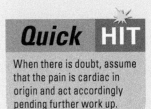

Quick HIT

When there is doubt, assume that the pain is cardiac in origin and act accordingly pending further work up.

Cardiovascular Emergencies

TABLE 2-1 Typical Serum Marker Elevation after Acute Myocardial Infarction			
Markers	**Time of Initial Elevation**	**Time of Peak Elevation**	**Time to Return to Normal**
CK-MB	4–8 h	12–24 h	72–96 h
Myoglobin	2–4 h	8–10 h	24 h
Troponin I (cTnI)	4–6 h	12 h	3–10 d
Troponin T (cTnT)	4–8 h	12–48 h	7–10 d

Total CK: 0–120 ng/mL or 0–120 μg/L
CK-MB: 0–3 ng/mL or 0–3 μg/L
CK index: 0–3
Myoglobin: <55 ng/mL or <55 μg/L
Values will vary depending on the testing method used. Check with your laboratory for reference values.
(From Fischbach FT, Dunning MB. A. *Manual of Laboratory and Diagnostic Tests*, 9th ed. Philadelphia: Lippincott Williams & Wilkins, 2014.)

E. **Disposition**
  1. **Admission**
     a. Patients with chest pain due to life-threatening causes require admission to an intensive care unit (ICU) and in some instances will require emergent cardiac catheterization or surgery. Early subspecialty consultation in the emergency department (ED) is indicated.
     b. Patients with serious but not life-threatening causes of chest pain will most likely require admission to the hospital for further evaluation and treatment. Discussion with the patient's primary physician provides additional historical information and ensures coordinated outpatient follow-up for those patients well enough for discharge.
  2. **Discharge.** Patients with benign or chronic causes of chest pain can, in most instances, be safely discharged with a prescription for analgesics and arrangements for outpatient follow-up.

II. MYOCARDIAL ISCHEMIC DISEASE

Myocardial ischemic disease encompasses angina, MI, acute coronary syndrome, and cardiogenic shock.
A. **Angina**
  1. **Discussion**
     a. **Definition.** Angina means pain, understood to refer to pain of cardiac origin, and implies myocardial ischemia.
     b. **Mechanisms.** Ischemia results from an imbalance between myocardial oxygen demand and supply.
        i. **Decreased myocardial oxygen supply**
           a) **Coronary artery occlusion** resulting from **atherosclerosis** of coronary arteries is the most common cause of ischemic heart disease and is the focus of this section. Other causes of coronary artery occlusion include **coronary artery spasm, dissection, arteritis,** and **embolism.**
           b) **Decreased coronary artery perfusion pressure** (e.g., as a result of hypotension, shock, or aortic regurgitation) can lead to decreased myocardial oxygen supply.
        ii. **Increased myocardial oxygen demand** can be due to many causes, including hypertension, hypertrophy, aortic stenosis, and emotional or physical stress.
     c. **Pathogenesis of coronary occlusion**
        i. **Atherosclerotic narrowing** of the coronary arterial lumen occurs gradually and will usually give rise to a pattern of stable anginal symptoms related to exertion and recognized by the patient. Angina typically

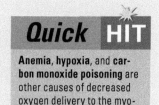

Quick **HIT**

Anemia, hypoxia, and carbon monoxide poisoning are other causes of decreased oxygen delivery to the myocardium.

occurs with exercise when the artery is 75% occluded and at rest when the artery is 90% occluded.

  ii. **Acute coronary occlusion** may be caused by thrombus formation or embolization. These acute events can cause unstable angina or MI.

  iii. **Vasospasm.** Myocardial ischemia or infarction, usually in proximal artery at the site of an atherosclerotic plaque. Prinzmetal (variant) angina often causes angina with no obstructive coronary lesions.

2. Clinical features

  a. Patient history

    i. **Symptoms.** Patients typically describe the pain of angina as "dull," "pressure-like," "heavy," "squeezing," and poorly localized. Patients may demonstrate Levine sign (i.e., the clenching of a fist in front of the sternum to describe the pain). Associated symptoms include nausea, vomiting, diaphoresis, shortness of breath, syncope, and palpitations. Pain can radiate to the arms, neck, or jaw.

      a) Anginal equivalent symptoms do not fit the strict definition of angina. Examples include jaw, neck, or epigastric pain, shortness of breath, and eructation. Patients may recognize their own anginal equivalent, and a high index of suspicion should be maintained for patients complaining of these symptoms.

      b) Vague symptoms in elderly or diabetic patients (e.g., dizziness, syncope, confusion, symptoms of peripheral emboli, or unexplained hypotension) may represent silent ischemia or infarct. In patients older than 75 years, 50% of infarcts occur without chest pain.

    ii. **Patterns.** Details of the history of chest pain should be obtained (see I.B.1).

      a) **Stable angina** occurs in a pattern of frequency, intensity, and associated level of exertion that is recognized as "usual" by the individual patient. The pain should also have an identifiable pattern of relief with rest and nitroglycerin.

      b) **Unstable angina** is characterized by symptoms that are different from the "usual" pattern and is frequently a prelude to infarction. Patients with a first episode of angina, or without prior evaluation, have unstable angina.

      c) **Prinzmetal (variant) angina** often occurs with an explosive onset, waking patients from sleep.

    iii. **Risk factors** must be elicited and include a personal history of ischemic heart disease, a family history of ischemic heart disease before age 55, smoking, hypertension, male sex, increasing age, and elevated serum cholesterol.

  b. Physical examination findings are rarely contributory.

    i. The blood pressure and respiratory rate are typically elevated, but otherwise, the vital signs are usually normal.

    ii. The patient may be diaphoretic and pale, with cool, clammy extremities.

    iii. Signs of CHF may be present (see III.B.2).

3. Differential diagnoses include those discussed in I.C.

4. Evaluation

  a. Electrocardiography. An ECG should be performed to risk-stratify patients. The ECG is normal in 50% of patients with angina who are pain-free. In patients who are experiencing pain, acute ischemia may be represented by ST-segment and T-wave abnormalities.

    i. Classically, ST-segment depression and T-wave inversion suggest non-transmural (subendocardial) ischemia (Figure 2-1), whereas Prinzmetal angina and transmural ischemia cause ST-segment elevation similar to the pattern of acute infarction (Figure 2-2).

    ii. The leads in which ST-segment abnormalities are seen suggest the area of ischemic myocardium (Table 2-2).

  b. Radiography. A chest radiograph should be performed to search for signs of CHF or lung disease.

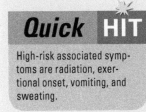

Quick HIT

High-risk associated symptoms are radiation, exertional onset, vomiting, and sweating.

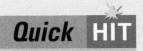

Quick HIT

HIV, rheumatoid arthritis, chronic cocaine abuse, and radiation therapy are under-recognized risk factors for coronary artery disease.

Cardiovascular Emergencies

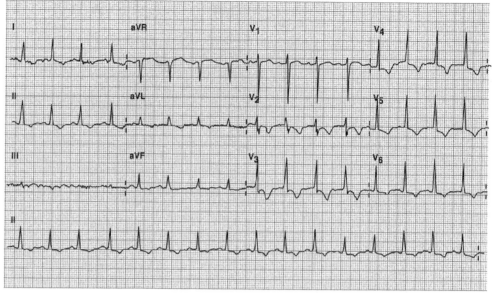

FIGURE 2-1

Electrocardiogram strip showing anterior, septal, and lateral nontransmural (subendocardial) ischemia. Symmetrical T-wave inversion and ST-segment depression are noted in leads I, II, aVL, and V_2 to V_6.

   c. **Laboratory studies.** A blood sample should be evaluated for cardiac markers (troponin, CK-MB), electrolytes, and blood urea nitrogen (BUN) and creatinine levels. A complete blood count (CBC) and baseline coagulation studies should be performed as well.

5. **Therapy.** Patients should be placed on a monitor and receive oxygen by nasal cannula, and on an intravenous line with normal saline at a keep vein open rate in the ED, after determining that immediate instability and deterioration are not present.

   a. **Stable angina.** A patient who has had an episode of stable angina, and is now pain-free, should be monitored for a period to ensure that there is

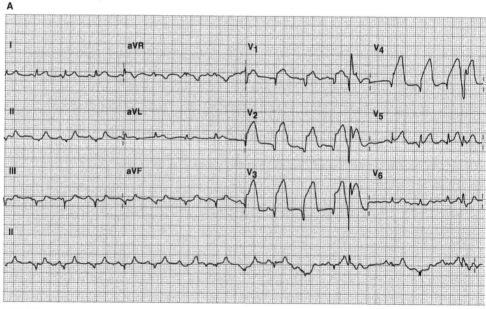

FIGURE 2-2

(A) Electrocardiogram showing anterior septal myocardial infarction. Transmural ischemia is evidenced by ST-segment elevation and hyperacute T waves seen in leads V_1 to V_5. (B) Electrocardiogram from the same patient, 24 hours later. Q-wave development, resolution of the ST-segment elevation, and T-wave inversion in leads V_1 to V_5 are evident.

B

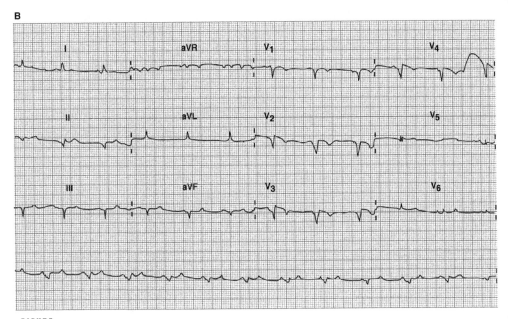

FIGURE 2-2 *(continued)*

no recurrence of pain. An ECG should be obtained, and some advocate checking cardiac enzyme levels (see II.B.4.c.i).

b. **Unstable angina.** Goals in the treatment of patients with unstable angina are to prevent further coronary thrombosis, to minimize workload, to maximize oxygenation of the myocardium, and to control pain. In most cases, these goals can be accomplished with oxygen, aspirin, heparin, nitrates, and β blockers.

   i. **Oxygen** should be provided by nasal cannula at a rate of at least 2 L/min.

   a) It should be given in high concentrations by face mask if the patient is cyanotic or has a pulse oximetry reading of less than 95%.

   b) If the patient has a history of chronic obstructive pulmonary disease (COPD), oxygen should not be withheld, but the patient should be monitored carefully for signs of respiratory depression (e.g., somnolence, confusion, lethargy).

   ii. **Aspirin** (325 mg) should be given. The patient should chew the tablets to accelerate the antithrombotic effect. Aspirin can be tolerated by patients with peptic ulcer disease unless they are actively hemorrhaging.

TABLE 2-2 Location of Cardiac Ischemia or Infarction as Suggested by Findings in Various Electrocardiogram Leads

Location of Ischemia or Infarct	Leads in Which Abnormalities Are Seen
Inferior wall	II, III, aVF
Lateral wall	I, aVL, V_5, V_6
Anterolateral region	V_1–V_6, I, aVL
Anterior wall	V_1, V_2
Anteroseptal region	V_1–V_4
Right ventricle	V_3R–V_6R
Posterior wall	V_1, V_2, V_7–V_9

Cardiovascular Emergencies

    iii. **Heparin** should be given in a bolus of 80 U/kg and started as an infusion. Also consider enoxaparin (Lovenox, Sanofi, Bridgewater, NJ) 1 mg/kg subcutaneously every 12 hours.

    iv. **Nitroglycerin** decreases cardiac preload and afterload and may dilate the coronary arteries. Sublingual nitroglycerin is preferred to intravenous nitroglycerin initially because a therapeutic blood level can be obtained much more rapidly with sublingual administration.

      a) **Sublingual.** If the patient is presently experiencing pain, 400 μg should be administered sublingually unless the patient's systolic blood pressure is less than 90 mm Hg.

        1) The dose should be repeated every 5 minutes until the pain is relieved, the systolic blood pressure decreases to below 90 mm Hg, or a total of three nitroglycerin tablets or sprays have been given, whichever occurs first.

        2) Patients who have never taken nitroglycerin can be very sensitive to its effects.

      b) **Intravenous.** If pain persists, intravenous nitroglycerin should be started and titrated to maintain the systolic blood pressure at 90 to 100 mm Hg.

      c) **Dermal.** Once the pain has been relieved, nitroglycerin paste is applied to the skin.

    v. **Morphine** can be given in 2-mg aliquots if the patient has persistent chest pain, elevated blood pressure, or both.

    vi. **β blockers.** Mortality benefit when given in first 24 hours of MI. Caution in hypotension, severe asthma, emphysema, CHF, high-grade heart block, severe bradycardia, or peripheral vascular disease with peripheral cyanosis.

      a) **Esmolol** is a $β_1$-selective agent with a half-life of 9 minutes.

      b) **Metoprolol,** also a $β_1$-selective agent, can be given by intravenous push in three separate 5-mg doses, titrating for effect on blood pressure and heart rate.

    vii. **Calcium channel blockers** are indicated in the treatment of Prinzmetal angina but are otherwise of controversial utility.

  6. **Disposition**

    a. **Admission.** Unstable angina requires admission to at least a telemetry unit. If the pain is ongoing or difficult to control, if there is significant ECG evidence of ischemia, or if the patient is in any other way unstable, admission should be to the coronary care unit.

    b. **Discharge.** Stable angina does not require admission. Because it is unusual for patients with stable angina to present to the ED, it is advisable to consult with the patient's primary care physician to ensure that the evaluation is consistent with the patient's known disease and to coordinate follow-up.

B. **Myocardial infarction**

  1. **Discussion**

    a. **Incidence.** In the United States, approximately 1.5 million patients each year experience acute MI; half of these MIs are fatal. The mortality rate is much lower for those patients reaching the ED alive.

    b. **Pathogenesis.** The risk factors and pathogenesis of MI are the same as those of angina. A number of complications can occur with MI and contribute significantly to morbidity and mortality rates. Complications include:

     i. Ventricular dysfunction, leading to shock, CHF, or chronically impaired cardiac output.

     ii. Conduction system damage, leading to bradycardia, heart block, and bundle branch blocks.

      a) Inferior wall MI frequently affects the sinoatrial (SA) node, atrioventricular (AV) node, or both.

      b) Anterior wall MI can damage the His-Purkinje system.

Quick HIT

Patients discharged with a missed MI have a 14% mortality rate.

   iii. Other dysrhythmias, caused by repolarization abnormalities and myocardial irritability.

   iv. Tissue necrosis, leading to papillary muscle rupture, acute valvular incompetence, and ventricular free wall or septal wall rupture. Most such complications are fatal but may be present in patients in shock.

   v. Intracardiac thrombus formation, leading to systemic emboli and arterial insufficiency.

   vi. Acute pericarditis, which can occur at any time during the 2 months following MI.

c. Types

   i. **ST elevation MI.** Transmural infarction. May follow transmural ischemia and is indicated by hyperacute T waves followed by ST-segment elevation (see Figure 2-2)

   ii. **Non-ST elevation MI.** May be transmural but more commonly caused by incomplete coronary artery occlusion, leading to subendocardial ischemia. ST-segment depression and T-wave inversion are common ECG findings (see Figure 2-1). The immediate mortality rate is lower than that of ST elevation MI, but the incidence of reinfarction is higher.

2. Clinical features

  a. History. The focus of the history is the same as that discussed in I.B.1. A clear history of the duration of continuous pain prior to ED presentation is essential for making decisions concerning revascularization.

  b. Physical examination findings

   i. Vital sign abnormalities are nonspecific but may reflect some of the acute complications noted in II.B.1.b.

   ii. Cardiac examination may reveal a third or fourth heart sound (S_3 or S_4) suggestive of decreased ventricular compliance, increased end-diastolic pressure, or early ventricular failure. The physician should search for signs of left- or right-sided CHF (see III.B.3).

3. Differential diagnoses. Because of the potential need for anticoagulation and thrombolytic therapy, it is essential to rule out aortic dissection, tamponade, and acute pericarditis.

4. Evaluation. The patient should be monitored for cardiac arrhythmias and oxygenation status, and an intravenous line should be placed. Continuous blood pressure monitoring is contraindicated with thrombolytic therapy, unless the patient is unstable.

  a. Electrocardiography. An ECG must be obtained immediately. The ECG abnormalities characteristic of infarction are (in decreasing order of specificity): ST-segment elevation, "hyperacute" T waves, Q waves, ST-segment depression, T-wave inversions, and conduction abnormalities. A normal ECG does not rule out MI.

   i. The **time course** of the MI is suggested by characteristic ECG changes (see Figure 2-2):

    a) Minutes after the onset of ischemia, peaked "hyperacute" T waves may develop.

    b) Minutes to hours after the onset of ischemia, ST segments become elevated in transmural ischemia.

    c) T-wave inversions and Q-wave development occur in the same leads over a period of hours to days.

   ii. The **location** of either ischemia or infarction is suggested by the ECG leads in which abnormalities are seen (see Table 2-1, Figure 2-1, and Figure 2-2).

   iii. The ECG abnormalities of MI persist despite ED interventions, whereas those of ischemia subside with appropriate therapy (e.g., oxygen, pain relief) (Figure 2-3).

  b. Cardiac ultrasonography may reveal acute valvular dysfunction, wall motion abnormalities, or pericardial fluid collections.

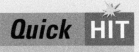

Quick HIT

A new systolic murmur is an ominous sign and may be indicative of either papillary muscle dysfunction or rupture or of interventricular septal rupture.

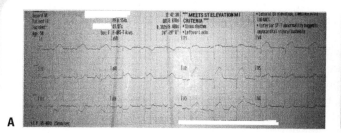
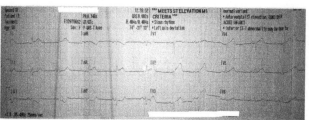
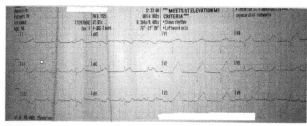
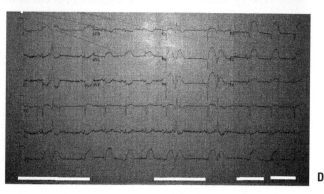

FIGURE
2-3 Schematic of electrocardiogram progression of myocardial infarction. (A) Initial pre-hospital ECG. (B) Five minutes later. (C) Ten minutes later. (D) Emergency department ECG showing obvious STEMI.

c. Laboratory studies
  i. **Cardiac markers. Troponin is the gold standard for diagnosis of MI. Creatine phosphokinase** is an enzyme released from damaged muscle. Elevations due to myocardial damage are distinguished by concomitant elevations of the MB isoenzyme fraction. Creatine phosphokinase elevations are found in 50%, 75%, and 90% of patients with MI at 3, 6, and 9 hours after the onset of pain, respectively.
  ii. **Assays for myoglobin, troponin, and lactate dehydrogenase** are still used (Table 2-3).
  iii. **Other laboratory studies** are similar to those for patients with angina (see II.A.4.c).
  iv. **Time course of serum markers.** Time course of serum markers is used to diagnose an acute MI. Early onset of elevations of CK, both total and MB fraction, and troponin permits early detection of MI, whereas the short duration of the elevation of CK permits identification of infarct extensions. The long duration of troponin permits the diagnosis to be established days after the acute event.
5. **Therapy.** Clinical assessment is ongoing in the ED to determine the efficacy of therapy.
   a. **Antianginal therapy** is initiated immediately (see II.A.5.b).
   b. **Reperfusion therapy.** In a patient with ischemic chest pain, it is essential to rapidly decide whether the pain is due to angina or infarction and assess the

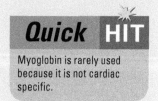

Quick HIT

Myoglobin is rarely used because it is not cardiac specific.

TABLE 2-3	Time Course of Serum Markers in Acute Myocardial Infarction		
Test	**Onset**	**Peak**	**Duration**
Creatinine	3–12 h	18–24 h	36–48 h
Troponin	3–12 h	18–24 h	Up to 10 d
Myoglobin	1–4 h	6–7 h	24 h
Lactate dehydrogenase	6–12 h	24–48 h	6–8 d

indications and contraindications for reperfusion therapy (i.e., thrombolysis or percutaneous transluminal coronary angioplasty [PTCA]). Minimizing the "door to balloon" interval so that reperfusion therapy is initiated within 90 minutes of ED presentation is the goal, or fibrinolysis within 30 minutes if PTCA is unavailable for 90 minutes.

  i. **PTCA** is indicated and preferable to thrombolytic agents when quickly available, especially in patients with MI who are in cardiogenic shock, who have contraindications to thrombolytic therapy, or who do not meet criteria for thrombolysis but have a high likelihood of infarction or intractable unstable angina. In most centers with active cath labs, PTCA is the treatment of choice.

  ii. **Thrombolysis**

  a) **Indications.** Thrombolytic therapy is indicated in eligible patients with signs and symptoms of acute MI, and in patients with ST-segment elevations of at least 0.1 mV in two ECG limb leads or 0.2 mV in two contiguous chest leads within 6 hours of the onset of symptoms, and where that ability to obtain PTCA is unavailable for 90 minutes.

  b) **Contraindications** for thrombolysis are listed in Table 2-4.

  c) **Thrombolytic agents.** Tissue plasminogen activator, streptokinase, and tenecteplase are all of similar administration and efficacy.

  d) **Complications of thrombolytic therapy**

  1) **Reperfusion arrhythmias** of any kind can occur, but accelerated idioventricular rhythms and sinus bradycardia are characteristic. These arrhythmias do not require treatment unless they are causing hemodynamic instability.

  2) **Reperfusion injury** is thought to be responsible for the increase in mortality rate observed on the first day after MI in patients given thrombolytics.

c. **Supportive therapy**

  i. **Morphine** should be given in 2-mg aliquots in patients who have persistent chest pain or elevated blood pressure.

  ii. **β blockers**, administered intravenously, are indicated within the first 24 hours for all patients with MI without overt CHF or other contraindications (see II.A.5.bvi).

  iii. **Nitroglycerin** (see II.A.5.b.vi) is indicated for careful reduction of hypertension. Lowering the blood pressure decreases the workload of

TABLE **2-4**	**Contraindications to Thrombolytic Therapy**
Absolute	**Relative**
Suspected aortic dissection or pericarditis	Cerebrovascular accident
Cerebrovascular accident	Conditions placing the patient at high risk of intra-cardiac thrombus (e.g., atrial fibrillation, mitral valve stenosis)
Cerebrovascular surgery within the previous 2 months	Major surgery within the previous 2 months
Cerebrovascular neoplasm or aneurysm	Puncture of, or recent injury to, a noncompressible vessel within the previous 2 weeks
Active bleeding in the gastrointestinal tract or other noncompressible site; hemorrhagic diathesis	Uncontrolled hypertension
Major surgery within the previous 2 weeks	Prolonged cardiopulmonary resuscitation
Pregnancy or 2 weeks postpartum status	Metastatic cancer
Allergy to thrombolytic agent	History of gastrointestinal bleeding
Unstable angina	Hemorrhagic retinopathy

the heart but also decreases coronary perfusion pressure. Elevations in blood pressure are better tolerated with lower heart rates. For these reasons, morphine and β blockers may be the first agents to consider in the treatment of MI accompanied by hypertension.

    iv. **Angiotensin-converting enzyme inhibitors** have been shown to improve outcome; the earlier they are administered, the more beneficial they are.

    v. **Antiplatelet medications** include aspirin, clopidogrel, and glycoprotein IIb/IIIa receptor inhibitors. These medications may be indicated. Protocols and doses are still in flux; consultation with the cardiologist is usually indicated. Recent literature has not shown clear benefit to starting these agents in the ED versus first dose in the cath lab.

  d. **Treatment of complications.** Complications are treated as they arise.

    i. **Dysrhythmias.** The treatment of dysrhythmias is described in section IV.

      a) **Lidocaine** is not indicated for routine prophylaxis in patients with acute MI or for patients with nonsustained runs of ventricular tachycardia (i.e., runs lasting less than 30 seconds). Sustained ventricular tachycardia should be treated as discussed in IV.B.2.b. Any ventricular dysrhythmia should prompt a search for recurrent ischemia or electrolyte imbalance.

      b) **Prophylactic pacemaker placement.** Transvenous pacemakers were routinely advocated prior to the development of reliable external pacemakers. In a stable, conscious patient, the latter, tested for capture, should be placed prior to making definitive decisions regarding the need for a transvenous pacemaker. Prophylactic pacemaker placement is indicated for the following rhythms in patients with acute MI:

        1) Bradycardia causing symptoms, hypotension, or both

        2) Second-degree Mobitz type II AV block or third-degree AV block (controversial in stable inferior MI)

        3) New bifascicular block or left bundle branch block with first-degree AV block

        4) Alternating bundle branch block

        5) Persistent atrial flutter or ventricular tachycardia

        6) New left bundle branch block or right bundle branch block (controversial)

    ii. **Free wall rupture.** Occurs in 10% of acute MI fatalities, usually 1 to 5 days after infarction. Rupture of the left ventricular free wall usually leads to pericardial tamponade and death in 90% of cases.

    iii. **Papillary muscle rupture** and **acute valvular incompetence.** Occurs in approximately 1% of patients with acute MI, is more common with inferior MI, and usually occurs 3 to 5 days after acute MI. These patients are usually in cardiogenic shock; treatment usually involves maximal afterload reduction.

  6. **Disposition.** Patients are admitted to an ICU or taken directly to cardiac catheterization.

C. **Cardiogenic shock**

  1. **Discussion**

    a. **Definition.** Cardiogenic shock occurs when the heart is unable to maintain perfusion adequate for the metabolic demands of the tissues.

    b. **Causes.** The cause of cardiogenic shock is usually acute MI, especially after extensive infarction of the anterior ventricular wall. Complications of acute MI, such as papillary muscle rupture, septal rupture, or right ventricular infarct, can precipitate cardiogenic shock in patients with smaller infarcts. Other causes include valvular stenosis, myocarditis, and cardiomyopathy.

  2. **Clinical features**

    a. **History.** Most patients are unable to give a history, but efforts should be made to gather information from fire-rescue personnel, family members, or other witnesses.

    b. **Physical examination findings** include hypotension and tachycardia. Diaphoresis, cool extremities, and poor capillary refill are usually present.

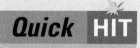

Quick HIT

Oral antiplatelet therapy also impacts downstream therapy, as patients should not undergo coronary artery bypass grafting within 5 days of receiving treatment.

Breath sounds may be clear initially, or rales from acute pulmonary edema may be present. An S$_3$ gallop or a murmur from a ruptured papillary muscle, acute mitral regurgitation, or septal rupture may be heard.

3. **Differential diagnoses** include other causes of shock, cardiac tamponade, primary CHF, adult respiratory distress syndrome, asthma, and pulmonary embolism. A cardiac etiology is suggested by a patient in shock with risk factors for ischemic heart disease and signs of acute CHF (see III.B).

4. **Evaluation**
   a. **Electrocardiography.** ST-segment elevation may be observed. Right-sided leads may show a right ventricular infarct pattern, which mandates therapy that differs from therapy for other causes of cardiogenic shock.
   b. **Radiography.** A chest radiograph may appear normal initially or show signs of acute CHF (see III.D.2).
   c. **Bedside echocardiography** is useful for demonstrating poor left ventricular function, assessing valvular integrity, and ruling out other causes of shock, such as cardiac tamponade.
   d. **Laboratory studies.** Blood studies are not of use in making the initial diagnosis but must be included in the overall evaluation. Cardiac enzyme studies, a CBC and serum electrolyte panel, BUN and creatinine levels, and coagulation studies should be ordered. The level of serum B-type natriuretic peptide is an indicator of CHF and is a prognostic indicator of survival.

5. **Therapy**
   a. **Emergent therapy** is aimed at hemodynamically stabilizing the patient with oxygen, airway control, and intravenous access. An effort should be made to maximize left ventricular function.
   b. **Volume expansion.** If there is no sign of volume overload or pulmonary edema, volume expansion with 100-mL boluses of normal saline every 3 minutes should be tried until either adequate perfusion is restored or pulmonary congestion occurs. Patients with right ventricular infarcts need significantly increased filling pressures to maintain adequate cardiac output.
   c. **Inotropic support**
      i. Patients with mild hypotension (i.e., a systolic blood pressure of 80 to 90 mm Hg) and pulmonary congestion are best treated with **dobutamine** (2.5 μg/kg/min, titrating upward by 2 to 3 μg/kg/min at 10-minute intervals). Dobutamine provides inotropic support while only minimally increasing myocardial oxygen requirements.
      ii. Patients with severe hypotension (i.e., a systolic blood pressure less than 75 to 80 mm Hg) should be treated with **dopamine.**
         a) This drug has varying effects dependent on dose. At doses of 2.5 to 10 μg/kg/min, it has positive inotropic and chronotropic effects. At dosages greater than 5.0 μg/kg/min, α-adrenergic stimulation gradually increases, causing peripheral vasoconstriction. At doses greater than 20 μg/kg/min, dopamine increases ventricular irritability without additional benefit. Not all patients have the characteristic dose-related effects of dopamine.
         b) A combination of dopamine and dobutamine is an effective therapeutic strategy for cardiogenic shock, minimizing the unwanted side effects of dopamine at high doses and providing inotropic support.
      iii. If additional support of blood pressure is needed, **norepinephrine,** which has much stronger α-adrenergic effects, can be tried. The starting dose is 0.5 to 1 μg/min.
      iv. Mechanical support (e.g., **aortic counterpulsation**) may be an option while arranging for more definitive management strategies.
   d. **Reperfusion therapy.** Reperfusion of the ischemic myocardium is the only effective therapy for patients with acute MI and cardiogenic shock. **Emergent PTCA** is the modality of choice.

6. **Disposition.** Facilities without angiographic support should consider transferring the patient to a facility with a cardiac catheterization laboratory and cardiac surgery services.

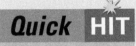

***Quick* HIT**

Because of its high negative predictive value, a normal B-type natriuretic peptide level (<100 picograms/mL) may effectively rule out cardiogenic shock. Conversely, an elevated level does not rule in the disease.

Cardiovascular Emergencies

III. CONGESTIVE HEART FAILURE AND PULMONARY EDEMA

A. **Discussion**

1. **Definition.** CHF is failure of the pumping organ in its role as a pump.

2. **Causes.** Most patients who present in acute CHF have chronic heart failure that has been exacerbated to a critical point of decompensation. It is important to identify the precipitating cause so that appropriate therapy can be carried out. Acute precipitating causes include the following.

   a. **Cardiac causes**

      i. **Myocardial disease** (e.g., ischemia, infarction, dysrhythmia, and myocarditis). Ischemia is by far the most common cardiac precipitating cause.

      ii. **Valvular disease** (e.g., stenosis, infection, rupture)

      iii. **Pericardial disease** (e.g., infection, restrictive cardiomyopathy)

   b. **Noncardiac causes** (e.g., noncompliance with diet or medications) are the most common precipitators of acute CHF. Other etiologies include hypertension, fluid overload, systemic infections, and pulmonary embolism.

3. **Pathogenesis**

   a. **Normal physiology.** In healthy people, there are three mechanisms by which cardiac output can be physiologically adjusted.

      i. **Frank-Starling mechanism.** Cardiac output is varied on a beat-to-beat basis according to the principles of the Frank-Starling mechanism. The myocyte generates a force proportional to its length in diastole, thereby providing instant correction for changes in the end-diastolic volume as a result of posture and activity.

      ii. **Neural, hormonal, and endocrine mechanisms.** Cardiac output is adjusted over a period of minutes to hours via vagal and sympathetic innervation of the SA and AV nodes, circulating catecholamines, the actions of antidiuretic hormone and atrial natriuretic peptide, and the renin-angiotensin-aldosterone system. These mechanisms adjust the chronotropic and inotropic state of the heart, the preload, and the afterload.

      iii. **Cardiac remodeling.** Over a period of weeks, the cardiac output can be adjusted by cardiac remodeling, which is growth or hypertrophy of cardiac muscle.

   b. **Pathophysiology.** Pathophysiologic effects occur when the cardiac output does not meet the body's metabolic needs. Some physiologic mechanisms cease to have any effect, whereas others become actively dysfunctional. Several processes at work in the heart in patients with heart failure are not present in the "healthy stressed" state.

      i. Progressive attempts to recruit the Frank-Starling mechanism cause cardiac dilatation, which leads to an increase in ventricular wall tension. In diastole, this increase in ventricular wall tension impairs coronary blood flow, and in systole, it ultimately leads to inadequate contraction with declining ejection fraction.

         a) This progressive failure of left ventricular function causes elevated pulmonary hydrostatic pressure, alveolar interstitial edema, and ultimately the accumulation of fluid in the alveoli (i.e., pulmonary edema).

         b) Pulmonary edema leads to decreased lung compliance, increased work of breathing, and impaired gas exchange, giving rise to the symptoms of shortness of breath and dyspnea.

      ii. Myocardial hypertrophy causes decreased diastolic compliance, while increasing oxygen requirements. In patients with CHF, the hypertrophied myocardium lacks normal architectural organization, leading to the additional loss of efficient systolic function.

B. **Clinical features**

1. **History.** The duration, pattern, and progression of the patient's symptoms should be investigated.

2. **Symptoms.** The primary symptom is usually shortness of breath or difficulty breathing (dyspnea). Dyspnea on exertion typically progresses to paroxysmal nocturnal dyspnea, then to orthopnea, and finally, to dyspnea while at rest.

   a. Symptoms of chronic "forward failure" result from hypoperfusion and include fatigue, weakness, and anorexia.

   b. Symptoms of "backward failure" include shortness of breath, anorexia, abdominal swelling and discomfort, and peripheral edema.

3. **Physical examination findings**

   a. **Vital signs**

      i. **Heart rate, blood pressure, and respiratory rate.** In patients with "compensated" CHF, the heart rate, blood pressure, and respiratory rate are elevated. As preterminal events, the patient's respiratory rate and then his or her heart rate start to decrease. A low heart rate can also be due to heart block, inferior wall MI, or both.

      ii. **Temperature.** An accurate rectal temperature should be obtained if concomitant infection is suspected.

   b. **Pulmonary examination.** Wheezing and rhonchi are heard early; in patients with left-sided CHF, rales are heard later. The lungs will be clear in patients with right-sided failure unless there is concomitant lung disease. Dullness suggests an effusion or infiltrate.

   c. **Cardiac examination** is likely to reveal tachycardia, with or without an S_3 gallop. An S_4 suggests chronic hypertension, hypertrophy, diastolic dysfunction, or acute MI. Murmurs and rubs might indicate specific precipitating causes. Jugular venous distention is seen in patients with right-sided heart failure.

   d. **General examination.** Hepatic enlargement and abdominojugular reflux may be seen with right-sided heart failure. Extremities should be checked for cyanosis, edema, jaundice, and cachexia.

4. **Clinical appearance.** Patients can be classified according to their clinical appearance.

   a. Patients with a normal or low blood pressure, often with signs of hypoperfusion (e.g., peripheral cyanosis, chest pain, impaired mentation), are in cardiogenic shock.

   b. Patients with severe CHF talk in short sentences, with words or gasps. They are too sick to give a full history but have normal or increased blood pressure.

   c. Patients with mild to moderate CHF are well enough to provide a history; they have a clear sensorium and speak in complete sentences.

C. **Differential diagnoses.** The following diagnoses should be differentiated from pulmonary edema.

   1. **Exacerbation of COPD** is suggested by the patient's history, medication list, and body habitus.

   2. **Right-sided MI** is a consideration in patients with chest pain, jugular venous distention, clear lung fields, and hypotension.

   3. **Cardiac tamponade** is suggested by Beck triad of jugular venous distention, hypotension, and pulsus paradoxus. Lung sounds are clear.

   4. **Pulmonary embolus** is suggested by jugular venous distention, the presence of risk factors, a precipitous onset, and the absence of rales. The patient may complain of chest pain and have wheezes.

   5. **Pneumonia** should be considered if there is a history of fever and productive cough.

D. **Evaluation** is indicated to rule in or rule out the differential diagnoses (see III.C), identify immediate precipitating causes, and detect underlying medical conditions. Treatment should not be delayed by tests if there is confidence in the clinical diagnosis. The patient should be placed on a cardiac monitor with a pulse oximeter and continuous blood pressure monitoring (the blood pressure should be checked every 5 minutes until the patient is stabilized).

   1. **Electrocardiography.** An ECG should be obtained to identify infarction, ischemia, and arrhythmias.

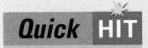

Quick HIT

The best physical finding suggestive of an elevated pulmonary capillary wedge pressure is an S_3 heard on auscultation of the chest, with a specificity of 99%.

Cardiovascular Emergencies

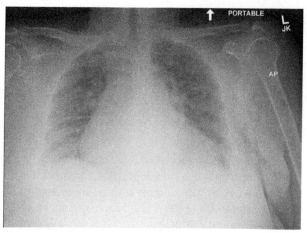

FIGURE 2-4 Chest X-ray image of patient with cardiomegaly and pulmonary edema from congestive heart failure.
(Used by permission of Martin Huecker, MD.)

2. **Radiography (Figure 2-4).** A chest radiograph may show signs of failure depending on the extent and duration of pulmonary capillary hydrostatic pressure elevations. The first finding is cephalization due to dilatation of the pulmonary vessels. As the left ventricular end-diastolic pressures increase, interstitial fluid accumulation is indicated radiographically by fluffy margins to vessels, peribronchial cuffing, and Curley A and B lines. With very high hydrostatic pressures, fluid is exuded into the alveoli, causing diffuse fluffy alveolar infiltrates.

3. **Laboratory studies**
   a. **Serum cardiac markers** should be obtained to evaluate the possibility of infarction.
   b. **CBC.** The CBC may show evidence of anemia or infection.
   c. **Serum electrolyte panel, serum BUN, and creatinine levels.** These studies will identify electrolyte imbalances and renal insufficiency. Many patients with CHF have an elevated BUN:creatinine ratio despite volume overload.
   d. **ABG.** ABGs rarely yield useful information in the initial evaluation and deflect attention from therapy to tests, as well as distress a patient whose only efforts should be directed to breathing. The decision to intubate is made clinically.
   e. **B-natriuretic peptide** elevation is highly suggestive of CHF although many other diseases may result in increased levels.

E. **Therapy**
   1. **Goals of therapy.** The goals of therapy are to optimize oxygenation and reverse the vicious cycle of decompensation. Therapy aims to:
      a. **Lower the preload,** allowing for lower end-diastolic volumes and pressures (thereby decreasing pulmonary edema)
      b. **Decrease the afterload,** improving ejection fraction and the perfusion of tissues, and minimizing the work of the heart
   2. **Treatment modalities.** In practical terms, the goals of therapy are accomplished via vasodilatation, blood pressure control, and diuresis. The ABCs are addressed first and continue to be monitored throughout.
      a. **Oxygen.** Patients with mild CHF can be administered oxygen via nasal cannula, but patients with moderate or severe failure should be given oxygen by 100% nonrebreather mask (see Clinical Pearl 2-1).
      b. **Nitroglycerin** is a venous and arteriolar dilator, with greater effect on the venous system.
         i. Sublingual nitroglycerin (every 5 minutes until the systolic blood pressure is less than 130 mm Hg or the symptoms are resolved) is administered first. Intravenous nitroglycerin is generally initiated if symptoms are not resolved with three sublingual tablets.

CLINICAL PEARL 2-1

Multiple trials have established the benefit in hospital mortality with noninvasive positive pressure ventilation for patients with decompensated congestive heart failure and concern for respiratory failure.

ii. Nitroglycerin should be used with caution in patients with conditions requiring high filling pressures (e.g., inferior wall MI with right ventricular infarct, cor pulmonale, hypertrophic cardiomyopathy, and tight mitral stenosis).

c. **Nitroprusside** is also a balanced preload and afterload reducer but with greater effect on afterload. It is less convenient to use than nitroglycerin because it is light sensitive, but it has a similarly rapid onset and short half-life. It is indicated in patients in whom hypertension is the cause of their acute pulmonary edema and in those patients who need rapid pressure control but have conditions that require high filling pressures.

d. **Furosemide and bumetanide.** Loop diuretics that help relieve acute pulmonary edema by diuresis of sodium and water, and prior to that by venodilation and preload reduction. A dose of 40 to 100 mg of furosemide (or 1 to 2 mg of bumetanide) is customary; patients already taking the drug usually require the higher doses. If the patient is in extremis, consider nitroglycerine and intermittent positive pressure ventilation prior to the administration of diuretics.

e. **Morphine.** Decreases sympathetic outflow; at the same time, it acts as a direct arteriolar and venous dilator. It is given as an intravenous push in 2-mg aliquots. Use of morphine in these patients is more dogma than evidence-based medicine.

f. **β_2-agonist nebulizer treatments.** Albuterol and terbutaline cause peripheral vasodilatation and help reduce the increased airway resistance caused by interstitial pulmonary edema and the release of inflammatory mediators. These agents are not routinely indicated but should be administered to patients with significant wheezing or history of airway disease.

g. **Rarely, digoxin, theophylline, milrinone, and amrinone** can be considered in certain circumstances.

h. **Intubation.** Almost all patients presenting with CHF and an elevated blood pressure respond to intensive therapy with the rapidly acting agents that are now available. However, those presenting in extremis or remaining hypoxic despite intensive therapeutic efforts will need to be intubated.

F. **Disposition**
1. **Admission**
   a. Patients with moderate or severe CHF generally require admission to a monitored setting. The decision to admit a patient to an ICU depends on the patient's response to therapy in the ED, the patient's baseline condition, and the precipitating cause.
   b. Patients with chronic CHF in whom no precipitating cause can be identified should probably be admitted to the hospital because of the high prevalence of serious medical conditions (including cardiac ischemia) in this group.
   c. Patients who have not been previously diagnosed as having CHF but who present with symptoms of acute CHF are likely to have an acute ischemic event as the underlying cause. These patients should be treated and admitted to a monitored bed as per unstable angina or infarction.
2. **Discharge.** Patients with an acute exacerbation of chronic CHF can be discharged if a benign precipitating event can be identified (e.g., medication noncompliance) and the patient's condition improves with treatment. The patient should be able to follow the discharge plans, discussion of which is advisable with the patient's primary physician. Outpatient therapy with diuretics, angiotensin-converting enzyme inhibitors, and/or other vasodilators should be initiated in concert with the private physician.

IV. RHYTHM DISTURBANCES

Rhythm disturbances can be classified as belonging to one of three major groups: supraventricular dysrhythmias, ventricular dysrhythmias, and disorders of cardiac conduction. Table 2-4 contains a summary of the drugs often used to manage dysrhythmias in the ED.

A. **Supraventricular dysrhythmias** arise in or above the AV node.
   1. **Sinus arrhythmia** occurs in young, healthy patients and refers to the cyclic variations of heart rate induced by respiration. Heart rate increases with inspiration and declines with expiration.
   2. **Sinus tachycardia** is a response to many pathologic processes, including fever, hypovolemia, hemorrhage, pain, hypoxia, and many drugs. It can also be a normal response to exertion or emotion.
      a. **ECG findings** include an atrial rate of greater than 100/min (even higher in infants and children) with a 1:1 ratio between atrial and ventricular contraction.
      b. **Therapy** consists of identification and treatment of the cause.
   3. **Multifocal atrial tachycardia and wandering atrial pacemaker.** Multifocal atrial tachycardia is usually seen in association with chronic lung disease. Wandering atrial pacemaker is seen in very young patients and in athletes.
      a. **ECG findings** include P waves of three or more different morphologies, with different PR intervals. Multifocal atrial tachycardia is characterized by an atrial rate of greater than 100/min, whereas wandering atrial pacemaker is characterized by an atrial rate of less than 100/min.
      b. **Therapy** is directed toward improvement of pulmonary function. If a high heart rate is contributing to the patient's distress and improvement of pulmonary function fails to reduce it, intravenous magnesium and diltiazem may be tried.
   4. **Atrial flutter** is seen in association with disorders that cause myocardial injury or inflammation (e.g., ischemic heart disease, MI) and pulmonary embolism. Specifically, this is a reentry tachydysrhythmia associated within the portalcaval isthmus.
      a. **ECG findings** include an atrial rate of 250 to 350/min. Classically, a ventricular rate of 150/min with a 2:1 AV block is seen (Table 2-5 and Figure 2-5), although 3:1 and 4:1 AV blocks are possible. Patients with accessory bypass tracts may have ventricular rates high enough to place the patient at serious risk of ventricular fibrillation (see IV.B.4).
      b. **Therapy**
         i. **Pharmacologic therapy.** Diltiazem, verapamil, digoxin, β blockers, and procainamide can all convert the patient to sinus rhythm by slowing AV conduction (and therefore, the ventricular rate).
         ii. **Direct current synchronized cardioversion** at 25 to 50 joules converts 90% of patients to sinus rhythm and is indicated for unstable patients.
   5. **Atrial fibrillation.** Several medical conditions are often associated with atrial fibrillation, especially cardiac ischemia, pulmonary embolism, hypertension, COPD, alcohol intoxication, mitral valve disease (often in patients with a history of rheumatic heart disease), pericarditis, and thyrotoxicosis.
      a. **Clinical findings.** The pulse is irregularly irregular. CHF can occur either as a result of a precipitating ischemic event or as a result of acute loss of the atrial contribution to ventricular filling (i.e., the "atrial kick").
      b. **ECG findings** include an irregularly irregular ventricular rhythm with fine fibrillatory waves that is seen best in the right chest leads. Ventricular rates are typically around 160/min. In patients who are not taking AV node blockers (e.g., digoxin), a slow ventricular response to acute atrial fibrillation indicates extensive heart disease.
      c. **Therapy**
         i. Hemodynamically unstable patients are cardioverted first with 100 joules and then with 200 joules.
         ii. In hemodynamically stable patients, ventricular rate control is obtained using intravenous diltiazem and β blockers. Chemical cardioversion with procainamide can then be effected, barring any contraindications.

TABLE 2-5 Commonly Used Drugs in the Emergency Treatment of Dysrhythmias

Antiarrhythmic Agent	Mechanism	Primary ED Indications	Contraindications	Dose	Side Effects	Dosing Considerations
Type 1a (e.g., procainamide)	Blocks fast sodium channels, thus slowing conduction (may increase PR and QRS duration) Prolongs action potential (increases QT interval) Decreases automaticity Increases refractory period	V tach, V fib not responsive to lidocaine, wide-complex tachycardia, SVT	Shock, second- or third-degree AV block, severe renal failure	Up to 1 g given IV over 50 minutes; stop for significantly decreased blood pressure, QT or QRS widening, control of arrhythmia	Hypotension, proarrhythmic effects (i.e., torsades), nausea, vomiting, CNS effects, seizures	Decrease maintenance infusion by half in patients with renal failure
Type Ib (e.g., lidocaine)	Blocks fast sodium channels selectively in injured cells, especially at a fast heart rate May shorten action potential duration	Arrhythmias, especially associated with MI (i.e., V tach, V fib, frequent multiform PVCs); wide-complex tachycardia	AV block, bradycardia, accelerated idioventricular tachycardia	1.5 mg/kg IVP (over 2 minutes if conscious); if no effect, 0.75 mg IVP every 5 minutes twice; infusion with 2–4 mg/min	Dizziness, numbness, speech disturbance	Decrease maintenance infusion in patients with liver disease
Type II (e.g., esmolol)	Increases SA automaticity Decreases AV conduction Increases AV refractory period Selective β₁ blocker	SVT or A fib (to achieve rapid control of heart rate); control of heart rate and blood pressure when CHF is of concern (e.g., in patients with acute ischemia); aortic dissection; hypertensive crisis	Severe CHF, severe asthma, severe peripheral vascular disease, bradycardia, AV block, prior calcium channel blocker administration	0.5 mg/kg IV bolus, then 0.05 mg/kg/min infusion; if no effect, repeat bolus and increase infusion by 0.05 mg/kg/min every 5 minutes up to 0.2 mg/kg/min maximum	Hypotension, CHF, dizziness, weakness	Complicated mixing and dosing can cause logistical problems in ED
Type IV (e.g., diltiazem)	Blocks slow calcium channels to decrease AV conduction velocity, increase the refractory period, and relax smooth muscle cells	SVT, ventricular rate control of A fib or flutter	Second- or third-degree AV block IV digoxin, IV β blocker, WPW syndrome with wide-complex tachycardia, V tach, hypotension	0.25 mg/kg bolus, repeated twice if needed, then 10–20 mg/hour infusion	Hypotension	Liver and kidney excretion

continued

Cardiovascular Emergencies

Cardiovascular Emergencies

TABLE 2-5 Commonly Used Drugs in the Emergency Treatment of Dysrhythmias (*Continued*)

Antiarrhythmic Agent	Mechanism	Primary ED Indications	Contraindications	Dose	Side Effects	Dosing Considerations
Adenosine	Significantly decreases AV node conduction	SVT; can be used in stable narrow-complex tachycardia for diagnostic purposes	Sick sinus syndrome, second- or third-degree AV block, severe asthma	6 mg IVP, may repeat at 12 mg IVP; IVP must be rapid by proximal vein, followed by rapid 20-mL saline flush	Atrial standstill, hypotension, syncope, transient chest pain, nausea, cough, flushing	Decrease dose if patient takes dipyridamole, increase dose if patient takes theophylline
Atropine	Acetylcholine blocker, blocks effects of vagus on the heart. Increases SA automaticity. Increases AV node conduction	Symptomatic bradycardia, bradycardia with PVCs, cholinergic overdose	Narrow-angle glaucoma	1 mg IV, may repeat up to a total of 4 mg	Tachycardia, palpitations, hypertension, dry mouth, blurred vision	Use with caution in patients with MI; ineffective post-cardiac transplant
Digoxin	Sodium-potassium pump inhibition leads to increased calcium and positive inotropy without increasing the heart rate. Vagotonic effects lead to decreased AV conduction, and increased AV refractory period. Inhibition of sympathetic outflow	Control of heart rate in SVT or A fib, especially with CHF	WPW syndrome with wide-complex tachycardia, AV block, hypokalemia, cor pulmonale	0.25 mg IVP, repeated in 30 minutes, then in 3 and 6 hours or until desired effect	Bradycardia	—
Magnesium sulfate	Intracellular calcium antagonist increases muscle relaxation and decreases neuromuscular irritability	SVT in digoxin toxicity, torsades de pointes, ± in acute MI, arrhythmias with hypomagnesemia, eclampsia	Renal failure with hypermagnesemia	1–2 g over 2 minutes followed by 0.5–1 g/hour infusion for torsades; 1–3 g in 50 mL D5W IV over 15 minutes, then infusion for digoxin toxicity (SVT)	Hypotension, flushing	—

A fib, atrial fibrillation; AV, atrioventricular; CHF, congestive heart failure; CNS, central nervous system; D5W, 50% dextrose in water; ED, emergency department; IV, intravenous; IVP, intravenous push; MI, myocardial infarction; PVCs, premature ventricular contractions; SA, sinoatrial; SVT, supraventricular tachycardia; V fib, ventricular fibrillation; V tach, ventricular tachycardia; WPW, Wolff-Parkinson-White.

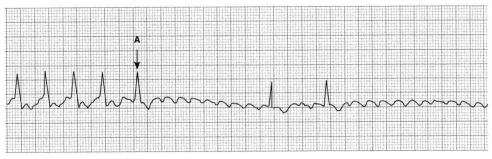

2-5 Rhythm strip from a patient with atrial flutter with 2:1 conduction. At point *A*, adenosine (12 mg) was administered, resulting in complete atrioventricular block and revealing flutter waves at a rate of 300/min.

    iii. A patient with symptoms suggestive of atrial fibrillation that last for more than 2 days is at risk of intracardiac thrombus formation and systemic embolization with cardioversion. These patients need ventricular rate control and systemic anticoagulation therapy for 2 weeks prior to cardioversion.

  6. Supraventricular tachycardia

    a. **Wide-complex supraventricular tachycardia** cannot reliably be distinguished from ventricular tachycardia, and is therefore treated as ventricular tachycardia (see IV.B).

    b. **Narrow-complex supraventricular tachycardia**

      i. **Reentrant supraventricular tachycardia**

        a) **Cause.** In the majority of patients with supraventricular tachycardia, the dysrhythmia is related to the mechanism of reentry. An abnormal loop of conductive tissue in the AV node or a bypass tract allows a circus rhythm to develop, with ventricular depolarization occurring at a rate of 140 to 200/min. Reentrant supraventricular tachycardia can occur in patients with normal hearts, and also in association with MI, pericarditis, mitral valve prolapse, or one of the preexcitation syndromes (see IV.C.5). The onset is usually sudden.

        b) **ECG findings.** Inverted, retrograde-conducted P waves are often buried in the QRS complex or found in the ST segment (Figure 2-6).

        c) **Therapy**

          1) **Unstable patients.** Direct current synchronized cardioversion should be carried out, starting with 50 joules.

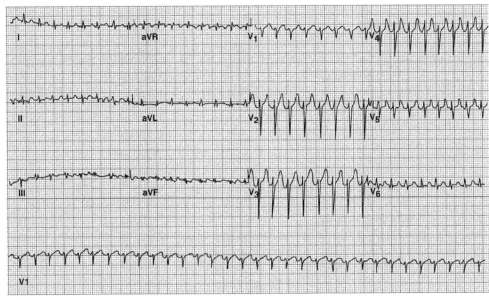

2-6 Electrocardiogram from a patient with supraventricular tachycardia (heart rate = 190 beats/min).

2) **Stable patients. Vagal maneuvers** (e.g., facial immersion in cold water, the Valsalva maneuver, carotid massage) can be attempted. Carotid massage is performed by applying steady pressure on the carotid for 10 seconds after first palpating for bilaterally intact carotid pulsations and auscultating for carotid bruits. If neither of these is present, the carotid on the side of the nondominant hemisphere should be massaged.

Adenosine, diltiazem, verapamil, digoxin, or **β blocker** therapy can be tried if vagal maneuvers are unsuccessful. If adenosine is used, it is essential that it be administered rapidly through a large vein (antecubital or more proximal), followed by a saline flush.

ii. **Ectopic supraventricular tachycardia**
   a) **Cause.** Ectopic supraventricular tachycardia is often caused by digoxin toxicity; in this situation, it is often associated with AV block. Ectopic supraventricular tachycardia also occurs with myocardial ischemia, lung disease, and alcohol abuse. The onset and resolution are usually gradual.
   b) **ECG findings.** Ectopic supraventricular tachycardia is characterized on the ECG by P waves before each QRS complex.
   c) **Therapy**
      1) If digoxin toxicity is suspected, treatment entails discontinuation of the drug and a stat drug level. If the patient is unstable, cardioversion is contraindicated, and digoxin-specific Fab may need to be given, in consultation with a toxicologist. Magnesium and phenytoin can also be used.
      2) In patients who have not been taking digoxin, treatment should be directed toward the underlying cause. Agents that decrease automaticity, AV conduction, or both (e.g., procainamide, β blockers, calcium channel blockers, digoxin) may also be administered.

7. **Sinus bradycardia**
   a. **Causes.** Sinus bradycardia occurs in three situations:
      i. As a normal finding in athletes
      ii. Secondary to drug therapy with sympatholytics, AV blockers, or vagotonics (e.g., β blockers, digoxin, calcium channel blockers, narcotics, miotic glaucoma medications)
      iii. Secondary to pathologic processes, especially myocardial ischemia, but also hypothermia, hypothyroidism, and increased intracranial pressure
   b. **ECG findings** include normal-width QRS complexes preceded by P waves at a rate less than 60/min.
   c. **Therapy** consists of atropine for hemodynamically unstable patients followed by elective pacemaker placement, depending on the clinical circumstances. Patients with signs of hypoperfusion may need immediate external or internal pacing if atropine is ineffective. Epinephrine and dopamine can be used as adjunctive therapy if there is difficulty achieving pacemaker capture or if the hypotension persists.

8. **Junctional arrhythmias** arise at the AV node and occur in situations of impaired sinus node discharge, impaired AV node conduction, and increased nodal automaticity. All of these mechanisms are associated with digoxin toxicity and diseases of the myocardium, especially ischemia, cardiomyopathy, and myocarditis.
   a. **Premature junctional beats** usually occur in patients with myocardial ischemia or in those with digoxin toxicity. The ECG reveals normal-appearing QRS complexes that occur prematurely, with no antecedent P wave. Treatment is of the underlying disease, or with procainamide.
   b. **Junctional rhythm** is characterized by a regular narrow-complex QRS morphology, at a rate of about 40 to 60 beats/min. Usually there is no evidence of atrial activity, which is the reason the junctional pacemaker cells have taken control. If P waves are seen, unrelated to the QRS complexes, the patient is in third-degree AV block (see IV.C.3; Figure 2-7).

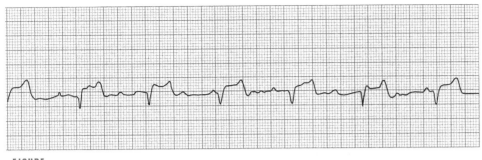

FIGURE

2-7 Rhythm strip from a patient with junctional rhythm at a rate of 60 beats/min and third-degree (complete) atrioventricular block.

    c. **Accelerated junctional rhythms** are characterized by normal-width QRS complexes at a rate of 60 to 100 beats/min and an absence of P waves.

    d. **Junctional tachycardia** is characterized by a rate greater than 100 beats/min.

B. **Ventricular dysrhythmias** arise below the AV node.

  1. **Premature ventricular contractions (PVCs)** are often observed in people with healthy hearts. However, they are more common in cardiac disease, especially ischemic states. They are also seen in conditions of increased myocardial irritability, such as severe electrolyte or acid–base imbalances or toxicity from stimulants or digoxin.

    a. **ECG findings** include premature, wide, bizarre-appearing QRS complexes, not preceded by a P wave. The QRS vector is usually opposite that of normally conducted complexes. There is typically a full compensatory pause because the SA node is not reset by the PVC.

    b. **Therapy.** In the setting of acute MI, PVCs should prompt a search for recurrent ischemia or metabolic abnormalities that need to be treated.

  2. **Ventricular (wide-complex) tachycardia** usually occurs in patients with serious heart disease. Other causes include severe electrolyte and acid–base disorders and toxicity from drugs, especially stimulant drugs of abuse, tricyclic antidepressants, and digoxin.

    a. **ECG findings.** Even experienced cardiologists cannot reliably distinguish supraventricular tachycardia with aberrant conduction (wide-complex supraventricular tachycardia) from ventricular tachycardia on the basis of the ECG.

      i. The ECG reveals a wide QRS complex (greater than 0.12 seconds, or 3 mm). The rhythm is usually regular (there may be beat-to-beat variation) and ranges from 100 to 200 beats/min. P waves independent of ventricular complexes (AV dissociation) may be noted, confirming the presence of ventricular tachycardia (Figure 2-8).

      ii. **Torsades de pointes** are runs of ventricular tachycardia, usually lasting 20 to 30 seconds, in which the amplitude of the QRS complexes waxes and wanes in any given lead. Torsades is associated with any condition that causes prolongation of cardiac repolarization, such as hypokalemia, bradycardia, or toxicity from antiarrhythmic agents.

Quick **HIT**

In the setting of acute MI, PVCs occur in most patients and are not predictive of which patients will develop ventricular fibrillation.

Quick **HIT**

Suppression of PVCs or non-sustained ventricular tachycardia with antiarrhythmic agents is not advocated by authorities in cardiology.

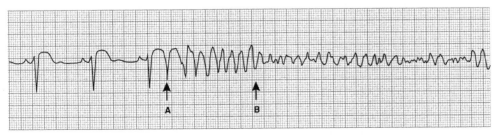

FIGURE

2-8 Electrocardiogram from a patient with an acute myocardial infarction. Ventricular tachycardia has developed at point *A*, rapidly degenerating into ventricular fibrillation (point *B*).

b. **Therapy**
   i. Unstable patients should undergo direct current cardioversion, starting at 50 joules. Pulseless ventricular tachycardia is treated like ventricular fibrillation, starting with 200 joules (see IV.B.4).
   ii. Stable patients are treated with amiodarone or procainamide. If the wide-complex tachycardia is suspected to be supraventricular tachycardia with abnormal conduction, adenosine can be used for both diagnostic and therapeutic effect.
   iii. Torsades de pointes is treated with intravenous magnesium sulfate. Type Ic and type Ia antiarrhythmic agents are contraindicated.

3. **Accelerated idioventricular tachycardia** is seen in association with acute MI. The QRS morphology is similar to that of ventricular tachycardia, but the rate is 40 to 100 beats/min. **Accelerated idioventricular tachycardia** should *not* be treated with lidocaine because it may represent the only functioning pacemaker in the heart.

4. **Ventricular fibrillation** is caused by chaotically disorganized electrical activity. Because there is no concerted electrical activity, there is no cardiac contraction and no perfusion.
   a. **ECG findings.** The ECG shows an irregular waveform of varying amplitude (see Figure 2-6).
   b. **Therapy.** The treatment is defibrillation, cardiopulmonary resuscitation, epinephrine, lidocaine, and procainamide, as per current Advanced Cardiac Life Support protocols.

C. **Disorders of cardiac conduction** are traditionally divided into those occurring in the AV node ("AV blocks") and those occurring in one or more of the main conduction fascicles of the His-Purkinje system ("bundle branch blocks"). However, AV blocks can occur in the bundle of His and the proximal Purkinje system as well as in the AV node.

1. **First-degree AV block** is really prolonged AV conduction and is usually found in patients with cardiac ischemia, rheumatic fever, myocarditis, or toxicity from digoxin or other AV blockers. First-degree AV block is diagnosed by finding a prolonged PR interval (i.e., greater than 0.20 seconds) on the ECG.

2. **Second-degree (intermittent) AV block.** Only some P waves are transmitted. Traditionally, second-degree AV block is classified as type I or type II; however, pathologically, the important distinction to make is between those conduction disturbances that are high in the ventricular conduction system and those that are low in the conduction system. The former, "low-grade" blocks, are less likely than the latter, "high-grade" blocks, to progress to complete heart block, and if they do, the rescue pacemaker is usually high in the conduction system, allowing for coordinated ventricular depolarization at a physiologically acceptable rate.
   a. **Mobitz type I (Wenckebach) block.** The same conditions that can cause first-degree AV block can cause a Mobitz type I block.
      i. **ECG findings.** The PR intervals become progressively longer until a P wave is completely blocked.
      ii. **Therapy.** If the patient is asymptomatic, no treatment is required. Symptomatic patients are treated as for bradycardia (see IV.A.7.c).
   b. **Mobitz type II block** is also associated with the same clinical conditions as first-degree AV block.
      i. **ECG findings.** Mobitz type II block is characterized by nonconducted P waves that are not heralded by progressive PR prolongation. It is often caused by disease of the distal bundle of His or proximal Purkinje system, so that there might be ECG evidence of concomitant fascicular or bundle branch blocks.
      ii. **Therapy.** For patients without antecedent MI, Mobitz type II block is treated as discussed in IV.A.7.c. Most patients with MI require prophylactic pacemaker placement.

3. **Third-degree AV block (complete heart block)** is characterized by AV dissociation with no relation between P waves and QRS complexes (see Figure 2-5). The causes and treatment are similar to those of Mobitz type II block.

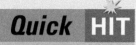

Quick HIT

Accelerated idioventricular tachycardia may be associated with large MIs, they can be the last effort of an otherwise damaged myocardium to elicit cardiac output and should be evaluated with caution.

Cardiovascular Emergencies

4. **Fascicular** and **bundle branch blocks** can be a sign of many forms of myocardial pathology but are most significant when they develop in association with acute MI. In patients with acute MI, the development of fascicular or bundle branch blocks signals extensive myocardial damage, the potential for unstable heart blocks, and the possible need for pacemaker placement.

   a. **Left anterior hemiblock** is identified by the presence of a normal-width QRS complex and a leftward QRS axis of less than −45 degrees.

   b. **Left posterior hemiblock** is suggested by a normal-width QRS complex and a rightward QRS axis of greater than 110 degrees.

   c. **Right bundle branch block** is diagnosed by a prolonged QRS complex (i.e., greater than 0.12 seconds) and a triphasic QRS complex in lead V_1—the RSR' pattern—and a prominent S wave in V_6. Right bundle branch block is seen in ischemic and valvular heart disease and may be idiopathic.

   d. **Left bundle branch block** causes a QRS complex of a duration greater than 0.12 seconds with wide, predominantly negative complexes in lead V_1 and positive complexes in V_6. Left bundle branch block is most commonly associated with ischemia, longstanding hypertension, cardiomyopathy, and severe aortic valve disease.

   e. **Bifascicular blocks** are identified by the presence of either left anterior or left posterior hemiblocks with right bundle branch block, or left bundle branch block alone.

5. **Preexcitation syndromes** are caused by abnormal bypass tracts between the atrial and ventricular conduction systems. These fibers can generate dysrhythmias by providing routes for the circus rhythms of reentrant tachycardias or by permitting abnormal retrograde conduction of ventricular impulses to the atria. **Wolff-Parkinson-White (WPW) syndrome** is the most common preexcitation syndrome; it is characterized by a high incidence of tachydysrhythmias—approximately 75% supraventricular tachycardias and 25% atrial fibrillation. Patients with WPW and atrial fibrillation may present with a rapid wide-complex ventricular response that can deteriorate to ventricular fibrillation if treated with AV nodal blockers (e.g., digoxin, calcium channel blockers, β blockers). Treatment is with intravenous procainamide.

V. HYPERTENSION

A. Overview

1. **Definition.** Hypertension, defined as a systolic blood pressure greater than 130 mm Hg or a diastolic pressure greater than 80 mm Hg, occurs in 20% to 40% of the population.

2. **Types**

   a. **Primary (essential) hypertension** does not have a cause that can be found on evaluation.

   b. **Secondary hypertension** occurs secondary to another disease process (e.g., a renal or endocrine disorder) in approximately 5% to 10% of patients.

3. **Assessment of hypertensive patients in the ED.** Elevated blood pressure is a common abnormal vital sign noted in the ED setting.

   a. **Transient hypertension** in the ED is quite commonly associated with acute anxiety, pain, drug intoxication, or overdose, and is not, in and of itself, a medical emergency. Treatment should be directed toward the underlying cause.

   b. **Uncomplicated hypertension** is frequently noted incidental to or in combination with many patient presentations to the ED. In most patients, the hypertension represents a chronic medical condition that requires long-term management. Isolated diastolic blood pressure elevations of less than 115 mm Hg, without evidence of acute end-organ damage, do not necessitate emergency medical treatment. Patients should be educated about their disease, encouraged to adhere to a low-sodium diet, and referred to a primary care physician for reevaluation.

   c. **Hypertensive urgency** and **hypertensive emergency** are characterized by diastolic blood pressure elevations of greater than 115 mm Hg and constitute medical emergencies. Although the degree of blood pressure elevation is

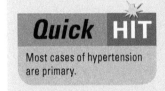

Quick **HIT**

Most cases of hypertension are primary.

useful in determining the need for emergent medical management, it should be remembered that, in the presence of signs of acute end-organ dysfunction, any elevation of blood pressure represents a medical emergency.

B. Hypertensive urgency

1. **Discussion.** Hypertensive urgency has been defined as an elevation of the diastolic blood pressure to greater than 115 mm Hg without evidence of acute end-organ damage. Elevations beyond this point place the patient at risk for vascular endothelial damage and disruptions in cerebral blood flow autoregulation.

2. **Clinical features**
   a. **History.** Noncompliance with medication is usually the precipitating event. A history of illicit drug or alcohol use should be sought as well.
   b. **Symptoms** are nonspecific. Patients may present to the ED for problems unrelated to their hypertension. Headache is a common presenting complaint. Focal neurologic complaints, visual symptoms, and chest pain or shortness of breath imply hypertensive emergency, not urgency.
   c. **Physical examination findings.** Signs of chronic hypertension may include the following:
      i. An elevated blood pressure
      ii. An S_4 or a prominent ventricular heave (or both) on cardiac examination
      iii. "Copper wiring" of arterioles and arteriovenous nicking on funduscopic examination

3. **Differential diagnoses.** Hypertensive urgencies must be differentiated from:
   a. **Transient, situational hypertension**
   b. **True hypertensive emergencies**
   c. **Pseudohypertension,** resulting from incorrect blood pressure cuff size or significant arteriosclerosis (leading to a noncompressible arterial system)

4. **Evaluation** must include an ECG, serum electrolyte panel, BUN and creatinine levels, and urinalysis to evaluate and exclude signs of acute end-organ damage.

5. **Therapy.** The goal of therapy is to reduce the patient's blood pressure within 24 to 48 hours.
   a. **Clonidine** is the most commonly used oral agent. It has an onset of action of approximately 30 minutes. Clonidine, 0.2 mg, can be given orally, with additional doses of 0.1 mg added every hour until the desired response is achieved or the maximum dose of 0.7 mg is reached.
   b. **Angiotensin-converting enzyme inhibitors, β blockers,** and **diuretics** are also useful in lowering the mean arterial pressure within 24 hours, especially if the patient has been prescribed one of these medications previously.

6. **Disposition.** Patients must be referred to their primary physician for reevaluation and should be discharged with a prescription for an antihypertensive medication.

C. Hypertensive emergency (malignant hypertension)

1. **Discussion**
   a. **Definitions.** Hypertensive emergency is an uncommon complication of hypertension and is defined as decompensation of brain, heart, or kidney function in the face of severe hypertension. Malignant hypertension is defined as an elevated blood pressure complicated by papilledema. The actual pressure at which end-organ dysfunction ensues is variable, but with the exception of pregnancy, this life-threatening situation does not occur unless the diastolic pressure exceeds 115 to 130 mm Hg.
   b. **Pathophysiology.** Consistently high pressure at the arteriole level overwhelms the normal autoregulatory mechanisms leading to dilatation, increases in capillary pressures, and leakage of fluid into the perivascular space. Tissue perfusion is compromised, resulting in areas of local ischemia.
      i. Endothelial damage, fibrinoid necrosis within vessel walls, rupture of the vessel, and tissue edema result in a microangiopathic hemolytic anemia.
      ii. Cerebral blood flow is especially compromised due to the limited space in the cranial vault. The sensitivity of brain tissue to increases in pressure causes cerebral edema, further compromising cerebral blood flow.

2. Clinical features
  a. **History** often reveals noncompliance with antihypertensive medications. Again, the use of illicit substances, especially cocaine, must be considered.
  b. **Symptoms**
    i. Headache, nausea, vomiting, visual complaints, or any change in mental status should be taken as evidence of encephalopathy.
    ii. Cardiac symptoms (e.g., ischemic chest pain, dyspnea due to CHF) may be present.
  c. **Physical examination findings**
    i. Funduscopic examination may reveal flame hemorrhages, exudates, and papilledema.
    ii. Cardiopulmonary examination may reveal evidence of acute CHF.
    iii. Neurologic examination may demonstrate alterations in mental status ranging from confusion and lethargy to coma. Focal findings may result from encephalopathy alone or be the result of concomitant cerebral vascular ischemia or hemorrhage, a common complication with dire consequences. Subarachnoid hemorrhage may be the result or the cause of malignant hypertension.
3. **Differential diagnoses** include hypertensive urgency, transient hypertension, and pseudohypertension.
4. **Evaluation**
  a. **Laboratory studies**
    i. **Serum electrolyte panel.** A serum electrolyte panel may reveal evidence of hypokalemia, present in 50% of patients with malignant hypertension.
    ii. **CBC.** Microangiopathic hemolytic anemia with schistocytes on peripheral smear is a common finding.
    iii. **BUN and creatinine levels.** End-organ damage to the kidneys may be reflected by an increased serum creatinine level.
    iv. **Urinalysis.** Renal abnormalities may be reflected by hematuria and proteinuria. A urine drug screen can be useful when cocaine toxicity is suspected.
  b. **Electrocardiography** and **radiography.** An ECG and chest radiograph are useful for assessing the degree of cardiac ischemia or the presence of CHF.
  c. **Computed tomography (CT).** A CT scan of the head to look for intracranial bleeding is appropriate.
5. **Therapy.** Emergent treatment should be initiated as soon as the diagnosis is made.
  a. **Goals of therapy.** The goal of therapy is to decrease the blood pressure so that the mean arterial pressure (i.e., the diastolic pressure plus one-third of the pulse pressure) is lowered by 20% to 25%.
  b. **Pharmacologic agents.** Oral agents are not useful in treating true hypertensive emergencies due to their delayed onset of action and the inability to closely titrate the medication based on effect.
    i. **Nicardipine** is a calcium channel blocker with properties similar to those of nifedipine, except that it is not a negative inotropic agent and it can be given intravenously. The onset of action is 15 to 30 minutes and the duration of action is 40 minutes.
    ii. **Nitroglycerin** has a rapid onset of action, is also consistent over the dose range, and has a duration of minutes. In patients with hypertensive crisis complicated by angina or pulmonary edema, nitroglycerin is the drug of choice. The initial dose is 20 to 30 μg/min and can be titrated up based on the response to therapy.
    iii. **Labetalol** is both an α and a β blocker that is available for intravenous use. It has an onset of action of less than 15 minutes and a duration of action of 2 to 8 hours. Although labetalol is useful in hypertensive patients with acute MI, the drug is not considered first-line therapy for most hypertensive emergencies.
    iv. **Sodium nitroprusside** has a rapid onset of action, consistency of effect over the dose range, and a duration of effect of only 1 to 3 minutes.

Quick HIT

Cerebral blood flow autoregulation is chronically altered in hypertensive states, and lowering the mean arterial pressure by more than 25% may result in a significant decrease in cerebral perfusion pressure, leading to cerebral ischemia.

Cardiovascular Emergencies

Cyanide or thiocyanate toxicity can develop in patients with hepatic or renal insufficiency and in those treated for more than 48 hours.

    v. **Benzodiazepines** are useful for controlling the hypertension and other adrenergic symptoms of cocaine overdose.

6. **Disposition.** Patients require admission to the ICU for further observation and treatment.

VI. SYNCOPE

A. **Discussion.** Syncope accounts for at least 1% to 2% of ED visits annually.

1. **Definition.** Transient loss of consciousness from which the patient has spontaneously recovered.

    a. **Presyncope** is a poorly defined term referring to symptoms of weakness, dizziness, or faintness, without complete loss of consciousness, which resolve spontaneously. The term can also be applied to symptoms preceding a full syncopal attack.

    b. Patients presenting with loss of consciousness followed by a partial recovery do not have true syncope, although the underlying mechanism may be similar to several of the causes of syncope.

2. **Causes.** The mechanism of syncope, in the vast majority of cases, is a shortfall in the supply of oxygen to the brain. This deficiency is usually due to disruption of cerebral circulation rather than inadequate oxygenation of blood in the lungs.

    a. **Autonomic dysfunction.** Adequate cerebral perfusion depends on adequate venous return, adequate peripheral resistance (maintained by arteriolar constriction), and adequate cardiac output (maintained by cardiac inotropy and chronotropy). Impairment of any one of these components of the circulatory system, which are largely under autonomic control, can cause a critical fall in cerebral perfusion.

      i. **Vasovagal syncope** usually occurs in the context of an emotionally disturbing situation, such as extreme fear or injury. The patient may report that the syncopal episode was preceded by nausea, warmth, dizziness, or "roaring in the ears," and that the episode resolved rapidly once the patient was placed in a recumbent position.

      ii. **Postural syncope**

        a) **Benign postural syncope** occurs in a percentage of healthy people after prolonged standing. A typical scenario is syncope after prolonged standing during a religious ceremony. Patients are always more susceptible to autonomic syncope while standing because the head is the hydrostatically lowest pressure zone of the body in a person who is standing erect.

        b) **Pathologic postural syncope** differs from benign postural syncope in that patients tend to be elderly and often have systemic disorders responsible for central or peripheral neuropathies. Pathologic postural syncope usually occurs after the patient rises from a seated or lying position. On examination, symptoms can often be reproduced by asking the patient to stand up; orthostatic blood pressure measurements are often abnormal. Medications are a common cause, and a careful history will often illicit the source of the problem.

      iii. **Carotid hypersensitivity** is associated with a history consistent with inadvertent carotid stimulation, such as a tight collar or head turning.

      iv. **Pain-induced syncope** is often associated with severe pain, especially pain of a visceral origin (e.g., abdominal aortic aneurysm, ruptured ectopic pregnancy).

      v. **Vasoactive drugs.** A vast number of drugs have vasoactive effects (e.g., antihypertensives, sedative-hypnotics, opiates, neuroleptics, cholinergics).

    b. **Inadequate venous filling**

      i. **Hypovolemia.** Syncope can be caused by inadequate intravascular volume, such as can occur with dehydration or hemorrhage. The patient shows signs of orthostatic hypotension.

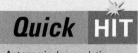

Quick HIT

Autonomic dysregulation is the most common single cause of identifiable syncope. However, in most cases of syncope the cause is undetermined.

Quick HIT

A first episode of syncope is unlikely to be attributable to benign vasovagal causes in patients older than 35 years.

ii. **Mechanical obstruction** of venous return to the heart (due to severe mitral or tricuspid valve stenosis or a ball-valve thrombus, atrial myxoma, pulmonary embolus, or prosthetic valve malfunction) may cause syncope.

iii. **Situational causes** are due to decreased venous return to the heart from Valsalva, which is exacerbated by increased vagal cardiopressor effects—for example, paroxysmal coughing ("tussive syncope"), voiding ("micturition syncope"), or defecation.

c. **Inadequate pumping action of the heart**

i. **Cardiac conduction problems**

a) **Tachydysrhythmia**, atrial or ventricular, is frequently associated with a history of palpitations or previous episodes. Syncope due to resolved ventricular tachycardia may be suggested by a prolonged QT interval or the murmur of hypertrophic cardiomyopathy (see X.B.3.b).

b) **Bradydysrhythmia** (usually characterized by a heart rate of less than 40 beats/min) can be due to injury to pacemaker cells or to the conduction system.

1) **AV nodal block** can cause syncope with no prodromal symptoms. Complete AV block, persistent or intermittent, that leads to syncope is known as **Stokes-Adams syndrome**. The diagnosis is suggested by the absence of prodrome and an ECG showing bradycardia, new fascicular or Mobitz type II blocks, or bundle branch block.

2) **Sick sinus (bradycardia–tachycardia) syndrome** can cause syncope by sinus arrest following paroxysmal supraventricular tachycardia. A history of prodromal palpitations should be sought.

ii. **Ischemic heart disease** can cause syncope by damaging the conduction system or the myocardium. In patients older than 65 years, syncope becomes an increasingly common presentation of MI; these patients often do not experience chest pain.

d. **Obstruction of pulmonary blood flow** due to pulmonary embolism, pulmonary outflow tract obstruction, or chronic pulmonary hypertension should be suspected in patients with increased respiratory rates, increased heart rates, or decreased oxygenation.

e. **Obstruction of cardiac outflow.** Aortic outflow tract obstruction often causes syncope associated with exertion.

i. **Aortic stenosis** can lead to syncope by both the mechanism of diminished arterial perfusion pressure and that of conduction system calcification (leading to heart block and arrhythmias).

ii. **Hypertrophic cardiomyopathy** can cause syncope via impairment of aortic outflow, but most commonly, the syncope is related to ventricular arrhythmias associated with the cardiomyopathy.

f. **Disturbances of arterial circulation**

i. **Cerebrovascular insufficiency** (due to embolic, atherosclerotic, or thrombotic phenomena) usually causes focal neurologic deficits rather than a loss of consciousness. Rarely, occlusion of the vertebrobasilar artery can lead to dysfunction of the reticular activating system, causing syncope.

ii. **Subclavian steal** is an unusual cause of syncope. It is suggested by syncope associated with exertion involving the upper extremities. An arterial blood pressure difference of 20 mm Hg or more is found between measurements taken in the left and right arm.

g. **Other causes**

i. **Hyperventilation** is a common cause of presyncope and can cause syncope. A history of anxiety or precipitating emotional stress should be sought. Patients may complain of numbness; tingling in the lips, face, or extremities; and spasms or dysfunction of the hands or feet. A provocative test with the patient carefully monitored can be performed.

Pulmonary embolism must be carefully excluded in any patient in whom hyperventilation is being considered as a cause of syncope.

    ii. **Intracerebral vascular catastrophe.** Subarachnoid hemorrhage or the sentinel bleed of a leaking saccular aneurysm can cause syncope, probably by autonomic mechanisms and cerebral vasospasm. However, intracerebral vascular catastrophe usually leads to coma, not syncope. Headache, photophobia, nausea, vomiting, neck pain, or meningeal signs suggest the diagnosis. A careful search for cranial nerve abnormalities might reveal signs of aneurysmal nerve compression.

    iii. **Drugs** can cause syncope by almost any of the mechanisms described. Any drug that has autonomic, vascular, cardiac, or central nervous system sedative or stimulant effects can cause or predispose to syncope.

    iv. **Psychogenic syncope** is a diagnosis of exclusion that cannot be reliably made with the time and resources available in the ED, especially because psychiatric or psychologic processes can precipitate organic causes of syncope.

B. Clinical features

  1. **History.** The history of events surrounding the syncopal episode may suggest the cause.

    a. Palpitations, chest pain, or shortness of breath may suggest an arrhythmic event, ischemia, or a pulmonary etiology.

    b. A change in posture or prolonged standing immediately preceding the episode may reflect a postural cause or orthostatic syncope.

    c. Emotional upsets usually precede vasovagal syncope or syncope caused by hyperventilation.

    d. Recent changes in medications as well as a current drug history may reveal drugs likely to precipitate syncope (e.g., β blockers, antiarrhythmic agents, antidepressive agents, diuretics, other antihypertensive medications, alcohol, cocaine).

    e. The patient should be questioned regarding recent illnesses that may have resulted in dehydration.

    f. A past medical history of ischemic or valvular heart disease, pulmonary disease, or prior syncopal episodes may help determine the cause.

  2. **Physical examination findings.** The physical examination must be focused on the cardiovascular system to assess the probability of a life-threatening cause; however, abnormal findings are usually absent.

    a. Evaluation of vital signs with testing of blood pressure in all extremities and orthostatic vitals is mandatory.

    b. Rectal examination with Hemoccult (Beckman Coulter, Brea, CA) testing may reveal gastrointestinal bleeding.

    c. Examination of the extremities may reveal evidence of thrombophlebitis as a source for pulmonary embolism.

    d. Neurologic examination may reveal subtle findings suggestive of cerebrovascular insufficiency.

C. Differential diagnoses

  1. **Hypoglycemia** usually causes a gradual impairment of consciousness that is not reversed until dextrose is administered. Hypoglycemia should be considered a reversible cause of coma rather than a cause of syncope.

  2. **Seizures** are a cause of spontaneously reversible loss of consciousness and must be distinguished from syncope. If, despite the clues listed below, the diagnosis is still unclear, the disposition should be based on the diagnosis of both possible syncope and possible new-onset (atypical) seizure.

    a. Seizures usually have a postictal period of impaired consciousness usually lasting 10 minutes. In syncope, there is a rapid and complete return to a clear sensorium.

    b. Patients rarely go limp during seizures. In syncope, there is usually a complete absence of motor activity. In the uncommon situation that transient tonic–clonic activity is witnessed during a syncopal episode, it will be

Cardiovascular Emergencies

described as following a short period of flaccid paralysis; in seizures, convulsive motor activity occurs simultaneously with the loss of consciousness.

    c. Most patients with seizures have a known history of the problem.

D. **Evaluation.** The cause of a given patient's syncope will not be found in 40% of patients despite extensive testing.

    1. **Electrocardiography.** An ECG is warranted in all patients without an unequivocal noncardiac diagnosis, and cardiac monitoring should be initiated in the ED in these patients.

    2. **Radiography.** A chest radiograph is indicated in any patient with abnormal vital signs, respiratory complaints, or suspected cardiac syncope.

    3. **Laboratory studies.** A CBC and serum electrolyte panel may reveal an anemia or electrolyte imbalance that may contribute to the cause of syncope.

    4. **Bedside echocardiography** can be useful in revealing cardiac tamponade, valvular abnormalities, abdominal aortic aneurysm, or ventricular wall motion abnormalities.

E. **Disposition**

    1. **Admission (see Clinical Pearl 2-2)**

        a. Patients with an identified serious cause of syncope will be admitted for urgent treatment or observation and monitoring.

        b. In the case of patients with an indeterminate cause of syncope (by far the largest group), clinical judgment is necessary to determine the likelihood of serious underlying illness.

    2. **Discharge.** Patients with a clearly benign cause for their syncope can be discharged from the ED to follow-up with their primary physician within several days.

VII. VALVULAR DISEASE

A. **Aortic valve disease**

    1. **Aortic stenosis**

        a. **Discussion**

            i. **Cause.** Stenosis of the aortic valve develops due to **abnormal valvular architecture**. The ordinary dynamic stress of blood flow across the defective valve progressively traumatizes the valve, resulting in thickening, calcification, and narrowing of the valve orifice.

                a) **Congenital.** A congenital bicuspid valve is the cause of aortic stenosis in 50% of symptomatic patients.

                b) **Rheumatic endocarditis** leads to commissural fusion of valve leaflets, often affecting the mitral valve as well.

                c) **Degenerative calcific aortic stenosis** occurs in elderly patients and appears to be part of the aging process. Degenerative calcific aortic stenosis is less likely to result in symptoms.

            ii. **Pathophysiology.** The obstruction to ventricular outflow that results from the stenotic valve stimulates concentric hypertrophy of the left ventricle to overcome the systolic pressure gradient and maintain cardiac output. The increased muscle mass of the ventricle leads to increased myocardial oxygen demands. The hypertrophied hyperdynamic ventricle loses its ability to compensate for hemodynamic changes and eventually fails, leading to increased atrial pressures and pulmonary congestion. The ventricle also loses its ability to increase cardiac output, leading to syncope or angina with exertion.

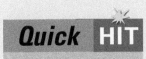

Quick HIT

Because patients with documented cardiac syncope have a 6-month mortality rate that exceeds 10%, timely and thorough evaluation is warranted.

Cardiovascular Emergencies

CLINICAL PEARL 2-2

The following criteria—age greater than 65 years, history or risk factors for serious underlying illness or advanced atherosclerosis (e.g., a history of transient ischemic attacks, cerebrovascular accident, CHF, or cardiac ischemia), a hematocrit <30, complaints of shortness of breath, and abnormal ECG, or systolic blood pressure <90—warrant a period of inpatient observation and workup.

b. Clinical features
  i. **Symptoms** usually do not occur until the valve orifice has narrowed to less than 1 cm^2. Patients may have been diagnosed previously or may present for the first time to the ED with dyspnea, angina, or syncope.
  ii. **Physical examination findings**
      a) The carotid arterial pulse is delayed and diminished in amplitude.
      b) The point of maximal impulse may be hyperdynamic and enlarged.
      c) Auscultation of the heart reveals a harsh systolic murmur that occurs just after the S$_1$ and is transmitted to the carotid arteries. The S$_2$ may diminish as the disease progresses and the contribution of the aortic component (A$_2$) is lost.
c. **Differential diagnoses.** The murmur of aortic stenosis must be differentiated from other systolic murmurs such as occur with mitral regurgitation, tricuspid regurgitation, pulmonic stenosis, and hypertrophic cardiomyopathy. Significant aortic stenosis must be differentiated from insignificant flow murmurs.
d. **Evaluation**
  i. **Electrocardiography.** Most patients show electrocardiographic evidence of left ventricular hypertrophy.
  ii. **Radiography.** A chest radiograph is usually normal until critical aortic stenosis develops. Later, this may reveal an increased cardiac silhouette and signs of CHF.
e. **Therapy.** Emergent management is guided by the presenting complaint. Valve replacement or repair will be necessary at some point in many of these patients.
f. **Disposition.** Patients with syncope, cardiac chest pain, CHF, or arrhythmias usually require admission to the hospital.

2. **Aortic regurgitation**
  a. **Discussion**
    i. **Causes** include **infective endocarditis, aortic dissection, rheumatic heart disease,** and **congenital valve abnormalities**.
        a) **Acute aortic regurgitation** is most often caused by infective endocarditis and aortic dissection.
        b) **Chronic aortic regurgitation** may also result from infective endocarditis but is more often secondary to rheumatic heart disease or congenital valve abnormalities. Rheumatic heart disease and congenital valve dysfunction usually cause both aortic stenosis and aortic regurgitation.
    ii. **Pathophysiology**
        a) **Acute aortic regurgitation** causes sudden increases in end-diastolic volumes and acute left ventricular failure with pulmonary edema.
        b) **Chronic aortic regurgitation.** The left ventricle dilates and hypertrophies to accommodate the regurgitant volume while maintaining cardiac output. Increasing the end-diastolic volume (i.e., the preload) is the primary hemodynamic compensation for aortic regurgitation. Eventually, the left ventricle fails, leading to signs of CHF. Myocardial oxygen demands are increased due to increased muscle mass, and coronary blood flow is diminished as a result of low diastolic blood pressures, leading to cardiac ischemia.
  b. **Clinical features**
    i. **Symptoms.** As with aortic stenosis, symptoms occur late in the course of the disease.
        a) Patients may complain of an uncomfortable awareness of their heartbeat or palpitations, especially in bed, for years before exertional symptoms develop.
        b) Chest pain may be present, either as a result of ischemia or as a result of chest wall discomfort from the hypertrophied hyperdynamic heart.
        c) As the ventricle fails, symptoms of left-sided, and then right-sided, heart failure develop.

Quick HIT

Patients are at risk for sudden death due to arrhythmia.

    ii. **Physical examination findings** include:
- a) A **widened pulse pressure**
- b) A **"water-hammer" pulse** that rises quickly, and then collapses in late systole
- c) **Head bobbing**, due to the jarring of the entire body with systole
- d) **Quincke pulse**, observed following the application of light pressure to the tip of the nail, which reveals pulsatile flushing of the nailbed at the root
- e) A **"pistol shot" sound** or **Duroziez sign** (a to-and-fro murmur), observed during auscultation of femoral pulses
- f) A **high-pitched, blowing, decrescendo diastolic murmur**, often accompanied by a loud systolic ejection sound or murmur due to the large volume of flow in early systole
- g) The **Austin Flint murmur**, a soft middiastolic rumble produced by displacement of the anterior leaflet of the mitral valve by the regurgitant stream

  c. **Differential diagnosis.** The murmur of aortic regurgitation may be confused with the Graham Steell murmur of pulmonic regurgitation.

  d. **Evaluation**
- i. **Electrocardiography.** The ECG is usually normal in patients with mild aortic regurgitation, but signs of left ventricular hypertrophy and ischemia may become evident as the disease progresses.
- ii. **Radiography.** A chest radiograph will usually show cardiac enlargement and pulmonary congestion. Dilatation of the ascending aorta and aortic knob may be seen.
- iii. **Echocardiography.** An echocardiogram reveals a hyperdynamic left ventricle, dilatation of the aortic annulus, and characteristic high-frequency fluttering of the anterior leaflet of the mitral valve during diastole.

  e. **Therapy.** Emergent stabilization is based on symptoms. Nitrates should be considered in patients with ischemia, despite the characteristically poor response. Arrhythmias are poorly tolerated and should be treated emergently.

  f. **Disposition** is the same as for aortic stenosis (see VIII.A.1.f).

B. **Mitral valve disease**
1. **Mitral stenosis**
  a. **Discussion**
- i. **Cause.** Mitral stenosis occurs mostly in women and is almost always the result of earlier **rheumatic heart disease**.
- ii. **Pathophysiology**
  - a) Stenosis of the mitral valve results in decreased left ventricle filling. As the valve orifice narrows, the atrium must generate more and more pressure to fill the ventricle, thus leading to marked atrial enlargement and elevated atrial pressures. The increase in atrial pressure is transmitted back to the pulmonary arterial system and eventually to the right side of the heart, leading to pulmonary hypertension and right-sided heart failure.
  - b) Cardiac output is maintained at the expense of dramatically increased pulmonary vascular pressures until late in the course of disease. Acute decompensation may be precipitated by conditions that increase the heart rate, such as fever, or conditions that increase circulating blood volume, such as pregnancy.

  b. **Clinical features**
- i. **Symptoms** develop after the hemodynamic compensatory changes begin to result in pulmonary hypertension.
  - a) Patients most commonly complain of **exertional dyspnea** and **cough** progressing to symptoms of CHF, and then right-sided heart failure.
  - b) **Hemoptysis** can occur due to rupture of bronchial vessels but is rarely fatal.

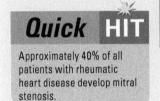

Quick HIT

Approximately 40% of all patients with rheumatic heart disease develop mitral stenosis.

      c) Embolic phenomena are a common complication of mitral stenosis; patients may present with **symptoms of cerebral, extremity, renal, or pulmonary embolism.**

  ii. **Physical examination findings**

      a) Patients have a normal or low blood pressure and a thin body habitus.

      b) The carotid pulse is brisk but diminished. The jugular venous pulse reveals a prominent *a* wave later in the course of illness.

      c) The first heart sound (S_1) is increased in intensity and, as pulmonary hypertension develops, the pulmonic component of the second heart sound (P_2) increases in intensity as well. An opening snap may be heard just after the second heart sound (S_2).

      d) A low-pitched diastolic rumble can be heard at the apex after the opening snap. Soft systolic murmurs are often associated with pure mitral stenosis. In severe forms of the disease, a pansystolic murmur of functional tricuspid regurgitation may be heard.

c. **Differential diagnosis.** Mitral stenosis must be differentiated from primary pulmonary hypertension and causes of secondary pulmonary hypertension, such as lung disease and recurrent pulmonary embolism.

d. **Evaluation**

  i. **Electrocardiography.** An ECG usually shows P mitrale (i.e., tall, notched P waves in lead II) and biphasic P waves in lead V_1 indicative of left atrial enlargement. Atrial fibrillation, which is poorly tolerated, may be seen.

  ii. **Radiography.** A chest radiograph reveals straightening of the left heart border, prominent pulmonary arteries and, later in the course of the illness, signs of CHF.

e. **Therapy**

  i. CHF and arrhythmias should be treated.

  ii. Hemoptysis is best controlled by bed rest in an upright position and by diuretics. Both of these measures help decrease pulmonary venous pressure.

  iii. Patients with embolic phenomena should be anticoagulated.

f. **Disposition** is as noted in VIII.A.1.f.

2. **Mitral regurgitation**

a. **Discussion**

  i. **Cause**

      a) **Acute mitral regurgitation** may be the result of **papillary muscle rupture in acute MI, infective endocarditis, or trauma.**

      b) **Chronic mitral regurgitation** is most commonly caused by **rheumatic heart disease** in association with mitral stenosis. Mitral regurgitation may be due to **mitral valve prolapse, hypertrophic cardiomyopathy, congenital valve deformity, or connective tissue disease.**

  ii. **Pathophysiology**

      a) **Acute mitral regurgitation** causes acute pulmonary edema due to the large volume of regurgitant blood flow and is a diagnosis to consider when a previously healthy person presents to the ED with pulmonary edema.

      b) **Chronic mitral regurgitation.** The left ventricle dilates to increase the end-diastolic volume in order to maintain cardiac output as a greater percentage of the ejection fraction is ejected back into the left atrium. The left atrium also progressively dilates. As the chambers dilate, closure of the mitral valve orifice is disrupted even more as the posterior leaflet is pulled away from the orifice. This progressive course of events has led to the saying, "mitral regurgitation begets mitral regurgitation." Enlargement of the atrium also begets atrial fibrillation, a common finding in patients with mitral regurgitation. Cardiac output is maintained until late in the course.

b. **Clinical features**
  i. **Symptoms**
    a) **Acute mitral regurgitation** is associated with **symptoms of acute pulmonary edema**. Acute mitral regurgitation may be catastrophic, leading to cardiogenic shock.
    b) **Chronic mitral regurgitation.** Patients remain asymptomatic until the mitral regurgitation becomes severe. At this point, patients may complain of **fatigue, dyspnea,** or **palpitations**. Patients are at risk for systemic emboli from the damaged valve leaflets and may present with **symptoms of embolic events**.
  ii. **Physical examination findings**
    a) Acutely, only a murmur may be heard in association with signs of CHF. The murmur is loud and holosystolic but may be a decrescendo murmur in patients with sudden valve failure. Often, the murmur can be heard through the back when auscultating breath sounds.
    b) The S_1 may be absent or lost in the murmur, and there is usually an S_3. A palpable systolic thrill and ventricular heave are usually present in patients with chronic mitral regurgitation.
c. **Differential diagnoses.** The murmur of mitral regurgitation must be differentiated from the murmurs of aortic stenosis, hypertrophic cardiomyopathy, and other systolic murmurs.
d. **Evaluation**
  i. **Electrocardiography.** The ECG is normal in acute mitral regurgitation, but signs of left ventricular hypertrophy and atrial enlargement will be evident in chronic disease. Atrial fibrillation may be seen.
  ii. **Radiography.** A chest radiograph may reveal an enlarged cardiac silhouette and evidence of pulmonary vascular congestion. Pulmonary edema with a normal heart size would be expected in patients with acute mitral regurgitation.
  iii. **Echocardiography** may demonstrate erratic movement of the valve leaflets in papillary or chordae rupture. Chamber enlargement will be evident in patients with chronic mitral regurgitation.
  iv. **Cardiac catheterization.** Although not an ED procedure, it may be necessary to diagnose acute mitral regurgitation emergently and evaluate for surgery.
e. **Therapy**
  i. Cardiogenic shock should be treated as outlined in II.C.5. Dopamine should be avoided because it increases afterload.
  ii. Counterpulsation devices may be necessary to stabilize the patient for catheterization and surgery.
  iii. Anticoagulant therapy may be a consideration if embolic events are suspected.
f. **Disposition.** Emergent surgical intervention may be indicated in patients with acute mitral regurgitation; consultation with a cardiothoracic surgeon should be considered.
3. **Mitral valve prolapse (systolic click–murmur syndrome, floppy valve syndrome, Barlow syndrome)**
  a. **Discussion.** Mitral valve prolapse varies from minimal prolapse of valve leaflets during systole to severe mitral regurgitation. (Mitral valve prolapse is the most common cause of isolated mitral regurgitation.) The cause of mitral valve prolapse is unclear, but the syndrome may be due to congenital collagen tissue disorders, Marfan syndrome, or cystic medial necrosis.
  b. **Clinical features**
    i. **Symptoms.** Most patients remain asymptomatic. Some patients develop chest pain, often vague in nature, palpitations, lightheadedness, and syncope. Neurologic symptoms from embolic events are rare but possible. Severe mitral valve prolapse with mitral regurgitation results in symptoms similar to those described in VIII.B.2.b.i.b.

      ii. **Physical examination findings.** A midsystolic click followed by a crescendo–decrescendo murmur is best heard at the apex with the patient in the left lateral decubitus position. Orthostatic hypotension is a common finding.

  c. **Differential diagnoses** include other causes of mitral regurgitation, such as hypertrophic cardiomyopathy and ischemic papillary muscle dysfunction.

  d. **Evaluation**

      i. **Electrocardiography.** The ECG is usually normal but may show T-wave abnormalities in leads II, III, and aVF. An ECG will also reveal any rhythm disturbances that may be present.

      ii. **Radiography.** A chest radiograph is usually unremarkable.

      iii. **Echocardiography** may reveal prolapse of the valve leaflet during systole.

  e. **Therapy**

      i. Chest pain often responds to treatment with β blockers.

      ii. Patients with more severe forms of the syndrome may require treatment for arrhythmia.

      iii. Aspirin is recommended for patients who develop symptoms suggestive of transient neurologic events, and anticoagulation may be considered for patients with more severe symptoms.

  f. **Disposition.** Uncomplicated mitral valve prolapse does not require admission.

C. **Tricuspid valve disease**

  1. **Tricuspid stenosis**

    a. **Discussion**

      i. **Cause.** Tricuspid stenosis is most commonly caused by **rheumatic heart disease**, often in association with mitral valve disease. The second most common cause is **infective endocarditis**.

      ii. **Pathophysiology.** Stenosis of the tricuspid valve is well tolerated. The normal valve area is 7 cm^2; adequate blood flow is possible through openings as small as 1.5 cm^2.

    b. **Clinical features**

      i. **Symptoms** of right-sided heart failure may be noted, especially after surgical correction of mitral lesions.

      ii. **Physical examination findings** include **jugular venous distention** with **giant a waves**, along with **signs of right-sided heart failure**. The **diastolic murmur** of tricuspid stenosis is best heard along the left lower sternal border and may be obscured by an accompanying murmur of mitral stenosis. The murmur is increased in inspiration when venous return to the heart is increased, and the murmur is diminished during expiration and with performance of the Valsalva maneuver.

    c. **Differential diagnoses.** Constrictive cardiomyopathy, which can also result in jugular venous distention, must be ruled out. The murmur of tricuspid stenosis is often confused with or obscured by the murmur of mitral stenosis.

    d. **Evaluation**

      i. **Electrocardiography.** An ECG will reveal evidence of right atrial enlargement with tall, peaked P waves in leads II and V$_1$.

      ii. **Radiography.** A chest radiograph may be unremarkable.

    e. **Therapy** entails fluid restriction, diuresis, and, if the stenosis is severe, surgical correction.

    f. **Disposition** is the same as that for aortic stenosis (see VIII.A.1.f).

  2. **Tricuspid insufficiency (tricuspid regurgitation)**

    a. **Discussion.** Tricuspid insufficiency is most commonly caused by a dilated right ventricle secondary to **left-sided heart failure** or **pulmonary hypertension**. It is also often the result of **infective endocarditis** arising from intravenous drug abuse. Tricuspid insufficiency is usually very well tolerated.

    b. **Clinical features**

      i. **Symptoms.** Intravenous drug abusers with endocarditis may appear ill and feverish. Other patients with tricuspid insufficiency may present with symptoms of systemic venous congestion (especially patients with pulmonary hypertension).

ii. **Physical examination findings** may include a blowing, holosystolic murmur along the left lower sternal border in addition to jugular venous distention and hepatomegaly with edema.

c. **Differential diagnoses.** Acute bacterial endocarditis with tricuspid insufficiency, progressive heart failure due to cardiac disease, acute pulmonary embolism, and other causes of pulmonary hypertension must be considered.

d. **Evaluation** should proceed as noted in the discussions of endocarditis (see XI.D), CHF (see III.D), and pulmonary embolism (see Chapter 3.VI.D).

e. **Therapy** should be directed toward the underlying cause (e.g., CHF, pulmonary hypertension, pulmonary embolism, endocarditis).

f. **Disposition** is as noted in VIII.A.1.f.

D. **Pulmonic valve disease**

1. **Pulmonic stenosis**

a. **Discussion.** Pulmonic stenosis is usually secondary to **congenital valve deformity**. The pulmonic valve is rarely affected by rheumatic heart disease or infective endocarditis.

b. **Clinical features**

i. **Symptoms.** Patients note **progressive fatigue** from decreased cardiac output and may present with **syncope**.

ii. **Physical examination findings** include evidence of systemic venous congestion. The murmur of pulmonic stenosis is a harsh, systolic ejection murmur often accompanied by a thrill at the upper left sternal border and a parasternal lift with a right ventricular heave on palpation. Severe pulmonic stenosis leads to tricuspid insufficiency, and the murmur of tricuspid insufficiency along with jugular venous distention may be evident.

c. **Differential diagnoses.** The murmur may be confused with the murmur of aortic stenosis.

d. **Evaluation.** Chest radiographs and ECGs are not usually helpful in the diagnosis of pulmonic stenosis.

e. **Therapy.** Fluid restriction and diuretics will alleviate the symptoms of systemic venous congestion.

f. **Disposition** is as noted in VIII.A.1.f.

2. **Pulmonic regurgitation**

a. **Discussion.** Pulmonic regurgitation is almost exclusively the result of **pulmonary hypertension**, which in turn can be caused by mitral valve disease, COPD, or pulmonary embolism.

b. **Clinical features**

i. **Symptoms.** Patients suffer from symptoms related to the underlying cause of the pulmonic regurgitation, which in and of itself is not clinically significant.

ii. **Physical examination findings.** The Graham Steell murmur of pulmonic regurgitation is a high-pitched, diastolic, decrescendo blowing sound heard along the upper left sternal border.

c. **Differential diagnoses.** The murmur may be confused with that of aortic regurgitation.

d. **Evaluation.** An ECG may reveal signs of pulmonary hypertension with right axis deviation and right atrial hypertrophy. A chest radiograph is usually unremarkable.

e. **Therapy.** Because pulmonic regurgitation is usually well tolerated, no specific therapy or surgical correction is indicated.

f. **Disposition** is as noted in VIII.A.1.f.

VIII. PERICARDIAL DISEASE

The pericardium is composed of a thin visceral layer adjacent to the epicardium and a loose parietal layer normally separated by approximately 15 to 50 mL of fluid. The parietal pericardium is composed of a dense collagen layer (approximately 1 mm thick)

Cardiovascular Emergencies

with very few elastic fibers. The parietal pericardium creates a minimally distensible sac that encases the heart.

A. **Acute pericarditis**

 1. **Discussion.** Pericarditis occurs when inflammation develops within the pericardium. Specific causes are listed in Table 2-6.

 a. **Postcardiac injury pericarditis** often involves blood in the pericardial space.

 i. **Post-MI pericarditis.** Patients with post-MI pericarditis can develop one of two syndromes:

 a) **Acute fibrinous pericarditis** develops in 20% of patients with acute transmural infarctions within days of the infarction. This type of pericarditis is usually of short duration.

 b) **Dressler syndrome** is less prevalent and may result from an autoimmune reaction that occurs when antimyocardial antibodies are produced following the infarction.

 ii. **Postpericardiotomy syndrome** occurs after cardiac surgery.

 iii. **Posttraumatic pericarditis** may be due to blunt or penetrating injury and is also thought to represent an autoimmune phenomenon due to circulating autoantibodies elicited after cardiac injury.

 b. **Uremic pericarditis** occurs in up to one-third of patients with end-stage renal disease and is most frequently seen in those on hemodialysis. Patients are often asymptomatic with serosanguineous effusions.

 c. **Idiopathic pericarditis** is most common and frequently follows an upper respiratory infection.

 2. **Clinical features**

 a. **Symptoms**

 i. **Chest pain** is typically severe and retrosternal, and it worsens with inspiration and when the patient is in the supine position. It is

TABLE 2-6	Causes of Pericarditis		
Noninfectious	**Infectious**	**Hypersensitivity**	
Postcardiac injury	Viral	Drug-induced	
Postmyocardial infarction	Coxsackie B virus infection	Procainamide	
Postpericardiotomy	Echovirus infection	Hydralazine	
Posttraumatic	HIV infection	Isoniazid	
Uremic	Epstein-Barr virus infection	Rheumatic fever	
Idiopathic	Bacterial	Kawasaki syndrome	
Malignancy	*Mycobacterium tuberculosis* infection	Collagen vascular disease	
Leukemia	β-Hemolytic *Streptococcus* infection	Rheumatoid arthritis	
Lymphoma	*Streptococcus pneumoniae* infection	Systemic lupus erythematosus	
Metastatic carcinoma	Syphilis	Scleroderma	
Metastatic melanoma	Lyme disease	Dressler syndrome	
Familial	Fungal		
Radiation-induced	Histoplasmosis		
Cholesterol pericarditis	Protozoal		
Myxedema	Chagas disease		
	Toxoplasmosis		

characteristically referred to the back and trapezius ridge. Pain is usually improved by sitting forward.

    ii. **Constitutional symptoms** such as fever and malaise are present as well as dyspnea and possibly dysphagia due to associated irritation of the distal esophagus.

  b. **Physical examination** may reveal the hallmark **pericardial friction rub**, described as a scratchy, leathery sound, with three components resulting from movement of the heart within the inflamed pericardium.

3. **Differential diagnoses.** Patients of all ages present to the ED with complaints of chest pain. The diagnosis of pericarditis must be differentiated from other causes of chest pain (see I.C).

4. **Evaluation**
  a. **Electrocardiography** (Figure 2-9)
    i. ST elevations in many leads are a classic finding that probably represents associated subepicardial inflammation. Downsloping PR-segment depression accompanies the ST elevation in the early stages of the disease and is specific for pericarditis. After several days, T-wave inversion is seen following normalization of the ST-segment elevation.
    ii. Differentiating these changes from benign early repolarization may be difficult. The PR depression is usually not present with benign early repolarization.
    iii. ECG changes usually resolve, but in a few patients, they may persist for years.
  b. **Radiography.** A chest radiograph may show an enlarged cardiac silhouette resulting from an associated effusion, but usually the chest radiograph is unremarkable.
  c. **Echocardiography** is useful for demonstrating a pericardial effusion and excluding tamponade.
  d. **Laboratory tests.** The white blood cell (WBC) count, sedimentation rate, and serum cardiac enzyme level may all be elevated.

5. **Therapy** consists of bed rest until the fever and pain subside. Anti-inflammatory agents are useful in controlling the pain, and specific therapy should be directed toward the underlying cause of the pericarditis, if it is known.

6. **Disposition.** Hospitalization is indicated for patients with intractable pain and for those in whom the diagnosis of MI or ischemia cannot be excluded. Some

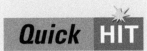

Quick HIT

Friction rubs tend to be intermittent over time and may change in intensity with position—they are heard best when the patient is leaning forward.

Cardiovascular Emergencies

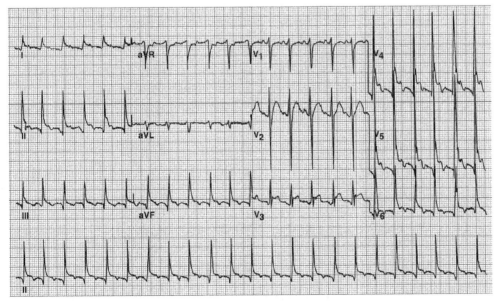

FIGURE 2-9 Electrocardiogram from a 38-year-old man with fever and chest pain caused by acute pericarditis. Diffuse ST-segment elevations are evident and PR-segment depression is noted.

authors recommend hospitalization of patients with moderate to large effusions to observe for signs of tamponade.

B. **Pericardial effusion**

1. **Discussion.** Effusion within the pericardial sac develops in response to inflammation or injury. Most commonly, an exudate, the fluid can also represent blood from an injury or a leaking thoracic dissection of the aorta. Causes are the same as those of pericarditis (see Table 2-6).

2. **Clinical features**
   a. **Symptoms** may be the same as in pericarditis, but most patients with small effusions are asymptomatic. Anxiety, dyspnea, or fatigue in patients with pericardial effusion may be early signs of tamponade.
   b. **Physical examination findings** include decreased heart sounds with or without a friction rub.

3. **Differential diagnosis.** Dilated cardiomyopathy may be difficult to distinguish from pericardial effusion on a chest radiograph. Differentiating a stable pericardial effusion from an evolving process that might result in cardiac tamponade is difficult and may require close observation in the hospital.

4. **Evaluation**
   a. **Electrocardiography.** An ECG may reveal low QRS voltage throughout or an alternating QRS amplitude, referred to as **electrical alternans**, caused by the swinging of the heart beat to beat within the pericardial effusion.
   b. **Radiography.** A radiograph may show an enlarged cardiac silhouette with a "water bottle" appearance. Lucent epicardial fat lines may be visible when displaced into the cardiac silhouette due to the fluid density surrounding the heart.
   c. **Bedside echocardiography** is very sensitive and specific for demonstrating an effusion and excluding tamponade.

5. **Therapy.** Emergent treatment may include pericardiocentesis and should be performed if symptoms of cardiac tamponade are present. Treatment of underlying conditions should be initiated in the ED.

6. **Disposition.** Patients with newly diagnosed pericardial effusions should be admitted to the hospital for close observation. Signs or symptoms of an enlarging effusion mandate admission to an ICU.

C. **Cardiac tamponade**

1. **Discussion.** Tamponade can occur when the effusion surrounding the heart exerts pressure sufficient enough to impair diastolic filling of the ventricles. Cardiac tamponade is usually fatal if untreated.
   a. **Factors contributing to the development of tamponade** include the rate of fluid accumulation, the mass of the ventricular muscle, and the total intravascular blood volume.
   b. **Causes.** In patients who are seen in the ED, tamponade is usually a complication of **trauma**. However, other causes of tamponade include **malignant effusions, idiopathic pericarditis, and uremia.** Patients with acute pericarditis are at risk for cardiac tamponade if treated with anticoagulants.

2. **Clinical features**
   a. **Symptoms** include dyspnea, fatigue, possibly chest pain, and other symptoms associated with the various causes of pericarditis. Patients may be moribund due to hemodynamic compromise.
   b. **Physical examination findings**
      i. **Beck triad** of neck vein distention, hypotension, and muffled heart sounds is classic.
      ii. **Pulsus paradoxus**, which is a decrease in arterial systolic pressure with inspiration that is greater than normal (i.e., greater than 10 mm Hg), is an important finding but is not pathognomonic.
      iii. **Kussmaul sign** (i.e., increased jugular venous distention with inspiration) is rare in tamponade.
      iv. Examination of the lungs often reveals normal breath sounds, and peripheral edema is usually absent.

Cardiovascular Emergencies

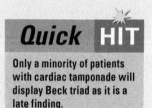

Quick HIT

Only a minority of patients with cardiac tamponade will display Beck triad as it is a late finding.

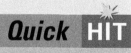

Quick HIT

The paradox in pulsus paradoxus is that, on clinical examination, one can detect beats on cardiac auscultation during inspiration that cannot be palpated at the radial pulse.

3. **Differential diagnoses.** Tamponade must be distinguished from constrictive pericarditis and restrictive cardiomyopathy; however, emergently, tamponade must be assumed to be present in patients with hypotension and jugular venous distention.

4. **Evaluation**
   a. **Electrocardiography.** Electrical alternans is often noted.
   b. **Radiography.** Cardiomegaly without evidence of pulmonary vascular congestion may be seen.
   c. **Bedside echocardiography** can confirm the diagnosis and will reveal an effusion with a hyperdynamic heart that demonstrates diastolic collapse of the right ventricle and atrium.

5. **Therapy** entails immediate pericardiocentesis; removal of as little as 10 mL of fluid can be lifesaving. Volume expansion with intravenous fluids and inotropic medications such as dobutamine may improve the stroke volume and cardiac output in patients in cardiogenic shock when combined with therapeutic pericardiocentesis.

6. **Disposition.** Patients with traumatic cardiac tamponade may require emergent surgery. Patients who are not treated surgically require admission to an ICU for close observation and definitive treatment.

D. **Constrictive pericarditis**
   1. **Discussion.** Constrictive pericarditis occurs when diffuse thickening and scarring with fibrinous adhesions develops within the pericardium following acute pericarditis, leading to impaired ventricular filling. Ventricular filling is unimpeded during early diastole but abruptly reduced when the elastic limit of the pericardium is reached. Causes are the same as those of pericarditis (see Table 2-6). Once caused predominantly by tuberculosis, chronic constrictive pericarditis now more commonly follows uremic pericarditis, postcardiac injury pericarditis, and viral pericarditis.

   2. **Clinical features**
      a. **Symptoms** include dyspnea on exertion, mild orthopnea, fatigue, and weakness. Complaints referable to right-sided heart failure may predominate. Frank pulmonary edema does not occur.
      b. **Physical examination findings**
         i. Jugular venous distention with Kussmaul sign may be seen. A paradoxical pulse is occasionally found.
         ii. Cardiac examination may reveal a diastolic shock on palpation and a pericardial knock on auscultation.
         iii. Hepatomegaly with hepatic tenderness and ascites, often more prominent than peripheral edema, is common.
         iv. A pericardial friction rub is not usually found.

   3. **Differential diagnoses.** Constrictive pericarditis is often confused with CHF and may mimic tamponade, restrictive cardiomyopathy, or tricuspid and pulmonic valvular disease. The diagnosis should be suspected in anyone with evidence of elevated venous pressure without prior myocardial dysfunction or in anyone with a clinical picture of hepatic cirrhosis accompanied by distended neck veins.

   4. **Evaluation**
      a. **Electrocardiography.** An ECG may show low QRS amplitude and atrial arrhythmias.
      b. **Radiography.** A chest radiograph reveals pericardial calcification (best seen on the lateral view) in 50% of patients. The cardiac silhouette is frequently normal in size, but some degree of cardiomegaly may be present.
      c. **Bedside echocardiography** is limited in its diagnostic utility but useful in excluding tamponade.

   5. **Therapy.** Emergent treatment includes fluid restriction, diuretics, and, possibly, inotropic agents. Mild cases may be followed with medical therapy alone; however, pericardiectomy is the definitive treatment in patients with elevated central venous pressure.

6. **Disposition.** Patients with evidence of decompensation due to decreased cardiac output or CHF require admission for improved medical management. Patients in whom the diagnosis is suspected require cardiac catheterization because constrictive pericarditis is a potentially treatable disease.

IX. PRIMARY MYOCARDIAL DISEASES

A. Myocarditis
   1. **Discussion**
      a. **Definition.** Myocarditis is an inflammatory process of the myocardium. Pathologically, myocarditis is characterized by focal inflammatory infiltration. The process frequently extends to the pericardium, causing a pericarditis.
      b. **Causes**
         i. **Infectious causes**
            a) **Viral causes** include infection with coxsackie B virus, echovirus, HIV, influenza B, parainfluenza, Epstein-Barr virus, and hepatitis B virus.
            b) **Bacterial causes** include Lyme disease and infection with *Corynebacterium diphtheriae*, *Neisseria meningitidis*, *Mycoplasma*, β-hemolytic streptococci, and *Staphylococcus aureus*.
            c) **Other infectious causes** include Chagas disease and toxoplasmosis.
         ii. **Immunologic causes** include rheumatic fever, giant cell myocarditis, and Kawasaki syndrome.
         iii. **Toxic causes** include cyclic antidepressants, hydrochlorothiazide, vaccines, cocaine, and radiation.
   2. **Clinical features**
      a. **Symptoms**
         i. Constitutional symptoms such as fever, fatigue, myalgias, and headache often accompany cardiac-specific symptoms.
         ii. Chest pain, often vague or pleuritic and accompanied by palpitations, is a common complaint.
            a) The pain may represent associated pericarditis.
            b) Myocardial irritability, conduction system involvement, or both are common and may be perceived as palpitations.
         iii. Dyspnea may be present in more severe cases in which myocardial dysfunction has progressed to heart failure.
      b. **Physical examination findings** may be normal in patients with mild disease. In patients with more moderate illness, a muffled S_1 along with an S_3 and a mitral regurgitation murmur may be elicited. A pericardial friction rub may be heard with associated pericarditis. Severe disease results in progressive systolic dysfunction and typical signs of CHF.
   3. **Differential diagnoses**
      a. Chest pain must be differentiated from that of acute MI or ischemia and other causes of chest pain as discussed in section I.C.
      b. Palpitations must be differentiated from benign palpitations and other arrhythmias as discussed in section IV.
      c. Dyspnea can be secondary to many primary pulmonary etiologies (e.g., pneumonia, pneumothorax, pulmonary embolism, obstructive lung disease). Patients with acute CHF, valvular disease, or pulmonary hypertension might also present with complaints of dyspnea.
   4. **Evaluation**
      a. **Electrocardiography.** An ECG most commonly reveals nonspecific ST-segment and T-wave changes. Elevations of the ST segments, due to accompanying pericarditis, along with conduction disturbances (e.g., AV block, prolonged QRS duration) reflect more severe disease. Arrhythmias, ectopy, or both may be noted.
      b. **Radiography.** A chest radiograph is not helpful unless the illness has progressed to heart failure, when pulmonary vascular congestion and cardiomegaly may be noted.

c. **Laboratory studies** reveal elevations of the WBC count and sedimentation rate as well as elevations in cardiac enzyme levels.

d. **Myocardial biopsy** is diagnostic and may be indicated after initial emergency management to direct continued therapy.

5. **Therapy.** Emergent treatment is supportive and symptom directed. Antibiotics should be administered if an acute bacterial cause is suspected. Steroids remain controversial, limited to the treatment of idiopathic disease, and are not part of the emergency management of myocarditis.

6. **Disposition**

a. Patients with evidence of more severe disease accompanied by myocardial dysfunction, CHF, or significant arrhythmias, or those suspected of having bacterial myocarditis, should be admitted to a monitored setting.

b. Most patients with idiopathic or viral myocarditis can be safely treated and followed as outpatients. Discussion of follow-up plans with a cardiologist or the patient's primary care physician is appropriate.

B. **Cardiomyopathies** are the third most common form of cardiac disease in the United States, after ischemic and hypertensive heart disease.

1. **Introduction**

a. **Definition.** This group of cardiac illnesses is characterized by primary abnormalities or dysfunction of the heart muscle.

b. **Cause.** By definition, the cause of true cardiomyopathy is unknown; however, viral infections may account for a subgroup of illnesses currently thought to be idiopathic. Contrary to this strict definition, however, the term "cardiomyopathy" is used to refer to a number of disorders of cardiac function (Table 2-7).

2. **Dilated (congestive) cardiomyopathy**

a. **Discussion.** Dilated cardiomyopathy is the most common type.

i. **Causes** (see Table 2-7). Alcohol is the most common cause of dilated cardiomyopathy in the United States.

ii. **Pathogenesis.** Systolic and diastolic dysfunction due to increased ventricular volume and pressure eventually leads to decreased cardiac output and overt heart failure. Cardiomegaly with chamber enlargement can result in arrhythmias and mural thrombi. Patients typically have a progressively downhill course; death usually occurs within 2 years of symptom onset unless cardiac transplantation is attempted.

b. **Clinical features**

i. **History.** The patient should be questioned regarding a recent pregnancy, substance abuse, a recent viral illness, and systemic illness.

ii. **Symptoms** suggestive of left- and/or right-sided heart failure predominate. Chest pain, often vague, may be present. Palpitations are common. Cerebral or systemic embolic phenomena secondary to mural thrombi occur with complaints of focal weakness, numbness, or a cold, painful extremity.

iii. **Physical examination findings**

a) Evidence of cardiac enlargement with an enlarged point of maximal impulse, an audible S_3 and S_4, and murmurs of mitral or tricuspid regurgitation (or both) are often present.

b) Findings of left- and right-sided heart failure may be evident.

c) Focal neurologic findings or a cold, pulseless extremity may be found when embolic phenomena occur.

c. **Differential diagnosis.** The differential diagnosis includes ischemic or hypertensive heart disease, acute ischemia or infarct, decompensation of valvular disease, and other causes of pulmonary edema.

d. **Evaluation**

i. **Radiography.** A chest radiograph reveals cardiomegaly with variable degrees of pulmonary congestion.

ii. **Electrocardiography.** An ECG most commonly shows nonspecific changes and may reveal sinus tachycardia, atrial fibrillation, AV conduction abnormalities, or ventricular arrhythmias.

TABLE 2-7	Classification of Cardiomyopathies	
Dilated	**Hypertrophic**	**Restrictive**
Idiopathic	Asymmetric septal hypertrophy	Endomyocardial fibrosis
Secondary	Friedreich ataxia	Löffler endocarditis
Infective		Secondary
Viral myocarditis		Infiltrative/granulomatous
Protozoal		Familial storage diseases
Spirochetal		Amyloidosis
Bacterial		Progressive systemic sclerosis
Fungal		Fibroelastosis
Toxic		Radiation
Ethanol		
Cocaine		
Heavy metals		
Radiation		
Drugs		
Doxorubicin		
Nutritional/metabolic		
Collagen vascular diseases		
Infiltrative/granulomatous		
Amyloidosis		
Sarcoidosis		
Malignancy		
Hemochromatosis		
Peripartum heart disease		
Neuromuscular disorders		
Familial storage diseases		

      iii. Bedside echocardiography will reveal chamber enlargement and decreased ventricular function.

    e. **Therapy**

      i. CHF should be treated as discussed in III.E.2.

      ii. Anticoagulation should be initiated if there are no contraindications.

      iii. Antiarrhythmic therapy may be necessary (see section IV). Rapid atrial fibrillation can usually be controlled with intravenous diltiazem, digoxin, or both. Implantation of automatic defibrillators or surgical ablation of arrhythmic circuits is gaining favor for treatment of rhythm disturbances.

      iv. Nonemergent, longer term treatment includes discontinuing any offending agents (e.g., alcohol, drugs). Maximizing known disease-specific therapies, such as nutritional supplementation or therapies for infiltrative malignancies, is essential. Cardiac transplantation may be a consideration.

    f. **Disposition** depends on the severity of symptoms, but most patients present to the ED in a decompensated state and require admission.

  3. **Hypertrophic cardiomyopathy**

    a. **Discussion.** Hypertrophic cardiomyopathy is characterized by muscular hypertrophy of a nondilated left ventricle. Most patients have regional variations in the extent of hypertrophy, but the majority demonstrate disproportionate septal hypertrophy.

    i. Hypertrophy of the left ventricle results from cardiac muscle cell disorganization and variable myocardial fibrosis. Diastolic dysfunction occurs secondary to stiffness of the hypertrophied muscle, which leads to increased end-diastolic pressures and restricted ventricular filling.

    ii. Outflow obstruction due to systolic motion of the anterior leaflet of the mitral valve has been demonstrated in up to 25% of patients and is dynamic in nature depending on the end-diastolic volume, the heart rate, and the afterload.

  b. **Clinical features**

    i. **Symptoms** vary depending on the extent of the disease and the patient's age and are related to the progressive diastolic dysfunction, not the presence or degree of outflow obstruction.

      a) Sudden death may be the first clinical manifestation and is more common in children or young adults. Syncope and near-syncope can occur.

      b) Dyspnea on exertion is a common complaint, and an exercise history must be obtained.

      c) Anginal chest pain is due to the increased oxygen requirements of the hypertrophied muscle that are not met by coronary blood flow.

      d) Palpitations due to arrhythmia may be a complaint. Atrial arrhythmia is usually poorly tolerated due to the loss of atrial contribution to ventricular filling.

    ii. **Physical examination findings** are often benign and unrevealing.

      a) Examination may reveal an audible S_4 as well as a double or triple atrial impulse palpable over the chest wall.

      b) Cardiac examination reveals the **hallmark systolic murmur**, which is harsh, occurs after the S_1, and is diamond-shaped in only 25% of patients. The murmur is best heard at the left sternal border and may be accentuated by performing a Valsalva maneuver. Passively raising the legs, squatting, or a sustained handgrip will decrease the intensity of the murmur. A blowing quality to the murmur may be heard at the apex and represents mitral regurgitation due to the poor apposition of the anterior mitral valve leaflet.

  c. **Differential diagnoses**

    i. Differential diagnoses include aortic or mitral valvular disease, hypertensive heart disease, ischemic heart disease, and other causes of diminished diastolic compliance such as restrictive cardiomyopathy or constrictive pericarditis.

    ii. Athlete's heart syndrome, in which ventricular hypertrophy is physiologic, is often accompanied by similar physical examination findings, ECG abnormalities, and benign arrhythmias, and may be confused with hypertrophic cardiomyopathy. However, a history consistent with that of an asymptomatic trained athlete is a clue to this diagnosis.

  d. **Evaluation.** The diagnosis of hypertrophic cardiomyopathy may be entertained in a patient with a history of exertional dyspnea, classic physical examination findings, and a family history of the disease; however, this diagnosis is not usually made based on the ED evaluation.

    i. **Radiography.** A chest radiograph is initially normal but may show a mild to moderate increase in the cardiac silhouette. Pulmonary vascular congestion is unusual.

    ii. **Electrocardiography.** An ECG demonstrates left ventricular hypertrophy and left atrial enlargement. Deep Q waves (septal Q waves) in multiple leads may mimic those that indicate an old MI (see Figure 2-10). Atrial and ventricular rhythm disturbances are common.

    iii. **Bedside echocardiography** is the diagnostic modality of choice and is useful for distinguishing athlete's heart syndrome from hypertrophic cardiomyopathy.

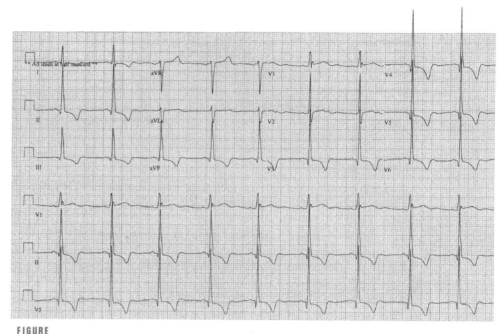

FIGURE 2-10 ECG in a patient with hypertrophic cardiomyopathy.

e. Therapy
   i. Emergent management of the acutely symptomatic patient, especially one with chest pain, is with β blockers to decrease the force of ventricular contraction and increase diastolic filling time. Calcium channel blockers may be of benefit in decreasing ventricular wall stiffness, thereby decreasing ventricular filling pressures. Amiodarone is effective in reducing supraventricular as well as ventricular arrhythmias. Digoxin, nitrates, diuretics, and β agonists should be avoided.
   ii. Longer term therapy may include implantation of a dual-chamber pacemaker and surgical myomectomy.
   iii. Endocarditis prophylaxis is indicated as discussed in XI.F.2.
f. **Disposition.** Patients who present with syncope or chest pain require admission to a monitored setting for further evaluation and treatment. Patients in whom the diagnosis is suspected but who do not demonstrate acute signs and symptoms should be advised to avoid strenuous activity until more thorough evaluation can be performed by a cardiologist.

4. **Restrictive cardiomyopathies**
   a. **Discussion.** Restrictive cardiomyopathies are also characterized by diastolic dysfunction, which results from noncompliance of the ventricles secondary to myocardial fibrosis, infiltration, scarring, or thrombus. The progressively rigid ventricle leads to impedance of filling, high filling pressures, and persistently elevated venous pressure.
   b. **Clinical features**
      i. **Symptoms** relate to the persistently elevated venous pressures from a small, rigid ventricular cavity and include those of right- and left-sided heart failure.
      ii. **Physical examination findings** may include jugular venous distention, often with Kussmaul sign, findings of right-sided heart failure, and findings of CHF. Heart sounds may be distant, and an S_3 and an S_4 are common. A murmur of mitral regurgitation is also common.
   c. **Differential diagnoses** include constrictive pericarditis, cardiac tamponade, pulmonary hypertension, causes of right-sided heart failure (e.g., right ventricular infarct, valvular dysfunction), and causes of left-sided heart failure.

d. **Evaluation**

    i. **Radiography.** A chest radiograph may be unremarkable but may show evidence of pulmonary vascular congestion with a normal cardiac silhouette.

    ii. **Electrocardiography.** An ECG usually reveals nonspecific changes and may show low QRS voltages, also a finding in constrictive pericarditis.

    iii. **Echocardiography** typically reveals symmetric thickening of the ventricular walls with normal or mildly reduced systolic function.

e. **Therapy.** Emergent treatment is symptom-directed and entails the judicious use of diuretics, vasodilators, and antiarrhythmics as necessary. Patients with amyloidosis may be sensitive to digoxin; therefore, this medication should be used with caution.

f. **Disposition.** Depends on the severity of the presenting symptoms, but most patients will require admission for treatment of heart failure.

X. INFECTIOUS ENDOCARDITIS

A. **Discussion**

1. **Definition.** Infectious endocarditis is an infection of the endothelial surface of the heart, most commonly affecting the heart valves.

2. **Pathogenesis**

a. Platelet and fibrin thrombi form on areas of endocardium with damaged endothelium. Endothelial damage can result from scarring (e.g., following rheumatic fever), turbulent blood flow (e.g., such as occurs with ventricular septal defect or patent ductus arteriosus), direct trauma (e.g., caused by pacemaker wires or pulmonary artery catheters), or cachectic states (e.g., malignancy).

b. Transient bacteremia occurs as a result of everyday activities (brushing teeth, chewing hard food, straining during defecation). Iatrogenic procedures can also induce a transient bacteremia.

    i. Bacteria in the bloodstream colonize the thrombus, where they multiply to form an infectious or inflammatory vegetation on the heart valve.

    ii. Aggressive pathogens, such as *S. aureus*, can infect previously undamaged valves, often with rapid local tissue invasion and destruction, leading to symptoms of acute valvular dysfunction, heart failure, and shock.

3. **Classification of infectious endocarditis.** Infectious endocarditis is classified by course, predisposing factors, and the side of the heart affected. These classification systems are predictive of typical infecting organisms, clinical syndromes, and prognosis and thus provide a basis for empiric therapy.

a. **Classification by course**

    i. **Acute** infectious endocarditis has a fulminant presentation, characterized by a high fever and systemic toxicity. Acute infectious endocarditis is usually caused by *S. aureus* and is more often seen in younger patients.

    ii. **Subacute** infectious endocarditis has a more indolent course with nonspecific symptoms and signs. It is most often caused by *Streptococcus viridans* and enterococci (group D streptococci), which usually infect previously damaged valves.

    iii. **Chronic** infectious endocarditis is now included as part of the subacute category.

b. **Classification by predisposing factors**

    i. **Prosthetic valves** are present in 10% to 20% of patients with infectious endocarditis. In such patients, fever without a source mandates admission and empiric antibiotics pending the results of blood cultures.

    ii. **Intravenous drug abuse.** Intravenous drug abusers are at high risk for infectious endocarditis, which is usually acute.

    iii. **Prior valvular lesions.** Approximately two-thirds of patients with native valves who develop infectious endocarditis and do not use intravenous drugs have a prior valvular lesion. Most of these patients have a history of **rheumatic fever. Congenital heart disease** (including mitral valve prolapse and hypertrophic cardiomyopathy) and **degenerative**

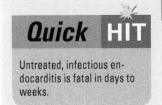

Quick HIT

Untreated, infectious endocarditis is fatal in days to weeks.

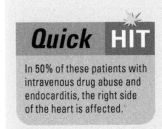

Quick HIT

In 50% of these patients with intravenous drug abuse and endocarditis, the right side of the heart is affected.

Cardiovascular Emergencies

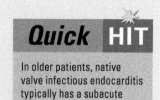

Cardiovascular Emergencies

problems (e.g., calcific aortic stenosis) can also predispose to native valve endocarditis.

  iv. **No identifiable antecedent risk factors.** In patients with infectious endocarditis without a prosthetic valve or a history of intravenous drug abuse, approximately one-third will have no identifiable antecedent risk factors.

4. **Microbiology of infectious endocarditis.** An understanding of the typical pathogens in various clinical settings provides the basis for empiric therapy. Table 2-8 lists typical pathogens in various clinical settings in order of frequency.

  a. The streptococci, staphylococci, and enterococci listed in Table 2-8 are responsible for more than 90% of cases of infectious endocarditis; however, almost any organism can cause infectious endocarditis.

  b. *S. aureus* usually causes fulminant disease, whereas *Staphylococcus epidermidis* and *S. viridans* typically have a more indolent presentation.

B. **Clinical features**

1. **Symptoms** are nonspecific. Fever is the most common symptom, occurring in 80% of patients. Other symptoms include chills, weakness, malaise, sweats, weight loss, neurologic symptoms (especially focal weakness and change of mental status), headache, pain (in the chest, back, abdomen, or joints), cough, shortness of breath, and hemoptysis.

2. **Physical examination findings** are inconsistently present.

  a. In retrospective review, fever and heart murmur are present at some time during the course of 80% to 90% of cases of infectious endocarditis.

  b. Signs of chronic infection, vasculitis, and circulating immune complexes occur in various combinations.

  i. **Osler nodes** are painful nodules on the fingers and toes.

  ii. **Janeway lesions** are nontender hemorrhagic nodules on the palms and soles.

  iii. Splinter hemorrhages and clubbing may be seen.

  iv. Petechiae can occur in any part of the body but are most characteristically seen in the mouth, on the conjunctivae, and on the upper extremities.

  v. Splenomegaly and cachexia may be noted.

  c. Emboli can give rise to signs caused by occlusive and septic phenomena.

  i. Embolic occlusion can cause infarction in any organ without rich collateral circulation, especially the kidneys (causing flank pain and hematuria), the brain (giving rise to neurologic findings in 33% of patients with infectious endocarditis), and the heart. Less commonly, occlusion of large arteries (e.g., the femoral artery) can be caused by fungal emboli.

  ii. Septic emboli can cause pneumonia with multiple infiltrates in patients with right-sided infectious endocarditis. In patients with left-sided

TABLE 2-8	Common Causes of Infectious Endocarditis	
Predisposing Condition	**Typical Pathogens**
Prosthetic valve	
Less than 60 days postoperative	*Staphylococcus epidermidis, Staphylococcus aureus,* gram-negative bacilli, fungi
More than 60 days postoperative	*Streptococcus viridans* (40%), *Staphylococcus epidermidis* (30%), *Staphylococcus aureus,* gram-negative bacilli
Intravenous drug abuse	*Staphylococcus aureus* (more than 50%), group D streptococci (enterococci), *Pseudomonas aeruginosa,* other gram-negative bacilli, *Streptococcus viridans,* fungi
Prior history of valvular disease	*Streptococcus viridans* (40%), enterococci, *Staphylococcus epidermidis, Staphylococcus aureus*
No prior history of valvular disease	*Staphylococcus aureus,* group A and group B streptococci

infectious endocarditis, foci of infection in the brain (abscesses), meninges (meningitis), heart (myocarditis, myocardial abscesses, pericarditis), kidneys (pyelonephritis), and arteries (mycotic aneurysms) may be seen.

d. Local tissue destruction of valves and myocardium can cause signs and symptoms of heart failure, acute valvular insufficiency, myocarditis, heart blocks, dysrhythmias, and myocardial abscesses.

C. **Differential diagnoses.** The diagnosis of infectious endocarditis should be considered in all febrile patients when the source of the fever cannot be identified, especially if the patient has predisposing factors or a heart murmur. Early subacute infectious endocarditis is frequently misdiagnosed as a urinary tract infection or viral syndrome. Other considerations include Lyme disease, malignancy (predisposing to nonbacterial endocardial thrombosis), disseminated gonococcemia or meningococcemia, acute rheumatic fever, valvular myxoma, and collagen vascular disease (especially systemic lupus erythematosus).

D. **Evaluation.** The diagnosis is made by blood culture. Other tests are of limited use in the ED.

1. **Blood cultures.** Detection of bacteria becomes almost impossible after administration of antibiotics. For this reason, and because infectious endocarditis is a disease with high morbidity and mortality rates if inadequately treated, it is necessary for the emergency physician to ensure that optimal blood cultures are obtained.

2. **Other tests**

a. **CBC.** A CBC may reveal an increased WBC count with a left shift in patients with acute infectious endocarditis. In patients with subacute infectious endocarditis, the WBC count is usually normal, with a mild normochromic normocytic anemia. The erythrocyte sedimentation rate is usually elevated.

b. **Urinalysis** is abnormal in the majority of cases, showing some combination of proteinuria, hematuria, and pyuria.

c. **ECGs, chest radiographs, and blood chemistries** may reveal signs of damage to the heart, lungs, or kidneys, respectively; however, these test results are nonspecific and may actually detract attention from the correct diagnosis.

d. **Echocardiography.** Routine transthoracic echocardiography, even in the hands of a cardiologist, is only 50% to 80% sensitive in detecting valvular vegetations. Transesophageal echocardiography is the gold standard diagnostic test.

E. **Therapy.** The following regimens for empiric therapy are based on American Heart Association recommendations.

1. **Prosthetic valve endocarditis.** In all cases, patients with prosthetic valve endocarditis are treated with **vancomycin**, plus **gentamicin**, plus **rifampin**.

2. **Native valve endocarditis**

a. **Sick or unstable patients.** Patients with acute infectious endocarditis are often thought to have undifferentiated sepsis at the time of their ED presentation. If endocarditis is recognized as a possible cause for the patient's clinical presentation, the patient should be treated with **nafcillin** and **gentamicin**, unless he or she is an intravenous drug abuser in an area of methicillin-resistant *S. aureus*, in which case **vancomycin** is added.

b. **Patients with a subacute presentation and a strong suspicion for native valve endocarditis.** Intravenous drug abusers should be treated as described in XI.E.2.a. Other patients are treated with **ceftriaxone** or **vancomycin** plus **gentamicin**.

c. **Patients with a subacute presentation and a low suspicion for native valve endocarditis.** These patients should undergo three or more blood cultures over 6 hours, with or without initiating antibiotic therapy, as determined in consultation with the admitting physician or the patient's private physician.

F. **Prevention.** Infectious endocarditis is more easily prevented than cured.

1. **Conditions requiring antibiotic prophylaxis.** Recommendations for antibiotic prophylaxis against endocarditis change often upon review of evidence. Antibiotic prophylaxis against endocarditis should be administered for patients with highest risk factors for endocarditis as listed below (see Clinical Pearl 2-3).

CLINICAL PEARL 2-3

High-risk Conditions for Endocarditis: prosthetic heart valves, prosthetic material used for valve repair, a history of endocarditis, unrepaired cyanotic heart disease, repaired cyanotic heart disease, and cardiac transplant recipients.

2. **Prophylactic regimens** and some of the ED procedures that necessitate them are summarized in Table 2-9.
G. **Disposition.** Diagnosis is not possible in the ED. Therefore, clinical judgment is required to weigh the likelihood of infectious endocarditis against the risks and expenses of unnecessary treatment. The diagnosis must at least be considered in any patient with a fever. Risk of infection is increased if the patient has a murmur of undetermined etiology, or any of the predisposing conditions listed in XI.A.3.b.
   1. **Admission**
      a. Patients with prosthetic valves are at risk for devastating complications if endocarditis is misdiagnosed, so those with unexplained fever should have blood cultures and be admitted for empiric treatment.
      b. Clinical assessment of intravenous drug abusers with fever has been shown to be unreliable in ruling out dangerous bacteremic states. It is prudent to obtain blood samples for culture and admit these patients to the hospital.
      c. Patients with a high likelihood of infectious endocarditis or those who are deemed unlikely to comply with follow-up arrangements should be admitted for observation and transesophageal echocardiography studies, pending culture results.
   2. **Discharge.** Patients who may have infectious endocarditis, but in whom the diagnosis is unlikely, can be discharged after blood cultures are obtained if the physician is reasonably sure that the patient will comply with follow-up arrangements.

XI. VASCULAR DISEASE

A. **Thoracic aortic dissection**
   1. **Discussion**
      a. **Cause.** Causes include the following:
         i. **Hypertension,** the most common cause of thoracic aortic dissection
         ii. **Congenital conditions** (e.g., Marfan syndrome, Ehlers-Danlos syndrome, Turner syndrome)

TABLE 2-9 Common Endocarditis Prophylaxis Regimens for High-Risk Patients[a]

Procedure	Targeted Organism	Antibiotic
Ear, nose, and throat procedures (e.g., nasal packing, incision and drainage of abscesses)	*Streptococcus viridans*	Amoxicillin or clindamycin or ceftriaxone
Minor procedures (e.g., urethral catheterization anoscopy)	Enterococci	Ampicillin
Major procedures (e.g., preoperative for abdominal or genitourinary surgery)	Enterococci	Ampicillin + gentamicin *or* vancomycin + gentamicin
Dermal procedures (e.g., incision and drainage of abscesses)	*Staphylococcus aureus, Staphylococcus epidermidis*	Cephalexin or dicloxacillin or clindamycin

[a]For example, history of infectious endocarditis or prosthetic valve.

      iii. **Pregnancy** (the most common cause of dissection in women younger than 40 years)

      iv. **Trauma**

  b. **Pathogenesis.** The affected aorta is usually not aneurysmal. The aging process combined with dynamic stress of persistently elevated pressures results in loss of structural integrity with weakening of the medial and intimal layers. Tears in the intima most commonly occur just distal to the aortic valve or at the level of the ligamentum arteriosum. Blood then dissects between the layers of the arterial wall forming a false lumen, reentering the true lumen through another intimal tear.

      i. Dissection can proceed proximally, distally, or in both directions, accounting for the various associated problems such as acute aortic valve insufficiency, coronary artery occlusion, and neurologic deficits due to affected carotid arteries.

      ii. Occasionally, the vessel can rupture outward into the pleural space, esophagus, or pericardium, causing massive hemorrhage, cardiac tamponade, or both.

2. **Clinical features**

  a. Patients complain of severe pain, often radiating to the back or abdomen, and usually of sudden onset. Pain may be described as ripping or tearing and may be associated with diaphoresis, nausea, and vomiting. A positive family history may be elicited.

  b. Physical examination often reveals hypertension.

      i. A systolic blood pressure difference of more than 15 mm Hg between measurements taken in each arm or a unilateral absence of pulses suggests dissection.

      ii. Hypotension suggests rupture of the dissection, possibly into the pleural space (causing a hemothorax) or into the pericardium (causing tamponade).

      iii. Cardiac examination may reveal a musical, diastolic murmur of aortic insufficiency.

      iv. Neurologic deficits are common and are due to cerebral or spinal ischemia from decreased blood flow or occlusion of affected arteries.

3. **Differential diagnoses.** The chest pain of thoracic aortic dissection must be differentiated from that of acute MI and esophageal rupture.

4. **Evaluation**

  a. **Electrocardiography.** An ECG will demonstrate left ventricular hypertrophy and may be helpful in differentiating thoracic aortic dissection from acute MI, but up to 40% of patients with thoracic aortic dissection may have evidence of ischemia or infarction on ECG.

  b. **Radiography.** A chest radiograph is abnormal in 80% of patients and may show mediastinal widening, obliteration of the aortic knob, tracheal displacement to the right, a double-density appearance of the aorta, or pleural effusion (usually on the left).

  c. **Laboratory studies.** Blood tests are of little value emergently, but a CBC, BUN and creatinine level, serum electrolyte panel, coagulation studies, and type and cross match should be sent.

  d. **Transesophageal echocardiography** or **CT** of the chest helps establish the diagnosis, but **CT angiography** is the gold standard and is needed in preparation for surgical repair (see Figure 2-11).

5. **Therapy** initially entails controlling the blood pressure and heart rate.

  a. Afterload reduction with nitroprusside or nicardipine must be combined with a β blocker to control heart rate and decrease the shearing forces in the aorta. Esmolol is often used because this agent can be given intravenously and closely titrated.

  b. Labetalol, with both α and β blocker activity, has been advocated as a single agent, but lacks the flexibility of nitroprusside and esmolol administration.

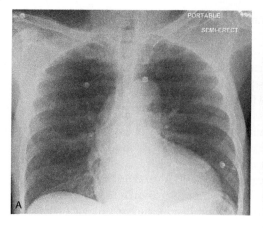
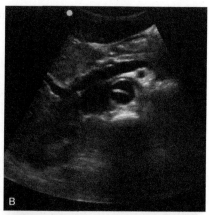
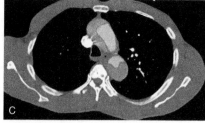

FIGURE
2-11 (A) Chest X-ray with mildly widened mediastinum. (B) Bedside ultrasound image of aorta with intimal flap. (C) CTA chest redemonstrating aortic dissection.
(Courtesy of Hugh W. Shoff, MD.)

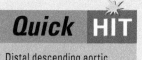

Quick HIT

Distal descending aortic dissections can be treated medically with antihypertensive medications and observation.

6. **Disposition.** Surgery is indicated for patients with a dissection involving the ascending aorta and aortic arch, ruptured dissections, aortic regurgitation, cerebral complications, and uncontrollable pain.

B. **Peripheral artery disease**
1. **Chronic arterial insufficiency**
   a. **Discussion.** Chronic arterial insufficiency is usually caused by advanced atherosclerosis but may be caused by Buerger disease and vasculitis (especially systemic lupus erythematosus). Advanced atherosclerosis is more likely to affect the aortic arch, the bifurcation of the common carotids, the infrarenal aorta, the common iliac bifurcation, the bifurcation of the common femorals, the adductor canal, and the trifurcation of the popliteal arteries. The upper extremities are usually spared.
   b. **Clinical features**
      i. **History.** Arterial insufficiency often occurs in patients with "panatherosclerosis." A history of myocardial ischemia, cerebrovascular disease, or renal insufficiency should be sought. Chronic arterial insufficiency shares the risk factors of smoking, hypertension, diabetes, hypercholesterolemia, and obesity with these disorders.
      ii. **Symptoms.** Pain on exertion, referred to as claudication ("limping"), progresses to pain at rest and then to cellular injury and frank gangrene.
         a) Occlusion in the aortoiliac region ("inflow disease") suggests Leriche syndrome: buttock or thigh claudication accompanied by impotence in men.
         b) Occlusion in the infrainguinal region ("outflow disease") causes symptoms in the calf and foot.
      iii. **Physical examination findings**
         a) Cool, shiny, atrophic skin with thickened nails, poor capillary refill, and cyanosis is seen. As the ischemia progresses, muscle atrophy occurs. Ulcers develop over the bony prominences of the toes, the metatarsophalangeal joints, and the heels.
         b) Pulses should be palpated and evaluated for strength and symmetry. If not palpable, they should be sought by Doppler. In healthy

Cardiovascular Emergencies

patients, the Doppler signal has a sharp, "whipping," triphasic sound, which becomes progressively less distinct as the occlusion worsens.

  c) The **ankle–brachial index** is the ratio between the highest systolic blood pressures as measured in the posterior tibial and brachial arteries. The ankle–arm index should be > 0.9; a value less < 0.40 indicates severe disease (Table 2-10).

  d) **Buerger sign** indicates advanced disease. With the patient supine, the extremity becomes white and painful when the foot is elevated 12 inches. When the extremity is placed in a dependent position, the foot regains color abnormally slowly, and then an intense hyperemia ("dependent rubor") occurs.

c. Differential diagnoses

  i. Chronic arterial insufficiency must be distinguished from acute arterial occlusion (see XII.B.2) on the basis of the patient history.

  ii. Poorly defined pain of the hips and pelvis, sometimes associated with exertion ("pseudoclaudication"), can be a sign of spinal cord disease.

  iii. Lower extremity ulcerations caused by venous insufficiency have a different location and appearance (see XII.B.3.c.ii.b). Other causes of lower extremity ulcerations include diabetes, vasculitis, vasospasm, pyoderma gangrenosum, carcinoma, spider bites, and infections.

d. Disposition

  i. Chronic arterial insufficiency that has progressed to loss of motor or sensory function must be treated as an acute occlusion (see XII.A.2.e).

  ii. Patients with chronic arterial insufficiency (diagnosed on the basis of the history) require no further ED evaluation and should be referred to primary care or a vascular surgeon for continued treatment. Smokers should be counseled on cessation.

2. Acute arterial occlusion

a. Discussion. Acute arterial occlusion can be caused by emboli or in situ thrombosis.

  i. **Embolic disease.** Embolism is suggested by a precipitous onset, asymmetrical extremity examination, or sharp demarcation of ischemia, in the context of dysrhythmias, recent MI, or ventricular aneurysm.

  a) **Sources of emboli**

  1) The **heart** is the source of 85% of emboli, at least 66% of which originate in the ventricles (even in the presence of atrial fibrillation). Ventricular thrombi are associated with MI and ventricular aneurysm.

  2) Approximately 15% of emboli are **arterioarterial**, originating from ruptured atheromatous plaques (**atheroemboli**), or **mural thrombi**, which typically form in arterial aneurysms. Atheroemboli tend to be small and can occur in showers, leading to focal, asymmetric areas of ischemia and necrosis in regions dependent on a single end-arterial arcade—typically the digits (e.g., "blue toe syndrome").

  b) **Sites.** The most common site of embolic occlusion is the femoral bifurcation. A bounding "water hammer" pulse can be heard at that site initially; the water hammer pulse then disappears as the thrombus propagates proximally.

TABLE 2-10	Interpretation of Ankle–Brachial Index
1.30	Noncompressible
0.91–1.30	Normal
0.41–0.90	Mild-to-moderate peripheral arterial disease
0.00–0.40	Severe peripheral arterial disease

Cardiovascular Emergencies

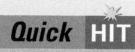

Quick HIT

Pain is the first symptom to develop; the rest of the "six P's" are late findings and their absence should not delay consultation and therapy.

ii. **In situ thrombosis** is usually seen as an acute deterioration of limb function in patients with chronic arterial insufficiency. These patients have usually developed extensive collateral circulation so that symptoms are less severe, and signs of chronic disease are present bilaterally.

b. **Clinical features** are summarized by the "**six Ps**": **pain, pallor, pulselessness, paresthesia, paralysis,** and **poikilothermia.** A thorough extremity examination should be performed (see Figure 2-12).

c. **Differential diagnoses** are the same as for chronic arterial insufficiency. A search for a possible cardiac source should be made.

d. **Evaluation.** As soon as acute arterial occlusion or limb-threatening chronic ischemia has been clinically identified, a vascular surgeon should be consulted. Preoperative laboratory studies, including a CBC, coagulation studies, blood type and screen, an ECG, and a chest radiograph, should be obtained. There are several options for vascular imaging.

   i. **Ultrasound** can demonstrate an intra-arterial clot. If ultrasound is available in the ED, definitive information about femoral thromboembolism may be available, precluding the need for time-consuming radiologic studies. **Duplex ultrasound** provides color representation of blood flow.

   ii. **Angiography** provides definitive anatomic information about the vascular tree and is essential for most decisions about vascular bypass. However, it is time-consuming, invasive, and subject to several complications, including allergic reactions, intrinsic endothelial toxicity from radiocontrast agents, direct arterial damage, and renal failure.

   iii. **CT angiogram** has similar sensitivity as compared to angiography and is easily performed in the ED. It is indicated to evaluate the possibility of abdominal aorta or popliteal artery aneurysm and to help guide surgical intervention.

e. **Therapy**

   i. **Supportive measures**

      a) **Aspirin.** The patient should be administered aspirin (325 mg, to be chewed) immediately to inhibit propagation of the platelet-rich "white thrombus" characteristic of arterial occlusion.

      b) **Heparin.** The patient should be administered heparin as per the protocol described in XII.C.1.e.i.

   ii. **Definitive therapy.** If complete occlusion is suspected (on the basis of loss of sensation or motor function), emergency revascularization is required within 4 hours if the limb is to be salvaged. Options include the administration of thrombolytic agents, Fogarty catheter embolectomy, endarterectomy, PTCA, bypass grafting, and primary amputation. Which therapy is used depends on the time course, site, and cause of the occlusion, as well as surgical preferences.

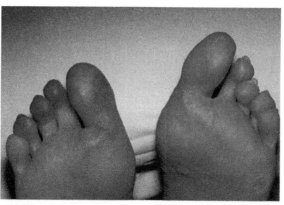

FIGURE
2-12 Blue toes/foot in embolic disease.
(Courtesy of Lawrence B. Stack, MD.)

f. **Disposition.** Patients with limb-threatening chronic arterial insufficiency or acute arterial occlusion must be admitted to the hospital for emergency revascularization. Patients with acute partial occlusion may be admitted and observed at the discretion of the vascular surgeon.

3. **Arterial trauma** is an obvious consideration whenever a patient presents with blunt or penetrating extremity trauma and any or all of the "six Ps" of acute insufficiency. However, arterial trauma can also occur without any immediate sign of arterial insufficiency. Arterial trauma must be considered with trauma in the proximity of a major neurovascular bundle, even in the presence of normal pulses and perfusion. The decision regarding whether to perform emergent arteriography or to observe the patient expectantly is usually made in consultation with a vascular or trauma surgeon.

C. **Venous disease**

1. **Deep venous thrombosis (DVT) of the lower extremities**

   a. **Discussion**

      i. **Normal physiology.** The anatomy and physiology of the venous system are such that blood is returned to the heart passively.

         a) **Venous valvular competence.** Venous valves work as a "water ladder," returning blood in a series of steps, pumped by the motion of surrounding muscles. Any process injuring the valves puts an additional stress on those that remain, causing them to fail sooner. Most of the blood in the superficial veins of the lower extremities passes via valved perforating veins through the muscles to the deep system (i.e., the tibial, peroneal, popliteal, and femoral veins). The rest passes via the lesser saphenous vein into the popliteal vein at the knee, or the greater saphenous vein to the femoral vein at the foramen ovale.

         b) **Coagulation.** The ideal coagulation system rapidly arrests hemorrhage with specificity of action (i.e., clotting is tied temporally and spatially to sites of hemorrhage), forms blood clots that permit blood-borne agents of inflammation and healing access to the site of injury, and initiates clot lysis as soon as tissue repair is completed. Physiologically, these functions are accomplished by means of a dynamic equilibrium between procoagulant/thrombotic and anticoagulant/thrombolytic agencies.

            1) **Procoagulant mechanisms** are effected primarily through endothelial cells, platelets, and the clotting cascades.

            2) **Anticoagulant mechanisms.** Agents include **antithrombin III,** which inactivates factors XIIa, XIa, Xa, IXa, and IIa in a reaction catalyzed by heparin, and **proteins C and S,** which act together to inhibit factors VIIIa, Va, and IIa. **Thrombolysis** (fibrinolysis) is mediated primarily by plasmin, which is formed from plasminogen by tissue plasminogen activator and urokinase. **Active blood flow** dilutes and removes activated clotting factors, platelets, and platelet aggregates, and provides access to coagulation inhibitors.

      ii. **Pathophysiology.** Dysfunction of the venous valves leads to stasis of blood and endothelial injury, two of the three components of **Virchow triad: stasis, hypercoagulability, and endothelial injury.** Pathologic clotting occurs when procoagulant forces predominate in intravascular sites where there is no acute injury. Disruption of thrombolysis can occur as a result of decreased levels of plasminogen activators, or abnormal configurations of fibrin or plasmin. Conditions that predispose to DVT are summarized in Table 2-11.

      iii. **Types of DVT**

         a) **Distal DVT.** Most venous thromboses of the lower extremities are thought to originate in the veins of the calf. Distal DVT does not pose a significant risk of pulmonary embolus.

TABLE 2-11	Clinical Conditions Associated with Deep Venous Thrombosis
Predisposing Condition	**Examples**
Medical conditions associated with significant inflammation	Acute MI, DIC, ulcerative colitis
Surgical conditions	Burns, multiple trauma, CNS trauma, orthopedic surgery
Hypercoagulable states	Antithrombin III deficiency, protein C deficiency, dysfibrinogenemia, lupus anticoagulant
Venous stasis	Rheologic (e.g., polycythemia vera)
	Immobilization (e.g., illness, long journeys)
	Local (e.g., chronic venous insufficiency)
	Systemic (e.g., CHF)
Endothelial injury	Vasculitis, especially SLE
Drug therapy	Oral contraceptives, estrogens
Other conditions	Previous DVT, age, obesity, cerebrovascular accident, blood type A, pregnancy, malignancy, intravenous drug abuse, sepsis

CHF, congestive heart failure; CNS, central nervous system; DIC, disseminated intravascular coagulation; DVT, deep vein thrombosis; MI, myocardial infarction; SLE, systemic lupus erythematosus.

    b) **Proximal DVT.** Twenty percent of calf thromboses extend to the popliteal, femoral, or iliac veins. DVT in these locations mandates therapy because pulmonary embolism occurs in as many as 50% of these patients.

    c) **Phlegmasia alba dolens** is an advanced and clinically identifiable syndrome of DVT in which iliofemoral thrombosis is so severe as to cause massive edema of the extremity. The leg is pale, cool, and in jeopardy.

    d) **Phlegmasia cerulea dolens** is a syndrome in which occlusion has progressed from the iliofemoral system to include all of the collateral veins of the lower extremity. Arterial ischemia and cyanosis are present. The patient and the limb are in immediate jeopardy.

b. **Clinical features**

    i. **Symptoms** include pain, tenderness, and leg swelling. Of these, the most specific symptom is swelling. With such nonspecific symptoms, DVT must be considered in every patient with nontraumatic leg pain.

    ii. **Physical examination findings** are similarly nonspecific and include leg swelling, edema, tenderness in the calves and thighs, and fever. Homan sign and palpable "cords" are neither sensitive nor specific.

        a) A ballpoint pen should be used to mark both legs at the same point, at midcalf and midthigh (usually approximately 7 cm below and 22 cm above the tibial tubercle). The circumference of the legs should be compared. A difference of more than 1.5 cm is considered significant.

        b) The location of leg tenderness cannot reliably distinguish proximal from distal thrombosis, although pain in areas distant from the anatomic location of deep veins suggests an alternative diagnosis.

c. **Differential diagnoses** include cellulitis, a ruptured popliteal (Baker) cyst, lymphedema, chronic venous insufficiency (with or without acute phlebitis), superficial thrombophlebitis, arterial insufficiency, and musculoskeletal disorders, including trauma, arthritis, and tendonitis. The most difficult distinction is between chronic postphlebitic inflammation and recurrence of acute DVT; the two can rarely be differentiated without diagnostic testing.

d. Evaluation
  i. Modalities
   a) **Duplex ultrasound** combines ultrasonographic images of the veins with color representations of blood flow. Clots are imaged directly or indirectly at sites of impaired flow. Sensitivity is around 92%, with a specificity of 98% for femoral vein thrombi.
   b) **Doppler testing** measures venous flow of blood, the effect of respiration, and distal and proximal compression. Sensitivity and specificity are 85% to 90% for proximal DVT. The test is noninvasive, can be performed in the ED, and can diagnose superficial thrombophlebitis. Its main disadvantage is that it is highly operator-dependent.
   c) **Venography** is often considered the gold standard for diagnosis of DVT because of its high degree of sensitivity and specificity. It is the only modality that reliably demonstrates DVT in the calf. However, venography is time-consuming, technically difficult (5% of studies are "inadequate"), invasive (2% to 4% of studies actually cause venous thrombosis), and, in most institutions, available only on a limited basis.
   d) **Laboratory studies** prior to treatment are limited to a CBC, platelet count, D-dimer, and coagulation studies (e.g., prothrombin time, partial thromboplastin time). Therapy should not be withheld pending laboratory test results unless coagulopathy is suspected on clinical grounds.
  ii. Approach to the patient
   a) Patients with leg symptoms of DVT should first be evaluated using Well criteria for pretest probability of DVT (Table 2-12). In most institutions, diagnostic testing is focused on duplex ultrasound of the lower extremities. In patients without contraindications to heparin who are clinically suspected of DVT, anticoagulation therapy should be initiated and the patient should be admitted for inpatient work up.
   b) Patients who are moderate or high risk for DVT (Well score >1) require a diagnostic study emergently to establish the diagnosis and determine the relative risk of heparin therapy versus surgical intervention. When imaging is performed, the results generally put the patient in one of the three following categories:
    1) An unequivocally positive result is indication for starting heparin therapy or intervening surgically.
    2) A patient with a venogram showing calf DVT or with a negative duplex ultrasound scan requires a D-dimer. Patients with a

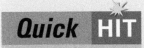

Quick HIT

The D-dimer has a half-life of approximately 8 hours and remains elevated for 3 days in symptomatic DVT. The sensitivity and specificity approach 95%.

TABLE **2-12** Wells Score for Deep Venous Thrombosis	
Clinical Feature	**Points[a]**
Active cancer	1
Paralysis, paresis, or immobilization of lower extremities	1
Bedridden for 3 days due to surgery (within 4 weeks)	1
Tenderness along distribution of deep veins	1
Entire leg swollen	1
Unilateral calf swelling	1
Unilateral pitting edema	1
Collateral superficial veins	1
Alternative diagnosis more likely than DVT	−2

DVT, deep venous thrombosis.
[a]Risk score interpretation (probability of DVT): >3 points: high risk (75%); 1–2 points: moderate risk (17%); <1 point: low risk (3%).

negative duplex ultrasound of the lower extremities and a negative D-dimer require repeat imaging in 1 week.

3) An unequivocally negative result with duplex ultrasound and D-dimer rules out DVT.

c) **Patients who are low risk for DVT (Well score <1) should undergo D-dimer testing.**

1) An unequivocally positive result is indication for Duplex imaging and if positive starting treatment with heparin.

2) A positive D-dimer with negative duplex ultrasound in a low risk patient rules out DVT.

3) An unequivocally negative D-dimer rules out DVT.

e. **Therapy.** Therapeutic options include the following:

i. **Heparin** is given in an initial bolus followed by an infusion. The activated partial thromboplastin time is checked in 6 hours and the heparin rate adjusted accordingly. As an alternative, consider enoxaparin (Lovenox) 1 mg/kg subcutaneously every 12 hours.

ii. **Surgical therapy** is indicated for those with contraindications to anticoagulation. A filter can be placed in the inferior vena cava fluoroscopically, without the need for general anesthesia. Thrombectomy is indicated for patients with phlegmasia cerulea dolens.

iii. **Thrombolytic therapy** for proximal DVT of the lower extremities is controversial but recommended by some for the treatment of phlegmasia cerulea dolens and acute-onset DVT in young patients.

f. **Disposition.** Patients with a possible or established diagnosis of DVT are still often admitted to the hospital. Patients in whom proximal DVT has been ruled out, but distal DVT is still possible, can be discharged with follow-up for repeat diagnostic studies in 5 to 7 days; however, it is essential that the patient be compliant and motivated.

2. **DVT of the upper extremities**

a. **Discussion.** Thrombosis of the axillary or subclavian veins represents less than 2% of the cases of DVT. It is often associated with anatomic obstructions at the thoracic inlet. Other causes include excessive muscular activity of the arms (i.e., "effort thrombosis") and trauma (including intravenous catheters and drug abuse). Pulmonary embolism can occur in 10% to 15% of cases.

b. **Clinical features.** Symptoms and signs are similar to those of lower extremity DVT. Distended superficial veins are more easily identifiable and strongly suggest the diagnosis if they fail to collapse when the patient's arm is raised. Prominent superficial veins of the shoulder suggest that the thrombosis is chronic.

c. **Differential diagnoses** include cellulitis and lymphedema. Precipitating causes, including occult cancer, should be considered.

d. **Evaluation** is made by venography, implantable pulse generator, or duplex scanning.

e. **Therapy.** Axillary and subclavian vein thrombosis is usually an isolated event (i.e., not associated with preexistent venous insufficiency), and reestablishing venous patency is usually sufficient to prevent recurrence.

3. **Other venous system diseases**

a. **Varicose veins** (i.e., swollen, usually nontender, superficial veins) can be primary or secondary. Primary varicose veins are associated with female sex and increasing age. Secondary varicose veins can be caused by any process that causes sustained venous hypertension. Common causes include valvular incompetence, pregnancy, and DVT. Varicose veins are rarely of clinical significance except as a cause of hemorrhage from minor trauma to the overlying skin.

b. **Superficial thrombophlebitis** (i.e., thrombosis and inflammation of a superficial vein) is usually a diagnosis that can be made on clinical grounds. In the presence of varicose veins, superficial thrombophlebitis is generally a benign disease and can be treated with elevation, local heat, and nonsteroidal anti-inflammatory drugs for pain. In the absence of varicose veins, it is frequently a sign of DVT, occult malignancy, or both. DVT must be ruled out prior to discharge; occult malignancy can be worked up on an outpatient basis.

c. **Chronic venous insufficiency** refers to the skin and tissue changes seen with chronic venous hypertension.

  i. **Discussion.** With loss of venous valvular function, a state of chronic venous hypertension develops in the veins of the legs, causing direct endothelial injury. The endothelial injury leads to capillary leakage, increased interstitial oncotic pressure, and further edema. Chronic fibrosis further impedes cellular nutrition, whereas skin breakdown causes bacterial invasion and cellulitis, propagating the injury.

  ii. **Clinical features**

  a) **Symptoms** start at the ankles and progress proximally. The patient complains of a swelling, burning sensation of the skin, and, later, venous ulceration. Venous claudication, a bursting pain in the calves with exercise, is relieved by raising the leg. (This is in contrast to arterial claudication, where the leg is held dependently for relief.)

  b) **Physical examination findings** include hyperpigmented skin with pitting or brawny edema and loss of skin appendages, eventually progressing to beefy ulceration. Findings predominate on the ankle, anterior to the medial malleolus.

  iii. **Therapy** ultimately requires prolonged outpatient follow-up. In the ED, depending on the severity of the disease, a patient may need compression stockings or an Unna boot; admission may be necessary for some patients, especially if cellulitis is present.

  iv. **Disposition.** Admission is indicated if there is ischemia, significant necrosis, signs of systemic toxicity, or obvious inability of the patient to care for him- or herself. If the patient is to be discharged, cellulitis must be treated if present, and the patient must be educated about meticulous elevation of the extremity at all times while not active.

Cardiovascular Emergencies

3 PULMONARY EMERGENCIES

Thomas Cunningham • Peter Latino

I. ACUTE RESPIRATORY FAILURE

A. **Discussion**

1. **Definition.** Acute respiratory failure is defined as an acute impairment in oxygen or carbon dioxide exchange that results in, or has the potential to result in, patient morbidity or mortality. **Impaired gas exchange** (e.g., as a result of shunting, alveolar hypoventilation, ventilation–perfusion [$\dot{V}/\dot{Q}$] mismatch, or decreased pulmonary diffusion capacity) leads to hypoxemia (decreased arterial oxygen tension [PaO_2]) and possibly **hypoxia** (i.e., insufficient delivery of oxygen to tissues). **Impaired ventilation** causes **hypercapnia** (i.e., an elevated carbon dioxide tension [PCO_2]). Because the baseline respiratory status may vary greatly among patients, it is difficult to characterize acute respiratory insufficiency by purely numeric criteria.

   a. Generally, a patient who acutely develops a PO_2 below 60 mm Hg on room air or a PCO_2 greater than 50 mm Hg with an arterial blood pH less than 7.35 is considered to be in respiratory failure.

   b. Some patients (e.g., those with chronic obstructive pulmonary disease [COPD]) chronically have an elevated PCO_2 but a normal arterial blood pH. In these patients, respiratory failure is defined as a PCO_2 higher than baseline with a concurrent decrease in serum pH.

2. **Causes.** There are many causes of acute respiratory failure, including most pulmonary diseases as well as many cardiac diseases. Most commonly, one should consider airway obstruction, asthma, COPD, congestive heart failure (CHF), noncardiogenic pulmonary edema, pulmonary emboli, massive pleural effusion, pneumonia, hemothorax, pneumothorax, toxic inhalation, advanced lung cancer, and neurologic or muscular disorders that result in impaired respiratory abilities.

B. **Clinical features**

1. **Symptoms**

   a. **Cardiovascular. Dyspnea** is the most common symptom of acute respiratory failure.

   b. **Neurologic**

      i. **Confusion, agitation**, and **disorientation** can occur with marked hypoxia.

      ii. **Lethargy** or **somnolence** is commonly seen in patients with marked hypercapnia.

      iii. **Generalized seizures** or **coma** may result from profound central nervous system hypoxia.

   c. **Other signs** of respiratory failure include **cyanosis, diaphoresis**, and **severely labored breathing** (including the use of accessory muscles). Children may demonstrate nasal flaring, audible grunting, or retractions (i.e., intercostal, subcostal, suprasternal).

2. **Physical examination findings**

   a. **Tachycardia, tachypnea**, and **mild hypertension** are usually present.

   b. **Bradypnea** may be seen in patients with hypercapnia. **Wheezing, rales**, or **decreased breath sounds** may be noted on pulmonary examination, depending on the underlying disease.

C. **Evaluation.** In a patient with suspected acute respiratory failure, patient evaluation and treatment occur simultaneously.

1. **Patient history and physical examination.** A brief, focused history and physical examination, including vital signs, will often reveal the cause of respiratory failure prior to obtaining any diagnostic studies.

2. **Diagnostic tests**

   a. **Chest radiography** is helpful for determining the underlying cause of the acute respiratory failure. Radiographs should be obtained rapidly at the patient's bedside.

   b. **Arterial blood gas (ABG).** An ABG should be obtained in all patients with suspected acute respiratory failure. The most important elements of the ABG are the P_{O_2}, P_{CO_2}, and pH.

   c. **Pulse oximetry** may provide an immediate measurement of the patient's oxygen saturation.

   d. **Ancillary tests** may be indicated, depending on the cause of the respiratory failure (e.g., ABG with co-oximetry for dyshemoglobinemias, an electrocardiogram [ECG] for a patient with suspected CHF, a $\dot{V}/\dot{Q}$ scan or computed tomography [CT] pulmonary angiogram for a patient with suspected pulmonary embolism, a urine toxicology screen for a patient with suspected narcotic overdose).

D. **Therapy**

1. **Airway, breathing, circulation (ABC)**

   a. **Airway.** Airway management, usually **orotracheal intubation**, is required for patients who do not have an intact airway or who are unable to protect their airway.

   b. **Breathing.** After an airway has been established, ensuring adequate oxygenation and ventilation is the mainstay of treating respiratory failure.

      i. **Oxygenation.** Patients should be administered supplemental oxygen in order to maintain a serum oxygen saturation of at least 90%.

         a) In **intubated patients**, it is best to start with an inspired oxygen concentration (FIO_2) of 100% and then reduce this percentage, depending on the ABG results.

         b) In **nonintubated patients**, supplemental oxygen can be administered via **nasal cannula** or **face mask**.

      ii. **Ventilation** should be addressed in addition to oxygenation. Patients with a P_{CO_2} greater than 50 mm Hg and an arterial blood pH below 7.30 require intubation and mechanical ventilation if their condition cannot be quickly improved.

         a) Following intubation, ventilator settings for respiratory rates and tidal volumes should generally be adjusted to gradually normalize the blood pH. In general, the initial respiratory rate should be 12 to 16 breaths/min, with a tidal volume of 6 to 8 mL/kg.

         b) As a general rule, oxygenation is more important than ventilation. For this reason, it is acceptable to have a mild respiratory acidosis (e.g., a pH less than 7.35) if necessary to maintain adequate oxygenation or to minimize peak airway pressures.

   c. **Circulation.** The placement of **two peripheral intravenous lines** allows the administration of fluids and medications to the patient.

2. **Specific therapy** that addresses the cause of the acute respiratory failure should be undertaken after the ABCs have been addressed. In some cases, aggressive treatment of the underlying condition may reverse the respiratory failure and eliminate the need for intubation (e.g., nitroglycerin and afterload reduction for CHF, inhaled β_2 agonists for asthma or COPD, chest tube placement for a large pneumothorax or hemothorax).

E. **Disposition.** All patients with acute respiratory failure should be admitted to an intensive care unit (ICU). Patients who are clinically stable but have the potential for developing respiratory failure should be admitted to an ICU or another closely monitored unit.

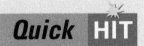

Quick HIT

Chest radiographs lag behind in their appearance when compared to the clinical course.

Quick HIT

In situations where hemoglobin is unable to bind oxygen (e.g., methemoglobinemia and carboxyhemoglobinemia), pulse oximetry analysis overestimates the oxygen saturation.

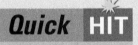

Quick HIT

Although the concentration of oxygen delivered by each of these methods is variable, it is best to start with a method that delivers a high oxygen concentration (e.g., a nonrebreather face mask).

Pulmonary Emergencies

II. ASTHMA

A. **Discussion**

   1. **Definition.** Asthma is defined as the presence of intermittent symptoms from airway hyperactivity and reversible airway obstruction due to multiple stimuli. Airway obstruction is usually caused by smooth muscle contraction and airway inflammation.

      a. **Extrinsic asthma** is immunologically mediated and tends to develop in childhood.

      b. **Intrinsic asthma** has no identifiable cause and tends to worsen with age.

   2. **Incidence.** Asthma affects approximately 5% of adults in the United States; approximately 1.5 million patients seek care for asthma in the emergency department (ED) each year.

B. **Clinical features**

   1. **Symptoms**

      a. **Wheezing, dyspnea,** and **cough** are most common. In cough-variant asthma, cough, which is often worse at night, is the prominent feature.

      b. **Pleuritic chest pain** is noted in some patients.

      c. **Accessory muscle use** may be seen in patients having moderate to severe attacks.

      d. **Altered mental status, severely labored breathing,** or **extreme fatigue** are signs of **impending respiratory arrest.**

   2. **Physical examination findings**

      a. **Tachypnea** and **tachycardia** are common.

      b. Pulmonary examination often demonstrates **wheezing,** a **prolonged expiratory phase,** and **decreased breath sounds.**

C. **Differential diagnoses** include CHF, upper airway obstruction, foreign body aspiration, pulmonary embolism, anaphylactic reactions, pneumonia, croup, bronchiolitis, COPD, and toxic inhalation.

D. **Evaluation**

   1. **Pulmonary function tests.** The **peak expiratory flow rate (PEFR)** can be used to evaluate the degree of obstruction (Table 3-1).

   2. **Pulse oximetry** can be used to evaluate the degree of hypoxia.

   3. **Chest radiographs** should be ordered for patients with hypoxia, fever, a focal lung examination, or symptoms not responsive to bronchodilator therapy.

   4. **ABG.** ABGs should not be ordered routinely but should be reserved for patients with severe attacks or suspected respiratory failure. Because a patient having an asthma exacerbation is breathing quickly, his or her arterial carbon dioxide tension ($PaCO_2$) should be less than 40 mm Hg (respiratory alkalosis).

E. **Therapy**

   1. **Oxygen** is indicated for all asthma patients to keep the oxygen saturation greater than 95%.

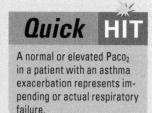

Quick HIT

In severe asthma, when airflow is very low, wheezing may be absent.

Quick HIT

A normal or elevated $PaCO_2$ in a patient with an asthma exacerbation represents impending or actual respiratory failure.

TABLE 3-1	Asthma Severity Assessment	
Severity	**Signs and Symptoms**	**Initial PEF Rate as % of Predicted**
Mild	Dyspnea with activity	PEF >70% predicted
Moderate	Dyspnea interferes with activity	PEF 40%–69% predicted
Severe	Dyspnea at rest	PEF <40% predicted
Life-threatening	Too dyspneic to speak	PEF <25% predicted

PEF, peak expiratory flow.

2. Pharmacologic therapy
   a. **Standard (first-line) agents**
      i. **Inhaled short-acting β_2 agonists** act as bronchial smooth muscle relaxants. Nebulized **albuterol** is administered every 15 to 20 minutes; in patients with severe attacks, these agents may be administered continuously.
      ii. **Corticosteroids** suppress the inflammatory component of asthma and are considered first-line agents for the treatment of patients with asthma that do not respond rapidly to inhaled β_2 agonists.
         a) Oral prednisone (60 mg in adults, 2 mg/kg in children) may be administered. Methylprednisolone (125 mg in adults, 2 mg/kg in children) may be administered intravenously if the patient is unable to tolerate oral prednisone secondary to vomiting or respiratory distress. Dexamethasone (0.6 mg/kg) is a viable alternative and allows for less frequent dosing than prednisone.
         b) Patients who have been administered steroids in the ED who are subsequently discharged to home should continue to take oral steroids for 5 days (e.g., prednisone, 40 to 60 mg once daily for adults or 1 mg/kg/day for children; dexamethasone one further dose 72 hours from the first dose) to reduce the rate of asthma relapse.
      iii. **Anticholinergic agents** relax bronchial smooth muscle, particularly in the more proximal airways. Although these agents are most useful in the treatment of COPD, they may also be used for patients with asthma exacerbations that do not rapidly respond to inhaled β_2 agonists.
         a) Metered-dose or nebulized **ipratropium bromide** can be administered for up to three doses.
         b) **Ipratropium** and **albuterol solutions** may be mixed together and administered in the same handheld nebulizer.
   b. **Second-line agents**
      i. **Magnesium sulfate** (2 g intravenously over 30 minutes) should be considered in adults with severe asthma exacerbations not responsive to initial therapy.
      ii. **Epinephrine** (0.3 mg subcutaneously in adults or 0.01 mg/kg in children, up to 0.3 mg) or **terbutaline** (0.25 mg subcutaneously in adults or 0.01 mg/kg/dose for children, maximum dose is 0.4 mg) can be considered for young patients with severe asthma not responsive to first-line agents.
   c. **Other pharmacologic options**
      i. **Inhaled general anesthetics** are potent bronchodilators. Their use in the treatment of asthma is reserved for patients with severe asthma exacerbations in whom previous therapy has not resulted in adequate oxygenation or ventilation.
      ii. **Ketamine** is a dissociative anesthetic agent that also causes bronchodilation and can be used for severe, refractory asthma.
         a) An initial bolus of 1 to 2 mg/kg is administered intravenously over 30 to 60 minutes, followed by an intravenous ketamine drip (1 mg/kg/hour).
         b) Ketamine is contraindicated in patients with ischemic heart disease, increased intracranial pressure, severe hypertension, or preeclampsia.
      iii. **Heliox**, a mixture of 80% helium and 20% oxygen, can be administered via face mask or nebulizer to patients with severe, refractory asthma. In nonintubated patients, heliox decreases the work of breathing by improving laminar gas flow and airway resistance. In intubated patients, heliox results in improved oxygenation and decreased peak airway pressures.
3. **Intubation and mechanical ventilation.** Intubation is indicated for patients with impending respiratory failure. Orotracheal intubation is preferred over nasotracheal intubation because orotracheal intubation allows for the placement

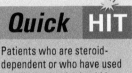

Quick HIT

Patients who are steroid-dependent or who have used steroids recently should be gradually tapered off the steroids over 10 to 14 days rather than discontinuing steroids after 5 days.

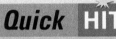

Quick HIT

Epinephrine should not be used during early pregnancy or in patients suspected of having coronary artery disease.

Pulmonary Emergencies

of a larger endotracheal tube, which decreases the work of breathing (by lowering airway resistance) and facilitates the management of pulmonary secretions.

   a. **Rapid sequence intubation** (see Chapter 1.III.B.3.c) should be considered for asthmatic patients requiring intubation.

      i. **Ketamine** (2 mg/kg intravenously), because of its bronchodilation properties, is a good choice of induction agent.

      ii. **Benzodiazepines**, rather than opiates, should be used for sedation in intubated patients with asthma because opiates may induce histamine release from mast cells, exacerbating the bronchospasm.

      iii. **Pancuronium** or **vecuronium** may be administered to induce muscle paralysis if ventilation is difficult following intubation.

   b. Complications

      i. **Barotrauma** is a common complication of mechanical ventilation in patients with asthma. To avoid this complication, the tidal volume should be 6 to 8 mL/kg, and the ventilator should be adjusted to increase the time allowed for expiration to minimize peak airway pressures.

      ii. **Hypotension** that develops rapidly after intubation and mechanical ventilation usually results from the auto–positive end-expiratory pressure (auto-PEEP) phenomenon or a tension pneumothorax.

         a) **Auto-PEEP phenomenon.** Air-trapping in the lungs can lead to increased intrathoracic pressure, which may result in decreased venous return and a resultant decrease in cardiac output. If air-trapping is suspected as the cause of hypotension, the respiratory rate on the ventilator should be decreased to allow adequate time for exhalation.

         b) **Pneumothorax.** A tension pneumothorax may develop as a result of air-trapping and increased airway pressures, leading to kinking of the mediastinal vessels, a decrease in venous return to the heart, and decreased cardiac output. If tension pneumothorax is suspected, immediate needle decompression of the affected side should be undertaken, followed by chest tube placement.

F. **Disposition**

   1. **Admission.** In a patient with asthma, evidence of pneumonia is generally an indication for hospital admission. Patients with persistent symptoms despite treatment and continued PEFR of <40% of predicted value should be admitted to the hospital.

   2. **Discharge**

      a. Patients may be discharged to home if they have made significant clinical improvement, have a PEFR greater than 70% of the predicted value (or equal to their baseline PEFR), have a normal respiratory rate, and are able to walk without recurring symptoms.

      b. Patients with a PEFR that is 40% to 60% of the predicted value may be discharged if they are otherwise stable, compliant, and have a good follow-up system.

III. CHRONIC OBSTRUCTIVE PULMONARY DISEASE

A. **Discussion**

   1. **Definition.** COPD is a syndrome characterized by chronic dyspnea and expiratory airflow obstruction as a result of increased resistance or decreased airway caliber throughout the small bronchi and bronchioles. There are two types of COPD.

      a. **Emphysema** is permanent, abnormal enlargement of the terminal bronchioles accompanied by destruction of the bronchoalveolar lining.

      b. **Chronic bronchitis** is defined by a productive cough on most days for at least 3 months per year for at least 2 consecutive years.

   2. **Incidence.** COPD is the fifth leading cause of death in the United States.

   3. **Causes.** Smoking is the leading cause of COPD. Cystic fibrosis, α_1-antitrypsin deficiency, and some occupational exposures predispose to the development of COPD.

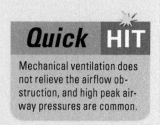

Quick **HIT**

Mechanical ventilation does not relieve the airflow obstruction, and high peak airway pressures are common.

Pulmonary Emergencies

B. **Clinical features.** Exacerbations are what bring most patients with COPD to the ED.
1. **Symptoms**
   a. **Wheezing, dyspnea on exertion,** and **cough** are the most common symptoms. Wheezing may not be audible if the patient's airflow is very poor.
   b. **Accessory muscle use** may be seen in patients with moderate to severe COPD exacerbations.
   c. **Pursed-lip breathing** may be present.
   d. **Altered mental status, severely labored breathing,** and **extreme fatigue** signal impending respiratory arrest.
2. **Physical examination findings. Signs of right-sided CHF (cor pulmonale)** may be present and include jugular venous distention, peripheral edema, and hepatomegaly.

C. **Differential diagnoses** include CHF, upper airway obstruction, foreign body aspiration, pulmonary embolism, an anaphylactic reaction, pneumonia, asthma, toxic inhalation, and pneumothorax.

D. **Evaluation.** The evaluation of a patient with COPD exacerbation is similar to that for patients with asthma.
1. **Pulmonary function testing.** The PEFR can assist in monitoring response to treatment; however, it is not as useful as an evaluation tool for patients with COPD (as compared with those with asthma) because acute bronchospasm contributes less to dysfunction in patients with COPD. Instead, forced expiratory volume in 1 second as a percentage of predicted is used (Table 3-2).
2. **Pulse oximetry** can be used to evaluate the degree of hypoxia.
3. **Chest radiographs** should be considered for patients with tachycardia, tachypnea, hypoxia, fever, a focal lung examination, age >65 years old, or symptoms not responsive to bronchodilator therapy.
4. **ABG.** An ABG should be obtained on patients who do not respond to bronchodilator therapy or in whom acute or serious respiratory failure is suspected. When interpreting the ABG, it is important to remember that patients with COPD may retain carbon dioxide on a chronic basis. If a patient has an elevated Pco_2 in the face of a normal blood pH, then this usually represents chronic carbon dioxide retention (with metabolic compensation) rather than acute respiratory failure. However, if the Pco_2 is elevated and the blood pH is low, the patient is in respiratory failure.
5. **Laboratory studies**
   a. The **hematocrit** may be elevated secondary to increased erythrocytosis.
   b. The **serum bicarbonate level** may be elevated, suggesting that a secondary metabolic alkalosis is compensating for the chronic respiratory acidosis.

E. **Therapy**
1. **Oxygen** should be administered to all patients with COPD. Some patients with COPD with a chronically elevated Pco_2 have lost their sensitivity to hypercarbia and thus depend on the hypoxic drive to stimulate their respirations. Therefore, the minimum amount of oxygen that is needed to maintain the oxygen saturation at 90% should be administered.

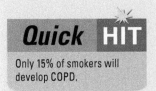

Quick HIT

Only 15% of smokers will develop COPD.

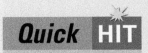

Quick HIT

If an excessive concentration of oxygen is administered to these patients in an attempt to normalize their oxygen saturation, it may depress their respiratory drive and lead to hypoventilation and respiratory failure.

TABLE 3-2	COPD Severity	
Stage	**Signs and Symptoms**	**Initial FEV₁ as % of Predicted**
I. Mild	Dyspnea with activity	$FEV_1 > 80\%$ predicted
II. Moderate	Dyspnea interferes with activity	FEV_1 50%–79% predicted
III. Severe	Dyspnea at rest	FEV_1 30%–49% predicted
IV. Life-threatening	Too dyspneic to speak	$FEV_1 < 30\%$ predicted

FEV_1, forced expiratory volume in 1 second.

2. Pharmacologic therapy
   a. **Inhaled β₂ agonists** are first-line agents for the treatment of acute exacerbations of COPD. Dosage and administration is the same as that for patients with asthma (see II.E.2.a.i).
   b. **Inhaled anticholinergic agents** are the second-line agents for the treatment of acute COPD exacerbations. Dosage and administration is the same as that for patients with asthma (see II.E.2.a.iii).
   c. **Corticosteroids** should be considered for patients with COPD who do not respond rapidly to inhaled β₂ agonists or anticholinergics. The dosing and administration is the same as that for patients with asthma (see II.E.2.a.ii).
   d. **Antibiotics** should be administered if there is evidence of infection, such as increased sputum production or change in sputum character. Choices should be directed at the common pathogens, namely, *Streptococcus pneumoniae*, *Haemophilus influenzae*, and *Moraxella catarrhalis*.
3. **Intubation and mechanical ventilation** are generally indicated for patients with impending respiratory failure. Unlike asthmatic patients, patients with COPD with mild acute elevations in Pco₂ and a decreased blood pH can sometimes be managed without intubation, as long as they do not demonstrate central nervous system or cardiovascular dysfunction and are not severely fatigued.
   a. **Noninvasive positive-pressure ventilatory support** can often assist ventilation and improve a patient's clinical condition enough to obviate intubation. Positive pressure is delivered through either a nasal or face mask using a ventilator or a bilevel positive airway pressure system.
   b. **Ketamine** is **not a preferred induction agent** in these patients because many of them have concomitant ischemic heart disease.

F. **Disposition.** Patients with COPD exacerbations are more likely to be admitted than patients with an asthma exacerbation because reversible disease accounts for a smaller part of their clinical presentation.
   1. **Admission.** Pneumonia, CHF, or other existing comorbid conditions are indications for hospital admission. Persistent hypoxemia or worsening hypercarbia with concomitant respiratory acidosis (pH <7.30) require ICU admission.
   2. **Discharge.** Patients may be discharged to home if they have made a significant clinical improvement and are near their baseline respiratory status.

IV. NONCARDIOGENIC PULMONARY EDEMA

Noncardiogenic pulmonary edema (NCPE) is also known as **acute respiratory distress syndrome**.

A. **Discussion**
   1. **Definition.** NCPE is a form of pulmonary edema resulting from an abnormal increase in the permeability of pulmonary vascular membranes.
   2. **Causes** of NCPE include sepsis, aspiration of gastric contents, near-drowning, thermal injury, trauma, high-altitude pulmonary edema, radiation, transfusions, eclampsia–preeclampsia, and selected drug reactions or overdoses, including narcotic and aspirin overdose.
   3. **Pathogenesis.** NCPE is not related to cardiac, hydrostatic, or hemodynamic edema. The proposed mechanism for the edema is damage to the vascular endothelium as a result of complement cascade activation or direct damage by bacterial endotoxin. Pulmonary surfactant is disrupted and lung compliance is decreased.

B. **Clinical features**
   1. **Symptoms. Dyspnea** with **rapidly progressive tachypnea** is common.
   2. **Physical examination findings** include **bilateral rales**.

C. **Differential diagnoses.** NCPE is most commonly confused with CHF or pneumonia. Asthma, COPD, pulmonary embolism, an anaphylactic reaction, and foreign body aspiration should also be considered.

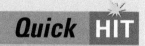

Quick HIT

Contraindications to noninvasive positive-pressure ventilatory support include obtunded patients, inability to handle secretions, hemodynamic instability, respiratory arrest, facial or gastrointestinal surgery, burns, or poor mask fitting.

Quick HIT

Oxygen saturation must be over 90% in discharged patients.

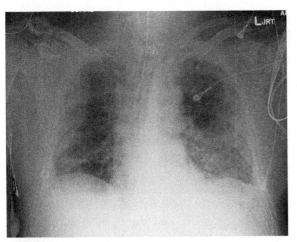

FIGURE
3-1 Diffuse patchy alveolar infiltrates typical of acute
respiratory distress syndrome.
(Used by permission of Martin Huecker, MD.)

D. **Evaluation**
1. **Chest radiographs**, **ABGs**, and an **ECG** should be obtained for all patients
suspected of having NCPE.
a. The chest radiograph demonstrates bilateral patchy alveolar infiltrates and
a normal heart size. In severe cases, the infiltrates may progress to a "white
out" of the lungs (Figure 3-1).
b. The ABG demonstrates hypoxia and an increased alveolar–arterial gradient
where PaO_2/FIO_2 is less than 300.
2. **Laboratory tests.** Pertinent laboratory tests include a **complete blood count
(CBC)**, **urinalysis**, an **electrolyte panel**, and **blood urea nitrogen (BUN)** and
creatinine levels.
E. **Therapy**
1. **Supplemental oxygen** should be administered to maintain the oxygen saturation above 90%. In intubated patients, the FIO_2 should be kept below 50%, if
possible, because of the potential for pulmonary oxygen toxicity.
2. **Intubation and mechanical ventilation** are indicated for patients who, despite
supplemental oxygen, have inadequate oxygenation or ventilation. **PEEP**
should be added if adequate oxygenation cannot be maintained with an FIO_2
of less than 50% in an effort to keep tidal volumes low at <6 mL/kg.
3. **Treatment of the underlying disorder** should be undertaken (e.g., antibiotics
for sepsis, alkalinization and dialysis for aspirin overdose).
4. The use of **corticosteroids, nonsteroidal anti-inflammatory drugs**, and **anticoagulants** is being investigated for the future treatment of acute respiratory
distress syndrome.
F. **Disposition**
1. **Admission.** The vast majority of patients with NCPE will need to be admitted
to the hospital and should be sent to a monitored bed.
a. Many patients who develop NCPE do so as a result of medical conditions
that often require hospitalization in and of themselves (e.g., sepsis, near-
drowning, thermal injury, trauma, aspirin overdose).
b. NCPE may be rapidly progressive, and patients may have a rapid deterioration in
their respiratory status. Intubated or critically ill patients require ICU admission.
2. **Discharge.** Overdose patients who are not hypoxic and are asymptomatic after
6 to 12 hours of observation are usually discharged home.

V. HEMOPTYSIS
A. **Discussion**
1. **Definition.** Hemoptysis is the expectoration of blood from the respiratory tract
when the source of the bleeding is below the level of the larynx. The degree of

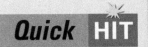

**The minimal amount of
PEEP to maintain adequate
oxygenation should be used
because high levels of PEEP
can result in pneumothorax
or hypotension secondary to
a decreased preload.**

Pulmonary Emergencies

CLINICAL PEARL **3-1**

Massive Hemoptysis is defined as the expectoration of more than 100 mL of blood per hour or more than 600 mL over 24 hours.

hemoptysis can range from blood-tinged sputum to massive hemoptysis (see Clinical Pearl 3-1).

   2. **Causes.** The most common cause of minor hemoptysis, <20 mL in 24 hours, is chronic bronchitis. Other causes of hemoptysis include pneumonia, tuberculosis, fungal infection, bronchiectasis, cystic fibrosis, pulmonary parasitic disease (e.g., ascariasis), lung abscess, bronchial malignancy, CHF, mitral stenosis, pulmonary embolism, pulmonary arteriovenous malformation, pulmonary hypertension, Wegener granulomatosis, Goodpasture syndrome, foreign body aspiration, and trauma. All of these conditions can be aggravated by a coagulopathy or thrombocytopenia.
   3. **Pathogenesis.** Death from hemoptysis results from suffocation, secondary to impaired gas exchange, rather than from exsanguination.
 B. **Clinical features.** The clinical presentation of hemoptysis depends on the underlying cause as well as the amount of bleeding.
   1. **Symptoms.** Patients may complain of a cough, chest pain, dyspnea, or systemic symptoms.
   2. **Physical examination findings.** Patients may appear well with normal vital signs, or they may demonstrate respiratory distress. Findings on pulmonary examination depend on the cause of hemoptysis but may include rhonchi in patients with bronchitis, rales in patients with CHF, decreased breath sounds in patients with pneumonia, or a pleural rub in patients with pulmonary infarction.
 C. **Evaluation.** It is important to first assess whether the bleeding represents true hemoptysis, or if the patient is actually bleeding from the stomach (hematemesis), the nose, or the oropharyngeal cavity.
   1. A **CBC** and **chest radiograph** should be obtained in all patients with hemoptysis.
   2. **Other laboratory studies.** Unless the patient is believed to have very minor hemoptysis secondary to bronchitis and is in no respiratory distress, it is prudent to obtain the following:
     a. **Prothrombin time** and **partial thromboplastin time**
     b. **Electrolyte panel**
     c. **BUN** and **creatinine level**
     d. **Glucose level**
     e. **Blood type** and **screen** (type and cross if the hemoptysis is massive)
     f. **Urinalysis**
     g. **ECG**
   3. **Specific tests** may be ordered depending on the suspected disease process. For example:
     a. If pulmonary embolism is suspected, pertinent studies include **pulse oximetry** or **ABG**, **lower extremity Doppler ultrasound**, $\dot{V}/\dot{Q}$ **scanning**, or **CT pulmonary angiography**.
     b. If malignancy is suspected, **bronchoscopy** or a **chest CT scan** would be appropriate.
     c. If mitral stenosis is suspected, an **echocardiogram** should be ordered.
     d. If tuberculosis is suspected, a **purified protein derivative skin test**, **sputum acid-fast bacillus stain**, or **mycobacterial culture** may be requested.
 D. **Therapy**
   1. **ABCs.** The management of hemoptysis begins with addressing the patient's airway, breathing, and circulation status.
     a. **Airway.** The patient should be intubated if he or she is having difficulty

maintaining airway patency secondary to bleeding. Oral intubation with a large endotracheal tube is best for ease of suctioning.

    i. If the patient is bleeding from the left lung, the right mainstem bronchus can be selectively intubated in order to maximize ventilation. This can be accomplished by advancing the tube 4 to 5 cm beyond the usual position.

    ii. If massive bleeding is occurring from the right lung, then selective intubation of the left mainstem bronchus is desirable but more difficult. If one rotates the endotracheal tube 90 degrees counterclockwise from the usual position and alters its concavity to face the left during intubation, there is an increased likelihood of left mainstem bronchus intubation.

    iii. Alternatively, a double-lumen endotracheal tube can be used to separately intubate the left and right mainstem bronchi.

  b. **Breathing.** Supplemental oxygen should be given to maximize oxygenation. The spread of blood can be minimized and ventilation improved by having the patient lie on the affected side, if known.

  c. **Circulation.** Intravenous access should be obtained to administer crystalloid or blood products as needed. The patient's vital signs should be monitored closely.

2. **Localization and control of the bleeding.** Once the ABCs have been addressed, localization and control of the bleeding are necessary.

  a. Anemia, thrombocytopenia, and coagulopathy should be corrected.

  b. Consultation with various specialists may be advisable:

    i. A pulmonologist may be called on to perform bronchoscopy in an attempt to localize and control the bleeding.

    ii. An interventional radiologist or vascular surgeon may be helpful if arterial embolization is needed.

    iii. A cardiothoracic surgeon should be consulted if surgical resection is being considered.

3. **Treatment for the cause of the hemoptysis** should be attempted.

E. **Disposition**

1. **Discharge.** Patients who meet the following criteria can be considered for discharge from the hospital, provided that they see a primary care physician for close follow-up care:

  a. Minor degree of hemoptysis

  b. Normal vital signs and near-normal hematocrit

  c. No additional hemoptysis over 2 to 3 hours of observation

  d. No other acute medical condition that requires hospitalization

2. **Admission.** All other patients should be admitted for further care and evaluation. Patients with unstable vital signs, life-threatening hemoptysis, respiratory compromise, or potential respiratory compromise should be admitted to the ICU.

VI. PULMONARY EMBOLISM

A. **Discussion**

1. **Definition.** Pulmonary embolism occurs when a venous thrombus (or, occasionally, another substance, such as fat or amniotic fluid) embolizes to the lung, causing occlusion of a pulmonary artery. Pulmonary emboli may be small, involving only a branch of the pulmonary artery, or large, causing an occlusion of both pulmonary arteries (a saddle embolus).

2. **Incidence.** Pulmonary embolism is the third most common cause of death in the United States.

3. **Predisposing conditions.** Heart disease (e.g., acute myocardial infarction, CHF, arrhythmia), venous stasis, pregnancy, obesity, prolonged immobilization, trauma, deep venous thrombosis, and conditions that lead to a hypercoagulable state (e.g., malignancy, oral contraceptive use, protein C or S deficiency). Risk factors are identifiable in approximately 90% of patients with pulmonary embolism (see Clinical Pearl 3-2; see Table 3-3).

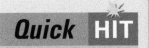

Quick HIT

Patients taking anticoagulants should receive fresh frozen plasma or prothrombin complex concentrates without waiting for coagulation study results.

Quick HIT

Even with minor hemoptysis, there is a 5% to 20% risk for occult neoplasms of the lungs, trachea, and pharynx. Follow-up is recommended.

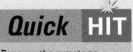

Quick HIT

Because the symptoms, history, and physical examination findings are often nonspecific, this often fatal disease is underdiagnosed and often missed.

Pulmonary Emergencies

The **Wells Score** is the most robust scoring system for categorizing the pretest probability for pulmonary embolism. Risk score interpretation (probability of pulmonary embolism): >6 points: high risk (78.4%); 2 to 6 points: moderate risk (27.8%); and <2 points: low risk (3.4%).

The **Pulmonary Embolism Rule Out Criteria (PERC)** can be combined with the Wells score to place a patient into a low risk pretest probability category (see Clinical Pearl 3-3). Most experts agree a low-risk Wells score and a PERC score of zero obviates further diagnostic testing for pulmonary embolism. However, a PERC score other than 0 has no prognostic or diagnostic utility.

B. **Clinical features**
   1. **Symptoms**
      a. The **classic triad** of **pleuritic chest pain, dyspnea, and hemoptysis** is present in less than 25% of patients.
      b. Other symptoms include **coughing** and **apprehension, diaphoresis, a low-grade fever**, or **symptoms of deep venous thrombosis**.
   2. **Physical examination findings**
      a. **Pulseless electrical activity** is often seen in patients with pulmonary embolism and cardiopulmonary arrest.
      b. **Tachypnea** is seen in approximately 70% of patients with pulmonary embolism and is the most common sign. **Tachycardia**, **rales**, and an **accentuated second heart sound** (S_2) are also common signs of pulmonary embolism. An S_3 or S_4 gallop may also be observed.
      c. **Lower extremity edema** may be observed.

C. **Differential diagnoses** include myocardial infarction, pneumonia, pleurisy, spontaneous pneumothorax, pericarditis, aortic dissection, esophageal perforation, costochondritis, asthma, COPD, rib fracture, and hyperventilation syndrome.

D. **Evaluation**
   1. **Laboratory studies.** A CBC, electrolyte panel, BUN and creatinine level, glucose level, prothrombin time/partial thromboplastin time, D-dimer, and urinalysis should be performed for patients with suspected pulmonary embolism. In women of reproductive age who have not had a hysterectomy, urine pregnancy test results should be obtained.
   2. **Chest radiograph.** A chest radiograph should be obtained for all patients with suspected pulmonary embolism. The chest radiograph is usually not completely normal, but the findings are not specific for pulmonary embolism; therefore, chest radiographs are most helpful for excluding other diseases

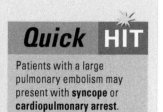

Quick HIT

Patients with a large pulmonary embolism may present with **syncope** or **cardiopulmonary arrest**.

TABLE **3-3**	Wells Score Calculation	
Factor	**Points**
Suspected deep vein thrombosis	3
Alternative diagnosis less likely than pulmonary embolism	3
Heart rate >100	1.5
Prior venous thromboembolism	1.5
Immobilization within prior 4 weeks	1.5
Active malignancy	1
Hemoptysis	1

CLINICAL PEARL 3-3

PERC score: Any of the following features deem the patient PERC positive and the PERC rule cannot be applied:
- Age >50
- Heart rate >100
- Room air O_2 saturation <95
- Unilateral leg swelling
- Prior history of deep vein thrombosis/pulmonary embolism, hemoptysis
- Exogenous estrogen
- Recent surgery or trauma

(e.g., pneumothorax, pneumonia, CHF). Specific signs associated with pulmonary embolism include Westermark sign and Hampton hump.

a. **Westermark sign** is a prominent central pulmonary artery with diminished distal pulmonary vessels in one lung field.

b. **Hampton hump** is a triangular or "wedge-shaped" pleural-based density that points toward the hilum, commonly seen at the costophrenic angle on the posteroanterior view.

3. **ECG.** An ECG should be obtained in order to evaluate for cardiac ischemia, and to assist in the diagnosis of pulmonary embolism. A completely normal ECG is found in only 5% to 15% of patients with pulmonary embolism.

a. **Sinus tachycardia** and **nonspecific ST-T wave changes** are the most common abnormalities in patients with pulmonary embolism.

b. Approximately 25% of patients with pulmonary embolism have some evidence of **right-sided heart strain**, such as right bundle branch block, right axis deviation, p-pulmonale, or a right ventricular strain pattern (see Figure 3-2).

c. The **classic finding** of a prominent S wave in lead I along with a Q wave and an inverted T wave in lead III ($S_1 Q_3 T_3$) is more specific to the diagnosis of pulmonary embolism but is seen in only 12% of patients (see Figure 3-3).

4. **ABG.** An ABG may demonstrate hypoxia, hypocapnia, or an elevated alveolar–arterial gradient. An abnormal ABG may help make the diagnosis of pulmonary embolism, but a normal ABG does not rule out the disorder.

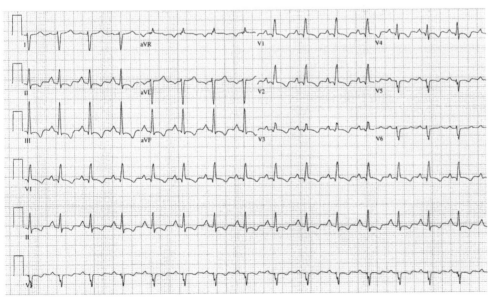

FIGURE 3-2 Electrocardiogram with inverted T waves V1 to V3 and right axis deviation.

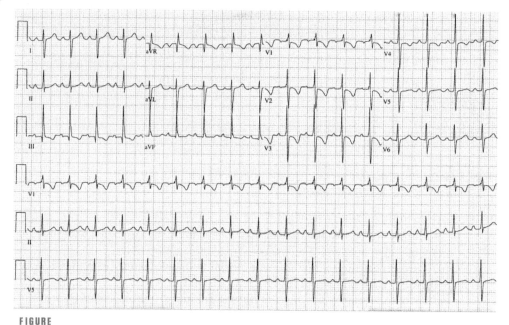

FIGURE
3-3 Electrocardiogram with S₁ Q₃ T₃ and inverted T waves leads V₁-V₄ indicative of right heart strain.

5. **CT-pulmonary angiogram.** Rapid CT evaluation is the most common and reliable method of diagnosing a pulmonary embolism. The diagnostic sensitivity and specificity of a technically adequate CT scan is 90% for each index (Figure 3-4).

6. **Noninvasive studies to evaluate the lower extremities** (e.g., **Doppler ultrasound**).

7. **$\dot{V}/\dot{Q}$ scan.** For patients with a contraindication to intravenous contrast, an elevation in serum creatinine, or glomerular filtration rate <60 mL/min a $\dot{V}/\dot{Q}$ scan may be obtained in the ED. The result of the $\dot{V}/\dot{Q}$ scan is reported as **normal, low probability, intermediate** (or **indeterminate**) **probability**, or **high probability**. The applicability of the $\dot{V}/\dot{Q}$ scan result depends on the clinical context and the degree of clinical suspicion for pulmonary embolism.

E. **Therapy.** Patients with pulmonary embolism may range from being mildly symptomatic to being in full cardiopulmonary arrest.

1. **ABCs.** Initial evaluation and support of airway, breathing, and circulation is the highest priority.

a. **Supplemental oxygen** should be administered to all patients with suspected pulmonary embolism.

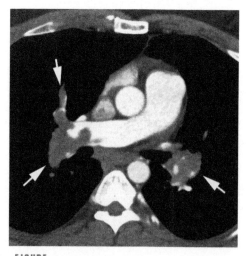

FIGURE
3-4 Bilateral pulmonary emboli (*arrows*) on computed tomography.

     b. Hypotension that is refractory to **crystalloid** should be treated with **pressors.**

  2. **Anticoagulation. Intravenous heparin** should be used for anticoagulation in most patients with pulmonary embolism. A loading dose of is administered via an intravenous bolus, followed by a maintenance infusion.

     a. Heparin therapy is justified prior to making a final diagnosis in patients with high clinical probability for pulmonary embolism.

     b. **Contraindications**

        i. **Absolute contraindications** include active bleeding, intracranial lesions, or severe uncontrolled hypertension.

        ii. **Relative contraindications** include recent stroke or major surgery, advanced liver or kidney failure, bacterial endocarditis, or a bleeding diathesis.

  3. **Thrombolytic therapy** (e.g., with **streptokinase, tissue plasminogen activator,** or **urokinase**) should be considered in patients with pulmonary embolism who are hypotensive or have evidence of right ventricular strain on echocardiography.

  4. **Inferior vena cava (Greenfield) filters** may be placed by a vascular surgeon or invasive radiologist in patients who are diagnosed with pulmonary embolism but have contraindications to anticoagulation therapy. They may also be used in patients who experience recurrent pulmonary embolism despite appropriate anticoagulation.

  5. **Surgical embolectomy** to remove pulmonary emboli is controversial and has largely been replaced by the use of thrombolytic therapy in hemodynamically unstable patients.

F. Disposition

  1. **Admission.** All patients suspected of having pulmonary embolism require admission to a telemetry bed for monitoring and anticoagulation therapy. Patients who demonstrate hemodynamic instability or potential respiratory compromise should be admitted to the ICU.

  2. **Discharge.** If clinical suspicion and diagnostic tests suggest that the patient does not have pulmonary embolism, he or she may be discharged unless another condition that requires hospital admission is responsible for his or her symptoms.

VII. PLEURAL EFFUSION

A. Discussion

  1. **Definition.** A pleural effusion is present when fluid in the pleural space is visible on a chest radiograph. Normally, the pleural space contains only a minimal amount of fluid that is not apparent radiographically.

  2. **Causes**

     a. **Intrathoracic causes** of pleural effusion include pulmonary infection (e.g., parapneumonic effusion, empyema), CHF, malignancy, pulmonary embolism, esophageal perforation, aortic dissection, collagen vascular disease, sarcoidosis, superior vena cava obstruction, and traumatic vascular disruption.

     b. **Systemic causes** include nephrotic syndrome, cirrhosis, pancreatitis, intraabdominal abscess, myxedema, and severe malnutrition.

B. Clinical features

  1. **Symptoms.** Pleural effusions may develop gradually and are **commonly asymptomatic.** Symptomatic patients may complain of **dyspnea, pleuritic chest pain,** or **cough.**

  2. **Physical examination findings.** Pulmonary examination reveals **decreased breath sounds** and **dullness to percussion.** A **friction rub** is sometimes heard. The patient's respiratory status may be impaired, depending on the size of the effusion.

C. Evaluation

  1. **Chest radiograph.** A chest radiograph may reveal the presence of an effusion, whether the effusion is free-flowing or loculated, and the cause of the effusion (e.g., malignancy, CHF, pneumonia).

     a. **Posteroanterior view.** A **blunted costophrenic angle** on the posteroanterior chest radiograph indicates that at least 150 to 200 mL of fluid is present.

b. **Lateral decubitus view.** The lateral decubitus view may help determine whether the effusion is free-flowing or loculated.

2. **Laboratory studies.** Routine laboratory analysis includes a CBC, an electrolyte panel, and BUN, creatinine, and glucose levels.

3. **Pulse oximetry** should be used to evaluate for hypoxia.

4. **Pleural fluid analysis.** Thoracentesis should be performed in patients with previously undiagnosed effusions or large effusions that compromise oxygenation or ventilation.

   a. As much as 1,500 mL of pleural fluid can be withdrawn and sent for laboratory analysis. Pleural fluid should be sent for **cell count and differential**; **pH determination**; **lactate dehydrogenase**, **protein**, and **glucose levels**; and **Gram staining**, **bacterial culture**, and **cytology**. **Amylase** should be ordered if pancreatitis or esophageal rupture is suspected to be the cause of the effusion. If the pleural fluid is serosanguineous or bloody, a **pleural fluid hematocrit** should be ordered.

   b. Pleural effusions are classified as either **exudates** or **transudates** according to pleural fluid characteristics (Table 3-4).

      i. Transudates are generally caused by CHF.

      ii. Exudates generally have less benign causes (e.g., infection, cancer, trauma).

5. **Other tests** may be indicated depending on the suspected cause of the pleural effusion (e.g., aortic angiography for suspected dissection, Gastrografin swallow [Bracco Diagnostics Inc, Cranbury, NJ] for suspected esophageal perforation).

D. **Therapy**

1. **Large effusions.** If the effusion is very large, patients should first be treated for impairment of oxygenation, ventilation, and circulation. Therapeutic thoracentesis should then be performed.

2. **Small effusions.** For smaller, non–life-threatening pleural effusions, treatment focuses on the underlying disease process. A diagnostic thoracentesis is usually performed after admission in well-appearing patients, unless an empyema, esophageal perforation, or a hemothorax is suspected. Each of these requires emergent placement of a chest tube and additional diagnostic studies.

E. **Disposition**

1. **Admission.** The need for hospital admission is determined by the presence of respiratory or circulatory impairment as well as the underlying cause of the pleural effusion. Most patients are admitted to the hospital for further evaluation of their medical condition and for observation following thoracentesis.

2. **Discharge.** If a patient is well-appearing, has no impairment in respiration or circulation, and has undergone thoracentesis (if the effusion is small and transudative), the patient may be discharged to home for outpatient follow-up after 4 to 6 hours of observation in the ED, provided that a repeat chest radiograph rules out a pneumothorax.

TABLE **3-4** Classification of Pleural Effusions		
Characteristic	**Transudate**	**Exudate**
Pleural fluid protein:serum protein ratio	<0.5	>0.5
Pleural fluid LDH:serum LDH ratio	<0.6	>0.6
Protein level	<3 g/dL	>3 g/dL
LDH level	<200 IU/mL	>200 IU/mL
Specific gravity	<1.016	>1.016

LDH, lactate dehydrogenase.

VIII. PNEUMONIA

A. **Discussion**

1. **Definition.** Pneumonia is defined as an infection of the pulmonary parenchyma.

   a. **Typical pneumonia** refers to pneumonia caused by bacteria; common causative organisms include *Streptococcus pneumoniae*, *H. influenzae*, *Staphylococcus aureus*, *Klebsiella pneumoniae*, anaerobes, and *Pseudomonas*.

   b. **Atypical pneumonia.** Common causative organisms include *Mycoplasma pneumoniae*, viruses, *Chlamydia pneumoniae*, *Mycobacterium tuberculosis*, *Pneumocystis carinii*, and *Legionella*.

2. **Incidence.** Pneumonia accounts for 10% of all hospital admissions and is a leading cause of death in the United States.

3. **Causes.** The causative agent of pneumonia depends, in part, on host factors.

   a. **Community-acquired pneumonia** is usually caused by *Streptococcus pneumoniae*, *M. pneumoniae*, viruses, *C. pneumoniae*, *H. influenzae*, and, occasionally, *Legionella* or *Staphylococcus aureus*.

   b. **Healthcare-associated pneumonia** is usually caused by gram-negative bacilli, *Staphylococcus aureus*, or anaerobic oral flora. Less often, *Streptococcus pneumoniae* or *Legionella* is involved.

   c. Patients with a history of travel, specific exposures, or certain risk factors may develop pneumonia caused by other agents (Table 3-5).

TABLE **3-5** Causes of Pneumonia in Patients with Selected Risk Factors	
Risk Factor	**Common Organisms**
Age	
Infants (1–4 months)	*Chlamydia trachomatis, Streptococcus pneumoniae, Haemophilus influenzae*
Infants and children younger than 5 years	Viruses, *S. pneumoniae, H. influenzae*
Older children and young adults	Atypical organisms (e.g., *Mycoplasma* or viruses) and *S. pneumoniae*
Elderly	*S. pneumoniae*, influenzavirus, *Legionella*
Health status	
Healthy patients	*S. pneumoniae, Mycoplasma*, viruses
Debilitated patients (e.g., those in hospitals and nursing homes), neutropenic patients, patients with cystic fibrosis	Gram-negative organisms, especially *Pseudomonas*
Patients with periodontal disease	Oral anaerobes
HIV-positive patients	*Pneumocystis carinii, Mycobacterium avium-intracellulare, Mycobacterium tuberculosis, S. pneumoniae, H. influenzae, Coccidioides immitis, Histoplasma*
Patients with sickle cell disease	*S. pneumoniae, H. influenzae*
Living conditions	
Patients in dormitories and barracks	*Mycoplasma pneumoniae, Chlamydia, Mycobacterium tuberculosis*, viruses
Exposures	
Contaminated water from air conditioning units	*Legionella*
Cows	*Coxiella burnetii*
Birds	*Chlamydia psittaci*
Geographical area	
Southeast Asia	*Mycobacterium tuberculosis, Paragonimus, Pseudomonas pseudomallei*
Ohio and Mississippi valleys	
Southwestern United States	*Histoplasma, Blastomyces*

Pulmonary Emergencies

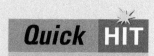

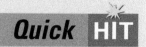

4. **Predisposing conditions** include those that impair host defense mechanisms.
   a. Failure of the gag or cough reflex may be secondary to **altered mental status, seizures, sedative use,** or **stroke.**
   b. Mucociliary clearance is affected by **smoking, smog inhalation, alcohol use, COPD,** and **viral infection.** Patients with **cystic fibrosis** and **chronic bronchitis** produce thick sputum that is difficult to expectorate.
   c. Cellular defense mechanisms can be impaired in patients with **AIDS, diabetes, asplenia, sickle cell disease, uremia,** or **malignancy. Chemotherapy** and **corticosteroid use** can also impair cellular defense mechanisms.

B. **Clinical features**
   1. **Symptoms**
      a. The clinical presentation of a patient with pneumonia depends, in part, on whether the patient suffers from typical or atypical pneumonia. However, there is considerable clinical overlap.
         i. **Typical pneumonia** is characterized by the abrupt onset of a **high fever, shaking chills, purulent sputum,** and significant respiratory complaints (e.g., **cough, dyspnea, pleuritic chest pain**). **Chest retractions** and **diaphoresis** may be evident.
         ii. **Atypical pneumonia** usually has an insidious onset accompanied by **mild respiratory complaints, low-grade fevers,** and **scant sputum.**
      b. Some patients may present predominantly with **abdominal complaints** (e.g., upper abdominal pain and vomiting), either from irritation of the diaphragm as a result of lower lobe infection or from the swallowing of purulent secretions.
      c. In elderly patients, the presentation of pneumonia may be more subtle (e.g., **weakness, fatigue,** or a **change in behavior**).
   2. **Physical examination findings**
      a. **Vital signs.** Fever, tachypnea, and tachycardia may be present.
      b. **Pulmonary examination** may reveal decreased or bronchial breath sounds, rales, dullness to percussion, increased tactile fremitus, and egophony.
      c. **Cyanosis** (if the patient is very hypoxic) may be noted.

C. **Differential diagnoses** include asthma, COPD, upper respiratory infection, bronchitis, pneumothorax, pulmonary embolism, foreign body aspiration, and an allergic reaction.

D. **Evaluation**
   1. **Pulse oximetry** is used to evaluate for hypoxia.
   2. **Chest radiograph.** A chest radiograph is used to diagnose pneumonia, and the radiographic pattern may be a clue to the causative organism.
      a. Classically, lobar infiltrates are seen with *S. pneumoniae* and *Klebsiella* infection. *Klebsiella* typically involves the right upper lobe and may cause bulging of the interlobar fissures.
      b. Patchy infiltrates, often multilobar and bilateral, are seen with *S. aureus* and *H. influenzae* infection.
      c. Interstitial infiltrates are seen with *Mycoplasma*, *Legionella*, and viral infections.
      d. Cavitation and pulmonary abscesses can be seen with infections caused by anaerobic organisms, *S. aureus*, *Klebsiella*, *Pseudomonas*, and *M. tuberculosis*.
      e. Pleural effusions are most commonly seen with *H. influenzae*, *Mycoplasma*, and *S. pneumoniae* infection.
   3. **Sputum Gram stain.** A sputum Gram stain is often helpful in identifying the causative organism, but its sensitivity is only 40% to 60%.
   4. **Sputum cultures** should be sent if an adequate specimen is available and for patients admitted to the hospital.
   5. **ABG.** An ABG does not need to be obtained routinely but may be useful in assessing patients with severe respiratory failure caused by the pneumonia.
   6. **Special tests** can be helpful in the diagnosis of certain types of pneumonia.
      a. Acute and convalescent *Legionella* **antibody titers** and **sputum direct fluorescent antibody** should be sent for patients with pneumonia thought to be caused by *Legionella*.

b. **Sputum acid-fast bacillus stain** and **culture** should be sent for patients with suspected pulmonary tuberculosis.

c. Acute and convalescent **serum titers** as well as **cold agglutinins** may be helpful in the diagnosis of *M. pneumoniae* infection. Acute and convalescent titers may also be helpful in diagnosing *Chlamydia* pneumonia.

d. The diagnosis of *P. carinii* pneumonia can be made by special **immunofluorescent stains of sputum** from induced specimens or bronchoscopy.

e. **Counterimmune electrophoresis** can help diagnose *S. pneumoniae*, *H. influenzae*, *Klebsiella*, and *Pseudomonas* as the cause of pneumonia.

E. **Therapy**

1. **ABCs.** Therapy begins with airway management, supplemental oxygen in all patients, mechanical ventilation in patients with respiratory failure, and cardiovascular stabilization.

2. **Antibiotic therapy** should be initiated early. Empiric choices depend on the patient's age, underlying medical conditions, specific exposures, clinical and radiographic presentation, and the results of sputum Gram staining. Recommended antibiotic regimens for the outpatient and inpatient treatment of common causes of pneumonia are given in Tables 3-6 and 3-7, respectively.

F. **Disposition**

1. **Admission**

a. Patients who are intubated or have the potential for respiratory failure should be admitted to the ICU.

b. Patients should be admitted to the hospital for intravenous antibiotic therapy if they meet any of the following criteria:

i. They have a serious underlying disease (e.g., COPD, AIDS, asplenia).

ii. They are older than 65 years or younger than 6 months.

iii. They show signs of toxicity or significant volume depletion.

iv. They are dyspneic or hypoxic on room air.

v. An empyema or abscess has developed.

vi. Dense multilobar involvement is present.

vii. Their living conditions are poor.

2. **Discharge.** Otherwise healthy adults who are not hypoxic and are well appearing may be discharged to home. Outpatient therapy with oral antibiotics should be initiated, and close follow-up is necessary.

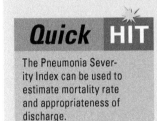

Quick HIT

The Pneumonia Severity Index can be used to estimate mortality rate and appropriateness of discharge.

TABLE 3-6	Outpatient Treatment of Community-Acquired Pneumonia[a]	
Patient Profile	**Drug**	**Dosage**
Children	Amoxicillin	40 mg/kg/day divided every 8 hours
	Amoxicillin-clavulanic acid	40 mg/kg/day divided every 8 hours
Healthy young adults	Erythromycin	500 mg four times daily
	Azithromycin	500 mg (initial dose), followed by 250 mg daily for 4 more days
	Clarithromycin	500 mg twice daily
Debilitated adults (smokers, alcoholics, patients > 65 years)	Levofloxacin	750mg daily for 5 days
	Azithromycin *plus*	500 mg (initial dose), followed by 250 mg daily for 4 more days
	Amoxicillin-clavulanic acid	500 mg three times daily
Patients with *Pneumocystis carinii pneumoniae*	Trimethoprim-sulfamethoxazole	Double strength, two tablets every 6 hours for 21 days

[a]10 days of treatment unless stated otherwise.

TABLE 3-7	Inpatient Treatment of Community-Acquired Pneumonia	
Suspected Cause	**Antibiotic Regimen**
Typical organism	Levofloxacin or moxifloxacin
Atypical organism	Ceftriaxone + azithromycin *or* fluoroquinolone
Aspiration	Clindamycin
Gram-negative organism (e.g., *Klebsiella, Pseudomonas*)	Ceftriaxone + piperacillin-tazobactam
Pneumocystis carinii	Sulfamethoxazole–trimethoprim or pentamidine; consider prednisone for severe cases
Mycobacterium tuberculosis	Isoniazid + rifampin + pyrazinamide + ethambutol *or* streptomycin

IX. MYCOBACTERIAL PULMONARY DISEASE

A. Discussion

1. **Causes.** *M. tuberculosis* and *Mycobacterium avium-intracellulare* are the most common causes of mycobacterial pulmonary disease in humans.

2. **Incidence**

a. **Tuberculosis.** The number of tuberculosis cases was decreasing at a rate of 5% per year until the mid-1980s, when the number of cases stabilized and then began to rise again. A higher incidence of tuberculosis is seen among individuals who are:

i. HIV-positive

ii. Foreign-born

iii. Residents of nursing homes, prisons, or shelters

iv. Homeless

v. Intravenous drug users

b. **Pulmonary infection with *M. avium-intracellulare*** is seen predominantly in AIDS patients, although it is also seen in patients with COPD.

3. **Pathogenesis.** Tuberculosis is transmitted via infectious droplets.

a. Following primary infection, host defenses stop replication of the organism in 2 to 10 weeks. The patient then enters a **latent period**, during which he or she is clinically well, not infectious, and the chest radiograph is without infiltrate.

b. **Reactivation** of pulmonary tuberculosis occurs when cell-mediated immunity wanes. There is increased risk of reactivation with HIV infection, corticosteroid therapy, chemotherapy, malignancy, renal failure, diabetes, malnutrition, and other causes of immunosuppression.

B. Clinical features

1. **Symptoms**

a. **Pulmonary symptoms.** Patients with active pulmonary tuberculosis or *M. avium-intracellulare* infection typically complain of a **chronic cough** that is usually nonproductive or productive of scant sputum. **Hemoptysis** may be present and can range from blood-tinged sputum to massive bleeding (as a result of arteriolar rupture following erosion by a tuberculous cavity [Rasmussen aneurysm]).

b. **Systemic symptoms** are common with active tuberculosis and may include **fever**, **night sweats**, **weight loss**, and **anorexia**.

2. **Physical examination findings** may include **fever, tachypnea, lymphadenopathy,** or **generalized wasting**. Pulmonary examination may demonstrate **decreased breath sounds, rales,** or **bronchial breath sounds**, or it may be normal.

C. **Differential diagnoses** include bacterial pneumonia, a lung abscess or tumor, and other atypical pneumonias.

D. **Evaluation**
   1. **Patient history and physical examination.** Emphasis should be placed on determining if the patient has risk factors for tuberculosis.
   2. **Pulse oximetry** should be used to determine if the patient is hypoxic.
   3. **Chest radiograph (see Clinical Pearl 3-4)**
      a. Reactivation of tuberculosis usually appears as an infiltrate in the upper lobes or superior segment of the lower lobes, often with cavitary lesions.
      b. The chest radiograph may also demonstrate a diffuse, patchy, interstitial, and alveolar pattern that represents endobronchial spread of tuberculosis.
      c. It is not possible to radiographically distinguish between *M. tuberculosis* and *M. avian-intracellulare* infection.
   4. **Intradermal skin tests** (e.g., the purified protein derivative test) may be helpful; however, many patients with active pulmonary tuberculosis or AIDS will have false-negative skin results as a result of anergy.
   5. **Sputum analysis.** Sputum should be obtained for acid-fast bacillus stain and culture, although a single acid-fast bacillus smear will be positive in only approximately 30% of tuberculosis cases.
   6. **Blood cultures** should be considered in critically ill or complicated patients.
E. **Therapy**
   1. **Isolation.** If a patient is suspected of having pulmonary tuberculosis, he or she should be asked to wear a surgical mask and placed in respiratory isolation for the protection of ED personnel and other patients. Any patient with AIDS or immunocompromised patient with pneumonia should be considered to have tuberculosis until proven otherwise. Health care workers should wear a particulate respirator-type mask while in the patient's room. All respiratory isolation precautions should be instituted as soon as possible, usually prior to obtaining a chest radiograph.
   2. **Supplemental oxygen** should be administered if the patient is hypoxic.
   3. **Antibiotic therapy.** Because the exact regimen varies depending on the patient's clinical situation, it is advisable to discuss treatment for mycobacterial disease with an infectious disease consultant.
      a. **Tuberculosis.** Patients with tuberculosis should usually be treated with isoniazid, rifampin, pyrazinamide, and either ethambutol or streptomycin for at least 6 months.
      b. *M. avium-intracellulare* infection is treated with clarithromycin and ethambutol.
F. **Disposition.** The criteria used to decide whether a patient with pulmonary mycobacterial infection requires hospital admission are generally the same as those for patients with other types of pneumonia.
   1. **Admission.** Patients who are admitted to the hospital for known or suspected tuberculosis should be placed in respiratory isolation initially.
   2. **Discharge.** Patients should be provided with a number of surgical masks and instructed to wear a mask if they will be in contact with other individuals. Patients should follow up within 1 week with a primary care provider. In order to be discharged, patients should meet the following criteria:
      a. Well-appearing
      b. Asymptomatic or minimally symptomatic
      c. Not hypoxic on room air
      d. Absence of significant hemoptysis
      e. Willing to comply with medical treatment and follow-up visits
      f. Acceptable living conditions

CLINICAL PEARL 3-4

Pneumonia patients with AIDS may have atypical chest radiographs, with infiltrates in the middle or lower lobes or mediastinal lymphadenopathy without any infiltrate. In approximately 10% of patients, the chest radiograph is completely normal.

X. PNEUMOTHORAX

A. **Discussion.** Pneumothorax is defined as an accumulation of free air in the pleural space.

1. **Simple pneumothorax**
   a. **Spontaneous pneumothoraces** can be secondary (i.e., occurring with underlying pulmonary disease) or primary (i.e., occurring in the absence of underlying pulmonary disease).
      i. Primary spontaneous pneumothoraces are more common in men (85%) and are often recurrent.
      ii. Risk factors for spontaneous pneumothorax include smoking, changes in ambient pressure (e.g., during scuba diving or aviation), inherited conditions (e.g., Marfan syndrome, mitral valve prolapse, α_1-antitrypsin deficiency), and underlying pulmonary disease (e.g., asthma, COPD, pneumonia, tumors).
   b. **Traumatic pneumothoraces** may be caused by blunt or penetrating chest trauma. Iatrogenic causes of pneumothorax (e.g., central venous line placement) are also included in this category.

2. **Tension pneumothorax** is a complication of pneumothorax that can occur if air continues to enter the pleural space but is unable to escape. Accumulating air collapses the lung and results in shifting of the mediastinum away from the pneumothorax, leading to kinking of the mediastinal vessels, a decrease in venous return to the heart, decreased cardiac output, and, ultimately, shock.

B. **Clinical features**

1. **Simple pneumothorax**
   a. **Symptoms.** Patients commonly complain of the sudden onset of **pleuritic chest pain** with **dyspnea** and **tachypnea**.
   b. **Physical examination findings**
      i. **Tachycardia** may result from impaired venous return.
      ii. **Decreased breath sounds** on the involved side of the chest and **hyperresonance to percussion** are evident on pulmonary examination.
      iii. **Crepitus** may be palpable in the neck or chest as a result of subcutaneous emphysema.

2. **Tension pneumothorax.** Patients with a tension pneumothorax are in severe respiratory distress and may be unconscious. Physical examination findings include **hypotension**, **jugular venous distention**, **tracheal deviation** away from the side of the pneumothorax, and **decreased breath sounds and chest movement** on the affected side. Tracheal deviation is a late sign of tension pneumothorax and may not always be present.

C. **Differential diagnoses** include pulmonary embolism, pneumonia, pericarditis, acute myocardial infarction, pleurisy, aortic dissection, esophageal perforation, costochondritis, and rib fracture.

D. **Evaluation**

1. **Simple pneumothorax.** If a simple pneumothorax is suspected, **pulse oximetry** should be used to evaluate oxygenation (Figure 3-5). A **chest radiograph** should be obtained to diagnose the pneumothorax as well as to look for the underlying cause.

2. **Tension pneumothorax.** Diagnosis of a tension pneumothorax is based on **history** and **physical examination** (see Clinical Pearl 3-5).

E. **Therapy**

1. **Oxygen** should be administered to all patients with pneumothorax. In addition to improving oxygenation, high oxygen concentrations increase the rate of resorption of air from the pleural space.

2. **Definitive therapy** for pneumothoraces is the release of air from the pleural space.
   a. **Tension pneumothorax.** If a tension pneumothorax is suspected, immediate **needle thoracostomy** should be performed, followed by **chest tube placement**. A needle thoracostomy is performed by placing a large-bore needle

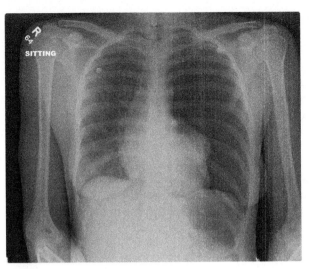

FIGURE 3-5 Pneumothorax.

into the pleural space through the anterior second intercostal space along the midclavicular line. An alternative site is the fourth or fifth intercostal space in the midaxillary line.

b. **Traumatic pneumothoraces** should be treated by placing a **large-bore thoracostomy tube** on the affected side in the fifth intercostal space along the anterior axillary line or midaxillary line.

c. **Spontaneous pneumothoraces.** The management of spontaneous pneumothoraces depends on the size of the pneumothorax, the presence of respiratory impairment, and the underlying cause of the pneumothorax.

   i. **Secondary spontaneous pneumothoraces** are treated by placing a **small-bore chest tube** for drainage.

   ii. **Primary spontaneous pneumothoraces** are managed variably.

   a) A **chest tube** should be placed if the pneumothorax involves more than 20% of the hemithorax or is recurrent.

   b) In a minimally symptomatic patient with a primary spontaneous pneumothorax that involves less than 20% of the hemithorax, **other techniques** may be attempted to avoid chest tube insertion.

   1) **Needle aspiration.** Simple aspiration of the pneumothorax may be attempted by placing a 16-gauge needle through the second intercostal space anteriorly along the midclavicular line or fifth intercostal space anterior or midaxillary line. A three-way stopcock is placed between the needle and the syringe. Air is drawn into the syringe and then released through the stopcock. If a repeat chest radiograph shows that this technique has failed to largely resolve the pneumothorax, a chest tube should be placed.

   2) **One-way catheter insertion.** A small catheter with a one-way valve (e.g., a Cook catheter) may also be used to treat small pneumothoraces. A one-way valve allows air to escape from the pleural space while preventing air from entering from outside of the body. The catheter is placed in the same location as that used for needle aspiration.

CLINICAL PEARL 3-5

If a tension pneumothorax is suspected, it should be treated immediately, rather than waiting to obtain a chest radiograph. Signs and symptoms include decreased breath sounds, distended neck veins, and painful respirations. Chest X-ray will show decreased lung markings over the side of incidence, deviation of the trachea away from the side of tension, shift of the mediastinum, and depression of the hemidiaphragm.

F. Disposition
1. Admission
   a. **All patients with tension pneumothorax** should be admitted to the ICU following chest tube placement.
   b. **Patients with traumatic pneumothorax** should be cared for in the ICU or another closely monitored setting, depending on other associated injuries.
   c. **Patients who have had a chest tube placed for a spontaneous pneumothorax** may be admitted to a medical ward, provided that the repeat chest radiograph shows resolution of the pneumothorax.
2. **Discharge.** Patients who have undergone successful needle aspiration or one-way catheter insertion in the ED to treat a small primary pneumothorax may be discharged to home, provided they are asymptomatic and without evidence of hypoxia. These patients should undergo a repeat evaluation and chest radiograph in 24 hours.

GASTROINTESTINAL EMERGENCIES

Daniel O'Brien • Kristine J. Krueger

4

I. ABDOMINAL PAIN

A. **Discussion**

1. Abdominal pain is the presenting complaint in approximately 5% of emergency department (ED) visits. Of these patients, 15% to 30% will have a condition requiring surgery.

   a. In patients complaining of abdominal pain, the most common discharge diagnosis is abdominal pain of unknown etiology (40% of patients).

   b. The next most common diagnosis is gastroenteritis (approximately 7% of patients).

   c. Pelvic inflammatory disease, urinary tract infection, nephrolithiasis, and appendicitis are the next four most common diagnoses in patients with abdominal pain.

2. **Types of abdominal pain.** Knowledge of the sources of abdominal pain is important in forming a differential diagnosis list. Visceral, somatic, and referred pain have been delineated elsewhere in the text.

B. **Evaluation**

1. Patient history

   a. **Characterization of the pain.** Any change in the character of the pain over time should be noted because changes may give a clue regarding the organ involved. For example, appendicitis often begins as a poorly localized cramping pain that becomes sharp and localizes in the right lower quadrant.

      i. Location

         a) **Epigastric pain** is associated with pancreatitis, peptic ulcer disease, myocardial infarction (MI), aortic aneurysms, and gastritis.

         b) **Right upper quadrant pain** is consistent with hepatitis, large liver (Glisson capsule stretch), gallstones, biliary colic, and cholecystitis.

         c) **Right lower quadrant pain** may be seen in patients with appendicitis, Crohn disease, diverticulitis, or gynecologic disorders.

         d) **Left lower quadrant pain** is associated with diverticulitis, ischemic colitis (most commonly affecting the splenic flexure) and gynecologic disorders.

      ii. Quality

         a) A **cramping pain** suggests obstruction of a hollow viscus, such as occurs in cholecystitis, small bowel obstruction, or renal colic.

         b) A **burning pain** is characteristic of gastroesophageal reflux and peptic ulcer disease.

         c) **Sharp, localized pain** suggests peritoneal irritation.

      iii. Radiation

         a) **Left shoulder.** Pain may radiate to the left shoulder in patients with a perforated peptic ulcer, subphrenic abscess, splenic rupture, or mononucleosis.

         b) **Chest.** Pain may radiate to the chest in patients with gastroesophageal reflux disease (GERD), hiatal hernia, or peptic ulcer disease.

107

       c) Back. Radiation of pain to the back is seen primarily in association with pancreatitis, abdominal aneurysms, and acute aortic dissection. Right subscapular pain is common in gallbladder disease.

  iv. **Timing**

      a) An **abrupt onset** of pain occurs with the perforation of a hollow viscus.

      b) A **waxing and waning** or colicky pain is indicative of obstruction (e.g., small bowel obstruction, cholecystitis).

  v. **Provocative and palliative factors**

      a) Movement. Patients with peritonitis find any movement painful.

      b) Position. Patients with pancreatitis often find that leaning forward improves the pain.

      c) Food may exacerbate the pain (as in pancreatitis and cholecystitis) or alleviate the pain (as in peptic ulcer disease).

      d) Medications. Antacids usually relieve the pain of peptic ulcer disease, gastritis, or esophagitis.

b. Associated symptoms. The order of appearance of associated symptoms may yield clues to the diagnosis. For example, vomiting most often precedes hematemesis in patients with a Mallory-Weiss tear of the esophagus.

  i. **Gastrointestinal symptoms**

    a) Vomiting

      1) Bilious or feculent vomitus suggests a bowel obstruction.

      2) "Coffee grounds" or **frank blood** in the vomitus suggests peptic ulcer disease, a Mallory-Weiss tear, bleeding esophageal varices, gastric varices, or significant erosive esophagitis.

    b) Anorexia and **nausea** are important to note because the diagnosis of appendicitis is of lower likelihood if anorexia is not present.

    c) Diarrhea

      1) Bloody diarrhea suggests inflammatory bowel disease, ischemic bowel, an invasive gastroenteritis, or bleeding from vessels within a diverticulum or arteriovenous malformation.

      2) Melena is consistent with an upper gastrointestinal source of bleeding and requires 150 mL or more blood loss.

    d) Severe constipation or **obstipation** suggests obstruction.

    e) Fever, sweats, and **chills** are hallmarks of an infectious process.

    f) Weight loss may be seen with cancer, inflammatory bowel disease, or chronic ischemic bowel syndromes.

  ii. **Gynecologic** or **urologic symptoms** should be noted because these symptoms may point away from a gastrointestinal process.

c. Past history

  i. **Surgical history.** Previous surgery may heighten suspicion for a bowel obstruction.

  ii. **Medication history.** Nonsteroidal anti-inflammatory drug (NSAID) use is associated with peptic ulcer disease. Any history of steroid use should be noted because symptoms may be masked, making the diagnosis much more difficult.

  iii. **Medical history.** A medical history should be taken, inquiring about any condition that can cause pain (e.g., diabetes, sickle cell anemia, porphyria, peptic ulcer disease, hepatitis, gallbladder disease).

  iv. **Gynecologic history.** A gynecologic history should be taken, including inquiring about the last menstrual period.

  v. **Social factors**

    a) Alcohol abuse raises the possibility of pancreatitis, hepatitis, cirrhosis, gastritis, and peptic ulcer disease. **Alcohol use** increases the probability of peptic ulcer disease or alcoholic gastritis.

    b) Smoking also increases the probability of peptic ulcer disease and pancreatitis. Nicotine is a potent vasoconstrictor and reduces healing.

2. **Physical examination**
   a. **General appearance.** Patients who are lying very still may have peritonitis, whereas a patient who is writhing in pain and who prefers to move about should be suspected of having biliary or renal colic.
   b. **Head, ears, eyes, nose, and throat.** The sclera and oropharynx should be evaluated for jaundice, which suggests biliary obstruction or liver disease.
   c. **Chest**
      i. An irregularly irregular heartbeat usually represents atrial fibrillation, which should increase suspicion for mesenteric ischemia.
      ii. The lungs should always be auscultated because a lower lobe pneumonia may present as abdominal pain.
      iii. Gynecomastia may be noted in men with liver disease due to decreased testosterone and increased estrogen effects.
   d. **Extremities.** The extremities should be examined for edema and palmar erythema, which suggest liver disease.
   e. **Skin.** The skin should be inspected for spider angiomata, which may appear in patients with portal hypertension.
   f. **Abdomen.** Serial abdominal examinations and repeat kidney, ureter, and bladder radiograph can be helpful as a key diagnostic aid (see Clinical Pearl 4-1).
   g. **Rectum.** A rectal examination is essential and may demonstrate focal tenderness or a mass. Gross or occult blood must be noted. Melena (black tarry stools with characteristic odor) indicates upper gastrointestinal tract bleeding.

CLINICAL PEARL **4-1**

Abdominal Evaluation: Appearance, Auscultation, Palpation, and Percussion

1. **Appearance**
   a. **Surgical scars** may be noted. In patients who have had abdominal surgery, the incidence of bowel obstruction from adhesions increases.
   b. **Distention** may result from a bowel obstruction or ascites.
   c. **Peristalsis** may be visible in a patient with a bowel obstruction or volvulus.
   d. **Cullen sign** (ecchymosis of the umbilicus) and **Grey-Turner sign** (flank ecchymosis) are consistent with retroperitoneal hemorrhage from pancreatitis or trauma.
   e. **Caput medusae** (dilated veins around the umbilicus) are seen in some patients with portal hypertension.
2. **Auscultation**
   a. **Short, high-pitched rushes of bowel sounds** are consistent with a bowel obstruction.
   b. **Hypoactive** or **absent bowel sounds** may be heard late in an obstruction and most often indicate an ileus from another intra-abdominal process, electrolyte imbalance, intra-abdominal infection, inflammation, or anticholinergic medication.
   c. **Bruits may be heard over aneurysms and hepatic tumors.**
3. **Palpation**
   a. **Masses**
      i. In patients with an abdominal aortic aneurysm, a pulsating mass may be palpated in the epigastrium.
      ii. In patients with acute cholecystitis, a tender right upper quadrant mass or splinting during inspiration may be detected (Murphy sign).
   b. **Organomegaly** may be noted.
   c. **Peritoneal signs** are indicative of peritoneal irritation and suggest that a condition requiring surgical intervention may be present.
      i. **Rebound tenderness** is pain elicited by the withdrawal of the examining hand.
      ii. **Guarding.** The patient may resist palpation to prevent pain (voluntary guarding). Involuntary guarding is a muscle spasm of the abdominal wall in response to peritoneal irritation.
      iii. **Rovsing sign** is referred pain felt in the right lower quadrant when the examiner palpates the left lower quadrant. It is one of the signs of peritonitis and appendicitis.
4. **Percussion**
   a. The liver span should be percussed. Shifting dullness and a fluid wave are indicative of ascites.
   b. Areas of tenderness should be percussed to elicit tenderness. Percussion tenderness is a very sensitive sign of peritoneal irritation.

Gastrointestinal Emergencies

   h. **Genitals**
      i. In women, a pelvic examination is mandatory in order to evaluate gastro-intestinal pathology and to rule out a disorder of the reproductive organs.
      ii. In men, the genitals should be examined to rule out epididymitis and torsion, which can cause referred abdominal pain.
      iii. In men and women, the inguinal and femoral regions should be examined to exclude an occult hernia.
   i. **Back.** The back should be percussed to reveal costovertebral angle tenderness, which is suggestive of pyelonephritis or nephrolithiasis.
3. **Laboratory studies** should be guided by the history and physical examination findings.
   a. **Urinalysis** should be performed, along with human chorionic gonadotropin level, in women of childbearing age.
   b. **Blood work**
      i. **Complete blood count (CBC).** The white blood cell (WBC) count is a nonspecific gauge of inflammation; however, it may be normal despite a serious medical or surgical condition. A leukemoid reaction (stress response) may often accompany a gastrointestinal bleed associated with a large volume loss.
      ii. **Electrolytes** may be abnormal due to losses from vomiting or diarrhea or decreased oral intake.
      iii. **Hemoglobin.** The hemoglobin level is an important parameter when evaluating hemorrhage, but it may take several hours to equilibrate.
      iv. **Amylase and lipase.** The amylase level is usually elevated in pancreatitis but may also be elevated in other conditions, such as perforated peptic ulcer, bowel necrosis, salivary gland disease, and a ruptured ectopic pregnancy.
      v. **Liver enzyme** (e.g., aspartate aminotransferase [AST], alanine aminotransferase [ALT], alkaline phosphatase [AP], γ-glutamyl transferase) and **bilirubin levels** should be ordered when hepatic or biliary disease is suspected. Elevated AST and ALT indicates hepatic cell injury or necrosis. Elevated AP, especially with elevated total bilirubin levels, suggests duct obstruction.
      vi. **Coagulation studies.** A prothrombin time (PT) and partial thromboplastin time should be ordered in patients with a suspected surgical abdomen or evidence of upper or lower gastrointestinal bleeding.
4. **Diagnostic imaging studies**
   a. **Radiography**
      i. **Abdominal films** may demonstrate cholelithiasis, nephrolithiasis, pancreatic calcification, or an appendicolith. They may show air–fluid levels or dilated bowel in a bowel obstruction. They may demonstrate calcification of the aorta in an abdominal aortic aneurysm.
      ii. **Chest films** may show free air, a pleural effusion, or a pulmonary process causing referred abdominal pain.
   b. **Ultrasonography.** Bedside ultrasonography is gaining acceptance and verification as research has demonstrated its usefulness for detecting cholelithiasis, abdominal aortic aneurysm, intra-abdominal fluid, hydronephrosis, ectopic pregnancy, and significant bowel wall edema. Formal ultrasonography can provide additional information in these areas and is also useful for identifying pelvic pathology.
   c. **Contrast imaging**, **computed tomography (CT)**, **angiography**, and **nuclear medicine studies** are useful. Abdominal CT has been shown to be extremely useful for detecting abdominal aneurysm, intra-abdominal fluid, traumatic injury, pancreatitis, and the identification of infectious and noninfectious diseases. It will also demonstrate ascites, liver cirrhosis, or hepatic lesions.
C. **Therapy.** General supportive measures include the following:
1. **Intravenous access** should be obtained and the patient hydrated as necessary. **The patient should not receive anything by mouth because he or she may need endoscopy or surgery.**

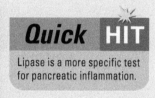

Quick HIT

Lipase is a more specific test for pancreatic inflammation.

2. **Pharmacologic management of symptoms** may involve the use of **antiemetics** (e.g., ondansetron, prochlorperazine), **antispasmodics** (e.g., dicyclomine, hycosamine), **antacids**, or **pain medication**.

   a. Adequate analgesia should be given to patients with renal colic or pain of aortic origin.

   b. Most data indicate that narcotic analgesia given in moderate doses will not mask true peritoneal signs and may improve the reliability of the physical examination in patients with peritoneal signs.

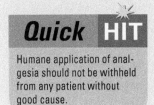

II. ESOPHAGEAL DISORDERS

Esophageal problems present with one of three predominant symptoms: pain, odynophagia/dysphagia, or bleeding.

A. **Esophageal pain**

1. **GERD**

   a. **Discussion**

      i. **Incidence.** Ten percent of the population experiences reflux symptoms daily, and 33% experience symptoms at least once a month. Reflux occurs in 70% of pregnant women and is very common in infants.

      ii. **Pathogenesis.** The reflux is caused by a decrease in the lower esophageal sphincter pressure. Pregnancy and drugs that cause smooth muscle relaxation (e.g., β agonists, peppermint, calcium channel blockers) may augment lower esophageal sphincter pressure. Physical conditions such as mid-body obesity or hiatal hernia may promote relaxation.

   b. **Clinical features.** The reflux of acidic gastric contents into the esophagus causes a **retrosternal, burning pain** that may radiate to the neck or jaw. More than 50% of "chest pain" seen in the ED may be reflux.

      i. The pain is often exacerbated by activities that overcome the lower esophageal sphincter resting pressure such as bending over, lying down, or consuming large meals.

      ii. Uncomplicated GERD is classically relieved within minutes by sitting up and drinking liquids or taking antacids.

   c. **Differential diagnoses.** Pain from GERD can be indistinguishable from **chest pain of cardiac origin**; therefore, a cardiac cause must be ruled out. The resolution of symptoms after a trial of oral antacids in the ED does not necessarily exclude a cardiac cause because many patients have both cardiac disease and GERD.

   d. **Evaluation** is primarily done on an outpatient basis and may include an upper gastrointestinal series, ambulatory acid reflux testing, endoscopy, or manometry to look for spasm as the cause of pain.

   e. **Therapy** entails the following supportive measures:

      i. Elevating the head of the bed 6 inches (or 30 degrees) and avoiding recumbency within 3 hours of eating

      ii. Eating smaller meals and avoiding fatty foods, chocolate, caffeine, peppermint, or alcohol

      iii. Smoking cessation

      iv. Weight reduction (in obese patients)

      v. Over-the-counter antacids, histamine-2 antagonists (e.g., ranitidine, cimetidine), or other agents such as proton pump inhibitors (PPIs; e.g., omeprazole, pantoprazole) are available for short-term use.

   f. **Disposition.** Patients at risk for coronary disease should be admitted. If a cardiac cause can be excluded, the patient may be safely discharged and further evaluated as an outpatient.

2. **Esophagitis**

   a. **Discussion**

      i. **Infectious esophagitis** occurs more commonly in immunocompromised hosts (e.g., patients with AIDS, patients with diabetes mellitus, patients receiving chemotherapy, organ transplant patients). Commonly implicated organisms include *Candida* and **herpes simplex virus and cytomegalovirus (CMV)**.

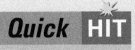

Gastrointestinal Emergencies

ii. **Pill esophagitis** occurs after taking caustic oral medications. The tablet adheres to the esophageal wall and dissolves, leading to local inflammation and irritation. Medications frequently responsible include **doxycycline** (the most common offender), **potassium chloride, quinidine, NSAIDs, ferrous sulfate**, and **oral bisphosphonates**.

b. **Clinical features.** Infectious or pill esophagitis presents as odynophagia (pain with swallowing). Unlike GERD pain, odynophagia predominates. Often the patients will drool or spit to avoid swallowing. Anorexia is common.

i. *Candida* **esophagitis.** Pain may be mild or severe. Oral candidiasis is often present (especially in patients with AIDS).

ii. **Herpes or CMV esophagitis.** The onset of pain is typically abrupt, and there may be a history of recent upper respiratory tract infection. Herpes or CMV esophagitis is associated with ulcerative lesions (distinct from the heaped plaques associated with oral candidiasis). Immunocompetent patients frequently demonstrate skin or oral lesions, but immunocompromised patients often do not.

c. **Differential diagnoses**

i. **Cardiac disease** must always be excluded.

ii. **Oropharyngeal odynophagia** can be caused by pharyngitis, retropharyngeal abscess, peritonsillar abscess, or epiglottitis and must be distinguished from esophageal odynophagia.

d. **Evaluation**

i. *Candida* esophagitis may be confirmed in the ED using an air-contrast barium swallow, which will reveal ulceration and plaques.

ii. Evaluation should include a soft tissue film of the neck if a retropharyngeal abscess or epiglottitis is suspected.

iii. Esophagoscopy with biopsy and culture is the definitive study.

e. **Therapy**

i. *Candida* **esophagitis.** Treatment is with oral ketoconazole or fluconazole. Granulocytopenic patients are at risk for dissemination; therefore, treatment with intravenous amphotericin B is warranted for these patients.

ii. **Herpes esophagitis** is self-limited in immunocompetent patients. Treatment with oral acyclovir may shorten healing time. Oral or intravenous acyclovir may be required for immunocompromised patients.

iii. **Pill esophagitis.** Symptoms usually resolve without any specific treatment. The offending medication should be discontinued if possible. If it is not possible to discontinue the medication, the patient should take the pills with plenty of water and remain in an upright position (sitting or standing) for 10 to 30 minutes immediately after taking the medication. A short course of antacids or acid-suppressing medications will provide symptom relief until the ulcer has healed.

f. **Disposition.** Immunocompetent patients with mild symptoms may be empirically treated with oral fluconazole and should be referred for outpatient follow-up within a week. Patients who are unable to maintain adequate oral fluid intake or those at risk for disseminated infection should be admitted.

3. **Boerhaave syndrome** is rupture of the esophagus during forceful emesis.

a. **Clinical features.** The patient reports an episode of severe, violent emesis and complains of severe chest pain with or without shortness of air.

b. **Evaluation**

i. **Physical examination**

a) **Hamman sign** is a crunching sound heard on auscultation of the heart. The crunching sound is due to mediastinal emphysema.

b) **Crepitation** may be found in the neck and signifies subcutaneous emphysema.

           c) **Signs of septic shock**, fever, hypotension, or altered mentation may be seen in late presentations.

     ii. **Diagnostic imaging**

         a) **Chest radiographs** may demonstrate mediastinal air, subcutaneous emphysema, a widened mediastinum, pneumothorax, or air–fluid levels.

         b) **Water-soluble contrast swallow** will show extravasation.

   c. **Therapy** entails fluid resuscitation, antibiotics, and emergent surgical repair. A chest tube may be needed if a pneumothorax is present.

  4. **Motility disorders** (see II.B.1.b and II.B.2.b) may produce esophageal pain.

B. **Esophageal dysphagia**

  1. **Discussion.** Dysphagia is defined as difficulty swallowing. It may or may not be accompanied by pain. Causes of esophageal dysphagia include:

   a. **Obstructive disorders** (e.g., aortic aneurysm, carcinoma, webs, and rings)

   b. **Motor disorders** (e.g., achalasia, diffuse esophageal spasm, and scleroderma)

   c. **Acute food impaction** (typically meat)

  2. **Clinical features**

   a. **Obstructive disorders.** Patients tend to have greater dysphagia for solids than for liquids.

   b. **Motor disorders.** Patients tend to have equal dysphagia for both solids and liquids. Dysphagia resulting from a motor disorder is often associated with pain.

   c. **Food impaction** often occurs in social situations and is often associated with alcohol. It may or may not indicate underlying esophageal disorders.

  3. **Differential diagnoses**

   a. **Cardiac disorders** must be excluded if the patient is experiencing chest pain.

   b. **Oropharyngeal dysphagia** is defined as difficulty passing food from the mouth to the esophagus and must be differentiated from esophageal dysphagia.

     i. **Common causes** include **cerebrovascular accident**, **multiple sclerosis**, **myasthenia gravis**, and **amyotrophic lateral sclerosis**.

     ii. **Clinical features** may include drooling, coughing, choking, nasal regurgitation, or aspiration. Patients with an acute sensation that something is stuck or who are unable to handle secretions most often have acute food impaction.

  4. **Evaluation**

   a. **Radiography.** A chest radiograph may demonstrate an aortic aneurysm, a tumor, a foreign body, or a dilated esophagus with an air–fluid level (characteristic of achalasia).

   b. **Other studies** are carried out on an outpatient basis for the nonemergent patient and may include endoscopy, a barium swallow, manometry, and motility studies.

  5. **Therapy**

   a. **Supportive therapy.** Intravenous hydration may be necessary.

   b. **Definitive therapy**

     i. **Obstructive disorders**

       a) **Medical treatment.** Acute esophageal obstruction may be treated medically with **glucagon**, **calcium channel blockers** (e.g., nifedipine) to induce smooth muscle relaxation, and **antispasmodics** (e.g., diazepam).

       b) **Acute endoscopy** is indicated if medical treatment fails to resolve the problem and complete esophageal obstruction persists. In these situations, endoscopy should be performed as soon as possible to avoid complications (perforation, mucosal necrosis, etc.).

     ii. **Motility disorders** (spasm) may be treated with nitrates, calcium channel blockers, or anticholinergic drugs to reduce symptoms pending definitive diagnosis

  6. **Disposition.** Most patients can be discharged for an outpatient work up. Dehydration or complete esophageal obstruction are the major indications for admission.

C. **Esophageal bleeding.** An esophageal source is responsible for approximately 25% of cases of upper gastrointestinal tract bleeding. Of these, nearly 80% are due

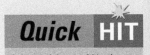

Quick HIT

It is crucial to avoid barium studies in patients suspected of having complete esophageal obstruction as barium may preclude the feasibility of urgent endoscopy.

Gastrointestinal Emergencies

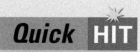

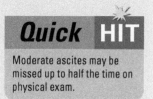

to esophageal varices and 20% are due to Mallory-Weiss tears or severe erosive esophagitis.

1. **Esophageal varices**
   a. **Discussion.** Varices are dilated submucosal veins that result from portal hypertension, which is most commonly caused by cirrhosis of the liver.
   b. **Clinical features.** Patients with esophageal varices commonly present with **painless** and **massive hematemesis**. The **stigmata of chronic liver disease** (e.g., spider angiomas, palmar erythema, ascites, gynecomastia, and testicular atrophy) may be present as well.
   c. **Therapy**
      i. **Supportive therapy.** Measures include:
         a) **Administration of intravenous fluids** through two large-bore intravenous lines
         b) **Administration of packed red blood cells (RBCs)** to a target hemoglobin of 7 gm/dL. Over-transfusion is associated with rebleeding or continuous bleeding due to increased portal pressure and should be avoided.
         c) **Fresh frozen plasma, platelet infusion, or recombinant factor VII may be administered** to correct any coagulopathy.
         d) **Nasogastric suction** to monitor bleeding is controversial and can provide misleading information.
         e) **Octreotide**, a synthetic somatostatin compound indicated for terminating upper gastrointestinal hemorrhage while not inducing vasoconstriction.
            1) **Dose.** Octreotide is administered as an intravenous infusion at a rate of 50 μg/hour for 72 hours or longer, which reduces rebleeding, transfusion requirements, and improves mortality.
            2) **Complications** of octreotide include hypoglycemia, hyperglycemia, and thrombocytopenia.
         f) **The use of ceftriaxone 1 gm intravenously daily or norfloxacin 400 mg daily for 7 days significantly reduces infectious sequelae and reduces portal pressure via gut decontamination reduction of endotoxemia.**
         g) **Erythromycin 250 to 500 mg given 30 minutes prior to endoscopy may aid in visualization by promoting gastric motility and emptying blood from the stomach.**
         h) **Intravenous PPI reduces transfusion requirements and helps stop bleeding because a pH of 7 is required for optimal platelet function and clot formation.**
      ii. **Definitive therapy**
         a) **Sengstaken-Blakemore** is an orogastric tube equipped with inflatable gastric and esophageal balloons. Inflation of the balloons applies direct pressure to the bleeding varices and is useful for acute hemorrhage control until definitive therapy is available.
            1) Endotracheal intubation should be performed prior to Sengstaken-Blakemore tube placement.
            2) Sengstaken-Blakemore tube placement controls hemorrhage in 85% of patients but is associated with a 65% re-bleed rate as well as a 30% incidence of significant complications including sepsis and esophageal perforation.
         b) **Endoscopic variceal ligation has replaced traditional sclerotherapy.** Bands are placed during a second endoscopy after diagnostic esophagogastroduodenoscopy reveals bleeding varices and is successful 98% of the time. After endoscopic variceal ligation, repeat banding at monthly intervals may be necessary to eradicate varices at risk for bleeding.
         c) Transvenous intrahepatic portosystemic shunt will lower portal pressure with the portal pressure gradient from the portal vein to the

hepatic vein reduced to less than 12 mm Hg. Although contraindicated in patients with high model for end-stage liver disease scores, it carries a significantly lower mortality that that of portosystemic shunt surgeries, which are associated with a 75% mortality rate and are rarely performed in the United States today.

2. **Mallory-Weiss tears**
   a. **Discussion.** Mallory-Weiss tears are partial-thickness lacerations of the gastroesophageal junction that result from forceful emesis.
   b. **Clinical features.** There is a history of vomiting in 85% of patients. Many patients also have a history of alcohol abuse.
   c. **Assess hemodynamics.** It is essential to obtain hemoglobin level and assess magnitude of bleeding by measuring hemodynamic and orthostatic parameters.
   d. **Therapy.** Bleeding usually stops spontaneously. When necessary, the condition can be treated with endoscopic clipping. Intravenous octreotide and intravenous PPI until urgent endoscopy is performed may be helpful.
   e. **Disposition.** Many patients can be discharged after urgent endoscopy is performed.

III. GASTROINTESTINAL FOREIGN BODIES

The ingestion of foreign bodies is responsible for approximately 1,500 deaths each year in the United States. Groups at risk include children, alcoholics, the mentally impaired, elderly with dementia, denture wearers, and prisoners.

A. **Esophageal foreign bodies**
   1. **Discussion.** Eighty percent of patients with esophageal foreign bodies are children. The child is typically brought to the ED by a caretaker after a witnessed ingestion. If the ingestion was not witnessed, the diagnosis can be difficult.
   2. **Clinical features**
      a. **Symptoms**
         i. **Adults** typically complain of a foreign body sensation in the throat or chest. The patient may appear anxious and experience retching or vomiting, choking, coughing, or drooling.
         ii. **Children.** Symptoms include refusal to eat, increased salivation, pain on swallowing, vomiting, choking, and referred respiratory symptoms (e.g., stridor, cough, and wheezing).
      b. **Physical examination** may reveal signs of infection. **Fever** and/or **subcutaneous emphysema** in the neck is suggestive of esophageal perforation.
   3. **Evaluation**
      a. **Laryngoscopy.** Direct or indirect laryngoscopy may be performed if the patient feels that the foreign body is in the throat or if respiratory symptoms are present.
      b. **Radiography**
         i. Radiographs can be used to pinpoint the location of radiopaque objects (e.g., coins, button batteries, sharp objects) (see Clinical Pearl 4-2).
         ii. Pneumomediastinum or air in the soft tissues suggests perforation.
      c. **Endoscopy** also allows localization of the object and is often therapeutic.
      d. **Esophagraphy.** An esophagram should be performed only after consulting with a specialist because the contrast material may interfere with later attempts at endoscopy.
   4. **Therapy**
      a. **Coins** and small smooth objects often pass through the gastrointestinal tract without difficulty. Coins that are too large to pass are removed by endos-

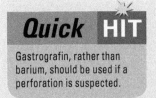

Quick HIT

Gastrografin, rather than barium, should be used if a perforation is suspected.

CLINICAL PEARL 4-2

1. Coins in the esophagus align themselves in the frontal plane and are therefore seen face-on in an anteroposterior view.
2. Coins in the trachea align themselves in the sagittal plane and are seen edge-on in an anteroposterior view.

Gastrointestinal Emergencies

copy. They can also be removed, by experienced physicians, using a Foley catheter guided by fluoroscopy.

b. **Button batteries** have the potential to cause chemical corrosion and perforation of the esophagus and must be endoscopically removed as soon as possible.

c. **Sharp objects** must be removed by endoscopy.

d. **Food impactions** can be treated expectantly if the patient is managing his or her secretions adequately. Medical interventions include the following:

   i. **Glucagon** (1 mg intravenously) may relieve the impaction. A second 2-mg dose can be administered in 20 minutes if the first dose is ineffective.

   ii. **Nitroglycerin** (administered sublingually) may also assist in relieving the impaction.

   iii. **Nifedipine** (10 mg sublingually) relaxes the lower esophageal sphincter and may allow passage of the food bolus.

   iv. **Diazepam** may be used as a last resort.

   v. **Endoscopy** should be performed if the bolus has not passed after several hours.

5. **Disposition.** All patients need follow-up to rule out underlying esophageal pathology.

B. **Nonesophageal foreign bodies**

1. **Discussion.** Once a foreign object has passed beyond the esophagus and into the stomach, most will pass without complications.

2. **Clinical features.** Typically, nonesophageal foreign bodies are asymptomatic unless perforation or impaction has occurred. Under these circumstances, the patient presents with signs of peritonitis or obstruction.

3. **Evaluation.** Abdominal radiographs should be obtained to localize the object.

4. **Therapy**

   a. **Peritonitis or obstruction.** Any patient with evidence of obstruction or perforation requires consultation with a surgeon.

   b. **Sharp objects** that are in the stomach should be removed endoscopically because they have a 15% to 35% chance of perforating the bowel if they are not removed. If the sharp object has passed the pylorus, consultation with a surgeon is required.

   c. **Other objects** can be managed on an outpatient basis.

      i. The stools should be checked for passage of the object, which usually occurs in 48 to 72 hours but may take as long as 6 to 14 days. A repeat radiograph should be obtained in 1 week if the object has not yet passed in the stool. If the object does not pass within 2 weeks, surgical removal may be necessary.

      ii. The patient should be advised to return immediately to the ED if he or she experiences fever, abdominal pain, or vomiting.

IV. PEPTIC ULCER DISEASE

A. **Discussion.** Peptic ulcers are localized erosions of the gastric or duodenal mucosa that produce pain and can perforate into a blood vessel (causing hemorrhage) or into the peritoneal cavity. Peptic ulcers used to be the most common cause of upper gastrointestinal hemorrhage; however, depending on the local incidence of hepatitis C liver disease with portal hypertension, variceal bleeding may predominate.

1. **Prevalence.** The prevalence of peptic ulcer disease is 1.7%. Approximately 350,000 new cases are diagnosed annually in the United States.

2. **Risk factors** include smoking, alcohol use, aspirin or other NSAID use, a family history of peptic ulcer disease, male gender, and age.

3. **Etiology.** *Helicobacter pylori*, a helical, gram-negative bacterium, has been found to be responsible for over 90% of duodenal ulcers and 65% to 70% of gastric ulcers.

B. **Clinical presentation.** Patients with peptic ulcer disease present to the ED for one of three reasons: pain, hemorrhage, or perforation.

1. **Pain.** Most frequently, the patient complains of a burning or gnawing epigastric pain that does not radiate. Physical examination may demonstrate

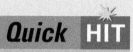

Quick HIT

Objects greater than 2 cm in diameter or longer than 12 cm may get hung up at the ileocecal valve or remain in the small intestine. It therefore becomes a significant early clinical decision whether to remove the object while it is still in the stomach.

Gastrointestinal Emergencies

CLINICAL PEARL 4-3

a. **Gastric ulcer pain** usually occurs immediately after eating. Nausea is also common. Up to 50% of persons may not have pain.

b. **Duodenal ulcer pain** occurs between meals, may awaken the patient from sleep, and is present in up to 75% of patients. It is often worse immediately before a meal and is relieved by eating due to buffering by pancreatic bicarbonate secretions into the duodenum.

epigastric tenderness but no peritoneal signs. The pain is typically relieved by over-the-counter antacids, histamine-2 blockers, or PPI (see Clinical Pearl 4-3).

2. **Hemorrhage** is the presenting complaint in 20% of patients with peptic ulcer disease.
   a. **Patient history.** The patient may or may not have a history of epigastric pain. Associated nausea is common.
   b. **Signs and symptoms.** Twenty percent of patients present with **melena**, 30% with **hematemesis**, and 50% with both.
   c. **Physical examination.** Epigastric tenderness may be present. Rectal examination will most likely be positive for occult blood, if not grossly melenic. Approximately 150 mL of blood is required for melena. Up to 10% of patients with peptic ulcer may present with **hematochezia**. These patients are often orthostatic, and 30% will require endoscopic intervention to stop the bleeding

3. **Perforation** occurs in 5% to 10% of patients with peptic ulcer disease.
   a. **Signs and symptoms.** Patients present with the abrupt onset of **severe epigastric pain** that may be associated with **vomiting** and **diaphoresis**.
   b. **Physical examination** reveals a diffusely tender abdomen with rigidity, rebound, guarding, and hypoactive bowel sounds.

C. **Differential diagnoses**
   1. **Pain.** Differential diagnoses for the pain of peptic ulcer disease include pancreatitis, cholelithiasis, abdominal aortic aneurysm, superior mesenteric artery syndrome, and cardiac causes.
   2. **Hemorrhage.** Differential diagnoses for upper gastrointestinal hemorrhage include esophageal or gastric varices, erosive gastritis, esophagitis, Mallory-Weiss tears, Dieulafoy lesions, arteriovenous malformations, or cancer.
   3. **Perforation.** Differential diagnoses include perforation of other organs, ruptured abdominal aortic aneurysm, and ruptured ectopic pregnancy.

D. **Evaluation**
   1. **Uncomplicated peptic ulcer disease.** In patients who are experiencing only pain, the **hemoglobin level** should be evaluated to rule out anemia due to chronic blood loss.
   2. **Hemorrhage.** In hemorrhaging patients, the evaluation should include a **CBC**, **PT**, and **blood typing and cross matching**.
   3. **Perforation**
      a. **Radiography.** A chest radiograph will reveal free air in 75% of patients. The radiographic yield is enhanced by instilling 100 to 200 mL of air via a nasogastric tube and keeping the patient in an upright position for at least 10 minutes prior to taking the radiograph.
      b. **Upper gastrointestinal series.** In some patients, an upper gastrointestinal series is necessary to demonstrate the perforation.

E. **Therapy**
   1. **Uncomplicated peptic ulcer disease.** If *H. pylori* has been confirmed to be the etiologic agent by biopsy or stool antigen, antibiotic therapy is indicated. Antibiotics coupled with high-dose PPI is highly effective in eradicating *H. pylori* and reduces ulcer recurrence rate from 70% to less than 5%. The patient is also advised to avoid alcohol, caffeine, and NSAIDs.

Gastrointestinal Emergencies

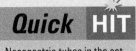

Quick HIT

Nasogastric tubes in the setting of gastrointestinal bleed are diagnostically misleading as they provide both false-positive and false-negative information.

2. **Hemorrhage.** A total of 70% to 80% of patients will cease bleeding spontaneously, but the mortality rate is still 7% to 10% percent overall.
   a. **Supportive therapy**
      i. **Fluid resuscitation** should be carried out through two large-bore intravenous lines.
      ii. **Administration of blood products** (e.g., packed RBCs to correct anemia, fresh frozen plasma for coagulopathy (international normalized ratio >1.8), or platelets for thrombocytopenia may be necessary.
      iii. **Intravenous administration of PPI** is often initiated, with studies showing reduced need for blood transfusion and reduced rebleeding.
      iv. **Administration of octreotide** may be useful for terminating the hemorrhage.
   b. **Definitive therapy**
      i. **Endoscopy** with **electrocautery** or **sclerotherapy** is the therapy of choice.
      ii. **Angiographic embolization** or **surgery** may be required.
3. **Perforation.** Therapy entails **nasogastric suction, intravenous fluids, antibiotics** (e.g., cefoxitin), and **surgery.**

F. **Disposition**
   1. Patients with no evidence of active bleeding, a normal hemoglobin, and normal vital signs may be discharged with a prescription for an histamine-2 blocker or PPI and instructions to follow up with a primary care physician.
   2. Patients with anemia or active bleeding should be admitted to the hospital and have a consultation with a gastroenterologist or surgical endoscopist.
   3. Patients with hemodynamic instability should be admitted to the intensive care unit, and a gastroenterologist should be consulted immediately.
   4. Patients with perforation must be evaluated by a surgeon.

V. GASTROENTERITIS OF INFECTIOUS ORIGIN

A. **Discussion**
   1. **Definitions**
      a. **Diarrhea** is the excretion of more than 250 g of stool per day.
      b. **Gastroenteritis** is acute enteritis (i.e., inflammation of the intestines manifested as diarrhea) accompanied by nausea and vomiting.
      c. **Food poisoning** is a gastroenteritis that occurs suddenly and is often associated with abdominal pain and cramping. It is caused by ingestion of food containing preformed toxins.
   2. **Etiology.** Gastroenteritis is caused by viruses in 50% to 70% of cases, bacteria in 15% to 20% of cases, and parasites in 10% to 15% of cases.
B. **Clinical features**
   1. **Viral gastroenteritis**
      a. **Norwalk agent.** The Norwalk agent is a parvovirus-like pathogen that is spread by the fecal–oral route and is often responsible for epidemic outbreaks of gastroenteritis (especially on cruise ships). The diarrhea is more prominent than the vomiting, and symptoms last 24 to 48 hours.
      b. **Rotavirus** is a major cause of gastroenteritis in children, but adults can also contract the virus. Infection is characterized by vomiting that lasts 24 to 36 hours and diarrhea that lasts 4 to 7 days.
   2. **Bacterial gastroenteritis**
      a. **Invasive organisms** induce bloody diarrhea by invading the intestinal mucosa.
         i. *Campylobacter* gastroenteritis. *Campylobacter* species are the most common cause of bacterial gastroenteritis in the United States. They are gram-negative organisms that cause an acute dysentery (i.e., diarrhea containing blood, pus, and mucus). The diarrhea can last for weeks, but most patients are ill for less than 1 week.
         ii. **Salmonellosis.** *Salmonella* is most often contracted from the ingestion of contaminated poultry products. It produces an acute gastroenteritis characterized by fever, abdominal pain, and diarrhea that may be bloody. Salmonellosis usually lasts less than 5 days.

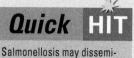

Quick HIT

Salmonellosis may disseminate and present with septic shock particularly in the immunocompromised host. Fever with a paradoxically low pulse is often seen.

iii. **Shigellosis.** *Shigella* produces a gastroenteritis similar to that produced by *Salmonella*, but bloody diarrhea is a less prominent feature. The gastroenteritis resolves within 1 week.

iv. *Vibrio parahaemolyticus* **gastroenteritis.** The most common route of infection is the ingestion of inadequately cooked seafood. Diarrhea lasting 24 to 48 hours is the predominant symptom. *Vibrio* may also disseminate in susceptible hosts with liver cirrhosis or with immunocompromise and present with septic shock.

b. **Toxigenic organisms** produce a toxin that induces diarrhea. These organisms do not invade the mucosa; therefore, the diarrhea is not bloody.

i. **"Traveler's diarrhea"** is most commonly caused by enterotoxigenic *Escherichia coli*. Enterotoxigenic *E. coli* produces a toxin that induces a mild diarrhea that typically lasts less than 1 week.

ii. *E. coli* **O157:H7** presents with bloody diarrhea and abdominal pain. It may be associated with hemolytic uremic syndrome, altered mental status, seizures, renal failure, sepsis, and death. The elderly and children younger than 5 years are at higher risk. Infections are more common in the summer and are related to undercooked hamburger meat.

iii. **Staphylococcal food poisoning.** *Staphylococcus aureus* produces a toxin in certain foods that are allowed to stand at room temperature (e.g., mayonnaise-based salads, cream-filled doughnuts). Ingestion of the toxin induces a gastroenteritis characterized by violent vomiting and diarrhea that lasts less than 24 hours.

iv. *Bacillus cereus* **gastroenteritis.** *B. cereus* produces a heat-stable toxin that can produce either an emetic syndrome similar to that produced by *S. aureus* or a diarrheal syndrome that is characterized by diarrhea and abdominal cramps lasting 24 to 36 hours. *B. cereus* is commonly contracted from contaminated rice.

v. **Pseudomembranous enterocolitis.** *Clostridium difficile* can cause diarrhea as a result of alterations in the intestinal flora following antibiotic therapy. The organism produces an enterotoxin that causes the enteritis.

3. **Protozoal diarrhea**

a. **Giardiasis** (see Chapter 6.VIII.A.2.j) is characterized by flatulence and loose, foul-smelling stools. However, symptoms vary and some patients may only complain of dyspepsia. *Giardia* cysts are usually acquired by ingestion of lake or stream water.

b. **Cryptosporidiosis** is characterized by a profuse, nonbloody diarrhea that lasts less than 3 weeks in immunocompetent individuals but may become chronic in immunocompromised patients.

C. **Differential diagnoses** include inflammatory bowel disease and, if pain is a prominent symptom, appendicitis, diverticulitis, small bowel obstruction, mesenteric infarction, and gynecologic disorders.

D. **Evaluation.** It is not usually possible, or necessary, to identify the causative organism in the ED. Rather, the focus should be on identifying whether the organism is invasive or toxigenic.

1. **Patient history**

a. The patient should be asked about the **onset of symptoms.** A sudden onset of nausea, violent vomiting, and diarrhea suggests a toxigenic cause, whereas a more gradual onset suggests an invasive cause.

b. The **duration of symptoms** can also provide valuable information. Toxigenic gastroenteritis from a preformed toxin (i.e., food poisoning) typically lasts less than 24 hours.

c. The patient should be asked about the **nature of the stool.** Blood, pus, or mucus in the feces is diagnostic of invasive diarrhea.

d. History of recent antibiotic use or hospitalization suggests *C. difficile* infection.

2. **Physical examination**

a. **Fever** is an uncommon manifestation of a toxigenic gastroenteritis and therefore points to an invasive cause.

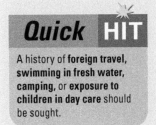

Quick **HIT**

A history of **foreign travel, swimming in fresh water, camping,** or **exposure to children in day care** should be sought.

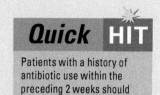

b. **Abdominal tenderness** may be prominent in an invasive gastroenteritis but is minimal in a toxigenic gastroenteritis.

3. **Laboratory studies.** If the patient is only mildly ill and there is no suspicion of invasive disease, then no further evaluation is necessary. However, if it is still unclear whether the cause is invasive or toxigenic, laboratory studies may be appropriate.

   a. **Fecal analysis.** Finding leukocytes in the stool sample is diagnostic for an invasive diarrhea.

   b. **Blood work.** The CBC is usually normal in toxigenic gastroenteritis but demonstrates an elevated WBC count and a left shift in patients with an invasive gastroenteritis.

E. **Therapy**

1. **Rehydration** and **correction of electrolyte imbalances** is indicated for dehydrated patients.

   a. **Intravenous rehydration** may be necessary for some patients.

   b. **Oral rehydration.** Patients who are able to tolerate oral fluids should be instructed to drink cold fluids containing sugars (e.g., fruit juice, nondiet soft drinks, Rehydralyte, sports drinks) because sugars assist in electrolyte absorption. Milk should be avoided because many patients experience a transient lactase deficiency (lactose intolerance) during a case of gastroenteritis.

2. **Antiemetics** (e.g., prochlorperazine) may be useful.

3. **Antidiarrheals** (e.g., loperamide, diphenoxylate) may be used in toxigenic gastroenteritis but are **contraindicated in invasive gastroenteritis or anyone who appears critically ill.**

4. **Empiric antibiotic therapy** is indicated for patients with invasive gastroenteritis, especially if the patient appears ill. However, antibiotics are **not useful in toxigenic gastroenteritis and may prolong infection.**

   a. **Ciprofloxacin** is the current drug of choice because it has good activity against the most common infectious agents. The dose is 500 mg twice a day for 3 to 4 days.

   b. **Metronidazole** or **oral vancomycin** is used to treat pseudomembranous enterocolitis. If *C. difficile* is confirmed, appropriate dose duration (10 to 14 days) and follow-up are essential.

F. **Disposition**

1. Patients who can tolerate oral hydration can be discharged with follow-up.

2. Patients who are severely dehydrated or severely ill should be admitted.

VI. INTESTINAL DISORDERS

A. **Inflammatory bowel disease**

1. **Crohn disease (regional enteritis)**

   a. **Discussion.** Crohn disease is a granulomatous inflammatory condition that can affect any portion of the digestive tract but most often involves the large and small bowel. In 87% of patients, the disease involves the terminal ileum.

      i. **Incidence and prevalence.** Men are more frequently affected than women, and the disease is more common in Jewish people. There are two peaks of incidence, between the ages of 12 and 30 years and 50 and 60 years.

      ii. **Etiology.** The cause is unclear, but infectious agents, immunologic factors, and genetic factors have all been implicated.

      iii. **Pathogenesis.** Crohn disease is characterized by areas of transmural inflammation interspersed with areas of normal bowel. The transmural nature of the inflammation predisposes to the formation of fistulae and strictures. Complications include bowel perforation, obstruction, hemorrhage, and abscess formation.

   b. **Clinical features** include **fever**, **weight loss**, **diarrhea** (possibly bloody), and **cramping abdominal pain** often in the right lower quadrant (terminal ileum location) that may be worse after meals. **Symptoms of complications** may be masked if the patient is taking corticosteroids or narcotic analgesics (see Clinical Pearl 4-4).

CLINICAL PEARL 4-4

Symptoms of hepatobiliary, renal, rheumatic, ocular, and cutaneous manifestations may be noted with Crohn disease

1. Biliary abnormalities (e.g., fatty liver, sclerosing cholangitis, cirrhosis, cholelithiasis)
2. Nephrolithiasis (resulting from calcium oxalate stones)
3. Arthritis and ankylosing spondylitis
4. Uveitis and episcleritis
5. Erythema nodosum and pyoderma gangrenosum

   c. **Differential diagnoses** include ulcerative colitis, lymphoma, gastroenteritis, and appendicitis.

   d. **Evaluation**

      i. **Known diagnosis.** In patients with known Crohn disease, studies should be performed to rule out complications suggested by the history and physical examination findings.

         a) **Laboratory.** A CBC may reveal evidence of hemorrhage, infection, or abscess. Electrolyte levels can be used to assess dehydration and secondary aberrations.

         b) **Liver studies** are indicated to evaluate suspected biliary pathology.

         c) **Radiographs.** An abdominal series can help rule out obstruction. A chest radiograph may reveal free air resulting from a perforation.

      ii. **Suspected diagnosis.** In patients who are suspected of having Crohn disease, a **contrast study** or **colonoscopy** may be indicated. These studies are usually performed on an outpatient basis. To limit radiation, avoid multiple repeat CT scans and consider bedside ultrasound or magnetic resonance imaging scanning instead.

   e. **Therapy**

      i. **Complications** such as perforation or obstruction must be treated with urgent admission and surgical consultation.

      ii. **Uncomplicated exacerbations** are ideally managed in consultation with the patient's gastroenterologist. Treatment measures may include administration of **antibiotics** (e.g., metronidazole), **steroids** (e.g., prednisone; 0.5 mg/kg orally daily), **sulfasalazine** (3 to 4 g four times daily), or mesalamine. Biologics such as anti–tumor necrosis factor infliximab (Remicade, Janssen Biotech, Inc, Horsham, PA) or immunomodulators such as azathioprine (Imuran, GlaxoSmithKline, Mississauga, Ontario, Canada) may be options for the patient's gastroenterologist to consider.

      iii. **Severe exacerbations** are treated with **bowel rest** and the intravenous administration of **fluids, antibiotics,** and **corticosteroids** (e.g., hydrocortisone; 100 mg every 8 hours or Solu-Medrol) if the patient is currently taking steroids.

   f. **Disposition**

      i. **Admission.** Indications for admission in patients in whom the diagnosis of Crohn disease has been established include:

         a) Complications (e.g., obstruction, perforation)

         b) Systemic symptoms (e.g., fever, weight loss)

         c) Severe symptoms (e.g., pain, symptomatic anemia, bloody diarrhea)

         d) Dehydration

      ii. **Discharge.** Patients with a definitive diagnosis who are discharged require careful instructions to return if the symptoms worsen or complications develop. Follow-up is essential. Patients in whom the diagnosis is suspected (on the basis of the history and examination), but who do not require hospitalization, must be referred to gastroenterology for follow-up to obtain a definitive diagnosis.

Gastrointestinal Emergencies

2. **Ulcerative colitis**
   a. **Discussion.** Ulcerative colitis is a chronic inflammatory condition affecting the mucosa and submucosa of the large bowel and rectum.
      i. **Incidence and prevalence.** Women are affected more than men. Peak incidence occurs between the ages of 15 and 30 years and 50 and 65 years.
      ii. **Pathogenesis.** Complications may include perforation, obstruction, hemorrhage, and toxic megacolon. Toxic megacolon occurs secondary to the loss of muscle tone in the affected portion of the colon with rapid dilatation due to gas produced by bacteria.
   b. **Clinical features** of ulcerative colitis include **watery diarrhea** containing blood, pus, and mucus; **crampy abdominal pain**; **fever**; and **weight loss**. In a patient with toxic megacolon, there may be a history of decreased stool output and the abdomen is distended, tender, and tympanitic. Symptoms or complications may be masked if the patient is taking steroids or narcotic analgesics.
   c. **Differential diagnoses** include Crohn disease, colon cancer, ischemic colitis, and diverticulitis.
   d. **Evaluation**
      i. **Known diagnosis.** In patients in whom a diagnosis of ulcerative colitis has been made, studies should be performed to rule out complications.
         a) **Radiography.** Dilatation of the large bowel to greater than 6 cm is evident on abdominal films in patients with toxic megacolon.
         b) **CT scan** with wall thickening of 4 mm or greater suggests severe colitis regardless of cause.
      ii. **Suspected diagnosis.** Patients in whom ulcerative colitis is suspected require **endoscopic** evaluation with mucosal biopsies, usually on an outpatient basis.
   e. **Therapy**
      i. **Toxic megacolon.** Therapeutic measures include admission, strict bowel rest, serial abdominal exams, administration of **intravenous fluids and electrolytes**, administration of broad spectrum **antibiotics** (e.g., fluoroquinolones), and quick look with flexible sigmoidoscopy to assess for pseudomembranes. Gastrointestinal and surgical consultation is advisable.
      ii. **Exacerbations** are managed similarly as for Crohn disease although response to therapies my differ (see VI.A.1.e).
   f. **Disposition** is as for Crohn disease (see VI.A.1.f).
B. **Bowel obstruction**
   1. **Discussion.** An obstruction of the normal flow of intestinal contents can occur in either the large or small bowel.
      a. **Causes** include adhesions from prior surgery (the most common cause), hernias, cancer, inflammatory conditions (e.g., Crohn disease, diverticulitis), foreign bodies, volvulus (i.e., twisting of the large bowel around its mesentery), and intussusception (i.e., invagination of one segment of the intestine into another).
      b. **Pathogenesis.** Obstruction leads to third spacing of fluid into the bowel wall and lumen, which can lead to hypovolemia and electrolyte abnormalities. If the circulation to a segment of the bowel is compromised, the bowel is said to be strangulated. Strangulation usually results from the twisting of the bowel on its mesentery and can lead to gangrene, sepsis, and perforation.
   2. **Clinical features**
      a. **Patient history.** The patient may describe **obstipation** (i.e., a lack of stool or flatus). Obstipation may not be a clinical feature if the patient presents early in the course of obstruction or if only a partial obstruction is present.
      b. **Symptoms**
         i. The patient complains of **cramping epigastric or periumbilical pain** that **waxes and wanes**.
         ii. **Vomiting** tends to be a prominent feature in patients with a proximal obstruction or obstruction of the small bowel but may be absent in patients with a distal colonic obstruction. The vomitus may become bilious and then feculent over time.

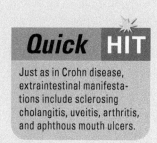

Quick HIT

Just as in Crohn disease, extraintestinal manifestations include sclerosing cholangitis, uveitis, arthritis, and aphthous mouth ulcers.

c. **Physical examination findings**
   i. The **abdomen tends to be diffusely tender** and without peritoneal signs. Peritoneal signs suggest that strangulation or perforation has occurred.
   ii. **Abdominal distention** tends to be more prominent with distal obstructions.
   iii. **Intermittent, high-pitched bowel sounds** may be auscultated, and the abdomen may be tympanitic to percussion.
3. **Differential diagnoses** include paralytic ileus (due to electrolyte abnormalities, trauma, uremia, or peritonitis), cholecystitis, pancreatitis, appendicitis, perforated peptic ulcer, and mesenteric ischemia.
4. **Evaluation**
   a. **Laboratory**
      i. An elevated WBC count with a left shift is suggestive of strangulation.
      ii. Electrolytes, blood urea nitrogen, and creatinine levels should be ordered to rule out an electrolyte abnormality and to further assess hydration status.
      iii. The amylase or lipase level may be elevated in the presence of strangulated or gangrenous bowel.
      iv. Serum lactate is elevated with advanced ischemia.
   b. **Abdominal radiographs**
      i. **Distention** of the large or small bowel or both may be evident.
         a) **Valvulae conniventes**, which are numerous, narrowly spaced (<1 mm), and cross the entire lumen, are seen in the small intestine.
         b) **Haustra**, which are less numerous, widely spaced, and do not cross the entire lumen, are seen in the large intestine. They may become wider spaced and thickened (thumb printing) with luminal dilatation greater than 6 cm.
      ii. **Air–fluid levels** in a **stepladder pattern** are consistent with small bowel obstruction.
      iii. A **dilated, looped large bowel** often pointing to the right side of the abdomen is characteristic of a sigmoid volvulus.
      iv. A **distended colon** in the left lower quadrant and absence of right-sided gas may indicate a cecal volvulus.
      v. The **"string-of-pearls" sign** (i.e., a line of small pockets of air in the fluid-filled lumen) may be observed.
      vi. **Free air** indicates that perforation has occurred.
   c. Other adjunct studies such as an **upper gastrointestinal series** or **diagnostic endoscopies** may be required for definitive diagnosis. The abdominal spiral CT scan is most helpful for determining the point of obstruction and assessing for the presence of focal bowel wall thickening (colitis) or pneumatosis intestinalis (ischemia).
5. **Therapy**
   a. **Supportive therapy**
      i. A nasogastric tube should be placed to decompress the bowel proximal to the obstruction. The patient should be on nothing by mouth orders.
      ii. Intravenous fluid hydration is indicated and electrolyte abnormalities should be corrected. Bladder catheterization may be used to monitor fluid status.
   b. **Definitive therapy**
      i. Intussusception is usually diagnosed and treated with a barium or air enema.
      ii. Small bowel obstruction may be managed expectantly or with surgical intervention.
      iii. Nonstrangulatory sigmoid volvulus is managed with decompression and detorsion using a rectal tube.
      iv. Cecal volvulus usually requires surgery.
6. **Disposition.** The patient should be admitted.
C. **Diverticular disease**
   1. **Discussion.** Diverticula are herniations of the colonic mucosa through the muscularis propria. They may be located throughout the colon although they are most frequently found in the sigmoid colon.
      a. **Incidence.** The incidence of diverticula is 30% in patients older than 50 years and increases to 50% in patients 70 years and older.

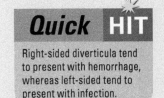

Quick HIT

Right-sided diverticula tend to present with hemorrhage, whereas left-sided tend to present with infection.

b. **Etiology and pathogenesis.** Diverticula are thought to be caused by a low-fiber diet, which leads to less stool mass and constipation. The diminished stool mass causes higher intracolonic pressures, which results in muscular hypertrophy as the colon attempts to move the stool along. Ultimately, the elevated intraluminal pressure promotes herniation of the mucosa.

  i. **Pain** is thought to result from the increased muscular contractions made necessary by the increased intraluminal pressure as well as from increased gas formation from stagnant bacteria.

  ii. **Diverticulitis** is an inflammatory condition resulting from microperforation of the diverticulum, which is often caused by feces lodging in the diverticulum.

  iii. **Bleeding.** Diverticula form near the perforating vessels of the colon. Bleeding results when the vessel ruptures into the diverticulum. Seventy percent of bleeding diverticula are found in the right colon.

2. **Clinical features.** Diverticula are most often asymptomatic, but 20% to 30% of patients eventually manifest some symptoms.

  a. **Diverticular pain.** The pain is a **dull, crampy left lower quadrant pain** that is **often relieved by the passage of stool or flatus**. A firm and tender cord, representing the hypertrophied sigmoid colon, may be palpable.

  b. **Diverticulitis**

    i. **Symptoms** include **left lower quadrant pain that is worse with bowel movements** and may radiate to the back, **fever**, and, possibly, **dysuria** (resulting from bladder irritation).

    ii. **Physical examination findings.** A **mass** may be noted on palpation of the left lower quadrant. Rectal examination may reveal a palpable mass or tenderness.

  c. **Bleeding. Massive, painless hemorrhage** is characteristic.

3. **Differential diagnoses**

  a. **Pain and diverticulitis.** Differential diagnoses include irritable bowel syndrome, Crohn disease, ulcerative colitis, gynecologic disorders (e.g., pelvic inflammatory disease, ovarian torsion), nephrolithiasis, urinary tract infection, colon cancer, and abdominal aortic aneurysm.

  b. **Bleeding.** Differential diagnoses include arteriovenous malformation, upper gastrointestinal hemorrhage, hemorrhoids, and cancer.

4. **Evaluation**

  a. **Pain**

  b. **Diverticulitis**

    i. **Laboratory studies**

      a) **Blood work.** A CBC and C-reactive protein and erythrocyte sedimentation rate may be helpful. The WBC count is usually increased with a left shift.

      b) **Urinalysis** may show microscopic hematuria.

    ii. **Radiography.** Abdominal films may demonstrate ileus or obstruction or a nonspecific bowel gas pattern. A chest radiograph may show free air in the event of a perforation.

    iii. **Other studies.** A **barium enema** or abdominal **CT scan** may be needed when the diagnosis is not clear.

  c. **Bleeding diverticula**

    i. **Nasogastric lavage** may be performed to rule out an upper gastrointestinal source of hemorrhage.

    ii. **Anoscopy** or **sigmoidoscopy** can be used to rule out a hemorrhoidal source of bleeding which also presents as painless hematochezia but with less blood volume.

    iii. **Other studies.** If the bleeding continues, the patient may require a tagged RBC study or colonoscopy to verify the source or angiography with embolization to stop the bleeding. Endoscopy is usually performed electively as an outpatient to confirm the diagnosis and exclude possible colitis or malignancy.

5. Therapy
   a. **Uncomplicated diverticular disease.** A high-fiber diet increases stool bulk, which decreases the intraluminal pressure and relieves the symptoms. An antispasmodic agent (e.g., dicyclomine) may also be helpful.
   b. **Diverticulitis.** Supportive measures include bowel rest and intravenous hydration. Antibiotic therapy (e.g., fluoroquinolones, sulfamethoxazole/trimethoprim, and/or metronidazole) is indicated. Surgery may be necessary if the patient develops perforation, obstruction, or abscess.
   c. **Bleeding diverticula**
      i. **Fluid resuscitation.** Two large-bore intravenous lines should be placed, along with a Foley catheter to monitor the resuscitation effort.
      ii. **Blood products** should be administered to maintain a hemoglobin level of 7 to 8 gm/dL.
      iii. **Octreotide,** 50 μg/hr, may reduce bleeding.
      iv. **Coagulopathy** in the 10% with persistent bleeding should be sought after and corrected.
      v. **Angiography** or urgent colectomy may be required in the 1% of patients that fail to respond to more conservative measures.
6. Disposition
   a. **Uncomplicated diverticula.** The patient should be carefully instructed to return if there is a worsening of the pain or the onset of fever. Follow-up colonoscopy is suggested to verify diagnosis and rule out cancer or colitis.
   b. **Diverticulitis**
      i. **Patients with mild disease** can be treated with oral antibiotics (trimethoprim–sulfamethoxazole and metronidazole or fluoroquinolones plus metronidazole) on an outpatient basis.
      ii. **Patients with more severe disease** should be admitted for intravenous antibiotic administration.
      iii. **Patients with suspected perforation**, **obstruction**, or **abscess** require immediate surgical consultation.
   c. **Bleeding diverticula**
      i. **Patients with significant blood loss** or **continuing hemorrhage** should be admitted to the intensive care unit.
      ii. **Patients with stable vital signs** and **no evidence of continuing bleeding** can be admitted to a general medicine unit.

VII. ANORECTAL DISORDERS
A. Hemorrhoids
   1. Discussion
      a. **Definition.** Hemorrhoids are dilatations of the veins of either the internal or external hemorrhoidal plexus. Internal hemorrhoids are found above the dentate line. There are four classifications of internal hemorrhoids (see Clinical Pearl 4-5).
      b. **Incidence.** Sixty to seventy percent of the population will experience a hemorrhoid at some time.
      c. **Etiology.** Contributing factors are thought to be constipation, diarrhea, straining at stools, prolonged sitting, pregnancy, and childbirth.
   2. Clinical features
      a. **History and symptoms.** Patients may report itching, pain, and blood on the toilet paper or in the toilet bowl.

CLINICAL PEARL 4-5

Classification of Internal Hemorrhoids
1. **First-degree:** simple internal hemorrhoids
2. **Second-degree:** prolapsed internal hemorrhoids that reduce themselves spontaneously
3. **Third-degree:** prolapsed internal hemorrhoids that must be reduced manually
4. **Fourth-degree:** prolapsed internal hemorrhoids that cannot be reduced

      i. Internal hemorrhoids present with painless rectal bleeding. They are painless because they originate above the dentate line.

      ii. External hemorrhoids present with rectal bleeding that becomes very painful if the vein becomes thrombosed.

  b. **Physical examination findings.** External and prolapsed internal hemorrhoids are visible on examination. Nonprolapsed internal hemorrhoids may be palpated as a hard mass on rectal examination if they are thrombosed or softer "cushions" when not. They may also be normal appearing when veins are decompressed.

3. **Differential diagnoses** include other causes of rectal bleeding, such as diverticular disease, arteriovenous malformations, cancer, and anal fissures.

4. **Evaluation.** Internal hemorrhoids are visualized using anoscopy or flexible endoscopy.

5. **Therapy**

  a. Conservative measures include a high-fiber diet, adequate fluid intake, stool softeners, sitz baths, topical analgesia (via an ointment or suppository), and application of hydrocortisone cream (either topically or via a suppository) to relieve itching. There may be systemic side effects from rectal steroids used for prolonged periods. Astringents such as Epsom salts or witch hazel relieve edema and reduce inflammation.

  b. An external thrombosed hemorrhoid may be resected in the ED. The packing may be removed by the patient while in a sitz bath or follow-up with a colorectal surgeon.

6. **Disposition**

  a. **External hemorrhoids** usually resolve in 1 to 3 weeks with conservative therapy. Incision and clot removal provides instantaneous relief.

  b. **Internal hemorrhoids.** Patients should be referred to a colorectal surgeon if symptoms persist.

B. **Anal fissures**

1. **Discussion.** Anal fissures, the most common cause of anal pain, are linear tears distal to the dentate line. Ninety percent occur in the posterior midline and most of the remaining ten percent are found in the anterior midline. Any other location should raise the suspicion of Crohn disease or ulcerative colitis.

2. **Clinical features** include burning or stinging pain associated with defecation and minimal rectal bleeding. The tears may be visible on examination of the anus. The patient, however, may resist the exam due to pain. High anal sphincter spasm is always a component of anal fissure disease.

3. **Therapy** involves a high-fiber diet and showers or sitz baths after bowel movements. Medical treatment of choice include nitropaste 0.125% to 0.250% compounded with petroleum jelly to reduce spasm. Botulinum toxin injection cures 90%. Patients with a chronic fissure or with a fissure in an unusual location (i.e., not the midline) should be referred to a gastroenterologist or colorectal surgeon.

C. **Anorectal abscesses**

1. **Discussion**

  a. A **perianal abscess** is a tender, red, fluctuant mass located near the anus. There is no usually induration or palpable mass on rectal examination.

  b. An **ischiorectal abscess** is deeper, has more lateral swelling, and may demonstrate induration on rectal examination.

  c. **Intersphincteric, intermuscular, and supralevator abscesses (deep abscesses)** are swollen and tender on rectal examination. Deep abscesses are usually associated with fever, chills, and the sense of rectal fullness or heaviness.

2. **Clinical features.** The pain tends to be steady, throbbing, and worse with bowel movements.

3. **Evaluation.** Patients with systemic signs and symptoms should have a WBC count and blood cultures sent.

4. **Therapy**

  a. **Perianal and ischiorectal abscesses** in patients with no evidence of deep abscess can be drained in the ED. The abscess is incised and packed with gauze, which should be removed or changed in 48 hours. Follow-up care

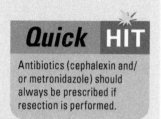

Gastrointestinal Emergencies

involves sitz baths and antibiotics (if the patient is immunocompromised or has systemic symptoms, or if evidence of cellulitis is present).

    b. **Deep abscesses.** Consultation with a surgeon is necessary.

D. **Anorectal fistulae** are abnormal tracts from the anal canal. Clinical manifestations may include a bloody or foul-smelling discharge, recurrent inflammation, or recurrent abscesses. Anorectal fistulae most often result from the external drainage of an anorectal abscess but may also result from diverticulitis, appendicitis, or inflammatory bowel disease. Patients should be referred to a surgeon for treatment.

VIII. HEPATITIS, PANCREATITIS, CHOLECYSTITIS, AND APPENDICITIS

A. **Hepatitis**

  1. **Discussion.** Hepatitis is most often caused by viruses, but it can also be caused by many medications, toxins, and other infectious agents.

    a. **Hepatitis A virus** is an RNA virus that is transmitted by the fecal–oral route. The incubation period is 2 to 6 weeks. The infection is self-limited and remains anicteric in 50% of patients. There is no chronic form or carrier state.

    b. **Hepatitis B virus (HBV)** is a DNA virus that is spread parenterally (i.e., via blood transfusion, intravenous drug abuse) or sexually. The incubation period is 1 to 6 months.

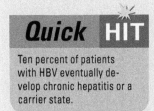

Ten percent of patients with HBV eventually develop chronic hepatitis or a carrier state.

    c. **Hepatitis C virus (HCV)** is a DNA virus that, until a screening test became available, was responsible for 90% of transfusion-related cases of hepatitis. HCV has an incubation period of 2 weeks to 6 months.

    d. **Hepatitis D virus (the delta agent)** is a defective virus that can only replicate in the presence of an acute or chronic HBV infection. Hepatitis D virus causes severe hepatitis in patients with an existing chronic HBV infection.

    e. **Hepatitis E virus** is a waterborne RNA virus that is endemic to Mexico, Asia, and Africa. It tends to cause fulminant hepatitis in pregnant women.

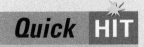

HCV tends to be milder than that caused by HBV, but 50% of patients eventually develop chronic hepatitis.

    f. **Herpes hepatitis** can present with fulminant liver failure, pneumonia, and encephalitis in immunocompromised hosts and in women in their third trimester of pregnancy. If suspected, intravenous acyclovir and consultation with an infectious disease specialist is required.

    g. **CMV Epstein-Barr virus leptospirosis** require serology and infectious disease consultation.

    h. **Third trimester pregnancy** associated with right upper quadrant pain, jaundice, elevated transaminases require admission and urgent gastroenterology consultation for definitive diagnosis. (HELLP syndrome [*h*emolysis, *e*levated *l*iver enzymes, and *l*ow *p*latelet count], acute fatty liver, biliary tract disease).

  2. **Clinical features**

    a. **Prodromal phase.** The prodromal phase occurs after the incubation period and is characterized by nonspecific symptoms such as anorexia, low-grade fever, nausea, and malaise.

    b. **Icteric phase.** Some patients then enter the icteric phase, which is characterized by jaundice, dark urine, and pale stools. The liver is usually enlarged and tender.

    c. **Extrahepatic manifestations** (e.g., urticaria, arthralgia, arthritis) may be seen in patients infected with HBV.

    d. **Fulminant hepatic failure.** Encephalopathy, coagulopathy, and jaundice are seen in a minority of patients who present in fulminant hepatic failure.

  3. **Evaluation**

    a. **Laboratory studies**

      i. **Liver enzyme studies.** ALT and AST levels are typically 10 times greater than their normal values. Elevations two or three times normal with a more significant increase in AST than in ALT suggest alcohol-induced liver damage. Significant elevation of the AP level is suggestive of biliary obstruction or gallbladder disease.

      ii. Low **serum albumin**, **glucose levels**, and prolonged **PT** are a better index of liver damage than liver enzyme studies.

Gastrointestinal Emergencies

      iii. **Ammonia level.** Patients with mental status changes should have a baseline ammonia level sent. The absolute level, however, may not correlate with mental status changes

   b. **Ultrasonography.** A right upper quadrant ultrasound should be ordered if there is suspicion of biliary obstruction, portal vein thrombosis, or underlying liver disease.

   c. **Serologic studies** are required to identify the causative agent, but these studies and results are not generally available in the ED.

   d. **Serum acetaminophen levels and a serum toxicologic screen are necessary to differentiate toxic/drug-induced hepatitis and to initiate therapy.**

4. **Therapy.** Asymptomatic patients do not require treatment.

   a. **Supportive measures**

     i. **Intravenous rehydration** is indicated for dehydrated patients.

     ii. **Antiemetics** may be given for vomiting. Ondansetron is the agent of choice.

     iii. **Vitamin K** should be given if the PT is elevated. Fresh frozen plasma should be reserved for patients with active bleeding

   b. **Prophylaxis** should be considered for household and sexual contacts.

     i. **Hepatitis A.** Immune globulin is administered intramuscularly within 2 weeks of exposure.

     ii. **Hepatitis B.** Immune globulin should be administered and vaccination started within 1 week of exposure to HBV.

5. **Disposition**

   a. Most patients can be treated as outpatients. Patients should be given a prescription for an antiemetic and be instructed to abstain from alcohol. Medication to attenuate alcohol withdrawal symptoms may be appropriate for some patients. Personal hygiene must be stressed to prevent spread of the infection to others. Hepatitis A and B, in particular, are very infectious, and intimate contact is discouraged.

   b. Indications for admission include intractable vomiting, dehydration, electrolyte derangement, a PT 3 seconds greater than normal, altered mental status, or encephalopathy.

   c. Patients with chronic hepatitis C can now achieve cure with sofosbuvir and simeprevir.

B. **Acute pancreatitis**

1. **Discussion**

   a. **Etiology.** Acute pancreatitis is most frequently caused by alcohol abuse in the United States with gallstones the most common cause worldwide. Alcohol abuse and cholelithiasis together account for 80% of all cases. Other causes include trauma, secondary to infection, medication induced, hyperparathyroidism/hypercalcemia, hyperlipidemia, or hereditary or congenital anomalies.

   b. **Pathogenesis.** Inflammation of the pancreas is thought to result from the inappropriate intrapancreatic activation of pancreatic proteolytic enzymes. Activation of these enzymes leads to coagulation necrosis of the pancreas and can progress to retroperitoneal hemorrhage, abscess formation, or organize into pseudocysts.

2. **Clinical features**

   a. **Symptoms** include nausea, vomiting, and epigastric pain that often radiates to the back and may be relieved by leaning forward.

   b. **Physical examination findings** include:

     i. **Epigastric tenderness**, which may or may not be associated with rebound tenderness and involuntary guarding, depending on the severity of the inflammation.

     ii. **Diminished bowel sounds**

     iii. **Fever** most often due to inflammatory cytokines with infection occurring as a late event (2 to 3 weeks)

     iv. **Jaundice** may be prominent in the case of a common bile duct stone or cysts that trap the bile duct.

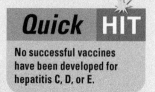

Quick HIT

No successful vaccines have been developed for hepatitis C, D, or E.

v. **Grey-Turner sign** (flank ecchymosis) or **Cullen sign** (periumbilical ecchymosis), if retroperitoneal hemorrhage has occurred.

3. **Differential diagnoses** include cholelithiasis, ascending cholangitis, peptic ulcer disease, abdominal aortic aneurysm, and MI.

4. **Evaluation**
   a. **Laboratory studies**
      i. **Serum amylase** rises first and is almost always elevated in acute pancreatitis but may not be elevated in patients with preexistent chronic pancreatitis.
      ii. **Serum lipase.** Rises later than amylase and may be persistently elevated, particularly if a pseudocyst develops.
   b. **Diagnostic imaging studies**
      i. **Radiography**
         a) **Abdominal plain films** may demonstrate:
            1) **Calcification** of the pancreas in patients with chronic pancreatitis
            2) **Blurring** of the psoas shadow
            3) The **"cutoff" sign** (i.e., abrupt ending of the transverse colon gas shadow at the pancreas)
            4) The **"inverted three" sign** (i.e., localized ileus of the duodenum and jejunum)
         b) **Chest radiograph.** A left pleural effusion may be seen.
      ii. **Ultrasonography** may show pancreatic edema, a pseudocyst, or an abscess. It can also be used to rule in suspected biliary pathology or an aortic aneurysm. Ultrasound is very sensitive for detecting gallstones, biliary ductal dilatation, and gallbladder wall edema. It may miss common duct stones, however, in more than half of patients. In addition, ileus may prevent adequate visualization.
      iii. **CT** is the study of choice for imaging the pancreas and detecting complications such as pseudocysts (Figure 4-1).
   c. **Ranson criteria** are prognostic indicators. Patients who fulfill less than three criteria have less than a 1% risk of mortality; the mortality rate increases

> **Quick HIT**
>
> Neither amylase or lipase are pancreas specific. Isoenzymes may be ordered to identify the organ of origin. However, the appropriate pain history with lipase two or three times elevated is usually diagnostic for pancreatitis.

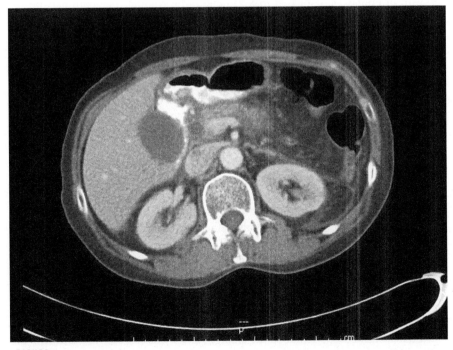

FIGURE 4-1 CT abdomen with IV contrast showing acute pancreatitis with fat stranding with intropentomeal fluid.

Gastrointestinal Emergencies

with more than three criteria. Ranson criteria are most often used for clinical trials and are not as helpful as Apache criteria or organ failure criteria, particularly at admission.

   d. **Apache II or III** criteria have higher predictive value than Ranson.
   e. **Multisystem organ failure** by identifying number or organs and degree of failure can predict mortality.

5. **Therapy**
   a. **Nasogastric suction** may help decompress if the patient has an ileus but is otherwise not useful.
   b. **Intravenous fluid hydration** should be initiated immediately.
   c. **Analgesics** may be necessary. All opioids may cause contraction of the sphincter of Oddi; however, fentanyl or hydromorphone are preferred over morphine.
   d. **Antibiotics** are no longer empirically given and may be associated with increased risk of *C. difficile* infection or resistance.

6. **Disposition**
   a. Patients with very mild pancreatitis and no evidence of biliary disease can be discharged if they are able to tolerate oral liquids. Outpatient therapy entails oral analgesics, effective hydration, and a diet high in carbohydrates and lower in long-chain triglycerides. Protein and healthy fats (olive oil, fish oil) need not be restricted.
   b. Patients with hemodynamic instability, evidence of hemorrhagic pancreatitis, or any evidence of organ failure (e.g., creatinine >2 mg/dL) warrant an intensive care unit admission. Surgical and gastroenterology consultation should be obtained for patients with severe pancreatitis.

C. **Cholecystitis**
1. **Discussion.** Cholecystitis is inflammation of the gallbladder that results from the impaction of a gallstone in the cystic duct.
   a. **Incidence.** Gallstones are present in 15% to 20% of the population, but in the majority of cases, they remain asymptomatic.
   b. **Risk factors** for gallstones include age, female sex, pregnancy, obesity, oral contraceptive use, family history of gallstones, diabetes mellitus, Crohn disease, rapid weight loss, Asian race, and sickle cell anemia.

2. **Clinical features**
   a. **Symptoms.** Patients complain of a **constant, cramping right upper quadrant** or **epigastric pain** that may radiate to the scapula. The pain may be postprandial, particularly after consuming a high-fat meal. The pain may be accompanied by **nausea** and **vomiting**.
   b. **Physical examination**
      i. **Right upper quadrant tenderness** with or without rebound tenderness is present.
      ii. **Murphy sign**, an abrupt halt in inspiration when the examiner palpates the right upper quadrant, may be present.
      iii. The **gallbladder may be palpable**.
      iv. **Fever** may be present.
      v. **Jaundice** suggests a common duct stone but may be present even if there is no stone in the common duct.

3. **Differential diagnoses**
   a. **Cardiac causes.** MI or angina must always be considered.
   b. **Biliary colic** is severe colicky "labor-like" pain that usually lasts several hours. There is no fever, and the WBC count, liver chemistries, and bilirubin levels are often normal.
   c. **Ascending cholangitis** is a bacterial infection of the biliary system that results from the impaction of a gallstone in the common bile duct. It is characterized by **Charcot triad** (right upper quadrant pain, fever and chills, and jaundice). Severe cases are characterized by the **pentad of Reynold**, which is Charcot triad plus mental status changes and hypotension. AST and ALT are usually two or three times normal. A persistent total bilirubin greater than 3 mg/dL indicates a high likelihood of retained common bile duct stones.

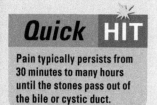

Quick HIT

Pain typically persists from 30 minutes to many hours until the stones pass out of the bile or cystic duct.

Gastrointestinal Emergencies

    d. **Hepatitis.** AST and ALT elevations are usually greater in hepatitis reflecting hepatocellular necrosis versus cholecystitis which presents with normal to mild AST and ALT levels often associated with elevated AP related to cystic duct obstruction.

    e. **Pancreatitis** is discussed in VIII.B.

    f. **Peptic ulcer disease** is discussed in IV.

    g. **Mesenteric ischemia** is discussed in X.A.

4. **Evaluation**

    a. **Laboratory studies**

        i. **CBC.** The WBC count is elevated with a leftward shift.

        ii. **Liver enzyme studies.** AST and ALT are usually mildly elevated. The AP level is mildly elevated; a significant elevation suggests a common bile duct stone.

        iii. **Bilirubin.** The bilirubin level is usually only slightly elevated or normal unless a common bile duct stone is present. The direct (conjugated) fraction is higher than the indirect (unconjugated) fraction.

    b. **Diagnostic imaging studies**

        i. **Radiography.** Plain films are useful to rule out other diagnoses such as bowel obstruction or perforation. Approximately 15% of gallstones are radiopaque.

        ii. **Ultrasonography** can detect gallstones, thickening of the gallbladder wall, or pericholecystic fluid, all of which suggest the diagnosis. Emergency bedside ultrasound is usually limited to evaluation for the presence or absence of cholelithiasis.

        iii. A **hepatobiliary radionuclide scan** should be performed if the ultrasound examination is equivocal. Nonvisualization of the gallbladder is consistent with cholecystitis, but false positives can occur.

5. **Therapy**

    a. **Cholecystitis** is treated with bowel rest and intravenous hydration. Surgical consultation is advisable for timing of definitive therapy. Antibiotics are not routinely indicated and should be used only after consulting with the surgeon.

    b. **Biliary colic** can be treated with antispasmodics (e.g., dicyclomine). The patient should be referred to a surgeon and instructed to return if he or she notices fever, persistent pain, acholic (light) stools, or darkening of the urine.

    c. **Ascending cholangitis** should be treated promptly with antibiotics that penetrate the biliary system (third-generation cephalosporins, piperacillin/tazobactam, or fluoroquinolone), with urgent endoscopic cholangiogram with drainage of infected bile. After infection resolution, stone removal and cholecystectomy may be performed.

6. **Disposition.** Patients with uncomplicated biliary colic may be discharged, but all other patients should be admitted.

D. **Appendicitis**

1. **Discussion.** Appendicitis is an acute inflammation of the appendix that is caused by the obstruction of its lumen.

    a. **Incidence.** The annual incidence is 1 in 1,000, with the peak incidence occurring between the ages of 10 and 19.

    b. **Etiology.** The most common cause of obstruction of the lumen is a fecalith. Less common causes include lymphoid hypertrophy, cancer, and parasites.

    c. **Pathogenesis.** Obstruction of the lumen leads to distention, inflammation, bacterial overgrowth, and ischemia. If left untreated, the ischemia will progress to gangrene and, ultimately, perforation.

2. **Clinical features**

    a. **Symptoms.** The presentation tends to be atypical in pediatric and geriatric patients; therefore, higher morbidity and mortality rates due to delayed diagnosis are seen in these populations.

        i. **Pain.** Typically, the pain begins epigastric or periumbilical and then localizes to the right lower quadrant. In pregnant women, the pain localizes to the area of the appendix, which rises as the pregnancy progresses. The pain is typically described as crampy or gassy and may be confused with that of indigestion.

ii. **Anorexia** is present in 92% of patients.

iii. **Nausea** and **vomiting** are present in 78% of patients and invariably follow the onset of pain.

b. **Physical examination findings**

i. **Fever** is present in only 21% of patients.

ii. **Right lower quadrant tenderness** is classically located at **McBurney point**. Later in the course of the illness, the patient will have **involuntary guarding** and **rebound tenderness** in the right lower quadrant due to local peritonitis. In the event of perforation, the patient may present with an **acute surgical abdomen** (i.e., rigidity, rebound, involuntary guarding), fever, chills, and vomiting.

iii. **Rovsing sign** is right lower quadrant pain elicited by palpation in the left lower quadrant.

iv. The **psoas sign** is pain elicited by extending the patient's right hip while the patient is lying on his or her left side.

v. The **obturator sign** is pain elicited by internal rotation of the right hip while the hip and knee are held in flexion.

vi. **Right-sided tenderness** or a **mass** may be demonstrated by rectal or pelvic examination.

3. **Differential diagnoses** include mesenteric lymphadenitis, Crohn disease, gastroenteritis, cecal diverticulitis, urinary tract infection, nephrolithiasis, and gynecologic conditions (e.g., pelvic inflammatory disease, ovarian torsion, tubo-ovarian abscess, ectopic pregnancy).

4. **Evaluation**

a. **Laboratory studies**

i. **CBC.** The WBC count is usually only moderately elevated, typically in the 10,000 to 16,000/mm^3 range.

ii. **Urinalysis** may show some RBCs as a result of ureteral irritation.

b. **Diagnostic imaging studies**

i. **Radiography.** Abdominal films may demonstrate a right lower quadrant ileus, a fecalith, or loss of the psoas shadow. A barium enema can be used to demonstrate nonfilling of the appendix, but false positives do occur.

ii. **Ultrasonography** has a sensitivity of 75% to 89% and a specificity of 86% to 100% when performed by an experienced sonographer.

iii. **CT scan** is very sensitive and specific and is the standard of care in evaluating most patients with suspected appendicitis. However, concerns about radiation are prompting more centers to use ultrasound as a rule in method prior to CT.

5. **Therapy.** The patient should have nothing by mouth. Intravenous hydration should be initiated along with antibiotics that cover enteric pathogens, and the patient should be seen by a surgeon immediately.

6. **Disposition.** Patients should be admitted if the diagnosis is confirmed. If the diagnosis is unclear, the patient should be either admitted or kept in the ED for serial abdominal examinations.

IX. HERNIA

A. **Discussion**

1. **Definition.** A hernia is the protrusion of a viscus through an opening into an abnormal location. Hernias are present in approximately 5% of the population. Approximately 75% are inguinal, 10% are incisional, 5% are umbilical, and 5% are femoral. Hiatal hernia is present in at least one-third of the population and refers to the herniation of the proximal stomach above the diaphragm.

a. **Inguinal hernias**

i. **Indirect inguinal hernias** are the most common type of hernia in both men and women. They occur when the bowel travels down a patent

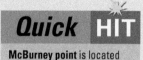

Quick HIT

McBurney point is located two-thirds of the distance along the line drawn from the umbilicus to the anterior-superior iliac spine.

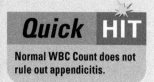

Quick HIT

Normal WBC Count does not rule out appendicitis.

processus vaginalis into the inguinal canal. The bowel may also progress into the scrotum.

  ii. **Direct inguinal hernias.** The bowel protrudes through a defect in the abdominal wall in Hesselbach triangle. The incidence increases with advancing age and physical exertion.

  b. **Incisional hernias** occur at sites of previous abdominal surgery.

  c. **Umbilical hernias** are 10 times more common in women than in men, and they are often associated with pregnancy or with ascites.

  d. **Femoral hernias.** The bowel protrudes into the femoral canal.

  2. **Complications**

  a. **Incarceration.** An incarcerated hernia is one in which the protruding abdominal contents cannot be returned to the abdominal cavity. Left untreated, an incarcerated hernia can progress and become strangulated. Thirty to forty percent of femoral hernias become incarcerated or strangulated.

  b. **Strangulation.** A strangulated hernia is one in which the tissue becomes necrotic due to obstruction of its blood supply.

B. **Clinical features**

  1. **Uncomplicated hernias**

  a. **Symptoms.** The patient may complain of a bulge or mass that grows and shrinks over time. The hernia may spontaneously reduce or be reducible by the patient.

  b. **Physical examination findings.** The patient should always be examined in both recumbent and standing positions.

  i. **Palpation.** The hernia may not be visible or palpable without provocative maneuvers (e.g., coughing or a Valsalva maneuver).

  a) **Femoral hernias** may be palpable below the inguinal ligament.

  b) **Inguinal hernias**

  1) **Direct inguinal hernias** are palpable in Hesselbach triangle superior to the inguinal ligament. In men, the examining finger should be placed in the inguinal canal by invaginating the scrotum, allowing palpation of the direct hernia at the floor of the inguinal canal.

  2) **Indirect inguinal hernias** can be palpated by moving the examining finger down the inguinal canal.

  ii. **Auscultation.** Bowel sounds may be heard in the area of the mass.

  2. **Incarceration.** An incarcerated hernia cannot be reduced with gentle pressure by either the patient or physician. Otherwise, the findings are the same as for uncomplicated hernias.

  3. **Strangulation**

  a. **Symptoms.** The patient may demonstrate symptoms of bowel obstruction (i.e., vomiting, obstipation, abdominal tenderness).

  b. **Physical examination findings.** The hernia will usually be tender to palpation. Fever is a consistent finding in patients with necrosis of the bowel.

C. **Differential diagnoses** include hydrocele, lipoma, lymphadenopathy, abscess, and tumor.

D. **Evaluation.** In patients who have a tender, irreducible mass or symptoms of strangulation, additional studies, including abdominal films, a WBC count, and amylase levels, should be performed.

E. **Therapy**

  1. **Relief of obstruction.** Patients with symptoms of strangulation or small bowel obstruction should be treated for bowel obstruction (see VI.B.5).

  2. **Reduction** is achieved through the application of continuous gentle pressure, often in conjunction with postural positioning. Pain or anxiolytic medications are often administered.

  3. **Surgery.** Patients with irreducible hernias require surgical consultation.

F. **Disposition.** Patients with reducible hernias may be discharged with instructions to avoid strenuous activities and to return to the ED if any symptoms of incarceration or strangulation develop. Surgical follow-up is mandatory. Patients with irreducible hernias or ascites associated with painful umbilical hernia require admission.

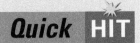

Quick HIT

Over 80% of femoral hernias occur in women, and they are thought to be related to pregnancy and physical exertion.

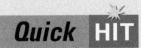

Quick HIT

Indirect inguinal hernias are more likely than direct inguinal hernias to become strangulated.

Gastrointestinal Emergencies

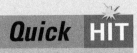

Quick HIT

The abdomen is no place for dead bowel. If necrosis or signs of acute strangulation are present, it is inappropriate to attempt to reduce the hernia.

X. VASCULAR DISORDERS

A. **Mesenteric ischemia**

1. **Discussion.** Mesenteric ischemia is inadequate oxygen delivery to some portion of the intestinal tract, which can ultimately result in necrosis and perforation. Mesenteric ischemia is associated with a mortality rate of 80%.

   a. **Etiology.** Ischemia can result from embolism, thrombosis, or low flow states. Acute ischemia is due to embolic obstruction of the superior mesenteric artery in most cases.

   b. **Risk factors** include atrial fibrillation and atherosclerosis. The mean age of occurrence is 60 to 80 years.

2. **Clinical features**

   a. **Patient history.** The patient may have a history of "**abdominal angina,**" a crampy, dull periumbilical pain commencing 15 to 30 minutes after eating and resolving over hours. The patient may have developed a fear of eating because of the pain and may have experienced weight loss. Often, the patient will have loose postprandial stools that are heme positive.

   b. **Symptoms**

      i. **Severe periumbilical pain.** Mesenteric ischemia most often presents as the acute onset of severe periumbilical pain "out of proportion" to physical findings.

      ii. Nausea, **vomiting,** and **diarrhea** may be present.

   c. **Physical examination findings.** Occult blood may be present on rectal examination, but hematochezia is not common.

3. **Differential diagnoses.** The list of differential diagnoses is long and includes essentially every other cause of abdominal pain.

4. **Evaluation**

   a. **Laboratory studies** are nonspecific.

      i. The hemoglobin may be elevated due to hemoconcentration.

      ii. The WBC count is usually elevated.

      iii. The amylase level may be mildly elevated.

      iv. Lactic acidosis may be present, but this is usually a late sign.

   b. **Diagnostic imaging findings**

      i. **Radiography.** Plain films are usually normal but may demonstrate an ileus. Gas in the portal system is a very late sign and an ominous finding.

      ii. **CT angiography** is the definitive diagnostic study. This can be followed by formal angiography.

5. **Therapy.** Acute measures include intravenous fluid resuscitation. Consultation with a surgeon is imperative.

B. **Abdominal aortic aneurysm**

1. **Discussion.** An abdominal aortic aneurysm is not a gastrointestinal emergency but may easily be misdiagnosed as a gastrointestinal problem. The mortality rate is 1% to 5% if elective repair of an abdominal aortic aneurysm is performed, but it increases to 75% after rupture occurs.

   a. **Definition.** An aneurysm is defined as dilatation of a blood vessel by 50% or more. Given an average normal aortic diameter of 2 cm, a diameter greater than or equal to 3 cm is an aneurysm.

   b. **Incidence.** Abdominal aortic aneurysms are found in 2% to 5% of the population older than 65 years.

   c. **Risk factors** include age greater than 65 years, male sex, smoking, chronic obstructive pulmonary disease, hypertension, atherosclerotic peripheral vascular disease, a family history, and collagen vascular diseases (e.g., Ehlers-Danlos syndrome, Marfan syndrome).

   d. **Complications.** The risk of rupture is directly related to the size of the aneurysm. Aneurysms 4 to 5 cm in diameter are associated with a 3% to 12% chance of rupturing in 5 years, whereas larger aneurysms are associated with a 25% to 41% chance of rupture.

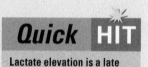

Quick HIT

Lactate elevation is a late finding in mesenteric ischemia and has varying level of sensitivity.

Gastrointestinal Emergencies

2. **Clinical features**
    a. **Symptoms** may be produced by expansion of the aneurysm or by rupture.
        i. **Pain.** Abdominal, back, or flank pain is usually the chief complaint. The pain is not affected by movement and may radiate to the testicle or leg.
        ii. **Syncope** may be the presenting symptom.
        iii. **Lower extremity claudication** or **neurologic symptoms** may be noted.
    b. **Physical examination findings**
        i. A **pulsatile abdominal mass** is usually palpable. Because the aortic bifurcation occurs at the level of the umbilicus, the mass will be palpated above the umbilicus.
        ii. An **abdominal bruit** may be audible.
        iii. **Decreased pulses** may be noted in the lower extremities. In the case of rupture, **hypotension** may be present.
3. **Differential diagnoses**
    a. **Renal colic** is the most common misdiagnosis. The patient may even have microscopic hematuria due to irritation of the ureter. Abdominal aortic aneurysm must be ruled out in any patient older than 60 years with symptoms of renal colic and no history of nephrolithiasis. Twenty-five percent of patients with an abdominal aortic aneurysm have hematuria.
    b. **Diverticulitis**
    c. **Pancreatitis**
    d. **MI**
    e. **Musculoskeletal back pain**
4. **Evaluation**
    a. **Laboratory studies.** The blood should be typed and cross-matched. Serum blood urea nitrogen and creatinine levels should be obtained. A CBC and PT should be sent. Electrocardiographic monitoring should be established.
    b. **Diagnostic imaging studies**
        i. **Radiography.** Plain abdominal films show calcification of the aorta in 60% of cases.
        ii. **Ultrasonography** is 100% sensitive in detecting an abdominal aortic aneurysm but is less helpful in assessing leaking or rupture.
        iii. **CT** is the most accurate study to assess rupture, but it takes time to perform and requires that the patient leave the ED. A CT scan is helpful to the surgeon if the patient is stable enough to tolerate the study.
5. **Therapy**
    a. **Asymptomatic patients.** An ultrasound study should be performed. If the aneurysm is less than 4 cm in diameter and has no evidence of dissection or rupture, the patient can be discharged with follow-up. Patients with larger aneurysms should be seen by a surgeon.
    b. **Symptomatic patients without hemodynamic catastrophe**
        i. Two large-bore intravenous lines should be established for the administration of crystalloid and blood products.
        ii. Hypertension should be pharmacologically managed, ideally with short-acting titratable agents.
        iii. Surgical and interventional radiology consultation should be arranged.
    c. **Unstable patients** need emergent surgery, which should not be delayed to obtain radiologic studies. The patient should be aggressively resuscitated while awaiting surgical intervention.

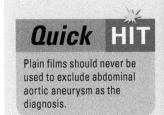

Quick HIT

Plain films should never be used to exclude abdominal aortic aneurysm as the diagnosis.

Gastrointestinal Emergencies

I. URINARY TRACT INFECTIONS (UTIs)

A. **Discussion.** UTIs are commonly evaluated in the emergency department (ED).

  1. **Causes.** Most UTIs are caused by pathogens that normally inhabit the perineum and gastrointestinal tract.

     a. *Escherichia coli* is responsible for 80% to 90% of UTIs.

     b. *Klebsiella*, *Proteus*, *Enterobacter*, and *Pseudomonas* species account for 10% to 20% of cases.

     c. Group D *Streptococcus*, *Chlamydia*, and *Staphylococcus* are responsible in fewer than 5% of cases.

  2. **Predisposing factors**

     a. **Women** are affected more often than men because the shorter female urethra facilitates bacterial access to the bladder.

        i. **Sexual intercourse** and the **use of nonoxynol-9–containing spermicides** predispose to the development of UTIs.

        ii. **Pregnancy** is associated with a high incidence of asymptomatic bacteriuria.

        iii. **Postmenopausal state**

        iv. **Immunosuppression**

     b. **Men**

        i. **Predisposing conditions** (e.g., anatomic abnormalities, tumors, calculi, prostatitis, enlarged prostate) are found in up to 80% of men with UTIs.

        ii. **Catheterization** accounts for many cases of UTIs in men.

        iii. **Uncircumcised men** (and women who have intercourse with uncircumcised men) are more prone to UTIs.

        iv. **Immunosuppression**

B. **Clinical features**

  1. **Symptoms.** Presenting symptoms may include **urinary urgency, frequency, nocturia, dysuria, a sensation of incomplete voiding**, and **suprapubic pain**. Patients with upper tract involvement may also have **fever, chills, nausea**, and **vomiting**.

  2. **Physical examination findings.** Flank pain, **mild suprapubic midline tenderness**, and **costovertebral angle tenderness** may be associated with pyelonephritis and cystitis.

C. **Differential diagnoses**

  1. **Vaginitis** resulting from *Candida albicans*, *Trichomonas vaginalis*, or *Gardnerella* infection must be considered.

  2. **Urethritis** is a particularly important consideration in men who present with urethral discharge. The most common pathogens are *Chlamydia trachomatis* and *Neisseria gonorrhoeae*.

  3. **Prostatitis** (see VI.D.)

D. **Evaluation**
1. **Urinalysis** should be performed on a midstream clean-catch specimen. Patients with certain clinical conditions (e.g., vaginal discharge, vaginal bleeding, obesity) may need to be catheterized to obtain a urine specimen.
   a. **Microscopic analysis**
      i. **Hematuria** may represent lower or upper tract involvement.
      ii. **Bacteriuria.** More than 10 to 15 organisms per high-power field on a centrifuged specimen is suggestive of UTI. Finding any bacteria on an uncentrifuged specimen correlates with a positive urine culture (see I.D.2).
      iii. **Pyuria** is defined by the presence of more than 10 white blood cells (WBCs) per high-power field.
   b. **Dipstick analysis**
      i. **Leukocyte esterase test.** The leukocyte esterase test is a reliable screen for pyuria, although false-negative results may occur with low-level pyuria.
      ii. **Detection of nitrites** is indicative of infection with a gram-negative organism.
2. **Urine cultures**
   a. **Indications.** Urine cultures are not routinely ordered on uncomplicated infections but may be indicated in some patients. Examples include immunosuppressed patients, suspected pyelonephritis, indwelling catheters, patients who fail to respond to therapy, patients requiring hospitalization, or a history of drug-resistant infections.
   b. **Interpretation.** The growth of 10^5 colonies/mL of urine is considered a positive culture.
3. **Complete blood count (CBC).** The CBC may reveal leukocytosis in patients with suspected pyelonephritis. The leukocyte count is not generally elevated or indicated in patients with only cystitis.
E. **Therapy**
1. **Cystitis.** Specific regimens are given in Table 5-1.
   a. **Uncomplicated cases.** In patients without constitutional symptoms or complicating medical conditions and a short duration of symptoms, uncomplicated cystitis can be treated with a 5-day course of nitrofurantoin, or a 3-day course of **oral trimethoprim–sulfamethoxazole.**
   b. **Complicated cases.** In patients with complicating medical conditions, a longer duration of symptoms, or a relapse of infection, 7 to 10 days of therapy is required.

TABLE **5-1**	Antibacterial Regimens for the Treatment of Lower Urinary Tract Infections		
Type of Infection	**Drug**	**Dosage**	**Dosage Frequency and Duration**
Uncomplicated cystitis	Trimethoprim–sulfamethoxazole	160/800 mg	Twice daily for 3 days
	Ciprofloxacin	500 mg	Twice daily for 3 days
	Nitrofurantoin	150 mg	Twice daily for 5 days
Complicated cystitis	Trimethoprim–sulfamethoxazole	160/800 mg	Twice daily for 7–10 days
	Ciprofloxacin	500 mg	Twice daily for 7–10 days
	Ofloxacin	300 mg	Twice daily for 7–10 days
Uncomplicated cystitis in pregnancy	Amoxicillin	250–500 mg	Three times daily for 7–10 days
	Nitrofurantoin	100 mg	Twice daily for 7–10 days
	Cefpodoxime	100 mg	Twice daily for 7–10 days

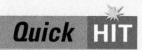

c. **Pregnant patients.** Uncomplicated cystitis and asymptomatic bacteriuria in pregnant women can be treated with **oral amoxicillin**, **nitrofurantoin**, or **cefpodoxime**.

2. Pyelonephritis
   a. **Outpatient treatment**
      i. **Parenteral antibiotics** should be given prior to discharge. **Ceftriaxone** (1–2 g) or **gentamicin** (1.0 mg/kg) **with ampicillin** (1–2 g).
      ii. **Oral antibiotics.** A 10- to 14-day course of **trimethoprim–sulfamethoxazole** (160/800 mg, twice daily by mouth) or a **fluoroquinolone** (e.g., ciprofloxacin, 500 mg twice daily) is required. **Nitrofurantoin** is not indicated for the treatment of pyelonephritis.
   b. **Inpatient management** entails the intravenous administration of the same **antibiotics noted in I.E.2.a.i, or aztreonam** (0.5–2 g two to four times daily), **imipenem** (600 mg three to four times daily), or **ciprofloxacin** (200–400 mg intravenously twice daily).

F. **Disposition**
   1. **Admission** to the hospital is indicated for the following patients:
      a. Those with clinical toxicity (e.g., fever, vomiting, ill-appearing)
      b. Those who are unable to tolerate oral medications or fluids
      c. Elderly, pregnant, or very young patients with pyelonephritis
   2. **Discharge.** Most patients are treated as outpatients. Prior to discharge, patients should be advised regarding the prevention of UTIs. Commonly accepted means of preventing UTIs include:
      a. Practicing postcoital voiding
      b. Urinating frequently and completely
      c. Increasing fluid intake
      d. Practicing local hygiene (including wiping from front to back)

II. NEPHROLITHIASIS

A. **Discussion** (see Clinical Pearl 5-1)
   1. Frequent sites of calculus obstruction
      a. **Ureteropelvic junction**
      b. **Pelvic brim.** The ureter crosses the iliac vessels and narrows to 4 mm in diameter at the pelvic brim.
      c. **Ureterovesical junction.** The most common site of obstruction
      d. **Renal pelvis.** Struvite stones commonly form large **staghorn calculi**, which are too large to enter the ureter and, instead, fill the renal pelvis.
   2. Predisposing factors
      a. **Certain clinical conditions** may predispose to stone formation (e.g., inflammatory bowel disease, immobilization, gout, hyperparathyroidism). Struvite stones are associated with **chronic infection** of the urinary tract by **urea-splitting bacteria** (e.g., *Proteus, Pseudomonas, Klebsiella*).
      b. **Dietary conditions.** Excess dietary oxalate, vitamin C abuse, or excess dietary purine can predispose the patient to the development of renal calculi.
      c. **Medications**
         i. **Acetazolamide, antacids**, and **ascorbic acid** may predispose to the development of calcium stones.
         ii. **Hydrochlorothiazide** therapy can lead to the development of uric acid stones.

CLINICAL PEARL 5-1

Types of Renal Calculi (Stones)
1. **Calcium oxalate** and **calcium phosphate** stones account for 70% to 80% of all renal calculi.
2. **Struvite (magnesium–ammonium phosphate)** stones account for 10% to 15% of all renal calculi.
3. **Uric acid** stones account for 5% to 10% of all renal calculi.
4. **Cystine** and **xanthine** stones account for a small number of renal calculi.

Urogenital Emergencies

iii. **Allopurinol** therapy has been associated with the development of xanthine stones.

B. **Clinical features**

1. **Symptoms**

   a. **Pain.** The sudden onset of **acute, severe, colicky pain** is most commonly observed. The pain is located in the **flank** or **abdominal area** and radiates to the corresponding testicle or labia. The patient is in obvious pain and is often moving around the bed trying to find comfortable position.

   b. **Nausea, vomiting**, and **diaphoresis** are commonly present.

2. **Physical examination findings**

   a. **Tachycardia, tachypnea**, and **hypertension** are commonly observed secondary to pain.

   b. **Costovertebral angle tenderness** and mild **abdominal tenderness** without peritoneal findings are often present.

   c. **Fever** should raise suspicion of infection.

C. **Differential diagnoses** include appendicitis, cholecystitis, diverticulitis, salpingitis, pelvic inflammatory disease, tubo-ovarian abscess, ovarian cyst or torsion, ectopic pregnancy, abdominal aortic aneurysm, and pyelonephritis.

D. **Evaluation**

1. **Laboratory studies**

   a. **Urinalysis. Hematuria** is usually present but not always.

   b. **CBC.** A CBC may reveal leukocytosis stemming from pain or infection.

   c. **Basic metabolic panel.** Paying close attention to creatinine

2. **Computed tomography (CT) (Figure 5-1)**

3. **Radiographs.** A kidney-ureter-bladder can be obtained in some patients instead of CT. Much less sensitive and specific than CT, however drastically less radiation exposure to patient. Generally should consider in patients with a known history of uncomplicated kidney stones.

4. **Ultrasound.** Maybe useful in pregnant patients, children, or patients with a known history of uncomplicated stones. Ultrasound is becoming more of a first line test for hydronephrosis and/or calculus due to superior safety profile for patients.

E. **Therapy**

1. **Parenteral analgesia** with **narcotics** and a **nonsteroidal anti-inflammatory drug** is often required.

2. **Antibiotic therapy.** Warranted if infection is present.

3. **Intravenous hydration** with an isotonic fluid (e.g., normal saline or lactated Ringer solution) may be beneficial.

4. **Antiemetics** such as ondansetron are often needed.

5. **Alpha blocking drugs** such as tamsulosin can be used to increase stone passage rate.

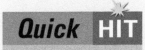

A spiral computed tomography of the abdomen and pelvis without contrast is the gold standard in diagnosis of urolithiasis.

Urogenital Emergencies

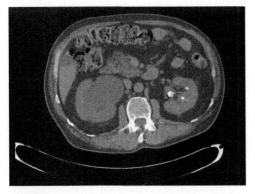

FIGURE
5-1 **Abdominal CT showing multiple non-obstructing left renal stones, one left proximal ureteral stone, and severe hydronephrosis on the right.**
(Courtesy of Chris Goshorn, MD.)

CLINICAL PEARL 5-2

1. Stone size
   a. 90% pass if less than 4 mm
   b. 50% pass if 4 to 6 mm
   c. 10% pass if greater than 6 mm
2. **Stone location.** The more proximal the stone is, the less likely it is that the stone will pass.

F. Disposition
   1. **Admission**
      a. Patients with **uncontrolled pain**, **persistent emesis**, or **concomitant infection** should be admitted to the hospital.
      b. Patients who have only **one kidney** should be admitted.
      c. Patients with **large** or **proximal stones** may require admittance to the hospital (see Clinical Pearl 5-2).
   2. **Discharge.** Patients should be discharged with a prescription for an oral analgesic and instructions to strain the urine in an effort to recover passed stones for analysis. They should be advised to follow up with a urologist or primary care physician and to return to the ED if symptoms of increased pain, vomiting, or fever occur. Studies have shown a short course of tamsulosin to be of benefit as well.

III. URINARY RETENTION

Urinary retention is the inability to void, resulting in bladder distention.
A. Obstructive
   1. **Causes**
      a. **Prostate enlargement.** Urinary retention in adult men is often due to an enlarged prostate gland.
      b. **Urethral strictures** (see VI.A.8.)
      c. **Urethral foreign bodies** (see VI.A.7)
      d. **Paraphimosis** and **phimosis** (see VI.A.1–2)
   2. **Clinical features**
      a. **Symptoms.** Urinary symptoms include **hesitancy, frequency, nocturia, urgency**, and a decrease in the amount and force of the urine stream, resulting in "**dribbling**."
      b. **Physical examination findings** include increased pain to suprapubic palpation and dullness to percussion over the distended fluid-filled bladder.
   3. **Differential diagnoses** include neurogenic causes, drug-induced retention, urinary retention secondary to pain, psychogenic causes, renal failure, abdominal aortic aneurysm, bowel obstruction, and a gravid uterus.
   4. **Evaluation**
      a. **Physical examination** readily identifies an obstructive etiology. A rectal examination should be performed to identify prostatic enlargement.
      b. **Urinary catheterization.** A postvoid residual of more than 300 mL of urine confirms the diagnosis.
      c. **Laboratory studies**
         i. **Urinalysis** should be performed to rule out infection.
         ii. **Renal** and **electrolyte panel.** Blood urea nitrogen, creatinine, and electrolyte levels should be assessed to rule out renal insufficiency.
      d. **Imaging.** Ultrasound can reveal a distended bladder. CT of abdomen and pelvis is often obtained in search of a kidney stone or other potential cause (malignancy).
   5. **Therapy**
      a. **Acute relief.** Catheterization should provide acute relief.
      b. **Definitive therapy.** The source of the obstruction should be treated.
   6. **Disposition.** Most patients with a mechanical obstruction may be discharged home with an indwelling catheter and a leg bag (and antibiotics). Follow-up with an urologist should be arranged.

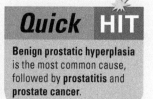

Quick HIT

Benign prostatic hyperplasia is the most common cause, followed by **prostatitis** and **prostate cancer**.

Urogenital Emergencies

B. **Neurologic**
1. **Causes.** Urinary retention may occur secondary to spinal cord trauma or compression, neuropathy (e.g., multiple sclerosis, diabetes mellitus, Guillain-Barré syndrome, tabes dorsalis), or viral infection.
2. **Clinical features**
    a. **Spinal cord injury** or **spinal shock**
        i. **Areflexia (atonic) bladder** is seen with spinal pathology at or below the second lumbar vertebra.
        ii. **Reflex (hypertonic) bladder** is seen with pathology above the second lumbar vertebra.
    b. **Spinal cord compression.** Back pain, gait disturbance, and hyperreflexia accompanying urinary retention may be indicative of spinal cord compression (e.g., by a tumor, herniated disk, or abscess).
3. **Differential diagnoses** are the same as those for obstructive retention.
4. **Evaluation.** A CT scan or magnetic resonance imaging scan should be obtained to evaluate spinal cord trauma or suspected compressive etiologies.
5. **Therapy**
    a. **Acute relief**
        i. **Atonic bladder** may be relieved with **self-catheterization** or **urecholine therapy.**
        ii. **Hypertonic bladder** may be relieved with **self-catheterization** or **flavoxate or oxybutynin therapy.**
    b. **Definitive therapy** depends on the underlying cause. Consultation with a specialist (e.g., a neurosurgeon, orthopedic surgeon, or neurologist) may be necessary.
C. **Pharmacologic**
1. **Causes** include **antihistamines**, **antidepressants**, and **α-adrenergic medications**, including over-the-counter preparations, and many illicit drugs.
2. **Differential diagnoses** include urethral obstruction, neurogenic retention, urinary retention secondary to pain, psychogenic causes, renal failure, abdominal aortic aneurysm, bowel obstruction, and a gravid uterus.
3. **Evaluation**
    a. **Patient history.** A thorough patient history, including recently prescribed medications, often suggests the etiology.
    b. **Physical examination** should rule out other causes.
4. **Therapy.** Catheterization will provide acute relief. The offending medication should be discontinued following consultation with the patient's primary care physician.

IV. RENAL FAILURE

A. **Acute renal failure**, now referred to as **acute kidney injury (AKI)**, is a sudden decline in renal function resulting in azotemia with an accumulation of nitrogenous waste products (creatinine and urea) over hours to weeks. AKI causes derangements in electrolyte, volume, and metabolic status. Patients may be either **oliguric** (i.e., producing less than 500 mL urine/day) or **nonoliguric** (i.e., producing more than 500 mL urine/day). **Anuria** is defined as the production of less than 100 mL urine/day.
1. **Causes.** There are three general mechanisms of AKI.
    a. **Prerenal causes. Hypoperfusion of the renal parenchyma**
        i. **True intravascular volume depletion** (e.g., from hemorrhage, severe dehydration, or overzealous diuresis) can lead to AKI.
        ii. **Peripheral vascular changes leading to vasodilatation** or **a decreased cardiac output** may result from cardiac failure, sepsis, or anaphylaxis, leading to AKI.
    b. **Renal (intrinsic) causes** involve direct injury to the renal parenchyma.
        i. **Tubule injury** (e.g., from acute tubular necrosis) is the most common cause of AKI in adults. Acute tubular necrosis can occur secondary to ischemia, toxins (e.g., intravenous contrast dye or aminoglycoside antibiotics), or rhabdomyolysis; fortunately, in many cases, the damage is reversible.
        ii. **Interstitial injury** (e.g., from acute interstitial nephritis) is most often caused by an adverse drug reaction and is often associated with systemic manifestations, such as fever, rash, and joint pain.

iii. **Glomerular injury** (e.g., from glomerulonephritis) is also an intrinsic cause of acute renal failure.

c. **Postrenal causes** (i.e., obstructive nephropathy) must be bilateral in order to induce renal failure (unless the patient has only one kidney). The obstruction may be intrinsic or extrinsic in origin and located anywhere along the urinary tract from the urinary meatus to the renal collecting system.

2. **Clinical features.** No specific constellation of symptoms is typical of AKI.

a. Patients may be asymptomatic or have complaints of fatigue, confusion, weakness, or shortness of breath.

b. Sometimes, patients present with complaints related to secondarily involved organ systems.

i. **Central nervous system symptoms** include **confusion, a diminished level of consciousness, and altered mental status.**

ii. **Cardiovascular symptoms** include **symptoms associated with congestive heart failure or pulmonary edema** secondary to volume overload, **hypertension,** and **arrhythmias** secondary to hyperkalemia.

iii. **Hematologic symptoms. Anemia** may be seen but is more common in chronic renal failure.

iv. **Metabolic symptoms** include **acidosis** and **uremia.**

3. **Differential diagnoses** include chronic renal failure (see IV.B.).

4. **Evaluation**

a. **Patient history and physical examination.** A thorough history and physical examination may offer insight into the cause of the acute renal failure (e.g., dehydration, drug toxicity) as well as reveal any associated sequelae (e.g., congestive heart failure, ascites, edema, altered mental status).

b. **Laboratory studies**

i. **Hematologic analysis** should include:

a) A **CBC** (anemia is more commonly associated with chronic renal failure)

b) An **electrolyte panel** (to screen for acidosis and hyperkalemia)

c) **Blood urea nitrogen** and **creatinine levels** (to assess renal function)

d) **Glucose, calcium,** and **phosphorus levels**

ii. **Urinalysis** findings are summarized in Table 5-2.

c. **Electrocardiography.** An electrocardiogram is appropriate if hyperkalemia is present.

TABLE 5-2 Urinalysis Findings in Patients with Acute Renal Failure			
	Prerenal Cause	**Renal (Intrinsic) Cause**	**Postrenal Cause**
Microscopic analysis	Unremarkable	Granular, hyaline, and cellular casts; red blood cell casts; proteinuria	Unremarkable
Urine sodium	<40 mEq/L	>40 mEq/L	Nondiagnostic
Urine specific gravity	>1.020	<1.010	<1.010
Urine osmolality	>500 mOsm/kg H_2O	<300 mOsm/kg H_2O	Nondiagnostic
Urine creatinine:serum creatinine ratio	>40:1	<20:1	<20:1
Serum urea nitrogen:serum creatinine ratio	>20:1	≈10:1	<10:1
Fractional excretion of sodium (FENa)[a]	<1%	>2%	

[a] $FENa = \dfrac{Urine\ Na/Serum\ Na}{Urine\ Cr/Serum\ Cr} \times 100$

5. Therapy
   a. **Emergent therapy.** Potentially life-threatening complications (e.g., hyperkalemia, hypertensive crisis) should be treated accordingly. **Dialysis**, performed under the supervision of a nephrologist, may be warranted for patients with severe acidosis, severe hyperkalemia, or volume overload.
   b. **Definitive therapy.** The cause of the AKI should be treated accordingly.
      i. **Prerenal causes**
         a) Intravascular volume levels should be restored by administering **isotonic fluids.**
         b) The cause of the intravascular volume depletion should be treated.
      ii. **Renal causes.** If the patient has rhabdomyolysis, aggressive **saline diuresis** with **alkalinization of the urine** to attain a pH greater than 6.5 should be instituted.
      iii. **Postrenal causes.** Elimination of the obstruction with a Foley catheter (for outlet obstruction) or with urethral stents (for urethral blockage) may be required. Consultation with an urologist may be advisable.
B. **Chronic kidney disease** is defined as a reduction of renal function (as measured by the glomerular filtration rate) over months to years to less than 20% of normal.

V. GENITAL LESIONS (TABLE 5-3)
A. **Primary syphilis**
   1. **Cause.** Syphilis is caused by *Treponema pallidum* infection.
   2. **Clinical features**
      a. **Lesion.** Chancre forms at the site of inoculation (e.g., the genitalia, anus, rectum, mouth, or perioral region). The painless papular lesion erodes to form an ulcer with a raised border, serous exudate, and a crusted surface (Figure 5-2).
      b. **Regional lymphadenopathy** may be present.
   3. **Differential diagnoses** include herpes simplex virus-type 1 infection, chancroid, lymphogranuloma venereum (LGV), traumatic ulcer, furuncle, and carcinoma.
   4. **Evaluation.** The clinical diagnosis can be confirmed by **darkfield microscopic examination** or **serologic testing** (e.g., the Venereal Disease Research Laboratory test for screening and the fluorescent treponemal antibody-absorbed test for confirmation).
   5. **Therapy.** Primary syphilis can be treated with any of the following antibiotic regimens:
      a. **Benzathine penicillin G** (one dose of 2.4 million U administered intramuscularly)
      b. **Doxycycline** (100 mg twice daily for 2 weeks administered orally)

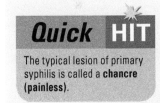

Quick **HIT**

The typical lesion of primary syphilis is called a **chancre (painless)**.

Urogenital Emergencies

TABLE 5-3	Summary of Genital Lesions		
	Lesion	**Lymphadenopathy**	**Average Incubation**
Primary syphilis	Painless ulcer (chancre)	Regional, painless	21 days (10–90 days)
Genital herpes	Painful vesicles and ulcerations	Unilateral, tender	6 days (2–20 days)
Chancroid	Painful ulcer	Buboes	4–7 days
Lymphogranuloma venereum	Painless ulcer	Suppurative, painful buboes	Primary stage: 3–12 days Secondary stage: 10–30 days
Condylomata acuminatum	Filiform, sessile, or cauliflower-like masses	None	Weeks to years
Molluscum contagiosum	Umbilicated papules	None	2–3 months

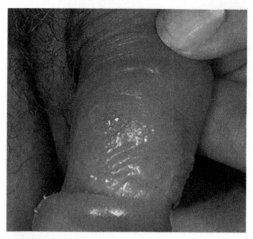

FIGURE
5-2 Chancre skin lesion.

c. Tetracycline or **erythromycin** (500 mg four times daily for 2 weeks administered orally)
d. **Ceftriaxone** (250 mg for 10 days administered intramuscularly)
6. **Disposition.** The patient should follow up with a physician in 1 month for serologic confirmation of cure.
B. **Genital herpes**
1. **Cause.** Genital herpes is caused primarily by **herpes simplex virus-type 2.**
2. **Clinical features**
a. **Lesion.** Genital herpes is characterized by **painful, recurrent, ulcerated lesions** on the genitalia, perineum, thigh, sacrum, buttocks, anus, or rectum. The lesions begin as erythematous papules that develop into groups of vesicles in a herpetiform arrangement. These vesicles become pustules, which erode to form ulcerations with a moist or crusted appearance.
b. **Lymphadenopathy.** The lesions are usually accompanied by **tender inguinal** or **femoral lymphadenopathy** that is usually **unilateral.**
3. **Differential diagnoses** include syphilis, chancroid, and gonococcal erosions.
4. **Evaluation**
a. **Tzanck smear.** A Tzanck smear is positive in 75% of cases.
b. **Viral culture** confirms the diagnosis in 1 to 10 days.
c. **Serologic evaluation** can detect the presence of antibodies to herpes simplex virus-type 1 or herpes simplex virus-type 2.
5. **Therapy.** Sexual contacts should be notified as well.
a. In most patients, **acyclovir** is administered orally to treat outbreaks and prevent recurrence.
i. Acyclovir (200 mg five times daily) is administered for 10 days to treat the first outbreak. An alternative is valacyclovir, which is more expensive but dosed three times daily.
ii. For recurrent episodes, patients begin treatment with acyclovir (400 mg three times daily for 5 days) at the beginning of the prodrome or within 2 days of the onset.
iii. Acyclovir, 400 mg twice daily, is administered to prevent recurrence of disease.
b. In patients infected with HIV, **acyclovir** or **foscarnet** may be administered intravenously to treat genital herpes.
6. **Disposition.** Patients who are being treated with acyclovir should schedule follow-up appointments with their primary care physicians. Patients should be advised to avoid sexual contact when ulcerations are present.
C. **Chancroid**
1. **Causes.** Chancroid is caused by *Haemophilus ducreyi* infection and is endemic in tropical and subtropical third world countries.

2. **Clinical features**
   a. **Lesion.** The characteristic lesion is a tender papule with an erythematous border that evolves from a pustule to an erosion and, eventually, to an ulcer with a friable base, granulation tissue, and exudate. Lesions are typically found on the genitalia, breasts, fingers, thighs, or oral mucosa.
   b. **Lymphadenopathy.** Chancroid is characterized by a **suppurative regional lymphadenopathy (bubo).**
3. **Differential diagnoses** include genital herpes, syphilis, LGV, and traumatic lesions.
4. **Evaluation.** Scrapings from the ulcer base or pus from a bubo will reveal clusters or parallel chains of Gram-negative rods. Culture of *H. ducreyi* is difficult, and no serologic tests are available.
5. **Therapy.** Appropriate antibiotic regimens include the following:
   a. **Erythromycin,** 500 mg orally four times daily for 7 days
   b. **Ceftriaxone,** one 250-mg intramuscular dose
   c. **Azithromycin,** one 1.0-g dose administered orally
   d. **Amoxicillin,** 500 mg, **plus clavulanic acid,** 125 mg, orally three times daily for 7 days
   e. **Ciprofloxacin,** 500 mg orally twice daily for 3 days
6. **Disposition.** Patients should be treated as outpatients. A follow-up appointment 1 week later with a primary care physician should be scheduled.

D. **LGV**
   1. **Cause.** LGV is caused by *C. trachomatis*, **immunotypes L^1, L^2, and L^3**, and is endemic in East and West Africa, India, South America, and the Caribbean.
   2. **Clinical features.** LGV is characterized by painless genital lesions and a suppurative, diffuse, painful lymphadenopathy.
      a. **Primary stage.** Any of the following types of lesions may be present on the genitalia or in the vagina or urethra during the primary stage: papules, shallow erosions, ulcers, or a herpetiform arrangement of lesions with a lymphangial nodule (bubonulus) that may rupture, causing deforming scars.
      b. **Secondary stage**
         i. **Inguinal syndrome.** The inguinal syndrome is characterized by **unilateral buboes** (one-third of which rupture) and the **groove sign** (i.e., the depression made by Poupart's ligament that separates inflamed femoral and inguinal nodes).
         ii. **Anogenitorectal syndrome** is characterized by proctocolitis that leads to perirectal abscesses, ischiorectal and rectovaginal fistulas, anal fistulas, and rectal strictures.
   3. **Differential diagnoses** include genital herpes, primary syphilis, and chancroid.
   4. **Evaluation**
      a. **Serologic studies.** *C. trachomatis* can be identified using a **complement-fixation test.**
      b. **Histologic identification** of *C. trachomatis* in a biopsy sample is also possible.
      c. **Culture** on tissue-culture cell lines is positive in approximately 30% of cases.
   5. **Therapy.** The following regimens are appropriate for the treatment of LGV:
      a. **Doxycycline,** 100 mg orally, twice daily for 21 days
      b. **Erythromycin** or **sulfisoxazole,** 500 mg orally, four times daily for 21 days
   6. **Disposition.** The patient should be reevaluated at the end of the antibiotic course.

E. **Condylomata acuminatum (genital warts)**
   1. **Cause.** Genital warts are sexually and nonsexually transmitted by skin-to-skin contact. The pathogen is **human papilloma virus.**
   2. **Clinical features**
      a. **Lesions** develop from papules to filiform, sessile, or cauliflower-like masses, usually located in clusters on the genitalia, perineum, urethra, anus, rectum, or perioral or perianal regions. The lesions are painless.
      b. **Lymphadenopathy.** No significant lymphadenopathy is associated with condylomata acuminatum.

3. **Differential diagnoses** include molluscum contagiosum, folliculitis, skin tags, and cancer.
4. **Evaluation.** Diagnosis is confirmed by outpatient biopsy but is suggested by whitening of the lesions when 5% acetic acid is applied for 5 minutes.
5. **Therapy.** Methods of wart removal include:
   a. Cryosurgery with **liquid nitrogen**
   b. Topical application of **podophyllin** (10% to 25%) in compound tincture of benzoin or **trichloroacetic acid** (80% to 90%)
   c. **Electrodesiccation, electrocautery,** or **laser surgery**
6. **Disposition.** The patient should be warned that the lesions are highly contagious and advised to follow up with a primary care physician for long-term treatment.

F. **Molluscum contagiosum**
1. **Causes.** Molluscum contagiosum is a sexually and nonsexually transmitted disease caused by **poxvirus.**
2. **Clinical features.** The lesions are painless, well-defined, umbilicated, pearly white papules (1 to 10 mm in diameter) on the neck, trunk, genitalia, or eyelids.
   a. HIV-positive patients are more likely to have multiple lesions.
   b. The lesions may be pruritic if they are secondarily infected.
3. **Differential diagnoses** include **keratoacanthoma** and **basal cell carcinoma.**
4. **Evaluation.** Microscopic examination of a **Giemsa-stained central core biopsy specimen** reveals "molluscum bodies." If sexual abuse is suspected, serotyping may be performed.
5. **Therapy.** Spontaneous remission occurs in the majority of cases. Curettage, topical application of liquid nitrogen, topical imiquimod, or electrocautery may be employed if spontaneous remission does not occur.
6. **Disposition.** The patient should be discharged with outpatient follow-up.

G. **Pediculosis pubis (phthiriasis, pubic lice, crabs)**
1. **Causes.** The pathogenic organism is the pubic louse, *Phthirus pubis.* Transmission is through close physical contact.
2. **Clinical features**
   a. **Lesions.** The lice appear to be brown specks, 1 to 2 mm in diameter. The eggs (nits) appear to be white specks attached to the hair. The area is pruritic.
   b. **Lymphadenopathy.** Secondary infection of excoriations may be associated with regional lymphadenopathy.
3. **Differential diagnoses** include eczema, tinea, and folliculitis.
4. **Evaluation.** Diagnosis is based on clinical assessment.
5. **Therapy**
   a. **Permethrin (1%) rinse** is applied topically.
      i. Shaving hair in the affected area may help.
      ii. Treatment of contacts is mandatory.
   b. **Antibiotics** may be indicated for infected excoriations.
6. **Disposition.** Patients should be reevaluated in 1 week if symptoms persist because retreatment may be necessary.

VI. MALE UROGENITAL PROBLEMS
A. Disorders affecting the penis
1. **Phimosis,** the inability to retract the foreskin proximally over the glans, rarely brings patients to the ED (Figure 5-3).
   a. **Cause.** Phimosis may occur secondary to chronic infection or as a consequence of poor hygiene.
   b. **Clinical features.** Patients may present with poor hygiene, painful erections, or urinary retention. If infection (balanoposthitis) is present, prepuce tenderness with associated erythema, edema, and purulent drainage may be seen.
   c. **Therapy.** Consultation with an urologist is advisable. Phimosis is usually treated surgically (e.g., by making an operative dorsal slit or circumcising the patient).

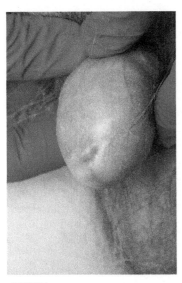

FIGURE
5-3 Phimosis.

(Courtesy of Lawrence B. Stack, MD.)

2. **Paraphimosis** results when the foreskin is retracted proximal to the coronal sulcus of the glans and cannot be reduced distally (Figure 5-4).
   a. **Clinical features.** The retracted foreskin becomes edematous leading to edema of the glans. Eventually, necrosis of the glans occurs when the venous congestion progresses to arterial compromise.
   b. **Therapy.** Applying pressure to the glans for 5 minutes may reduce the tissue edema, allowing reduction of the foreskin. If applying pressure is unsuccessful, making a dorsal slit following local infiltration with 1% lidocaine will allow for decompression of the glans and foreskin reduction.
3. **Balanoposthitis** is inflammation of the glans (balanitis) and of the foreskin (posthitis).
   a. **Cause.** If the condition is recurrent, diabetes mellitus should be considered as the cause.
   b. **Clinical features.** The foreskin and glans appear erythematous and are tender. A malodorous, purulent exudate is present.
   c. **Therapy** entails practicing local hygiene with soap and water and applying a topical antifungal cream. If bacterial infection is present, a broad-spectrum antibiotic should be prescribed.

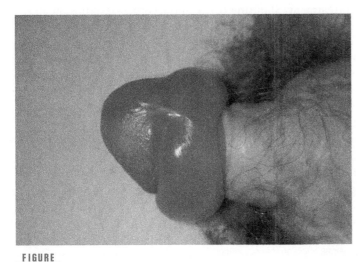

FIGURE
5-4 Paraphimosis.

(Courtesy of Lawrence B. Stack, MD.)

4. **Penile fracture** is disruption of the tunica albuginea of the penis.
   a. **Clinical features.** The patient usually describes experiencing a sudden, acute pain in the penis during sexual intercourse that is accompanied by a "cracking" sound. The penis is swollen and tender to palpation.
   b. **Evaluation.** A retrograde urethrogram should be obtained to rule out urethral injury.
   c. **Therapy.** Immediate urologic consultation should be obtained for penile hematoma evacuation and repair of the tunica albuginea.
5. **Zipper entrapment.** Local anesthesia is all that is usually required to allow the zipper to be unzipped.
6. **Urethral foreign bodies.** Patients of all ages may have various objects placed into the urethra. The placement of foreign objects in the urethra may be related to curiosity or sexual experimentation, but an abusive situation should also be considered.
   a. **Clinical features.** Patients may present with penile pain associated with dysuria and hematuria.
   b. **Evaluation**
      i. **Physical examination.** A physical examination, including a **rectal examination**, should be carried out.
      ii. **Laboratory studies.** Urinalysis and **urine culture** should be performed.
      iii. **Radiographs.** Views of the **penis** and **kidney-ureter-bladder** views should be obtained.
   c. **Therapy.** Immediate urologic referral for foreign body removal is required, followed by retrograde urethrography or endoscopy.
7. **Priapism** is a painful, prolonged penile erection (see Clinical Pearl 5-3).
   a. **Clinical features.** Patients present with a history of a painful erection that has lasted for several hours. The corpus cavernosum is firm and tender to palpation. The glans and corpus spongiosum are soft and uninvolved.
   b. **Evaluation**
      i. **Patient history.** A complete history is necessary to identify the possible etiology.
      ii. **Laboratory studies.** A CBC may be of benefit. Reticulocyte count in patients with sickle cell disease. Blood gas of penile aspirate may be used to determine the type of priapism.
   c. **Therapy.** Consultation with an urologist is necessary.
      i. **Acute therapy** entails the subcutaneous administration of **terbutaline** (0.25 to 0.5 mg) every 4 to 6 hours.
      ii. **Definitive therapy**
         a) **Identifiable causes** should be treated accordingly. For example, iatrogenic causes respond to corpus cavernosum blood aspiration followed by the intracorporeal injection of an α-adrenergic agent.
         b) **Surgical treatment. Shunting** between the corpus cavernosum and the glans or corpus spongiosum or dorsal vein may be required.
B. **Disorders affecting the testicles and epididymis**
   1. **Testicular torsion** occurs most commonly during the second decade of life.
      a. **Cause.** Testicular torsion occurs when the tunica vaginalis envelops the testis and attaches above the epididymis, rather than attaching at the posterior

CLINICAL PEARL 5-3

Causes of Priapism
1. **Medications** (e.g., trazodone, phenothiazine, Viagra [Pfizer, New York, NY], Cialis [Eli Lilly and Company, Indianapolis, IN])
2. **Spinal cord injury**
3. **Hematologic disorders** (e.g., sickle cell disease, leukemia)
4. **Iatrogenic causes** (e.g., papaverine injection for impotence)
5. **Idiopathic causes**

aspect of the testis. The anatomic defect (referred to as "bell-clapper deformity") is bilateral and allows the testicle to rotate within the tunica vaginalis.

b. **Clinical features**
   i. **Symptoms**
   ii. **Physical examination findings**
      a) The involved testicle is high-riding, may be positioned horizontally, and is markedly tender to palpation. The overlying scrotum is erythematous and edematous.
      b) Elevation of the scrotum to the symphysis does not relieve the pain (i.e., Prehn's sign is absent). The cremasteric reflex is often absent as well.

c. **Differential diagnoses** include acute epididymitis, orchitis, appendicitis, testicular or epididymal appendix torsion, hernia, tumor, and hydrocele.

d. **Evaluation**
   i. **Laboratory studies.** A **CBC** may reveal leukocytosis. Pyuria is absent on **urinalysis.**
   ii. **Doppler ultrasound** examination is rapid and should be arranged as soon as possible.

e. **Therapy.** An urologist should be consulted immediately, prior to ultrasound. **Manual** or **surgical detorsion** must occur within 4 to 6 hours; treatment should not be delayed to await ancillary test results.
   i. **Sedation and analgesia.** Often require intravenous opioids. Spermatic cord blocks, accomplished by the administration of 10 mL of 1% lidocaine high in the scrotum, may be beneficial.
   ii. **Reduction.** Initial attempts at reduction should be toward the ipsilateral thigh because the torsion usually occurs toward the midline (i.e., the patient's left testicle should be rotated clockwise and the patient's right testicle counterclockwise as the physician faces the patient).
   iii. **Bilateral orchiopexy** is necessary to prevent recurrence.

2. **Testicular** or **epididymal appendage torsion** occurs most commonly in prepubescent boys.

   a. **Clinical features.** The patient complains of the **sudden onset of pain** near the location of the appendage (e.g., at the head of the epididymis or the superior pole of the testicle). A **"blue dot" sign** is seen as the engorged, cyanotic appendage approaches the overlying scrotal skin.

   b. **Differential diagnoses** include testicular torsion, epididymitis, orchitis, and testicular trauma.

   c. **Evaluation.** Often the diagnosis is clear following physical examination. Doppler ultrasound should be obtained. If the diagnosis is still uncertain, urologic surgical exploration may be required.

   d. **Therapy.** Symptomatic relief is provided with oral analgesics. Some urologists may consider excision.

   e. **Disposition.** Following discharge from the ED, patients should see an urologist or primary care physician within 1 week.

3. **Acute epididymitis**

   a. **Causes**
      i. **Sexually transmitted epididymitis** is often associated with urethritis. The most common causative organisms include *C. trachomatis* and *N. gonorrhoeae.*
      ii. **Nonsexually transmitted epididymitis** is often associated with prostatitis or UTI. The most common causative organisms are *E. coli*, *Pseudomonas*, and *Klebsiella.*

   b. **Clinical features**
      i. **Symptoms.** Patients report the gradual onset of **scrotal pain** that becomes progressively more severe. The pain may radiate along the spermatic cord. **Urinary symptoms** are often present.
      ii. **Physical examination findings**
         a) **Epididymal swelling** and **tenderness** may prevent the examiner from distinguishing the testes from the epididymis.

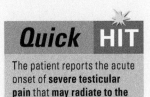

Quick **HIT**

The patient reports the acute onset of **severe testicular pain** that **may radiate to the abdomen. Nausea** and vomiting are common.

Urogenital Emergencies

   b) **Fever** and **urethral discharge** may be observed.
   c) **Prehn's sign** is present.
   c. **Differential diagnoses** include testicular tumor, testicular torsion, testicular appendix torsion, testicular trauma, and orchitis.
   d. **Evaluation**
      i. **Physical examination.** Prostate palpation (not massage) should be performed to rule out prostatitis.
      ii. **Laboratory studies**
         a) **Urinalysis** may reveal pyuria.
         b) **Urine culture** may identify the organism in cases of nonsexually transmitted infection.
         c) **Urethral swab.** A urethral swab for *C. trachomatis* and *N. gonorrhoeae* should be performed.
      iii. **Doppler ultrasound** is often obtained to differentiate epididymitis from testicular torsion.
   e. **Therapy**
      i. **Antibiotic therapy**
         a) **Sexually transmitted epididymitis** is treated with **doxycycline** (100 mg by mouth twice daily for 10 days) and **ceftriaxone** (one 250-mg dose administered intramuscularly). Treatment of sexual partners is required.
         b) Nonsexually transmitted epididymitis is treated with **trimethoprim–sulfamethoxazole** (160/800 mg), one tablet by mouth twice daily, or **ciprofloxacin** (500 mg by mouth twice daily for 10 to 14 days).
      ii. **Pain relief. Nonsteroidal anti-inflammatory drugs** or **narcotics** (e.g., acetaminophen with codeine) can be prescribed to relieve pain.
      iii. **Supportive care.** Bed rest for 2 days is advisable, and physical activity and heavy lifting should be minimized. Patients may be advised to wear an athletic supporter.
   f. **Disposition.** Outpatient therapy is usually sufficient, but admission may be required for an ill-appearing patient with severe pain and swelling, leukocytosis, and an elevated temperature.
4. **Orchitis**
   a. **Causes.** Orchitis is usually associated with a systemic infection, particularly mumps, and occurs only in postpubertal patients.
   b. **Clinical features.** Mumps orchitis occurs 3 to 4 days after the development of parotitis and is bilateral in up to 10% of cases. Physical examination reveals a tender, swollen testicle.
   c. **Differential diagnoses** include epididymitis, testicular torsion, testicular trauma, and testicular tumor.
   d. **Evaluation.** Urinalysis is usually normal. A **CBC** reveals a leukocytosis.
   e. **Therapy** entails bed rest, local application of heat, oral analgesics, and antipyretics as needed. Patients may be advised to wear an athletic supporter.
5. **Testicular masses**
   a. **Clinical features.** Only 10% of patients present with acute pain as a result of hemorrhage or infarction. Another 10% may present with complaints related to malignant disease.
   b. **Evaluation.** Any patient with a painless testicular swelling or mass must be referred to an urologist for evaluation. Misdiagnoses are not uncommon and include epididymitis, hydrocele, spermatocele, and orchitis.
C. **Disorders affecting the scrotum**
   Fournier gangrene is a rapidly spreading infection of the scrotum that progresses to gangrene. Patients with diabetes and immunocompromised patients are most often affected.
   1. **Causes.** The infection is polymicrobial; causative organisms originate from the integument, urethra, or rectum. Commonly isolated organisms include:
      a. Hemolytic streptococci and *Clostridium*
      b. *E. coli*
      c. *Bacteroides*

> **Quick HIT**
>
> Fournier gangrene is a surgical emergency.

2. **Clinical features.** Early in the course of the disease, the condition may be misdiagnosed as cellulitis or abscess.
3. **Therapy.** Patients should be admitted to the hospital. Immediate consultation with an urologist is necessary.
   a. **Broad-spectrum intravenous antibiotic coverage** should be initiated.
   b. **Wide surgical debridement** is required.
   c. **Hyperbaric oxygen** should be considered.
D. **Disorders affecting the prostate** include **acute prostatitis**, **chronic prostatitis**, **nonbacterial prostatitis** (Table 5-4), and **prostatodynia**.
   1. **Acute prostatitis**
      a. **Causes.** The most commonly infecting organisms are *E. coli* (80% of cases), *Pseudomonas*, *Klebsiella*, *Proteus*, and *Enterococcus*.
      b. **Clinical features**
         i. **Symptoms.** Patients present with an acute **febrile illness** characterized by chills, myalgias, arthralgias, and low back, perineal, or rectal pain. **Urinary frequency**, **urgency**, **nocturia**, **dysuria**, and varying degrees of **urinary retention** may exist.
         ii. **Physical examination findings.** Rectal examination reveals a prostate that is painful, swollen, firm, and warm to touch.
      c. **Differential diagnoses** include cystitis, pyelonephritis, diverticulitis, and perirectal abscess.
      d. **Evaluation**
         i. **CBC.** A CBC may reveal leukocytosis.
         ii. **Urine culture** usually identifies the offending organism.
         iii. **Prostate secretion analysis and culture.** Prostate massage should not be performed because of the risk of bacteremia.
      e. **Therapy.** Most patients with prostatitis may be managed as outpatients with appropriate antibiotic therapy and supportive measures. Patients who are febrile and present with urinary retention may require hospitalization and intravenous antibiotics.
         i. **Supportive measures** include hydration, antipyretics, analgesics, and stool softeners.
         ii. **Outpatient antibiotic therapy** must be continued for a minimum of 2 weeks.
            First-line agents. Fluoroquinolones are prescribed until culture and sensitivity testing results are known. Appropriate regimens might include oral **ciprofloxacin** (500 mg twice daily) or **ofloxacin** (200 to 300 mg twice daily).

TABLE **5-4**	Comparison of Findings in Acute, Chronic, and Nonbacterial Prostatitis		
	Acute Prostatitis	**Chronic Prostatitis**	**Nonbacterial Prostatitis**
Constitutional symptoms	Severe	Mild	Mild
Urinary symptoms	Severe	Mild	Mild
Rectal examination findings	Painful, swollen, firm, warm prostate gland	Normal or boggy prostate gland	Normal
Expressed prostate fluid analysis	Not performed	>10 WBCs per high-power field	>10 WBCs per high-power field
Expressed prostate fluid culture	Not performed	Positive	Negative
Urine culture	Positive	Positive	Negative
Complete blood count	Leukocytosis	Usually normal	Normal

WBCs, white blood cells.

iii. **Inpatient antibiotic therapy. Ciprofloxacin** (400 mg intravenously every 12 hours) or **gentamicin** (1 mg/kg every 8 hours) **plus ampicillin** (2 g every 6 hours) is continued for 1 week, followed by oral antibiotics.

2. Chronic prostatitis
   a. **Causes.** The most commonly infecting organisms are *E. coli*, *Pseudomonas*, *Proteus*, *Enterobacter*, *Staphylococcus*, and *Streptococcus*.
   b. **Clinical features**
      i. **Signs and symptoms.** Fever and chills are uncommon, except with acute exacerbations. **Urinary symptoms** of frequency, urgency, nocturia, and dysuria may be present and are associated with **low back, perineal, or suprapubic pain.**
      ii. **Physical examination findings.** Rectal examination may reveal a normal or boggy prostate gland.
   c. **Evaluation**
      i. **CBC.** Typically, the CBC is normal.
      ii. **Urine culture.** The offending organism can usually be cultured from the urine.
   d. **Therapy.** Supportive measures and antibiotic choices are similar to those for acute prostatitis, although the antibiotics must be continued for up to 12 weeks.

3. Nonbacterial prostatitis
   a. **Cause.** Nonbacterial prostatitis may be caused by *Mycoplasma*, *Chlamydia*, or *Ureaplasma*.
   b. **Clinical features.** The presenting signs and symptoms are similar to those of chronic prostatitis.
   c. **Evaluation**
      i. **Urine cultures** are negative.
      ii. **Prostate secretion analysis and culture.** Analysis reveals more than 10 WBCs per high-power field, but culture is negative.
      iii. **CBC** results are normal.
   d. **Therapy.** A clinical trial of antibiotics may be tried for a minimum of 4 weeks. Commonly used agents include **erythromycin** (500 mg by mouth four times daily) and **doxycycline** (100 mg by mouth twice daily for 14 days).

4. Prostatodynia
   a. **Cause.** The cause is unknown.
   b. **Clinical features** are similar to those of chronic noninfectious prostatitis.
   c. **Evaluation**
      i. **Urine cultures** are negative.
      ii. **Prostate secretion analysis** reveals fewer than 10 WBCs per high-power field, and cultures are negative.
   d. **Therapy.** α-Adrenergic blocking agents may provide relief.

INFECTIOUS DISEASE EMERGENCIES

Amanda Korzep • Nathan Berger

I. SEPSIS

A. **Discussion.** Sepsis should be considered a clinical syndrome. Sepsis is defined as meeting two of systemic inflammatory response syndrome criteria *plus* a source of infection (see Clinical Pearl 6-1). Over 1,665,000 cases of sepsis occur in the United States every year, with a mortality rate of up to 50% (see Clinical Pearl 6-2). Early goal-directed therapy has revolutionized sepsis management, and sepsis bundles have shown promise in improving mortality rates.

B. **Clinical features** vary considerably depending on whether the patient is in the early, intermediate, or late phase of the syndrome.

1. **General symptoms and physical examination findings**
   a. **Systemic findings** may include fever, chills, rigors, or hypothermia.
   b. **Neuromuscular findings** may include myalgias and arthralgias.
   c. **Neurologic findings** may include altered mental status.
   d. **Cardiopulmonary findings** may include tachycardia, arrhythmias, hypotension, hypertension, a widened pulse pressure, or tachypnea.
   e. **Dermatologic findings.** Dermal lesions that should increase clinical suspicion of sepsis include petechiae, embolic lesions, and ecthyma gangrenosum.

2. **Site-specific symptoms and physical examination findings**
   a. **Skin.** Findings that might be indicative of the initial focal source include erythema, a localized increase in temperature, lymphadenitis, induration, fluctuation, and pus.
   b. **Heart or lungs.** Findings may include a cough, sputum, dyspnea, chest pain, cyanosis, rales, or edema.
   c. **Urinary tract.** Findings may include urinary urgency, frequency, dysuria, tenesmus, flank pain, oliguria, or anuria.
   d. **Gastrointestinal tract.** Findings may include abdominal pain, nausea, vomiting, diarrhea, constipation, or jaundice.
   e. **Central nervous system (CNS).** Findings may include an altered sensorium, headache, stiff neck, focal neurologic signs, photophobia, retinal hemorrhages, cotton wool spots, conjunctival petechiae, endophthalmitis, or panophthalmitis.

C. **Differential diagnoses** include the following:

1. **Viral diseases** (e.g., influenza, dengue fever, coxsackie B virus infection)
2. **Spirochetal diseases** (e.g., syphilitic Jarisch-Herxheimer reaction, leptospirosis, relapsing fever caused by *Borrelia* infection)
3. **Rickettsial diseases** (e.g., Rocky Mountain spotted fever, endemic typhus)
4. **Protozoal diseases** (e.g., *Toxoplasma gondii* infection, *Trypanosoma cruzi* infection, *Pneumocystis carinii* infection, *Plasmodium falciparum* infection)
5. **Endocrine diseases** (e.g., adrenal insufficiency, thyroid storm)
6. **Nonseptic causes of shock** (e.g., cardiogenic shock, hypovolemic shock, neurogenic shock, pulmonary embolism, cardiac tamponade, anaphylaxis, dissecting aortic aneurysm)

***Quick* HIT**

In an immunosuppressed or neutropenic patient, a localized area of painful erythema may well indicate an initial focal source, even in the absence of localized warmth and swelling and irrespective of the absolute white blood cell count.

***Quick* HIT**

When the initial focus of infection is difficult to discern, one must strongly consider the probability of infection originating in the gastrointestinal tract (especially in patients on chemotherapy).

Infectious Disease Emergencies

153

CLINICAL PEARL **6-1**

Systemic Inflammatory Response Syndrome Criteria:
1. Temperature >38°C (101.4°F) or <36°C (96.8°F)
2. Heart rate >90
3. Respiratory rate >20 or PaCo2 <32 mm Hg
4. While blood cells >12,000/μL or <4,000/μL, or >10% bandemia

    7. Collagen vascular diseases
    8. Vasculitides
    9. Thrombocytic thrombocytopenic purpura/hemolytic–uremic syndrome
  D. **Evaluation.** There is no single reliable laboratory test for the diagnosis of sepsis. Although the **history** and **physical examination** form the basis of the presumptive diagnosis, the following additional testing is still considered essential.
    1. Laboratory studies
      a. **Blood cultures** and **site-specific cultures** (e.g., sputum, urine, cerebrospinal fluid [CSF]) should be obtained prior to initiating empiric antibiotic therapy.
      b. **Gram staining** of site-specific samples is indicated.
      c. **Serologic studies** (e.g., counterimmune electrophoresis, latex agglutination) are useful when infection with pneumococcus, *Haemophilus influenzae*, meningococcus, or group B streptococcus is suspected.
      d. **Complete blood count (CBC).** Findings compatible with a diagnosis of sepsis include leukocytosis, eosinopenia, anemia, leukopenia, and thrombocytopenia.
      e. **Urinalysis.** Proteinuria is a finding that supports a diagnosis of sepsis.
      f. **Urine *Legionella* antigen.** Positive result suggests current or past infection. May be detectable in the urine as early as 3 days after onset of symptoms
      g. **Urine *Streptococcus pneumoniae* antigen** is the most frequently encountered agent of community-acquired pneumonia.
      h. **Coagulation profile.** Findings that would support a diagnosis of sepsis include a prolonged prothrombin time and thrombocytopenia.
      i. **Arterial blood gas profile.** Findings in a patient with sepsis could include hypoxemia and metabolic acidosis.
      j. **Serum biochemical profile.** Supportive findings would include hypoferremia, hyper- or hypoglycemia, hypocalcemia, hyperbilirubinemia, and azotemia.
      k. **Lactic acid.** Mainly produced in the muscle and red blood cells under anaerobic conditions. Elevated levels (>1 mmol/L) can be a manifestation of organ hypoperfusion in the presence or absence of hypotension and is an important component of initial sepsis work-up. Note that elevated levels occur not only in sepsis, but in heart, liver, and pulmonary disease.
      l. **Procalcitonin** may be helpful to evaluate a seriously ill patient for systemic bacterial infection. This test is best used during the first day of presentation of illness and subsequently to monitor the response to treatment.

CLINICAL PEARL **6-2**

Factors Predisposing to Sepsis
a. **Extremes of age**
b. **Iatrogenic procedures** (e.g., indwelling catheters, surgical or invasive diagnostic procedures)
c. **Medical conditions** (e.g., cirrhosis, burns, multiple trauma, diabetes mellitus, cancer, complicated pregnancy or delivery)
d. **Social factors** (e.g., alcoholism, substance abuse, intravenous drug abuse)
e. **Immunosuppression** (e.g., neutropenia, complement deficiencies, hypo- or agammaglobulinemia, splenectomy, HIV infection)
f. **Malnutrition**

2. **Imaging studies.** Site-specific **radiographs**, **ultrasonograms**, **computed tomography (CT) scans**, or **magnetic resonance imaging scans** may be appropriate.
3. **Other studies.** Evaluation of site-specific samples obtained by **biopsy** or **aspiration** may be helpful.

E. **Therapy**
1. **Supportive measures**
   a. **Mechanical ventilation** is necessary for patients with respiratory insufficiency.
   b. **Volume replacement.** Serial 500 mL boluses of normal saline are indicated as initial therapy for sepsis or septic shock. Exercise caution and intubate early with coexisting heart failure.
   c. **Pressor agents** may also be required for patients who remain hypotensive despite adequate fluid resuscitation or develop cardiogenic pulmonary edema.
      i. **Norepinephrine** is the preferred vasopressor for the treatment of septic shock. Acting both on both alpha-1 and beta-1 adrenergic receptors, norepinephrine produces potent vasoconstriction as well as a modest increase in cardiac output.
      ii. **Phenylephrine (Neo-Synephrine, Bayer, Leverkusen, Germany)** has purely alpha-adrenergic agonist activity and therefore results in vasoconstriction with minimal cardiac inotropy or chronotropy. Useful for patients with severe hypotension such as hyperdynamic sepsis, neurologic disorders, or anesthesia-induced hypotension, or reserved for patients in whom norepinephrine is contraindicated due to arrhythmias or who have failed other therapies.
      iii. **Epinephrine** is most often used for the treatment of anaphylaxis, as a second-line agent after norepinephrine in septic shock.
      iv. **Dopamine** is most often used as a second-line alternative to norepinephrine in patients with absolute or relative bradycardia and a low risk of tachyarrhythmias.
   d. **Transfusion**
      i. **Pack red blood cell transfusion** is indicated if the patient has hemoglobin below 10 mg/dL or signs of hypoperfusion.
      ii. **Fresh frozen plasma transfusion** is necessary for patients with depleted levels of coagulation factors.
      iii. **Platelet transfusions** may be indicated when the patient has thrombocytopenia.
      iv. **Cryoprecipitate transfusions** are indicated for patients with hypofibrinogenemia.
   e. **Correction of metabolic abnormalities.** Acidemia, hypoxia, hyper- or hypoglycemia, electrolyte imbalances, and nutritional deficiencies must be corrected.
   f. **Supportive pharmacologic therapy**
      i. **Corticosteroids** (hydrocortisone) may be indicated in the presence of shock with poor response to fluids and vasopressors. Dexamethasone should be considered before antibiotic administration for patients with pneumococcal meningitis.
      ii. **Drotrecogin alpha (Xigris, Eli Lilly and Company, Indianapolis, IN):** Activated protein C is no longer used even in patients with severe sepsis.

2. **Specific measures**
   a. **Source control.** Focal causes of infection such as abscess or osteomyelitis must be treated locally.
   b. **Antibiotic therapy.** All patients with septic shock should receive empiric antibiotic therapy as soon as possible. Once the source of the infection has been identified, the spectrum of antibiotic coverage may be narrowed. Two to three antibiotics should be given in cases of sepsis, with goal of administration in less than 60 minutes from arrival.
      i. **Selecting empiric antibiotics.** Knowledge of preexisting immune dysfunction can be useful for targeting antibiotics for initial empiric

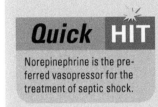

Quick HIT

Norepinephrine is the preferred vasopressor for the treatment of septic shock.

Infectious Disease Emergencies

TABLE 6-1 Organisms Commonly Associated with Infections in Patients with Immune Dysfunction		
Immune Dysfunction	**Potential Causes**	**Commonly Associated Microbes**
Granulocytopenia	Myelosuppressive therapy, irradiation	Gram-negative bacilli (e.g., *Pseudomonas aeruginosa*, staphylococci)
Cellular immune dysfunction	Congenital defects, Hodgkin disease, AIDS, antineoplastic therapy (e.g., for lymphoma), immunosuppressive therapy (e.g., to prevent transplant rejection)	*Mycobacterium*, fungi, *Listeria*, *Pneumocystis carinii*, herpesviruses
Humoral immune dysfunction	Splenectomy, untreated multiple myeloma	*Streptococcus pneumoniae*, *Haemophilus influenzae*

therapy (Table 6-1). Empiric therapy should be effective against gram-positive and gram-negative bacteria, and given intravenously in the maximum doses allowed.

ii. **Specific drug combinations** are summarized in Table 6-2.

F. **Disposition.** Clinically unstable patients must be treated in the intensive care unit (ICU). Chemistries and CBC should be monitored closely in all patients. **Serial lactate or serial mixed venous oxygen saturation** are used to follow response to therapy.

G. **Prevention**

1. **Gammaglobulin** should be administered to hypo- or agammaglobulinemic patients.

2. **Pneumococcal vaccination** and **vaccination against *H. influenzae*** are indicated for geriatric patients and patients with certain chronic diseases. Further reading is encouraged (Surviving Sepsis Campaign) at www.survivingsepsis.org.

II. AIDS

A. **Discussion**

1. **Etiology.** AIDS is caused by HIV, a cytopathic retrovirus. Transmission of HIV can occur via semen, vaginal secretions, blood or blood products, or transplacental transmission in utero. HIV has been isolated from saliva, urine, CSF, brain tissue, tears, breast milk, alveolar fluid, synovial fluid, and amniotic fluid. Transmission has not been documented via casual contact (see Clinical Pearl 6-3).

B. **Clinical features.** Because of the complexity of HIV infection, the role of emergency department (ED) personnel is to diagnose and treat those complications that arise in HIV infection that may lead to acute morbidity and mortality.

1. **Symptomatic HIV infection.** Fever, malaise, weight loss, and night sweats in the absence of any opportunistic disease in a previously asymptomatic HIV-positive patient mark the transition toward symptomatic disease. Once these symptoms appear, systemic infection and malignancy must be ruled out.

2. **Cutaneous manifestations.** Skin disorders secondary to HIV are commonly encountered in the ED.

   a. **Kaposi sarcoma** is one of the most common manifestations of AIDS, second only to *P. carinii* pneumonia (PCP) (Figure 6-1).

   b. **Xerosis (dry skin)** and **pruritus** are common.

   c. **Bullous impetigo**, **ecthyma**, or **folliculitis** may be seen with *Staphylococcus aureus* infection.

   d. **Ulcerations** and **macerations** may be seen with *Pseudomonas aeruginosa* infection.

   e. **Herpes simplex**, **herpes zoster**, **syphilis**, and **scabies** are all commonly seen.

TABLE 6-2	Drug Regimens Used in the Empiric Treatment of Sepsis
Patient Profile	**Regimen**
Adult without an obvious source of infection	Basic regimen: Third-generation cephalosporin *or* an antipseudomonal β-lactamase–susceptible penicillin + an antipseudomonal aminoglycoside *or* imipenem
Adult with a high probability of having a gram-positive infection (e.g., intravenous drug abuser, patient with toxic shock syndrome, patient with infection secondary to an indwelling vascular catheter)	Basic regimen + nafcillin or vancomycin[a]
Adult with a high probability of having an anaerobic infection (e.g., intra-abdominal or biliary tract infection, female genital tract infection, necrotizing cellulitis, aspiration pneumonia, dental infection, soft tissue infection)	Basic regimen + metronidazole or clindamycin
Adult suspected of having a *Legionella* infection	Basic regimen + levofloxacin or azithromycin
Neonate	Ampicillin or ticarcillin with clavulanic acid + an aminoglycoside[a]
Infant (1 to 3 months)	Ceftriaxone or cefotaxime
Child older than 3 months	Ceftriaxone *or* cefotaxime
Nonneutropenic patient with a nosocomial infection	Third-generation cephalosporin + metronidazole *or* ticarcillin, ampicillin, or piperacillin with the corresponding β-lactamase inhibitor + an aminoglycoside[a] *or* imipenem ± an aminoglycoside[a]
Neutropenic patient with a nosocomial infection	Third-generation cephalosporin + metronidazole + an aminoglycoside[a] *or* ticarcillin, ampicillin, or piperacillin with the corresponding β-lactamase inhibitor + an aminoglycoside[a] *or* imipenem + an aminoglycoside[a]
Patient with thermal injuries to >20% of the body surface area	Ceftriaxone + an aminoglycoside[a] *or* an antipseudomonal penicillin + an aminoglycoside + vancomycin[a]
Pregnant woman	β-Lactam or erythromycin; gentamicin is also considered appropriate under these circumstances[b]

[a]Peak and trough levels for aminoglycosides and vancomycin must be monitored.
[b]Amikacin should be used when gentamicin resistance is known or suspected.

CLINICAL PEARL 6-3

HIV infection progresses through four stages.
a. **Acute illness associated with seroconversion.** Within a few weeks of HIV infection, patients may present with malaise, fever, rash, arthralgias, lymphadenopathy, and weight loss secondary to the acute, initial, primary infection. This phase is self-limited.
b. **Asymptomatic stage.** An asymptomatic period that may last 10 years or more follows. During this phase, the patient's CD4 count is normal (greater than 800/mm^3), and he or she is fully immunocompetent. The virus is actively replicating, but the host's immune response is still capable of keeping the virus in check.
c. **Early symptomatic AIDS.** Eventually, however, the pendulum swings in favor of the virus, and the CD4 count gradually declines as the infection wins over the host's defenses. When the CD4 count falls to around 500/mm^3, the patient becomes more susceptible to opportunistic infections.
d. **Late symptomatic AIDS.** As the CD4 count falls below 100/mm^3, the immune system is severely compromised and all types of life-threatening opportunistic infections (e.g., toxoplasmosis, coccidioidomycosis, cytomegalovirus [CMV] infection, *Mycobacterium avium-intracellulare* infection) and neoplasms (e.g., Hodgkin disease, non-Hodgkin lymphoma) are likely to occur.

Infectious Disease Emergencies

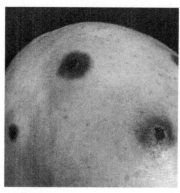

FIGURE 6-1 Kaposi sarcoma skin lesions.
(Courtesy of Lawrence B. Stack, MD.)

f. **Molluscum contagiosum, intertriginous infections** (often caused by candidiasis or *Trichophyton* infection), **seborrheic dermatitis, condylomata acuminata** (caused by human papilloma virus), **psoriasis, atopic dermatitis,** and **alopecia** are also commonly seen.

3. **Neurologic manifestations.** CNS disease occurs in 75% to 90% of patients with AIDS, and 10% to 20% of patients with AIDS initially present with CNS symptoms. The most common symptoms are seizures and altered mental status.

   a. **Toxoplasmosis** is the most common cause of focal encephalitis in patients with AIDS. Symptoms include fever, headache, focal neurologic symptoms, altered mental status, or seizures.

   b. **AIDS dementia complex** is a progressive dementia, with symptoms of impaired short-term memory and confusion. It is caused by the direct effect of HIV on neurons and occurs in over one-third of patients with AIDS.

   c. **Cryptococcal CNS infection** may be seen in up to 10% of patients with AIDS and may cause either focal cerebral lesions or diffuse meningoencephalitis. Symptoms may include headache, light-headedness, depression, seizures, or cranial nerve palsies.

   d. **Tuberculous meningitis** and **herpes simplex virus (HSV) encephalitis** are also common.

4. **Psychiatric manifestations**

   a. **Depression** is common among patients with AIDS and may initially manifest as a primary complaint or a suicide attempt.

   b. **AIDS psychosis** may present with hallucinations, delusions, or other abnormal behavioral changes.

5. **Ophthalmologic manifestations.** CMV retinitis occurs in 10% to 15% of patients and accounts for the majority of retinitis among patients with AIDS. It may be asymptomatic or patients may present with photophobia, scotoma, redness, pain, or diminished visual acuity.

6. **Pulmonary manifestations.** Lung infections are one of the most common reasons patients with HIV present to the ED. The most common pulmonary disorders in patients with HIV include PCP, *Mycobacterium tuberculosis* infection, CMV infection, *Cryptococcus neoformans* infection, *Histoplasma capsulatum* infection, and neoplasms.

   a. Nonproductive cough and the presence of a diffuse infiltrative process on chest radiography suggest PCP, CMV infection, or Kaposi sarcoma.

   b. Hilar adenopathy with a diffuse pulmonary infiltrate may be associated with *C. neoformans* infection, histoplasmosis, *M. tuberculosis* infection, or neoplasia.

7. **Gastrointestinal manifestations.** Approximately 50% of patients will present with gastrointestinal complaints at some time during their illness. The most common presenting symptoms include abdominal pain, bleeding, and diarrhea. Esophagitis may present as dysphagia or odynophagia. Common causes of gastrointestinal complications include *Candida* infection, Kaposi sarcoma, *Mycobacterium avium-intracellulare* infection, HSV type 1 or HSV

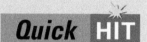

Quick HIT

CMV retinitis is characterized by **cotton wool spots** (Figure 6-2), fluffy white retinal lesions that are often perivascular.

Quick HIT

PCP is the most common opportunistic infection among patients with AIDS—over 80% will acquire PCP at some time during their illness.

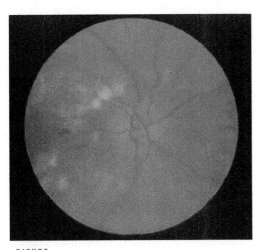

FIGURE
6-2 Cotton wool spots.

type 2 infection, CMV infection, *Campylobacter jejuni* infection, *Shigella* infection, salmonellosis, giardiasis, cryptosporidiosis, *Entamoeba histolytica* infection, and *Isospora* infection.

C. **Differential diagnoses.** The list of differential diagnoses for HIV and all of its manifestations is lengthy because virtually any disease process can mimic an illness associated with HIV infection.

D. **Evaluation**

1. **Confirmation of HIV infection.** A person suspected of being infected by HIV should be serologically tested using **enzyme-linked immunosorbent assay (ELISA)**. **Western blot assays** confirm the presence of the virus. These tests are usually not performed in the ED because of issues of confidentiality, counseling, and follow-up. If the patient's presenting complaint necessitates admission, then the testing should be performed as an inpatient. Otherwise, the patient should be given appropriate referrals for outpatient testing.

2. **Evaluation of presenting symptoms.** Additional tests depend on the symptoms at the time of presentation to the ED.

   a. **Systemic symptoms**

      i. **History and physical examination.** A complete history should be obtained and a thorough physical examination should be performed.

      ii. **Laboratory studies.** A CBC, serum biochemical profile, blood and urine cultures, urinalysis, liver function tests, chest radiographs, and serologic test results for syphilis, *Toxoplasma*, and *Coccidioides* should be obtained.

   b. **Neurologic symptoms.** For a patient infected with HIV presenting with headache, focal neurologic changes, or altered mental status, a CBC and serum biochemistry profile should be obtained, as well as a CT scan (with and without contrast). A lumbar puncture should be performed to obtain samples for serology to exclude toxoplasmosis, CMV infection, *Cryptococcus* infection, HSV infection, tuberculosis, and lymphoma.

   c. **Pulmonary symptoms.** The workup for any pulmonary complaint should include the following:

      i. Chest radiograph

      ii. Arterial blood gas analysis

      iii. Sputum culture, Gram stain, and acid-fast stain

      iv. Blood cultures

   d. **Gastrointestinal symptoms**

      i. **Diarrhea** is the most common gastrointestinal complaint. ED evaluation may include microscopic examination of a stool sample for leukocytes, acid-fast staining of a stool sample, and examination for ova and parasites, as well as bacterial culture of stool and blood.

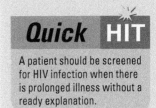

Quick **HIT**

A patient should be screened for HIV infection when there is prolonged illness without a ready explanation.

Infectious Disease Emergencies

ii. **Esophagitis.** Endoscopy, fungal stains, viral cultures, or biopsy may be necessary to establish the diagnosis. An air-contrast barium swallow may be necessary to confirm a diagnosis of *Candida* esophagitis.

E. **Therapy.** The role of the ED physician is rarely to treat directly the underlying HIV infection because the internist or infectious disease specialist is better able to follow the patient and monitor the efficacy and side effects of the drugs involved over a long-term basis. Instead, the ED physician's focus should be the acute presentations of the common opportunistic infections and how to treat them in order to avoid unnecessary morbidity.

1. **Primary disease**

   The ED physician should be aware that additional therapy is usually initiated when the patient's CD4 count drops below 500/mm^3.

2. **Complications of HIV infection**

   a. **Cutaneous complications**
      i. **Xerosis** can be treated with emollients; **pruritus** may respond to oatmeal baths or antihistamines.
      ii. ***S. aureus* infection**, ***P. aeruginosa* infection**, **herpes zoster**, **syphilis**, and **scabies** can all be treated with standard therapies.
      iii. **HSV lesions** can be treated with **acyclovir** (200 mg orally five times daily for 10 days or, for extensive disease, 30 mg/kg/day intravenously).
      iv. **Kaposi sarcoma** is generally not associated with significant morbidity or mortality. Chemotherapy (e.g., with vincristine, vinblastine, or doxorubicin) or radiation therapy is warranted only for extensive, painful, or cosmetically disfiguring lesions.
      v. **Molluscum contagiosum.** Cryotherapy or curettage can be used to remove the small, flesh-colored papules of molluscum contagiosum.
      vi. **Intertriginous infections** (e.g., such as can occur with *Candida* or *Trichophyton* infection) can be treated with **topical imidazole creams** (e.g., clotrimazole, miconazole, ketoconazole).
      vii. **Seborrheic dermatitis** is treated with **topical steroids**.
      viii. **Human papillomavirus infections** are treated for cosmesis with cryotherapy, topical therapy, or laser therapy.

   b. **Neurologic complications**
      i. **Toxoplasmosis** is treated with oral **sulfadiazine** (100 mg/kg/day) and **pyrimethamine** (25 to 50 mg/kg/day) with **folic acid** to reduce the incidence of hematologic toxicity. Short courses of **steroids** may be employed, and chronic suppressive therapy is needed after acute treatment.
      ii. **Cryptococcosis.** Treatment for cryptococcal infection includes **amphotericin B** (0.4 to 0.6 mg/kg/day IV) with or without **flucytosine** (75 to 100 mg/kg/day). Sixty percent of patients respond to this therapy. Initial therapy should continue for 6 weeks, and chronic suppressive therapy is often indicated.
      iii. **Other infections** (e.g., bacterial meningitis, brain abscess, CMV infection, HSV encephalitis, neurosyphilis) should be treated according to the standard therapies in place for each disease process.

   c. **Psychiatric complications.** Hospitalization should be instituted when necessary for patients with depression, acute delirium, or incapacitating dementia.

   d. **Ophthalmologic complications.** No specific therapy is indicated for cotton wool spots. CMV retinitis is treated with **ganciclovir** (5 mg/kg twice daily) for 2 weeks, followed by long-term maintenance therapy.

   e. **Pulmonary complications**
      i. **PCP.** Relapses are common—65% of patients will have a reinfection within 18 months.
         a) **Trimethoprim** (20 mg/kg/day) and **sulfamethoxazole** (100 mg/kg/day) should be administered either orally or intravenously for 2 to 3 weeks.
         b) **Pentamidine** (4 mg/kg/day) may be used as an effective alternate therapy.
         c) **Oral steroid therapy** should be instituted for those patients with an arterial oxygen tension less than 70 mm Hg, or an alveolar–arterial

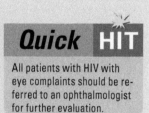

Quick HIT

All patients with HIV with eye complaints should be referred to an ophthalmologist for further evaluation.

Infectious Disease Emergencies

gradient greater than 35. The usual regimen consists of **prednisone**, 80 mg/day for 5 days, followed by 40 mg/day for 5 days, and then 20 mg/day for 11 days.

    ii. *M. tuberculosis* **infection** is treated with a triple drug regimen of **isoniazid, rifampin, and ethambutol.** This regimen may be supplemented with **pyrazinamide** and **streptomycin.**

  f. **Gastrointestinal complications**

    i. **Diarrhea.** Dehydration should be corrected. Antibiotic therapy should be initiated when appropriate.

    ii. **Oral candidiasis** is treated with **clotrimazole troches** five times daily until clear, or oral **ketoconazole** or **fluconazole.**

    iii. **Other oral lesions** (e.g., HSV infection, Kaposi sarcoma).

F. Disposition should be based on the ability to rule out any life-threatening complications of HIV infection.

1. **Discharge.** Many patients infected with HIV with fever may be managed as outpatients if the source of the fever does not dictate admission, appropriate laboratory studies have been initiated, the patient is able to function adequately at home (i.e., he or she is able to ambulate and maintain adequate oral intake), and appropriate medical follow-up can be arranged.

2. **Admission**

  a. Patients with a CD4 count below 500/mm^3 and an unknown source of fever are usually admitted for further observation and evaluation.

  b. If a life-threatening illness cannot be ruled out, or the patient is debilitated beyond the point where he or she can be cared for adequately at home, then the patient should be admitted for further treatment and evaluation.

III. CENTRAL NERVOUS SYSTEM INFECTIONS

A. **Meningitis**

1. **Discussion.** Meningitis is inflammation of the membranes of the brain and the spinal cord. The mortality rate ranges from 10% to 50%.

  a. **Etiology.** Infectious meningitis may be caused by bacteria, viruses, fungi, or parasites.

  b. **Pathogenesis.** Meningitis is usually caused by hematogenous bacterial seeding of the subarachnoid space, but direct inoculation via a dural defect (e.g., after trauma or neurosurgery) or direct spread of organisms from parameningeal infections (e.g., sinusitis or otitis media) can also occur.

  c. **Clinical syndromes**

    i. **Acute meningitis.** Onset of symptoms occurs within 24 hours, and patients have a rapidly progressive downhill course (the treated mortality rate is 50%). Most likely pathogens are *S. pneumoniae* and *Neisseria meningitidis*, or *H. influenzae* in the nonimmunized pediatric population.

    ii. **Subacute meningitis** presents in 1 to 7 days and is usually caused by viruses or fungi.

    iii. **Chronic meningitis.** Symptoms persist for longer than 1 week and the disease follows a prolonged, indolent course. Causes include some viral meningitides as well as *M. tuberculosis, Treponema pallidum, Cryptococcus,* and other fungi.

2. **Clinical features**

  a. **Bacterial meningitis.** The classic presentation of acute bacterial meningitis is fever, headache, photophobia, nuchal rigidity, lethargy, malaise, altered sensorium, seizures, vomiting, and chills. Complications include hyponatremia, hydrocephalus, and cerebrovascular accident.

  b. **Fungal meningitis** often has a more subacute course than bacterial meningitis, with the same range of symptoms but often to such a mild degree that the diagnosis may not be considered.

  c. **Tuberculous meningitis** often has a protracted course and a vague, nonspecific presentation of fever, weight loss, night sweats, and malaise, with or without headache and meningismus.

d. **Viral meningitis.** The presentation can range from acute to protracted with nonspecific findings.

3. **Differential diagnoses** include encephalitis, brain abscess, neoplasm, trauma, subdural hematoma, subarachnoid hemorrhage, systemic lupus erythematosus, sarcoidosis, rheumatoid arthritis, toxic encephalopathy, metabolic encephalopathy, multiple sclerosis, and granulomatous angiitis.

4. **Evaluation**
   a. **CSF analysis** for cell count and differential, Gram staining, and culture are the diagnostic procedures of choice. Increased intracranial pressure is a relative contraindication to performing a lumbar puncture.
      i. **Cell count and differential**
         a) **Bacterial meningitis.** An increase in the leukocyte count to greater than 5 cells/mm^3, a CSF:serum glucose ratio of less than 0.5 in normoglycemic subjects, and a CSF protein level greater than 45 mg/dL are all indicators of a bacterial infection.
         b) **Viral meningitis.** A marked lymphocytosis is evident on the differential, but this finding is not diagnostic for viral meningitis because 6% to 13% of all bacterial meningitides are also characterized by a marked lymphocytosis.
      ii. **Staining.** A Gram stain can rapidly detect the presence and type of bacterial organism, and an India ink preparation can identify cryptococcal organisms, but cryptococcal antigen testing, when available, is more sensitive and specific.
   b. **CT scan.** If there are any signs of focal neurologic deficits or altered mental status, a head CT scan should be obtained prior to a lumbar puncture, to rule out mass lesions or other evidence of increased intracranial pressure.

5. **Therapy**
   a. **Antibiotics.** Patients with an acute presentation should receive antibiotics within 30 minutes of presentation. Studies have shown that early antibiotic therapy will not significantly affect CSF analysis results or CSF cultures drawn within 6 hours of antibiotic administration, but failure to promptly administer antibiotics may dramatically affect patient morbidity and mortality.
      i. In the absence of knowledge of the offending organism, empiric therapy could be initiated with a **third-generation cephalosporin** (current practice favors ceftriaxone or cefotaxime). Dosages are as follows:
         a) **Ceftriaxone** (2 g intravenously for adults; 50 to 75 mg/kg/day every 12 to 24 hours for children)
         b) **Cefotaxime** (2 g intravenously every 4 to 6 hours for adults; 200 mg/kg/day every 8 hours for children)
      ii. If infection with *Staphylococcus* or a gram-negative bacillus is a concern (e.g., in a patient with a history of recent neurosurgery, head trauma, or a CSF shunt), **vancomycin** (25 mg/kg administered as an intravenous bolus) plus **ceftazidime** (2 g intravenously every 8 hours for adults; 90 to 150 mg/kg every 8 hours for children) should be used.
      iii. If the host is immunocompromised or infection with *Listeria monocytogenes* is a concern, **ampicillin** should be added.
   b. **Steroids.** The use of steroids in the pediatric population is controversial, but many authors favor steroid use to decrease inflammation and possibly decrease the incidence of long-term sequelae (e.g., hearing loss associated with bacterial meningitis caused by *S. pneumoniae* or *H. influenzae*). Current guidelines are to administer **dexamethasone** (0.15 mg/kg intravenously) at the time of antibiotic administration.

6. **Disposition.** All patients with suspected meningitis should be admitted to the hospital for further evaluation.
   a. If the results of CSF analysis are normal but the patient still shows clinical signs of infection, a repeat lumbar puncture should be performed in 8 to

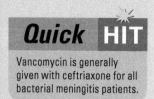

Quick HIT

Vancomycin is generally given with ceftriaxone for all bacterial meningitis patients.

12 hours and antibiotics should be initiated empirically before the second lumbar puncture is performed.

b. The diagnosis of aseptic or viral meningitis should be made only after hospital admission and the appropriate CSF cultures have proven negative for other forms of meningitis.

B. Encephalitis

1. **Discussion.** Encephalitis is an infection of the cerebrum, cerebellum, and brain stem. Two thousand cases of encephalitis are reported in the United States annually. Encephalitis may be caused by a number of organisms, including HSV type 1 and arboviruses (e.g., Eastern equine encephalitis virus, Western equine encephalitis virus, St. Louis encephalitis virus, California encephalitis virus), *Mycoplasma, Toxoplasma, Coccidioides, Cryptococcus, T. pallidum, Borrelia burgdorferi, Naegleria,* and *Mycobacterium.*

2. **Clinical features** are very similar to those of meningitis. An altered level of consciousness ranging from lethargy and irritability to frank obtundation and coma is common. Seizures and gait ataxia also occur. Personality change is generally a key factor to differentiate encephalitis from meningitis.

3. **Differential diagnoses** include meningitis, brain abscess, neoplasm, trauma, subdural hematoma, subarachnoid hemorrhage, systemic lupus erythematosus, toxic encephalopathy, and metabolic encephalopathy.

4. **Evaluation.** CSF analysis and a head CT scan form the cornerstone of diagnosis. The diagnosis of encephalitis is usually made by first ruling out the presence of meningitis using Gram staining, antibody titers, India ink preparations, and CSF cultures.

a. **CSF analysis.** A CSF sample obtained via a lumbar puncture usually shows a normal glucose level, an elevated protein level, and marked pleocytosis in patients with encephalitis, but these signs are nonspecific. When HSV or *Naegleria* is the causative organism, an elevated CSF red blood cell count is common. Specific CSF and blood serum titers for specific encephalitides (e.g., *Toxoplasmosis*) are available and useful for identifying the causative agent.

b. **HSV polymerase chain reaction** should be ordered when considering herpes encephalitis.

5. **Therapy.** Because differentiating encephalitis from meningitis is very difficult, presumptive therapy should be initiated for bacterial meningitis even before the initiation of the workup. Treatment is generally supportive. HSV is treated with acyclovir with goal of early administration.

6. **Disposition.** All patients suspected of having encephalitis should be admitted to the hospital for further evaluation and treatment.

C. Brain abscess

1. **Discussion**

a. **Incidence.** Brain abscesses are rare. The greatest incidence is seen in patients between the ages of 20 and 40 years; men are affected twice as often as women.

b. **Pathogenesis**

i. Abscesses usually occur secondary to a focus of infection outside the CNS.

a) Brain abscesses arise from the middle ear, mastoid, and paranasal sinuses 40% of the time.

b) Hematogenous spread of bacteria from remote sites causes 30% of infections.

c) Thirty percent of brain abscesses have no clear cause.

ii. Inflammation of the cerebrum progresses to abscess formation and finally encapsulation. Three major complications can cause sudden deterioration: uncal or tonsillar herniation, spontaneous hemorrhage, and rupture of the abscess into the ventricular or subarachnoid space.

c. **Risk factors** for brain abscess include AIDS, immunosuppression, and intravenous drug abuse.

2. **Clinical features.** The clinical presentation may mimic that of a brain tumor, but the presentation of an abscess usually evolves more rapidly (e.g., within

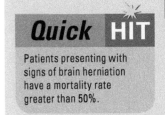

Quick HIT

Patients presenting with signs of brain herniation have a mortality rate greater than 50%.

Infectious Disease Emergencies

days to weeks). The classic presentation is one of headache, recent seizure, low-grade fever, and a focal neurologic deficit.

 a. **Headache** is the most common symptom; it is present in 70% to 90% of affected patients.

 b. **Focal neurologic deficits** are found in 75% of patients.

 c. **Seizures** are found in 30% of patients; **fever** in 50% of patients.

3. **Differential diagnoses** include a tumor, encephalitis or meningitis, cerebrovascular accident, subarachnoid hemorrhage, migraine, and an extradural abscess.

4. **Evaluation.** A head CT scan is the procedure of choice, with and without contrast. Laboratory values are rarely helpful, although the WBC count is elevated in 30% of patients.

5. **Therapy.** Definitive care entails surgical intervention and antibiotic therapy.

 a. **Supportive therapy.** If there are signs of increased intracranial pressure, the physician may need to elevate the bed 30 degrees, intubate the patient, and institute dexamethasone therapy (10 mg intravenously followed by 4 mg every 6 hours for adults; 0.6 mg/kg every 6 hours for children).

 b. **Antibiotic therapy.** Drugs should be selected using susceptibility testing as a basis (Table 6-3), and therapy should be continued for 4 to 6 weeks.

6. **Disposition.** Patients with brain abscesses require hospital admission and immediate neurosurgical consultation.

 D. **Rabies**

 1. **Discussion**

 a. **Etiology.** Rabies is caused by an RNA-carrying reovirus and is transmitted by infectious saliva.

 2. **Clinical features**

 a. Initial symptoms are nonspecific: fever, malaise, headache, nausea, sore throat, cough, and pain and paresthesias at the inoculation site. Incubation periods average 35 to 64 days.

TABLE **6-3**	Antibiotic Therapy for Brain Abscess		
		Regimen	
Type of Infection	**Drug**	*Adult dosage*	*Pediatric dosage*
Staphylococcus aureus or coagulase-negative staphylococci	Nafcillin	2 g intravenously every 4–6 hours	50 mg/kg/day intravenously every 4 hours
	Vancomycin (for MRSA)	1 g intravenously every 12 hours	15 mg/kg/day intravenously every 4–6 hours
Streptococcus	Penicillin G	2–4 million U intravenously every 4 hours	250,000 U/kg/day intravenously every 4 hours
Enteric Gram-negative bacilli or *Pseudomonas*	Piperacillin	4 g intravenously every 4–6 hours + an aminoglycoside	—
Mixed anaerobic/aerobic	Ticarcillin + clavulanic acid	3.1 g intravenously every 6 hours	200–300 mg/kg/day intravenously every 4–6 hours
	Ampicillin + sulbactam	3 g intravenously every 6 hours	—
	Piperacillin + tazobactam	3.375 g intravenously every 6 hours	—

MRSA = methicillin-resistant *Staphylococcus aureus.*

b. After 1 to 4 days, altered mental status, opisthotonos, painful visible spasms, and motor paresis occur. In 20% of patients, an ascending, symmetric, flaccid areflexia paralysis similar to that seen in Landry syndrome and Guillain-Barré syndrome may occur.

c. Hypersensitivity to secondary stimuli and hydrophobia occur in the later stages. Death usually occurs within 4 to 7 days in untreated patients; coma, convulsions, and apnea occur immediately prior to death.

3. **Differential diagnoses** include encephalitis, polio, tetanus, meningitis, brain abscess, septic cavernous virus thrombosis, cholinergic poisoning, Landry syndrome, and Guillain-Barré syndrome.

4. **Evaluation.** The diagnosis of rabies in animals and humans is made by **analysis of biopsied brain tissue**. Histologic examination will reveal Negri bodies; fluorescent antibody testing can also be performed.

5. **Therapy**
   a. **Postexposure immunoprophylaxis** should be instituted as soon as possible. Both of the following therapies are safe for pregnant women.
      i. **Rabies immune globulin** is administered as follows: 20 IU/kg daily, with half the dose infiltrated locally at the exposure site and the other half administered intramuscularly.
      ii. **Human diploid cell vaccine** is given in five 1-mL doses on days 0, 3, 7, 14, and 28.
   b. **Prompt cleansing and debridement of the wound** and **tetanus prophylaxis** should also be initiated.
   c. Any person who is bitten by a bat or who wakes up in a room with a bat should have **postexposure immunoprophylaxis**.

6. **Disposition.** Any patient suspected of having rabies should be admitted to the ICU for supportive management.

7. **Prevention.** Preexposure rabies prophylaxis should be considered for people involved in wildlife trapping or rabies vaccine production, animal handlers, and travelers to underdeveloped countries.

E. **Tetanus**
   1. **Discussion**
      a. **Etiology.** Tetanus is an acute, frequently fatal illness that results from infection of a wound with *Clostridium tetani*, an anaerobic, gram-positive rod that can exist in either a vegetative or sporulated form.
         i. The incubation period is 24 hours to 1 month. The shorter the incubation period, the more severe the disease.
         ii. *C. tetani* produces an exotoxin, **tetanospasmin**, which is transported to the CNS by retrograde axonal transport and via the bloodstream. Tetanospasmin acts on the motor endplates of the skeletal muscles and on the spinal cord, brain, and sympathetic nervous system to prevent transmission at inhibitory interneurons in the CNS.
      b. **Incidence.** In the United States, approximately 60 cases of tetanus are reported each year, with an overall fatality rate of 21%. Most of these cases occur in individuals older than 50 years who are inadequately immunized.
   2. **Clinical features** include muscular rigidity, violent muscular contractions, and autonomic dysfunction (see Clinical Pearl 6-4).
   3. **Differential diagnoses** include strychnine poisoning, neuroleptic malignant syndrome, meningitis, encephalitis, hypocalcemia tetany, rabies, and temporomandibular joint disease.
   4. **Evaluation.** The diagnosis is purely clinical.
   5. **Therapy**
      a. **Treatment of complications.** Respiratory compromise may require immediate neuromuscular blockade and orotracheal intubation.
      b. **Minimizing the spread of toxin**
         i. **Wound debridement.** All wounds into which spores were potentially introduced must be identified and débrided. A wound may not be identified in up to 20% of patients.

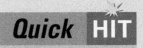

Quick HIT

In developing countries, dogs are the primary reservoir; in the United States, skunks (60%), bats (15%), raccoons (10%), and cows (4%) predominate.

Infectious Disease Emergencies

Infectious Disease Emergencies

CLINICAL PEARL 6-4

Clinical tetanus has four forms.
a. **Local tetanus** is persistent rigidity of the muscles in close proximity to the site of injury.
b. **Generalized tetanus** begins as pain and stiffness in the jaw muscles and progresses to involve muscular contractions and rigidity of the whole body.
c. **Cephalic tetanus** follows injuries to the head, involves cranial nerve dysfunction, and has a particularly poor prognosis.
d. **Neonatal tetanus** is an important cause of infant mortality in developing countries and carries an extremely high mortality rate.

      ii. **Tetanus immune globulin** is administered as a single intramuscular dose of 3,000 to 5,000 U to neutralize circulating toxin. Although tetanus immune globulin does not ameliorate the patient's symptoms, studies have shown that it does significantly decrease mortality.

      iii. **Metronidazole** (500 mg intravenously every 6 to 8 hours) is the preferred treatment for tetanus, but **penicillin G** (2 to 4 million U intravenously every 4 to 6 hours) is a safe and effective alternative.

   c. **Treatment of autonomic dysfunction.** Autonomic dysfunction can be successfully treated with **labetalol** (0.25 to 1 mg/min continuous intravenous infusion), **magnesium sulfate** (a loading dose of 70 mg/kg intravenously followed by infusion of 1 to 4 mg/hour to maintain a serum level of 2.5 to 4 mm/L), and **morphine sulfate** (5 to 30 mg intravenously every 2 to 8 hours) or **clonidine** (300 μg every 8 hours per nasogastric tube).

   d. **Immunization.** Patients who recover from tetanus must undergo active immunization because the disease does not confer immunity. **Tetanus toxoid** (0.5 mL) should be administered at 1 and 6 weeks and at 6 months after injury.

  6. **Disposition.** All patients suspected of having tetanus must be admitted to the ICU for further treatment and evaluation.

IV. SEXUALLY TRANSMITTED DISEASES (OTHER THAN AIDS)

  A. **Gonorrhea**

    1. **Discussion**

      a. **Etiology.** Gonorrhea is caused by *Neisseria gonorrhoeae*.

      b. **Incidence.** The highest incidence is in men between the ages of 20 and 24 years.

    2. **Clinical features**

      a. **Local disease**

        i. **Acute urethritis** is the most common presentation in heterosexual men. Symptoms begin within 1 to 14 days of exposure and consist of dysuria and penile discharge. Three to ten percent of men with gonorrhea may be asymptomatic.

        ii. **Cervicitis.** Primary gonorrhea in women is **usually asymptomatic**, and when symptoms do occur, they are usually mild and nonspecific. Up to 20% of women with primary gonorrhea develop **pelvic inflammatory disease**, and 33% to 81% of women with pelvic inflammatory disease have gonorrhea.

        iii. **Pharyngeal gonorrhea** can be **asymptomatic**. The pharynx is colonized in 3% to 7% of heterosexual men, 5% to 20% of women, 10% to 25% of homosexual men and 39% to 96% of pregnant women.

        iv. **Anorectal gonorrhea** is common in both heterosexual women and homosexual men and is **often asymptomatic**. When symptoms occur, they are usually **mild pruritus** and **rectal discomfort**.

      b. **Disseminated gonorrhea** may complicate the disease course in 1% to 3% of patients with localized disease and is manifested most commonly as a **monoarticular arthritis** or **pustular dermatitis syndrome**.

    3. **Differential diagnoses**

      a. **Gonococcal urethritis** must be differentiated from nongonococcal urethritis caused by *Chlamydia trachomatis*.

b. **Disseminated gonorrhea.** *N. meningitidis* infection, acute rheumatic fever, and Reiter syndrome must be ruled out. Differential diagnoses for skin lesions include syphilis, HIV infection, and condyloma acuminata.

4. **Evaluation.** Gram stain and culture of discharges are the cornerstone of diagnosis. All patients evaluated for gonorrhea should also have blood drawn for syphilis serology.

5. **Therapy.** For uncomplicated cervicitis or urethritis:
   a. **Ceftriaxone** (250 mg intramuscularly) and **doxycycline** (100 mg orally twice daily for 14 days, to cure possible concomitant *Chlamydia* infection) are the standard therapy.
   b. **Cefixime** (400 mg orally in a single dose) is no longer an accepted alternative due to resistance.
   c. **Azithromycin, 2 g** one-time dose, is an alternative for cephalosporin allergic patients.

6. **Disposition**
   a. Uncomplicated gonorrhea is managed on an outpatient basis. All sexual contacts must be identified and treated, and HIV testing should be considered by the patient with his or her primary physician at a later date.
   b. Patients with disseminated gonorrhea require hospitalization.

B. **Syphilis**
   1. **Discussion**
      a. **Etiology.** Syphilis is caused by *T. pallidum*.
      b. **Incidence.** There are 29,000 new cases of syphilis each year. This figure represents probably only 10% of actual cases.
   2. **Clinical features**
      a. **Primary syphilis.** After an average incubation period of approximately 3 weeks, a smooth, painless ulcer called a *chancre* appears at the site of primary inoculation. The chancre heals without treatment in approximately 3 to 6 weeks; at about the same time, a painless uni- or bilateral regional **adenopathy** develops.
      b. **Secondary syphilis** represents disseminated disease and occurs in all patients with untreated primary infection. The lesions of secondary syphilis are **papulosquamous lesions** that occur over the entire trunk, extremities, penis, and buttocks. **Fever and weight loss** occur in 70% of patients (Figure 6-3).
      c. **Tertiary syphilis** occurs at least 10 years after the primary infection in at least 30% to 35% of untreated patients. The two most important manifestations of tertiary syphilis are **cardiovascular syphilis**, causing thoracic aneurysms, and **neurosyphilis**, causing meningitis, stroke, seizures, dementia, general weakness, and posterior column dysfunction.
   3. **Differential diagnoses** include chancroid, HSV type 1 infection, lymphogranuloma venereum, tinea, sarcoid, lichen planus, seborrhea dermatitis, molluscum contagiosum, traumatic ulcer, furuncle, and carcinoma.
   4. **Evaluation.** The clinical diagnosis can be confirmed by **darkfield microscopic examination** or more commonly **serologic testing** (see Chapter 5.V.A.4).
   5. **Therapy**
      a. The standard treatment for **primary, secondary,** and **early tertiary syphilis** is **benzathine penicillin G** (2.4 million U administered intramuscularly as a single dose).
      b. For **late tertiary syphilis** or **neurosyphilis, benzathine penicillin G** (2.4 million U, three doses administered intramuscularly 1 week apart) is used. **Doxycycline** (100 mg orally twice daily for 14 days) can be given to patients who are allergic to penicillin.
   6. **Disposition**
      a. Primary and secondary syphilis can be treated on an outpatient basis.
      b. Patients with neurosyphilis or major cardiovascular manifestations require admission for intravenous therapy.

Infectious Disease Emergencies

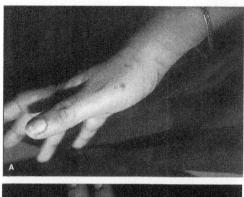
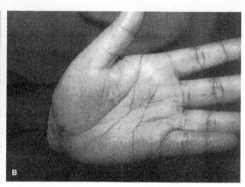
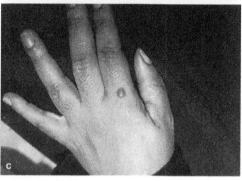

FIGURE

6-3 Secondary syphilis.

C. **Chlamydia**
1. **Discussion**
   a. **Etiology.** Chlamydia is caused by *C. trachomatis*, an obligate intracellular bacterium. Chlamydia is the most prevalent sexually transmitted infection in the United States.
   b. **Pathogenesis.** The incubation period is typically 1 to 3 weeks and symptoms, if present, can range from mild burning or irritation to those of peritonitis.
2. **Clinical features.** Chlamydia infections present a wide range of clinical manifestations.
   a. In **men**, infection causes **urethritis**, **epididymitis**, and **proctitis**.
   b. In **women**, **urethritis**, **cervicitis**, and **pelvic inflammatory disease** are common.
   c. The incidence of **asymptomatic infection** is high, from 3% to 20%.
3. **Differential diagnoses** include gonorrhea and urinary tract infection.
4. **Evaluation.** Although the organism can be cultured, the yield is relatively low. Chlamydia **antigen testing** can be performed on urine or cervical swabs.
5. **Therapy. Doxycycline** (100 mg orally twice daily by mouth) has been the standard therapy, but **azithromycin** (1 g orally in a single dose) is effective in noncomplicated infection.
6. **Disposition.** Once treated, patients can be discharged with strict instructions to have their partners checked and to follow up for culture results.
D. **Chancroid** is discussed in Chapter 5.V.C.
E. **Trichomoniasis**
1. **Discussion.** Trichomoniasis is caused by the protozoan *Trichomonas vaginalis*. It is contracted through contact with genital secretions.
2. **Clinical features.** After an incubation period of 4 to 20 days, women develop vaginitis characterized by a **copious, foamy, yellow discharge with a foul odor**. Men are usually asymptomatic.
3. **Differential diagnoses** include *Gardnerella* vaginitis, candidiasis, gonorrhea, syphilis, and HSV infection.

4. **Evaluation.** Diagnosis is by microscopic identification of the motile, flagellated parasites on a wet-mount slide.

5. **Therapy. Metronidazole** (250 mg orally three times daily for 7 days or 2 g orally as a single dose) is recommended. In pregnant women, a 7-day course of **1% clotrimazole vaginal cream** is used.

F. **Herpes**

1. **Discussion.** Herpes is the most common ulcerative sexually acquired lesion in the United States.

   a. **Etiology.** There are two clinically indistinguishable forms of the virus, HSV type 1 and HSV type 2. Although HSV type 2 more commonly causes lesions in the genital area and HSV type 1 more commonly causes lesions on the face, the two forms can exist (together or separately) anywhere on the body (Figure 6-4).

   b. **Pathogenesis.** Infants may acquire the infection while passing through the birth canal, leading to meningitis and ophthalmic involvement. The incubation period is 2 to 21 days.

2. **Clinical features.** HSV causes recurrent, painful, vesicular ulcerations most commonly on the cervix and vulva in women and the glans and prepuce in men. The initial episode may last several weeks and be accompanied by a flu-like illness, but subsequent recurrences are usually shorter in duration and less intense than the initial episode.

3. **Differential diagnoses** include chancroid, lymphogranuloma venereum, and syphilis.

4. **Evaluation.** Diagnosis is usually made by history and physical appearance of the lesions and confirmed by culture of the serous fluid from the lesions.

5. **Therapy.** There is currently no cure.

   a. Initial episodes may be treated with **acyclovir** (200 mg five times daily for 7 days), which usually decreases the duration and the intensity of the episode.

   b. Treatment of recurrent episodes is usually not very effective unless initiated early in the presentation of the episode. Early initiation of therapy may shorten the course of the illness by 1 to 2 days. Suppressive acyclovir therapy has been used with some success for those patients who have multiple recurrent episodes, although the episodes usually return once suppressive therapy is discontinued.

6. **Disposition.** Herpes is treated on an outpatient basis.

V. UPPER RESPIRATORY TRACT INFECTIONS

A. **Streptococcal pharyngitis**

1. **Discussion.** Pharyngitis (infection of the pharynx and tonsils) is commonly caused by viruses and bacteria. **Group A β-hemolytic streptococci** are clearly the most important causative agents, accounting for half of all pharyn-

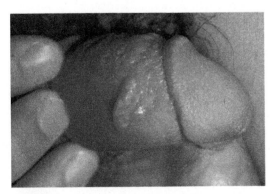

FIGURE
6-4 **Herpes genital lesions.**
(Courtesy of Lawrence B. Stack, MD.)

CLINICAL PEARL **6-5**

Centor criteria, used to diagnose streptococcal pharyngitis:
1. Tonsillar exudate
2. Fever or history of fever >38°C
3. Tender anterior cervical lymphadenopathy
4. Absence of cough
0–2 criteria: antibiotic treatment generally not indicated
3–4 criteria: consider antibiotic treatment

geal infections in patients between the ages of 5 and 15 years (see Clinical Pearl 6-5).

2. **Clinical features.** Although no set of symptoms is classic for streptococcal pharyngitis, the sudden onset of a fever and sore throat with enlargement of the cervical lymph nodes and red, swollen tonsils and palate are common. The presence of a scarlatiniform rash in the presence of pharyngitis practically identifies a group A β-hemolytic streptococcus as the causative agent. Headache, vomiting, abdominal pain, meningismus, and torticollis can occur as well.

3. **Differential diagnoses** include viral illnesses, diphtheria (*Corynebacterium diphtheriae* infection), *N. gonorrhoeae* infection, and Epstein-Barr virus infection.

   a. **Pharyngeal diphtheria** is characterized by tissue necrosis and the creation of a **pseudomembrane** over the tonsils, soft palate, uvula, or pharyngeal wall that can lead to airway obstruction (see V.B).

   b. **Pharyngeal gonorrhea.** *N. gonorrhoeae* causes a mild or asymptomatic pharyngitis seen in some sexually active adults and victims of child abuse (see IV.A.2.a.iii).

   c. **Infectious mononucleosis.** Epstein-Barr virus usually causes asymptomatic infections early in childhood and adolescence but has been associated with isolated tonsillopharyngitis characterized by malaise, fatigue, and sore throat. There is an increase in the number of atypical lymphocytes on peripheral blood smear and the heterophil antibody is present in over 90% of patients older than 5 years. Infectious mononucleosis is generally a benign, self-limited, somewhat prolonged illness.

4. **Evaluation**

   a. **Throat culture** is the mainstay of diagnosis.

   b. **Serology.** Rapid streptococcal antigen sensitivity of 50% to 90% and specificity of 98% to 100% when compared with throat culture (the gold standard).

5. **Therapy.** The objectives of management are to prevent rheumatic fever and suppurative complications and to hasten recovery.

   a. **Antibiotic therapy**

      i. A single dose of intramuscular **penicillin G benzathine** (600,000 to 1.2 million U for an average-sized adult) is very effective.

      ii. Oral **penicillin V** (250 mg four times daily for 10 days) is equally effective.

      iii. **First-** and **second-generation cephalosporins** and **erythromycin** are popular alternatives for patients who are allergic to penicillin.

   b. **Symptomatic therapy** includes acetaminophen, over-the-counter throat sprays and lozenges, and warm fluids.

6. **Disposition.** Pharyngitis is managed primarily on an outpatient basis.

B. **Diphtheria** is an acute infectious disease characterized by the formation of a fibrinous pseudomembrane on the respiratory mucosa. Cutaneous diphtheria lesions are also common.

   1. **Discussion**

      a. **Etiology.** Diphtheria is caused by *C. diphtheriae*.

      b. **Pathogenesis.** Transmission is via the secretions of infected individuals or carriers or via contaminated fomites.

c. **Complications**

  i. Myocarditis (days 10 to 14), congestive heart failure, and arrhythmias

  ii. Peripheral nerve palsies (weeks 3 to 6), bilateral flaccid weakness or paralysis, decreased deep tendon reflexes, ptosis, strabismus, and the inability to accommodate

d. **Predisposing factors.** Crowded habitats and low socioeconomic status predispose to the spread of diphtheria. The most significant risk factor is inadequate immunization.

2. **Clinical features**

a. **Symptoms.** Patients complain of a sore throat, dysphagia, and fever accompanied by nausea, vomiting, chills, and a headache. The patient's breathing may be labored as a result of upper airway edema or sudden detachment of the pseudomembrane, leading to sudden respiratory obstruction.

b. **Physical examination findings** include tachycardia and the pseudomembrane. Attempts to remove the pseudomembrane usually result in bleeding.

3. **Differential diagnoses** include streptococcal pharyngitis, viral pharyngitis, gonococcal pharyngitis, oral syphilis, epiglottitis, and (in the late stages of disease) Guillain-Barré syndrome.

4. **Evaluation.** The diagnosis is largely based on the clinical appearance of the membrane.

a. **Culture.** If antibiotic therapy has not been initiated, growth on Loeffler agar will reveal an aerobic, motile organism in 8 to 12 hours.

b. **Gram staining** of the membrane may show gram-positive, club-shaped rods.

5. **Therapy.** Spontaneous reversal occurs slowly over many weeks, but prompt treatment is essential to avoid complications. Recovery is slow, and too rapid a return to even "normal" levels of physical activity may worsen toxin-induced myocarditis.

a. **Diphtheria antitoxin** is derived from horse serum (therefore, sensitivity testing is recommended) and administered intramuscularly to neutralize the toxin. Antitoxin neutralizes only that toxin that is not yet bound to cells and should be administered immediately, without waiting for culture results.

b. **Antibacterial therapy.** Penicillin G eliminates the carrier state but has not been shown to alter the course, complications, or outcome of diphtheria. Erythromycin, ampicillin, clindamycin, and rifampin may be useful.

c. **Supportive therapy.** If oxygenation is impaired or obstruction appears imminent secondary to dislodgement of the membrane, tracheostomy is preferred over endotracheal intubation.

6. **Disposition.** Patients require immediate admission to the ICU.

7. **Prevention**

a. Contacts of patients with negative cultures and no symptoms should maintain adequate immunization status.

b. Asymptomatic carriers (those with positive cultures but no symptoms) should be treated with a full course of antibiotics and isolation at home.

c. Symptomatic carriers should be treated with antibiotics and antitoxin.

C. **Epiglottitis**

1. **Discussion.** Inflammatory disorders of the laryngeal region may be either supraglottic (i.e., affecting the supraglottis or epiglottis) or infraglottic (i.e., affecting the larynx or trachea).

a. **Etiology.** Epiglottitis can result from:

  i. **Chemical damage** (e.g., aspiration of gasoline)

  ii. **Mechanical injury** (e.g., trauma, burns)

  iii. **Sarcoidosis** (causes chronic epiglottitis)

  iv. **Infection**

    a) **Viruses** (e.g., parainfluenza virus, adenovirus, respiratory syncytial virus, herpes virus)

    b) **Bacteria** (e.g., *H. influenzae*, group A β-hemolytic streptococci, *S. pneumoniae*, *Haemophilus parainfluenzae*, *Klebsiella pneumoniae*, *Fusobacterium necrophorum*, *Pasteurella multocida*)

    c) **Fungi** (e.g., *Aspergillus*, *Candida*)

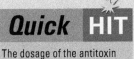

Quick **HIT**

The dosage of the antitoxin is based on the patient's clinical presentation, not on age or weight.

Infectious Disease Emergencies

2. **Clinical features.** Epiglottitis is characterized by a sudden, fulminant course.
   a. **Patient history.** Usually, there is no history of a prodromal upper respiratory tract infection. (This is in contrast to what is normally observed in patients with croup.)
   b. **Symptoms** include a disproportionately sore throat, fever, a muffled voice (versus the hoarseness seen in croup; see Chapter 15.V.A), minimal coughing (versus the bark-like cough seen in croup), dysphagia, and respiratory distress.
   c. **Physical examination findings** include:
      i. Drooling, dyspnea, tachypnea, inspiratory stridor (softer and less prominent than that seen with croup), and use of the accessory respiratory muscles
      ii. Cervical adenopathy
      iii. Tripod position (patient leans forward, supporting him- or herself with both hands, and hyperextends his or her neck)
      iv. Toxic or septic appearance
3. **Differential diagnoses** include croup, sepsis, aspirated foreign body, peritonsillar or retropharyngeal abscess, diphtheria, lingual tonsillitis, angioedema, pharyngitis, drug allergy, inhalation or ingestion of toxic substances, acute thyroiditis, and epiglottic hematoma.
4. **Evaluation.** Examination of the pharynx and administration of sedatives should be avoided when evaluating a patient with suspected epiglottitis.
   a. **Laryngoscopy** can be used to view the pharynx and larynx in adults.
      i. **Indications.** Oral instrumentation (e.g., indirect laryngoscopy) is indicated in the following circumstances:
         a) Patients in whom epiglottitis is only suspected and with mild to moderate signs and symptoms
         b) Patients without any indicators of potential airway compromise
      ii. Extreme caution should be employed. The procedure should be performed only in EDs with immediately accessible complete resuscitation equipment by a physician experienced in laryngoscopy.
   b. **Radiography.** A portable lateral neck radiograph is adequate for the diagnosis of epiglottitis and is much safer than allowing the patient to leave the ED. Most radiographic studies are inconclusive and should not be performed until experts on airway intervention are onsite. However, soft tissue lateral neck radiographs may demonstrate enlargement of the epiglottis (greater than 8 mm) and aryepiglottic folds (greater than 7 mm) and/or ballooning of the hypopharynx with air (Figure 6-5).

Quick HIT

No patient in respiratory distress or with any indication of potential airway compromise should ever be transferred to another institution until the airway is protected.

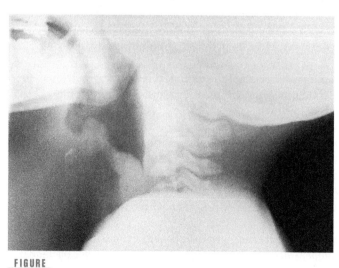

FIGURE 6-5 Radiograph of epiglottis "thumbprint."

5. **Therapy**
   a. **Intubation** (in a controlled setting, ideally in the operating room, by an anesthesiologist, otolaryngologist, or pediatric surgeon) is necessary.
      i. Venipuncture, injections, arterial blood gas analysis, the use of oxygen masks, and the taking of radiographs should be avoided until the patient is successfully intubated.
      ii. Blind nasal or orotracheal intubation should never be attempted.
   b. **Administration of racemic epinephrine is contraindicated.**
   c. **Antibiotic therapy** should be initiated immediately after blood and epiglottic cultures are taken and successful intubation has occurred.
      i. The antibiotic of choice is **cefotaxime** (50 mg/kg every 8 hours) or **ceftriaxone** (50 mg/kg/day administered intravenously in four equal doses).
      ii. As an alternative, **ampicillin** (200 mg/kg/day administered intravenously in four equal doses) together with **chloramphenicol** (100 mg/kg/day administered intravenously in four equal doses) can be used until the results of cultures and sensitivities are available.
   d. **Surgical intervention.** Bedside cricothyrotomy or tracheostomy may be necessary. Transtracheal needle jet ventilation in children younger than 8 years old may be done as a temporizing measure until the tracheostomy can be performed in the operating room.
6. **Disposition.** Laryngoscopy should be repeated prior to extubation, which is usually accomplished in 24 to 48 hours with appropriate treatment. ICU monitoring is indicated for 24 hours following extubation.
7. **Prevention**
   a. **Rifampin prophylaxis** (20 mg/kg/day once daily for 4 days, maximum 600 mg/day) is indicated for all family members and household and daycare contacts.
   b. **Vaccination against** *H. influenzae* is an excellent prophylactic measure but obviously is not 100% effective.

D. **Laryngitis**
1. **Discussion.** Laryngitis in the adult is usually synonymous with hoarseness.
   a. **Etiology**
      i. **Acute laryngitis.** Causes of acute laryngitis include:
         a) **Trauma** (e.g., laryngeal hematoma, edema secondary to exposure to heated gasses or liquids, dislocation or disruption of an arytenoid)
         b) **Infection**
            1) **Viruses** (e.g., adenoviruses, coronaviruses, parainfluenza viruses, respiratory syncytial viruses)
            2) **Bacteria** (e.g., *Staphylococcus*, *H. influenzae*, *C. diphtheriae*, mycobacteria)
            3) **Fungi**
      ii. **Chronic laryngitis**
         a) **Intralaryngeal causes** include benign laryngeal disease (e.g., benign polyps, vocal fatigue) and malignant laryngeal disease.
         b) **Extralaryngeal causes**
            1) **Perilaryngeal causes** include infiltrating thyroid carcinoma, lymphoma, and deep neck infection.
            2) **Remote causes** include recurrent entrapment from lung cancer and stroke.
            3) **Systemic causes** include neuromuscular disorders, rheumatoid disorders, and infiltrative processes.
2. **Clinical features.** Hoarseness is the most common manifestation of laryngeal disease regardless of its cause.
   a. **Symptoms** include dysphagia, odynophagia, and hoarseness. If the hoarseness presents as a part of the self-limited coryza syndrome (the most common form of adult laryngitis), it usually develops 2 to 4 days into the illness and lasts from 1 to 3 weeks.

b. **Physical examination findings** may include stridor; aspiration; a gray pseudomembrane attached to the posterior pharynx; lesions on the nose, pharynx, larynx, skin, penis, vagina, or bladder; peripheral neuritis or cranial nerve dysfunction; and signs of myocarditis (e.g., heart failure, dysrhythmias).

3. **Differential diagnoses**
   a. **Epiglottitis.** Laryngitis must be differentiated immediately from epiglottitis.
      i. Clinically, findings such as the tripod position, drooling, reluctance to speak, extreme apprehension, stridor, and retractions clearly indicate impending airway obstruction.
      ii. Radiographic findings may help (see V.D.4.b).
   b. **Aspiration**

4. **Evaluation**
   a. **Laboratory studies** are generally not helpful diagnostically but may be useful for baseline and follow-up. Diphtheria may be an exception (see V.B.4).
   b. **Radiography.** Compared to epiglottitis, laryngitis calls for no specific radiologic testing.

5. **Therapy**
   a. **Coryza syndrome.** Treatment is symptomatic and includes voice rest.
   b. *Staphylococcus* or *H. influenzae* **infection.** Treatment with a third-generation cephalosporin is effective.

6. **Disposition**
   a. **Discharge.** Most patients are discharged for follow-up with their family physician. Patients with hoarseness persisting more than 4 to 6 weeks should be referred to an otorhinolaryngologist for further evaluation.
   b. **Admission.** Patients with a clinical presentation suggestive of impending airway obstruction are admitted to the hospital and treated as described for epiglottitis.

VI. SKIN AND SOFT TISSUE INFECTIONS

A. **Staphylococcal scalded skin syndrome (SSSS)** is an acute, widespread, erythematous process characterized by peeling of the epidermis. Neonates, infants, young children, and immunosuppressed patients are most often affected.
   1. **Clinical features**
      a. In neonates and infants, the syndrome usually begins as a localized crusted (impetigo-like) infection at the umbilical stump or in the diaper area. In children, it usually starts as a superficially crusted lesion around the nose or ear.
      b. Within 24 hours, tender scarlet areas appear around the crusted lesions. The areas become painful and rapidly progress to large, flaccid blisters that break easily, producing erosions. The epidermis peels off easily in large sheets, leaving moist, glistening surfaces and progressing rapidly (within 36 to 72 hours) to widespread desquamation of the skin. Minor pressure produces skin separation (Nikolsky sign; Figure 6-6). Systemic symptoms, including fever, chills, and malaise, ensue.
   2. **Differential diagnoses**
      a. **Toxic epidermal necrosis (TEN; see Chapter 11.XI.A).** A rapid and accurate differential diagnosis between SSSS and TEN is essential because the approach to treatment is completely different.
         i. SSSS occurs in infants, children, and immunocompromised patients and begins with a staphylococcal infection (which may not have been noted initially).
         ii. TEN usually occurs in older patients and is usually associated with an adverse reaction to a medication. TEN usually has an acute onset and is symmetric.
      b. **Drug hypersensitivity rashes, viral exanthems,** and **the rash of scarlet fever** are usually acute, symmetrical, associated with systemic signs, and nonpainful.
      c. **Toxic shock syndrome (TSS)** presents with a diffuse sunburn-like erythroderma, followed several days later with desquamation of the skin and

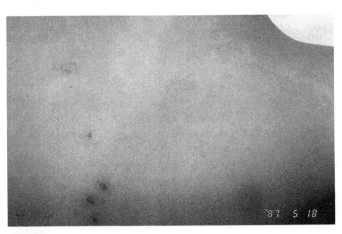

FIGURE
6-6 Nikolsky sign.

epidermal sloughing (especially of the palms and soles). The clinical course of the dermatologic lesions readily differentiates the two disease entities, but at a single point in time, the two may be difficult to differentiate.

    d. **Thermal burns, genetic bullous diseases, pemphigus vulgaris,** and **bullous pemphigoid** are also characterized by bullae, erosions, and easily loosened epidermis and must be differentiated from SSSS.

3. **Evaluation. Cultures** should be taken from the skin, nasopharynx, and blood.

4. **Therapy**

    a. **Antibiotic therapy.** Treatment with **systemic penicillinase-resistant anti-staphylococcal antibiotics** (e.g., **nafcillin,** 50 to 100 mg/kg/day) should be initiated immediately on the basis of the clinical diagnosis.

    b. **Supportive therapy. Intravenous fluids** should be administered to combat dehydration.

    c. Corticosteroids are contraindicated, and topical therapy and patient handling must be minimized.

B. **TSS** is a severe illness characterized by a high fever of sudden onset associated with vomiting, diarrhea, myalgias, and a rash. Hypotension rapidly progressing to shock follows.

1. **Discussion. Pathogenesis.** The organism has been isolated from mucosal surfaces (e.g., the nasopharynx, trachea, vagina) and the skin, empyemas, abscesses, and wounds.

2. **Clinical features** include the sudden onset of fever (102°F to 105°F), headache, intermittent confusion, lethargy, and an absence of focal neurologic findings. Patients may have a sore throat and nonpurulent conjunctivitis. The characteristic rash is a diffuse sunburn-like erythroderma, which between days 3 and 7 desquamates, leading to epidermal sloughing that is readily noticed on the palms and soles. Hypotension is associated with peripheral and pulmonary edema in the absence of an elevated central venous pressure.

3. **Differential diagnoses** include SSSS, TEN, streptococcal toxic shock–like syndrome, Kawasaki syndrome, meningococcemia, scarlet fever, and viral exanthems.

4. **Evaluation**

    a. **Laboratory studies**

        i. **CBC.** A CBC will reveal a mild nonhemolytic anemia, a moderate leukocytosis with a predominance of bands, and an early thrombocytopenia followed later by a thrombocytosis.

        ii. **Coagulation tests.** Mild prolongation of the prothrombin time and partial thromboplastin time may be observed (although clinically apparent bleeding is not).

        iii. **Serum biochemistry.** The blood urea nitrogen and creatinine levels are elevated in the presence of oliguria.

        iv. **Liver function tests.** Liver enzyme levels are elevated.

Infectious Disease Emergencies

Infectious Disease Emergencies

b. **Culture.** All probable and possible sources of infection should be cultured and Gram stained. *S. aureus* can be cultured from a wound or the vagina in 90% of patients. Rarely, a positive culture for *S. aureus* can be obtained from the blood.

c. **Serology.** Serum antibodies to TSST-1 are not detectable, but serology performed on an *S. aureus* isolate may be positive.

5. **Therapy.** Foreign objects (e.g., tampons, diaphragms, sponges, nasal packing) must be removed immediately, and hypotension or shock should be treated with fluids and electrolytes. Treatment with a **β-lactamase–resistant penicillin** or **cephalosporin** should be initiated immediately.

6. **Disposition.** Patients must be admitted to the ICU immediately. The mortality rate is 10% to 15%.

C. **Streptococcal toxic shock–like syndrome** is a life-threatening infectious syndrome characterized by fever, rash, rapidly progressive and destructive soft tissue infection, and hypotension.

1. **Discussion**

   a. **Etiology.** Streptococcal toxic shock–like syndrome is caused by *Streptococcus pyogenes*, a group A β-hemolytic streptococcus.

   b. **Pathogenesis.** Bacteremia is the pathogenic mechanism of the ensuing shock.

2. **Clinical features.** Streptococcal toxic shock–like syndrome presents in a fashion very similar to TSS except that the source of the soft tissue infection is exceedingly obvious.

3. **Differential diagnoses** include TSS, SSSS, and TEN.

4. **Evaluation.** Diagnosis is based on the clinical presentation and the dermatologic findings. Site and blood cultures will grow *S. pyogenes*.

5. **Therapy.** Antibacterial therapy must be effective against both *S. aureus* and *S. pyogenes* because until the culture results are available, the diagnosis cannot be made with absolute certainty on clinical grounds alone.

6. **Disposition.** All patients must be admitted to the ICU. In immunocompetent patients, the mortality rate is 30%; in immunocompromised patients, the mortality rate is 60% within 24 hours.

D. **Cellulitis** is a diffuse, spreading, acute inflammatory process affecting solid tissues and characterized by hyperemia, leukocytic infiltration, and edema without cellular necrosis or suppuration.

1. **Discussion**

   a. **Etiology.** *S. pyogenes* is the most common cause. Other less common causes include other serologic groups of β-hemolytic streptococci (B, C, and G), *S. aureus*, *P. multocida* (from cat or dog bites), *Aeromonas hydrophila* (from fresh water), *Vibrio vulnificus* (from warm salt water), and aerobic gram-negative bacilli (in patients with granulocytopenia, diabetic foot ulcers, or severe tissue ischemia).

   b. **Predisposing factors** include skin trauma or ulceration, preexisting infections (e.g., tinea pedis), scars (especially from saphenous vein removal), immunocompromise, and edema.

2. **Clinical features.** The major findings are local erythema and tenderness, often with lymphangitis and lymphadenopathy.

   a. The skin is hot, red, and edematous, and the borders of the lesions are usually indistinct. Peau d'orange and petechiae are frequently observed. Vesicles and bullae may develop and rupture. Occasionally, necrosis of the involved skin is noted. Rarely, there are large areas of ecchymosis.

   b. Systemic manifestations may include fever, chills, and tachycardia.

3. **Differential diagnoses** include erysipelas (spreading infection of the skin and mucous membranes that is usually observed on the face). The rash of **erysipelas** differs from that of cellulitis in that the raised margins are sharply demarcated.

4. **Evaluation.** The diagnosis depends mainly on the clinical findings.

   a. **Laboratory studies.** Leukocytosis is common.

   b. **Culture.** Culturing of the etiologic organism is difficult, even with aspiration or biopsy of the involved area, unless pus has formed or the wound is open. (One must also consider that a positive culture may be detecting a secondary pathogen.) Blood cultures are only occasionally positive.

5. Therapy
   a. **Supportive therapy**
      i. The affected area should be elevated and immobilized to help reduce the edema.
      ii. Cool, wet dressings should be applied to relieve local discomfort.
   b. **Antibacterial therapy**
      i. **Streptococcal cellulitis.** Penicillin is the drug of choice. Alternatives are erythromycin, clindamycin, or macrolides. Neutropenic patients should be started empirically on gentamicin and mezlocillin.
      ii. **Staphylococcal cellulitis.** Dicloxacillin is the drug of choice. Vancomycin, trimethoprim/sulfamethoxazole, or doxycycline should be considered if the infection is caused by a resistant strain (methicillin-resistant *S. aureus*).
      iii. ***P. multocida* cellulitis.** Penicillin is the drug of choice.
      iv. ***A. hydrophila* cellulitis.** An aminoglycoside should be used.
      v. ***V. vulnificus* cellulitis.** Tetracycline is the drug of choice.
      vi. **Recurrent cellulitis.** If the recurrent cellulitis affects a lower extremity, treatment for tinea pedis should be undertaken to eliminate a source of infection. If antifungal medication fails, or tinea is not present, recurrent cellulitis can be prevented by monthly administration of benzathine penicillin G, oral penicillin, or erythromycin.
6. **Complications** are rare but could be serious and include:
   a. Severe necrotizing subcutaneous infection
   b. Necrotizing fasciitis
   c. Bacteremia with or without metastatic foci
   d. Chronic lymphatic obstruction
   e. Chronic edema or elephantiasis
   f. Osteomyelitis underlying the infection or hematogenous spread.
E. **Lymphangitis** is an acute inflammation of the subcutaneous lymphatic channels.
   1. **Discussion**
      a. **Etiology.** *S. pyogenes* is the most common causative agent.
      b. **Pathogenesis.** The microbes usually enter the lymphatic channels from a wound or abrasion, or from a preexisting infection (e.g., a cellulitis).
   2. **Clinical features.** Red, warm, tender streaks extend proximally from a peripheral lesion toward regional lymph nodes, which may eventually also become enlarged and tender. Systemic manifestations (e.g., fever, chills, headache) may actually precede any obvious signs of cutaneous infection.
   3. **Differential diagnoses** include erythema marginatum (rheumatic fever), cutaneous larva migrans, and erythema chronicum migrans (Lyme disease).
   4. **Evaluation.** Diagnosis is clinical. Leukocytosis may be present.
   5. **Therapy.** Most patients respond readily to appropriate antibiotic therapy (e.g., penicillin for streptococcal infections, cephalosporin for staphylococcal infections). In addition, rest, elevation, and dressings will improve healing.

VII. BONE INFECTIONS (OSTEOMYELITIS)

A. **Discussion.** Osteomyelitis is microbial invasion and destruction of bone. The elderly, intravenous drug abusers, patients with sickle cell disease, and immunocompromised patients are at the most risk.
   1. **Etiology**
      a. *S. aureus* is the most common cause of osteomyelitis in adults.
      b. *P. aeruginosa* and *Serratia marcescens* are more frequently implicated in intravenous drug abusers.
      c. *Salmonella* infection is associated with osteomyelitis in patients with sickle cell disease.
   2. **Pathogenesis.** Infection can occur by hematogenous spread, by direct extension, from a retropharyngeal abscess, or by direct contamination.
B. **Clinical features.** Typical findings are fever and bone pain, but these symptoms occur in only approximately 50% of patients. Localized tenderness over the affected area of the bone or joint that is not relieved by rest is another major sign.
C. **Differential diagnoses** include malignancy, degenerative joint disease, and trauma.

D. **Evaluation**

1. **Laboratory studies.** An elevated erythrocyte sedimentation rate and C-reactive protein are typically found. The WBC count is also commonly elevated.

2. **Culture.** Blood cultures are positive in approximately 50% to 60% of patients.

3. **Imaging studies**

   a. **Plain radiographs** do not usually show the classic findings of lytic lesions, periosteal elevation, and cortical irregularity or destruction until 7 to 14 days after the onset of symptoms.

   b. **CT scans** and **magnetic resonance imaging scans** are more sensitive than radiographs. Magnetic resonance imaging is the best imaging technique, with a sensitivity of 96%, a specificity of 92%, and an accuracy of 94%. **Bone scan** may be used to help localize bone involvement but it is not specific to infection, as cancer and fractures may cause positive result.

4. **Bone biopsy or aspiration** is necessary to make the diagnosis if blood cultures are negative.

E. **Therapy.** The current regimen is 4 to 6 weeks of parenteral antibiotic therapy followed by a prolonged course of oral antibiotics. Because a wide variety of organisms can cause osteomyelitis, proper identification of the causative organism by blood cultures or bone biopsy is essential.

F. **Disposition.** All patients must be admitted to the hospital for administration of antibiotics and immobilization. An orthopedic or neurosurgical evaluation should always be sought.

VIII. OTHER INFECTIONS

A. **Parasitic infections**

1. **Discussion.** The incidence of parasitic disease is increasing in the United States due to immigration from other countries, increased travel, and an increase in immunosuppression caused by HIV.

2. **Clinical entities**

   a. **Ascariasis** is caused by *Ascaris lumbricoides*. The larvae hatch from ingested eggs and migrate through the bloodstream to the lungs, causing **fever**, **cough**, **dyspnea**, **hemoptysis**, and **eosinophilia**.

   b. **Pinworm infection** is caused by *Enterobius vermicularis* (Figure 6-7). The eggs hatch in the cecum, appendix, ileum, and ascending colon. The gravid

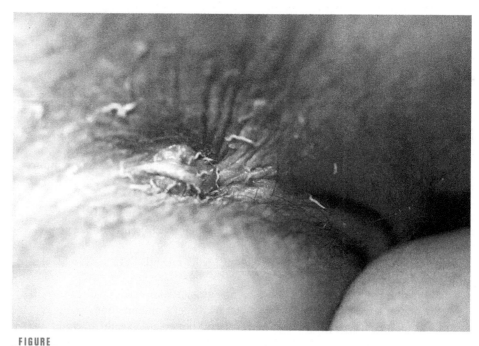

FIGURE
6-7 **Pinworm.**
(Courtesy of Lawrence B. Stack, MD.)

female migrates to the anus (usually at night), where it causes an intense pruritus (**pruritus ani**).

c. **Hookworm infection** is caused by *Necator americanus*, which is prevalent in Southern climates. Infection is associated with human waste used as fertilizer and the lack of shoes and latrines. Because each worm feeds on 0.03 to 0.2 mL of blood per day, chronic infection leads to **chronic anemia**, especially in children. Patients may present with a **cough, low-grade fever, abdominal pain, diarrhea, weakness, weight loss, guaiac-positive stools, and eosinophilia.**

d. **Threadworm infection** is caused by *Strongyloides stercoralis*, which infests the mucosa of the small intestine. The parasite invades the body by penetrating the skin, leading to **pruritus** and an **erythematous rash (cutaneous larval migrans)**. As the worms migrate through the lungs to the gastrointestinal tract, they also cause **cough, dyspnea,** and **pneumonia.** After they reach the intestine, they produce **abdominal pain** and **bloody mucoid diarrhea.** Fatalities have occurred in elderly and immunocompromised patients.

e. **Whipworm infection** is caused by *Trichuris trichiura*, a parasite most often found in rural communities in the United States. Children may become infected when playing in soil contaminated by ova. The adult worm resides in the cecum, causing **anorexia, insomnia, abdominal pain, fever, flatulence, diarrhea, weight loss, pruritus, eosinophilia, and microcytic hypochromic anemia.** *Trichuris* infestation can result in **colitis** and **rectal prolapse** in children.

f. **Trichinellosis** is caused by *Trichinella*. Transmission is by the ingestion of infected pork, beef, or walrus meat. Symptoms depend on the number of worms ingested, the number of larvae produced, and the site of invasion, although the primary lesions are in striated muscle; clinical manifestations include **acute myocarditis, nonsuppurative meningitis, bronchopneumonia,** or **catarrhal enteritis.** Patients may present with nausea and vomiting, diarrhea, fever, urticaria, periorbital edema (which is pathognomonic), splinter hemorrhages, myalgia, muscle spasms, a stiff neck, headache, and psychiatric disorders.

g. **Schistosomiasis** is caused by *Schistosoma*. The parasite penetrates the skin, creating a maculopapular rash, and the adult parasites then reside in the venous system.

   i. **Acute disease (Katayama fever)** is severe but rarely seen; **lymphadenopathy** and **hepatosplenomegaly** are characteristic.

   ii. **Chronic disease.** More typically, patients present in the chronic state with granulomas in the liver (leading to portal hypertension) and bladder (leading to obstructive hydroureter). Patients may present with **diarrhea, abdominal pain, melena, hepatosplenomegaly, hematemesis, ascites, and liver failure.** With *S. haematobium* infection, **dysuria** and **hematuria** may be found.

h. **Tapeworm infections** are caused by *Taenia solium* (pork tapeworm), *Taenia saginata* (beef tapeworm), and *Diphyllobothrium latum* (fish tapeworm).

   i. **Pork tapeworm** is indigenous to Central America and the Middle East. *T. solium* larvae may encyst in the subcutaneous tissues, eye, brain, and heart, causing **seizures, myocarditis, periorbital edema,** and sometimes morbidity.

   ii. **Beef tapeworm** is more common. Adult worms live in the small intestine. Infected patients can present with **nausea, vomiting, headache, abdominal pain, pruritus, constipation, diarrhea, and intestinal obstruction,** or they may be **asymptomatic.**

   iii. **Fish tapeworm.** Consumption of raw or undercooked fish (e.g., sushi; sashimi; pickled, salted, or smoked fish) is the most common method of transmission to humans. The parasite resides in the intestine and absorbs vitamin B_{12}, causing a **pernicious anemia.**

i. **Amebiasis** is caused by *E. histolytica*. The amoebae inhabit the cecum and large intestine, causing ulcers and diffuse inflammation that generally mimic ulcerative colitis. A total of 50% of infected patients are **asymptomatic**; the remaining 50% may experience **nausea, vomiting, anorexia, diarrhea, fever, abdominal pain, and leukocytosis.** Rarely, amebiasis can develop in the liver and produce an abscess.

j. **Giardiasis** is caused by *Giardia lamblia* and is the most common parasitic intestinal infection in the United States. Cysts are ingested in fecally contaminated water or are passed by hand-to-mouth transmission; once ingested, the parasite inhabits the host's duodenum and upper jejunum. Symptoms include **explosive, foul-smelling diarrhea, flatus, abdominal distention, fatigue, fever, weight loss, and malaise.**

k. **Trypanosomiasis** is caused by *Trypanosoma* species.
    i. *T. cruzi*, the American variety, causes **Chagas disease.** The acute phase of illness can last 2 to 3 months and consists of **fever, headache, anorexia, conjunctivitis, and myocarditis.** Infants can develop **meningoencephalitis**, and heart involvement can lead to **congestive heart failure** and **ventricular aneurysms.** The organism can attack the myenteric plexus of the gastrointestinal tract, resulting in **megacolon.**
    ii. *T. brucei rhodesiense* and *T. brucei gambiense*, the African varieties, cause **sleeping sickness.**

3. **Differential diagnoses** include bacterial or viral infection, collagen vascular disease, and neoplasia.

4. **Evaluation** is mainly by **fecal analysis** and **serology.**
    a. **Ascariasis** is diagnosed by finding eggs of the adult worm in the stool sample. Serologic tests (e.g., bentonite flocculation, ELISA, indirect hemagglutination) may also be useful.
    b. **Pinworm infection** is diagnosed by finding eggs or worms on a cellophane tape swab of the anus. Accuracy is improved by examination and testing in the early morning.
    c. **Hookworm infection** is diagnosed by finding ova in the stool sample.
    d. **Threadworm infection** is diagnosed by finding ova in a stool sample or a duodenal aspirate.
    e. **Whipworm infection** is diagnosed by finding ova in the stool sample.
    f. **Trichinellosis** is characterized by leukocytosis, eosinophilia, elevated serum creatine phosphokinase levels, and nonspecific electrocardiogram charges. The diagnosis can be confirmed with a latex agglutination skin test and a complement fixation or bentonite flocculation test (available from the Centers for Disease Control). ELISA is very sensitive and specific after the third week, and biopsy of tender muscle may be helpful after the fourth week of infection.
    g. **Schistosomiasis** is diagnosed by observing eggs in the feces or on rectal biopsy.
    h. **Tapeworm infection, amebiasis,** and **giardiasis** are diagnosed by ova and parasite stool examination and ELISA.
    i. **Chagas disease** is characterized by anemia, leukocytosis, an elevated erythrocyte sedimentation rate, and electrocardiogram changes (PR- and R-wave changes, heart block, arrhythmias).

5. **Therapy**
    a. **Ascariasis, pinworms,** and **hookworms** are treated with **mebendazole** or **pyrantel pamoate.**
    b. **Whipworms** and **trichinellosis** are treated with **mebendazole.**
    c. **Threadworms** are treated with **thiabendazole.**
    d. **Schistosomiasis** and **tapeworms** are treated with **praziquantel.**
    e. **Amebiasis** is treated with **metronidazole** followed by **iodoquinol.**
    f. **Giardiasis** can be treated with **quinacrine** or **metronidazole.**
    g. **Chagas disease** is treated with **nifurtimox.**

6. **Disposition.** Most parasitic infections are treated on an outpatient basis, although complications such as dehydration secondary to gastritis or myocardial involvement may require inpatient therapy for supportive care.

B. **Tick-borne disease**
    1. **Lyme disease**
        a. **Discussion.** Lyme disease, caused by the spirochete *B. burgdorferi*, is the most frequently transmitted tick-borne disease. It is prevalent in 33 of the 50 states, with the highest incidence in the Northeast. The majority of cases occur in the late spring and late summer.

CLINICAL PEARL | 6-6

Lyme Disease Stages

1. **Stage I** is characterized by **erythema chronicum migrans** (an annular lesion) and **flu-like symptoms** of fever, chills, headache, malaise, and weakness. Symptoms appear 3 to 32 days after the tick bite.
2. **Stage II** begins 4 weeks later. Ten percent of untreated patients develop **neurologic disorders** (e.g., headache, meningoencephalitis, facial nerve palsy, radiculoneuropathy) and **cardiac disease** (e.g., first-, second-, or third-degree atrioventricular block).
3. **Stage III** occurs in 60% of patients with untreated Lyme disease several weeks or years after infection. Patients develop **migratory polyoligoarthritis** that most often involves the knee, shoulder, and elbow.

    b. **Clinical features.** Lyme disease has three stages (see Clinical Pearl 6-6).
    c. **Differential diagnoses** include viral syndromes, connective tissue disease, Guillain-Barré syndrome, and rheumatoid arthritis.
    d. **Evaluation.** Diagnosis is best made by careful history and physical examination.
        i. **Laboratory studies.** The erythrocyte sedimentation rate is usually elevated and the lymphocyte count slightly decreased.
    e. **Treatment**
        i. **Tick removal.** If the patient presents with stage I symptoms, a careful search for the tick should ensue. The tick is best removed by grasping the head with forceps and gently pulling it away from the skin (see Clinical Pearl 6-7).
        ii. **Antibacterial therapy**
            a) **Adults and nonpregnant women.** Treatment is with **doxycycline** (100 mg orally twice daily for 10 to 21 days).
            b) **Children, allergic patients, and pregnant women. Amoxicillin** (40 mg/kg/day three times daily), **penicillin**, or **erythromycin** (30 to 50 mg/kg/day five times daily for children) can be used.
            c) **Patients with stage II disease.** For patients with severe neurologic or cardiac symptoms, **ceftriaxone** (1 g intravenously every 12 hours for 10 to 14 days) is recommended.
    f. **Disposition.** Lyme disease can usually be treated on an outpatient basis, regardless of the stage of disease.
  2. **Rocky Mountain spotted fever**
    a. **Discussion.** Rocky Mountain spotted fever, caused by *Rickettsia rickettsii*, is the second most common tick-borne disease. Rocky Mountain spotted fever occurs primarily in the Northwest United States but has also been reported in the Southern and Eastern states.
        i. **Incidence.** There are 500 to 1,000 cases annually. Peak incidence occurs from late spring to early fall.
    b. **Clinical features.** Rocky Mountain spotted fever has a wide clinical spectrum. The triad of fever, headache, and rash is seen in 55% to 65% of patients.
        i. Initial symptoms are fever, followed by an erythematous, maculopapular, blotchy rash that ultimately becomes petechial. The rash is present in

CLINICAL PEARL | 6-7

Prophylaxis for Lyme Disease

All inclusion criteria should be met.
1. Correct tick: identified as Ixodes
2. Correct time: >36 hours attached and engorged tick and/or <72 hours since removal
3. Correct location: endemic area = Northeast United States, some of Midwest and Pacific Northwest
If criteria met, doxycycline 200 mg by mouth once.

75% to 80% of patients, begins at the flexor surfaces of the wrists and ankles, and spreads centripetally.

    ii. Other symptoms are vomiting (66% of patients), myalgia (85% of patients), cough (33% of patients), and signs of meningoencephalitic involvement (25% of patients).

  c. **Evaluation.** The diagnosis of Rocky Mountain spotted fever is difficult. In addition to the physical examination and history, **immunofluorescent antibody staining or polymerase chain reaction** can be performed on a skin biopsy specimen obtained from an area of rash.

  d. **Therapy** for Rocky Mountain spotted fever is **tetracycline** (10 to 70 mg/kg given intravenously in one dose for 10 days for adults and children older than 8 years) or **chloramphenicol** (80 mg/kg given intravenously in one dose for children younger than 8 years).

  e. **Disposition.** Patients usually require admission.

3. **Tick paralysis**

  a. **Discussion.** Tick paralysis is a relatively uncommon tick-borne disease resulting in an ascending paralysis.

    i. **Incidence.** Incidence is highest in late spring to late summer and is higher in girls than in boys. The mortality rate in untreated cases may exceed 12%.

    ii. **Pathogenesis.** Tick paralysis is believed to be caused by a venom secreted from the female tick salivary glands during feeding—most probably a neurotoxin that produces a block of the peripheral motor nerve endplate, resulting in a failure of acetylcholine release at the neuromuscular junction.

  b. **Clinical features.** Symptoms of tick paralysis develop within 4 to 7 days and consist of **restlessness** and **paresthesias of the hands or feet**. Within 1 to 2 days, the presenting symptoms are followed by a **symmetric, ascending, flaccid paralysis** accompanied by **loss of deep tendon reflexes**. Death can result from respiratory paralysis.

  c. **Evaluation.** Tick paralysis is diagnosed by symptoms and discovery of the tick.

  d. **Therapy.** Tick paralysis is treated by tick removal.

  e. **Disposition.** Admission to the hospital may be required if the patient's symptoms are severe.

4. **Relapsing fever**

  a. **Discussion.** Relapsing fever is an uncommon acute recurrent febrile illness caused by a spirochete of the *Borrelia* species. It is isolated to the Western and Southwestern United States, with peak incidence in the summer months.

  b. **Clinical features.** After an incubation period of 5 to 9 days, individuals with **relapsing fever** may experience a febrile episode lasting 3 days, followed by an afebrile period and a return of fever. The fever is accompanied by **chills, malaise, vomiting, headache, and myalgias.** Splenomegaly (40% of patients), hepatomegaly (20% of patients), and neurologic involvement (10% of patients) may also be noted.

  c. **Evaluation.** There are no helpful serologic tests for relapsing fever, but peripheral blood smears show spirochetes in up to 70% of patients. Clinical presentation usually points to the diagnosis.

  d. **Therapy.** Relapsing fever is treated with **tetracycline** (500 mg orally four times daily for 10 days) or **erythromycin** (250 mg orally four times daily for 10 days).

  e. **Disposition.** Admission to the hospital may be required if the patient's symptoms are severe.

5. **Q fever** is caused by *Coxiella burnetii* and presents as a flu-like illness characterized by fever, myalgias, headache, and cough. Q fever is diagnosed by complement fixing antibody titers and clinical presentation. The flu-like syndrome resolves spontaneously in 2 to 4 weeks, but treatment is with tetracycline. Hospital admission may be required in the presence of severe symptoms.

6. **Tularemia**
   a. **Discussion.** Tularemia is caused by the bacterium *Francisella tularensis*. Although it was originally thought that tularemia was spread by rabbits and rabbit meat, it is now recognized that ticks are the most frequent vector. Peak incidence occurs in the summer months; most cases occur in the Southern and Midwestern states.
   b. **Clinical features.** Tularemia has two major presentations.
      i. **Ulceroglandular tularemia** is the most common (occurring in approximately 50% of patients) and presents as lymphadenopathy, fever, and reddened nodules that indurate and then ulcerate.
      ii. **Typhoidal tularemia** presents with fever, chills, debility, abdominal pain, diarrhea, anorexia, and weight loss.
   c. **Evaluation.** Tularemia is diagnosed on the basis of history and physical examination findings. Acute specific agglutination titers greater than 1:160 are diagnostic.
   d. **Therapy.** Tularemia is treated with **streptomycin** (30 to 40 mg/kg given in one dose for 4 to 7 days). **Tetracycline** (50 to 60 mg/kg given in four divided doses daily for 14 days) is an alternative for patients who are sensitive to streptomycin.
   e. **Disposition.** Hospital admission is usually required.
7. **Babesiosis**
   a. **Discussion.** Babesiosis is caused by *Babesia*, an intraerythrocytic protozoal parasite that causes a malaria-like syndrome. The distribution is similar to that of Lyme disease; in fact, the two entities have been seen concurrently in the same patient. Babesiosis was originally reported in only splenectomized individuals, but since 1969, there has been an increased incidence in all patients.
   b. **Clinical features.** Babesiosis has a broad range of clinical presentations, from a brief febrile illness to severe disease characterized by hemolytic anemia, hemoglobinuria, and death.
      i. Fever, malaise, anorexia, and fatigue are almost universally present. Headache and mild to moderate hemolytic anemia are also commonly seen.
      ii. The physical examination is usually nonspecific, although splenomegaly is seen in 40% of patients.
   c. **Evaluation.** Thick and thin Giemsa-stained blood smears will usually show intraerythrocytic organisms. A presumptive diagnosis can also be made by using indirect immunofluorescent staining for antibody if the titers are greater than 1:256.
   d. **Therapy**
      i. **Antibacterial therapy.** Babesiosis can be treated with **clindamycin** (600 mg orally twice daily for adults; 20 to 30 mg/kg/day every 6 hours for children) and **quinine** (650 mg orally twice daily for adults; 25 mg/kg/day every 8 hours for children) for 14 days.
      ii. **Exchange transfusion** has been effective in severe cases.
   e. **Disposition.** Hospital admission is indicated for patients with severe disease.
8. **Colorado tick fever**
   a. **Discussion.** Colorado tick fever is caused by an orbivirus of the family Reoviridae. Only 200 cases are reported annually.
   b. **Clinical features.** Patients develop the sudden onset of fever, headache, lethargy, myalgias, and anorexia within 3 to 6 days of exposure.
   c. **Evaluation** is by the clinical presentation and history.
   d. **Therapy.** Colorado tick fever is a self-limited disease. Patients usually recover in 3 weeks and treatment is supportive.
   e. **Disposition.** Patients with severe symptoms may require hospital admission.

Infectious Disease Emergencies

I. SODIUM IMBALANCE

A. **Hyponatremia**

1. **Discussion**

a. **Definition.** Serum sodium level <135 mEq/L

i. **True hyponatremia.** Serum sodium concentration <125 mEq/L *and* a serum osmolality <250 mOsm/kg

ii. **Pseudohyponatremia.** Secondary to severe hyperglycemia, hyperproteinemia, or hyperlipidemia. Serum sodium level is decreased but the total body sodium level is unchanged.

b. **Causes**

i. **Hypovolemic hyponatremia**

a) **Extrarenal losses.** Hypovolemic hyponatremia as a result of extrarenal sodium loss, urinary sodium level <20 mEq/L.

b) **Renal losses.** Hypovolemic hyponatremia as a result of renal sodium loss, the urinary sodium level >20 mEq/L.

ii. **Euvolemic hyponatremia.** Occurs due to an increase in total body water; the *total body sodium level is normal.* Hypothyroidism and the syndrome of inappropriate antidiuretic hormone are causes of euvolemic hyponatremia.

iii. **Hypervolemic hyponatremia.** Occurs with renal failure, cirrhosis, congestive heart failure, and nephrotic syndrome

2. **Clinical features.** The influx of water into brain cells may lead to apathy, agitation, headaches, altered consciousness, seizures, coma, weakness, nausea, anorexia, and vomiting.

3. **Differential diagnoses.** Includes **pseudohyponatremia**, which can be caused by diabetic ketoacidosis and a hyperosmolar state (leading to hyperglycemia), multiple myeloma (leading to hyperproteinemia), or hypertriglyceridemia (leading to hyperlipidemia)

4. **Evaluation**

a. **Laboratory studies.** Include a serum electrolyte panel (i.e., sodium, potassium, chloride, and bicarbonate); serum glucose, blood urea nitrogen [BUN], and creatinine levels; and urinalysis (to determine the urine sodium level and osmolality)

b. **Electrocardiography.** An electrocardiogram (ECG) should be obtained to evaluate for arrhythmia.

5. **Therapy**

a. **Fluid restriction** or **replacement**

i. **Hypervolemic** and **euvolemic hyponatremia** usually result from hemodilution; **fluid restriction** is the initial treatment in stable, asymptomatic patients. Inhibition of water reabsorption caused by syndrome of inappropriate antidiuretic hormone can be treated on an inpatient basis using demeclocycline (600 to 1,200 mg/day) or furosemide.

ii. **Hypovolemic hyponatremia** can usually be treated with **isotonic saline.**

Quick HIT

Sweating, vomiting, diarrhea, and third-space sequestration (e.g., as a result of burns, peritonitis, or pancreatitis) are common sources of extrarenal sodium loss.

Quick HIT

Loop or osmotic diuretics, Addison disease, ketonuria, and renal tubular acidosis are sources of renal sodium loss.

Quick HIT

Syndrome of inappropriate antidiuretic hormone is associated with tumors, central nervous system (CNS) disease, pulmonary disease, hypopituitarism, medications, idiopathic causes, and a reset osmostat.

b. **Sodium replacement.** Sodium deficits can be calculated as follows:

Na^+ deficit (mEq) $= 0.6 \times$ (weight kg) $\times (140 -$ serum $Na^+)$

  i. If the hyponatremia is acute, is severe (i.e., the serum sodium level is less than 120 mEq/L), and results in CNS symptoms, administration of **3% (hypertonic) saline solution** at 25 to 60 mL/hour is indicated.

    a) The serum sodium concentration should not increase at a rate that exceeds 2 mEq/hour.

    b) Hypertonic saline should be discontinued when sodium levels increase to 120 mEq/L or when the patient shows significant clinical improvement.

  ii. In patients with chronic severe hyponatremia, the rate of serum sodium correction should not exceed 0.5 mEq/L/hour (12 mEq/L/day). If the hyponatremia is severe (i.e., serum sodium levels less than 120 mEq/L) **and develops rapidly** with CNS manifestations, 3% saline should be administered.

6. **Disposition**

  a. **Admission.** Symptomatic patients, serum sodium concentration below 125 mEq/L (with or without symptoms), patients who require intravenous or pharmacologic correction of the sodium imbalance, and patients who have significant comorbid factors (e.g., diabetes, advanced age, sepsis)

  b. **Discharge.** If the patient is being discharged, the case should be discussed with a primary care physician and a follow-up appointment should take place within 48 to 72 hours.

B. **Hypernatremia**

1. **Discussion**

  a. **Definition.** Serum sodium levels greater than 155 mEq/L

  b. **Causes**

    i. **Reduced water intake** can be caused by a defective thirst mechanism, unconsciousness, an inability to drink, or a lack of access to water.

    ii. **Increased water loss** can be caused by vomiting, diarrhea, sweating, fever, hyperventilation, diabetes insipidus, osmotic diuresis, thyrotoxicosis, and severe burns.

    iii. **Increased sodium intake** or **renal salt retention** is due to hypertonic saline ingestion or infusion, sodium bicarbonate administration, hyperaldosteronism, Cushing disease, and congenital adrenal hyperplasia.

2. **Clinical features**

  a. **Symptoms.** Confusion, weakness, muscle irritability, tremulousness, seizures, and coma

  b. **Physical examination findings.** Flat neck veins, orthostatic hypotension, tachycardia, poor skin turgor, dry mucous membranes, tonic spasms, and respiratory paralysis

3. **Evaluation**

  a. **Laboratory studies** should include a complete blood count (CBC); serum electrolyte panel; serum glucose, BUN, and creatinine levels; urinalysis, urine sodium level, and osmolality.

  b. **Electrocardiography.** An ECG should be obtained.

4. **Therapy**

  a. **Fluid replacement.** The amount of water needed to correct hypernatremia can be estimated as follows:

Water deficit (L) $= 0.6 \times$ (usual body weight in kg) $\times$ (measured Na^+ concentration $-$ desired Na^+ concentration) / measured Na^+ concentration

    i. When dehydration is severe, normal saline or lactated Ringer solution should be administered to improve blood pressure and tissue perfusion.

    ii. Once perfusion is reestablished, 0.45% saline is administered to maintain a urine output of 0.5 mL/kg/hour.

  b. **Sodium reduction.** The rate of sodium reduction should not exceed 10 to 15 mEq/L/day. The goal is to reach a normal serum sodium value in 48 to 72 hours.

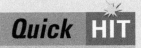

Quick HIT

Correcting the sodium deficiency too quickly could cause central pontine myelinolysis.

Quick HIT

Hypocalcemia, which is frequently seen in patients with hypernatremia, may contribute to the neurologic symptoms.

Metabolic Emergencies

5. **Disposition**
   a. **Admission.** Symptomatic patients, serum sodium concentration greater than 160 mEq/L (with or without symptoms), patients who require intravenous or pharmacologic correction of the sodium imbalance, and patients who have significant comorbid factors require admission.
   b. **Discharge.** Before discharging a patient, the case should be discussed with a primary care physician and arrangements should be made for appropriate follow-up.

II. POTASSIUM IMBALANCE
A. **Hypokalemia**
1. **Discussion**
   a. **Definition.** Most common electrolyte abnormality, serum potassium level that is less than 3.5 mEq/L
   b. **Causes**
      i. **Extrarenal causes.** Inadequate dietary intake, diarrhea, vomiting, and redistribution (e.g., as a result of insulin administration, epinephrine infusion, or acute alkalemia)
      ii. **Renal causes**
         a) **Drug-induced renal losses.** Loop diuretics, penicillin, aminoglycosides, and amphotericin B
         b) **Hormone-induced renal losses.** Can occur as a result of primary adrenal adenomas, adrenal hyperplasia, ectopic adrenocorticotropic hormone syndrome, renin-secreting tumors, renal artery stenosis, and malignant hypertension
         c) **Renal tubular acidosis, Bartter syndrome,** or **chronic magnesium depletion** can also lead to hypokalemia.
2. **Clinical features**
   a. **Symptoms.** Weakness, paresthesias, and polyuria
   b. **Physical examination findings.** Areflexia, orthostatic hypotension, ileus, paralysis, and arrhythmias
3. **Evaluation**
   a. **Laboratory studies** should include a serum electrolyte panel; serum BUN, creatinine, creatinine phosphokinase, phosphate, magnesium, and glucose levels; and urinalysis.
      i. **Serum evaluation** may show elevated creatinine phosphokinase levels.
      ii. **Urinalysis.** The urine specimen may be dipstick-positive for red blood cells. Formal urinalysis may reveal myoglobin, consistent with rhabdomyolysis.
   b. **Electrocardiography.** ECG findings include T-wave flattening or inversion, U waves (Figure 7-1), ST-segment depression, premature ventricular contractions, and a wide QRS complex.
4. **Therapy**
   a. **Potassium replacement**
      i. Serum potassium level is greater than 2.5 mEq/L, no ECG abnormalities; 40 to 80 mEq of potassium chloride should be administered per day until the imbalance is corrected, with no more than 40 mEq given as a single dose.
      ii. Severe hypokalemia, potassium level less than 2.5 mEq/L, is treated by infusing 10 mEq of potassium chloride per hour in 50 to 100 mL of 5% dextrose in water or normal saline by intravenous piggyback for 3 to 4 hours.
         a) No more than 40 mEq of potassium should ever be put in a single liter of intravenous fluid, and no more than 10 mEq should be given per hour.
         b) Continuous cardiac monitoring is required.
   b. **Magnesium replacement** with 2 g of magnesium sulfate in 50 mL of 5% dextrose in water administered over 20 minutes may be necessary.

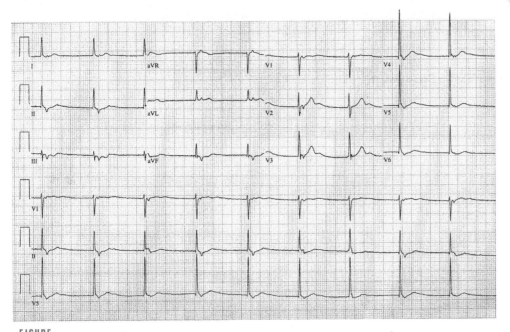

FIGURE
7-1 Electrocardiogram with U waves.

   c. **Phosphate replacement.** If the serum phosphate level is low, potassium phosphate may be used instead of potassium chloride. The recommended daily dose is 2.5 mg/kg.

5. **Disposition**
   a. **Admission**
     i. Patients with serum potassium concentrations of less than 2.5 mEq/L require admission to the hospital.
     ii. Patients with malignant cardiac dysrhythmias, digitalis toxicity, profound weakness with impending respiratory failure, rhabdomyolysis, hepatic encephalopathy, or a serum potassium level of less than 2.0 mEq/L require admission to the intensive care unit.
   b. **Discharge.** Patients with mild hypokalemia (serum potassium concentration = 2.5 to 3.5 mEq/L) can usually be managed as outpatients with gradual oral potassium repletion, provided they do not have ECG abnormalities, profound muscular weakness, ileus, or other serious effects. Patients who are discharged on oral supplementation should have a follow-up appointment within 48 to 72 hours.

B. **Hyperkalemia**
1. **Discussion**
   a. **Definition.** Serum potassium level that exceeds 5.5 mEq/L
   b. **Causes**
     i. **Extrarenal causes.** Insulin deficiency, acidemia, hyperosmolality, β blocker administration, oral or intravenous potassium supplements, penicillin potassium salts, massive blood transfusion, crush injuries, burns, mesenteric or muscular infarction, and tumor lysis syndrome.
     ii. **Renal causes.** Chronic renal insufficiency, acute renal failure, hypoaldosteronism, and drugs (e.g., nonsteroidal anti-inflammatory drugs, cyclosporine, heparin, angiotensin-converting enzyme inhibitors, potassium-sparing diuretics) can also cause hyperkalemia.
     iii. **Laboratory error** is the most common cause of hyperkalemia.

2. **Clinical features**
   a. **Symptoms.** Include weakness, paresthesias, and confusion
   b. **Physical examination findings.** Paralysis, areflexia, ileus, respiratory insufficiency, or cardiac arrest

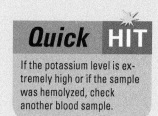

Metabolic Emergencies

3. **Differential diagnoses** include **pseudohyperkalemia**, which can occur as a result of hemolysis, extreme leukocytosis, acidosis, thrombocytosis, or cold agglutinins.

4. **Evaluation**
   a. **Laboratory studies** include a serum electrolyte panel, serum BUN, creatinine, glucose, and magnesium levels.
   b. **Electrocardiography.** The patient should be placed on a continuous cardiac monitor, and an ECG should be obtained. Early ECG findings include peaked T waves and a shortened QT interval. Later, widened QRS complexes, prolonged PR intervals, low-amplitude P waves, and elevation or depression of the ST segment are seen. Advanced changes include absent P waves, marked QRS complex widening, and tall T waves, resulting in a sine wave pattern, ventricular fibrillation, and asystole (Figure 7-2).

5. **Therapy**
   a. **Acute therapy**
      i. **Calcium chloride or calcium gluconate** is administered over 2 minutes and repeated in 5 to 10 minutes if necessary. By stabilizing cell membranes

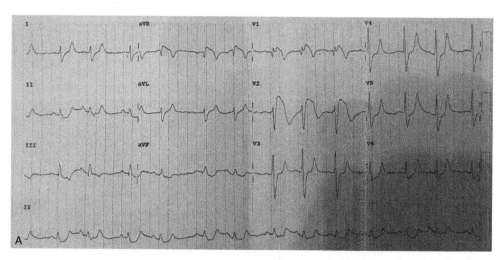

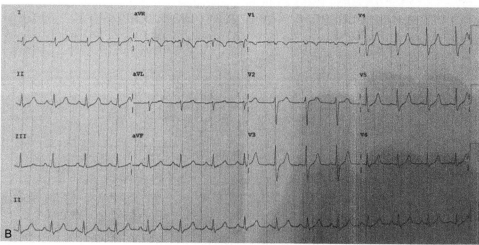

FIGURE 7-2 **(A) ECG findings of severe hyperkalemia. Peaked T waves with pseudoinfarction pattern. (B) Repeat ECG in the same patient after hyperkalemia treatment.**

(Used by permission of Martin Huecker, MD.)

without altering potassium levels, calcium protects the patient against malignant arrhythmia and is **the most important first step in treatment.** Calcium chloride should ideally be infused through a central line as it causes severe skin injury if accidentally infiltrated from peripheral intravenous lines.

  ii. **Sodium bicarbonate** (44 mEq [one ampule] administered intravenously over 5 minutes and repeated 10 to 15 minutes later if necessary) causes an intracellular influx of potassium. Onset of action occurs in approximately 15 minutes.

  iii. **Regular insulin** (10 to 20 U administered via an intravenous push) with **10% dextrose** (500 mL in water) administered over 1 hour, or 10 U of insulin administered via an intravenous push with one or two ampules (25 g) of 50% glucose administered over 5 minutes will lower potassium by causing an intracellular shift. Effects occur 30 to 60 minutes after administration.

  iv. **Furosemide, bumetanide,** and **acetazolamide** all increase potassium excretion.

  v. **Dialysis** should be considered for patients with severe hyperkalemia who have failed to respond to pharmacologic attempts at lowering the potassium level and for patients with acute or chronic renal failure.

  b. **Maintenance of potassium balance.** Potassium balance is maintained by:
    i. **Diuretics** and fludrocortisone
    ii. **Cation-exchange resins,** such as sodium polystyrene sulfonate
    iii. **Aldosterone,** either as **desoxycorticosterone acetate** or **fludrocortisone acetate**

6. Disposition
  a. **Admission.** When ECG abnormalities or clinical manifestations of hyperkalemia are present, admission to the intensive care unit with continuous cardiac monitoring is required.
  b. **Discharge.** Patients with mild serum potassium elevations in the absence of clinical and ECG abnormalities can be discharged, provided any identifiable predisposing factors have been corrected. Patients should have a follow-up evaluation within 48 to 72 hours.

III. CALCIUM IMBALANCE

A. Hypocalcemia
  1. Discussion
    a. **Definition.** Ionized calcium level below 2.0 mEq/L or a total serum level below 8.5 mg/dL.
    b. **Causes of hypocalcemia.** Shock, sepsis, renal failure, pancreatitis, hypomagnesemia, alkalosis, decreased serum albumin, hypoparathyroidism (idiopathic or as a result of irradiation or surgery), pseudohypoparathyroidism, osteoblastic metastasis, malabsorption, and excess phosphates.
  2. Clinical features
    a. **Symptoms.** Circumoral and distal extremity paresthesias, irritability, weakness, fatigue, muscle cramps, and seizures
    b. **Physical examination findings.** Hyperreflexia, carpopedal spasm, tetany, laryngospasm, Trousseau sign (carpopedal spasm after arterial occlusion of the arm for 3 minutes), and Chvostek sign (contraction of the facial muscles after percussion over the facial nerve)
  3. Evaluation
    a. **Laboratory studies** should include serum albumin, calcium, magnesium, phosphate, BUN, and creatinine levels; liver studies; amylase and lipase levels; ionized calcium levels; a serum electrolyte panel; and a CBC.
    b. **Electrocardiography.** ECG findings may include a prolonged QT interval, sinus bradycardia, complete heart block, ventricular arrhythmias, and ventricular fibrillation.
    c. **Radiology.** When hypocalcemia occurs in the context of osteomalacia, radiographic findings can include craniotabes, frontal skull bossing, rachitic

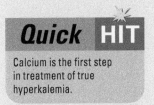

Quick HIT

Calcium is the first step in treatment of true hyperkalemia.

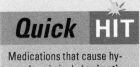

Quick HIT

Medications that cause hypocalcemia include **cimetidine, phosphate laxatives, phenytoin, phenobarbital, gentamicin, heparin, theophylline, loop diuretics,** and **glucocorticosteroids.**

Metabolic Emergencies

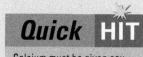

Quick HIT

Calcium must be given cautiously to patients receiving digitalis because calcium can worsen digoxin toxicity or cause sudden death.

rosary ribs, a widened rib cage (Harrison groove), bowed legs, demineralization, and thinning of the cortical bone.

4. **Therapy**
   a. **Acutely symptomatic hypocalcemia.** Administer 10 mL of 10% calcium gluconate infused intravenously over 10 to 15 minutes, followed by a maintenance infusion of 1 to 2 mg/kg/hour over 6 to 12 hours.
   b. **Asymptomatic.** Oral therapy with elemental calcium (with or without vitamin D) may be all that is required. The rapid intravenous administration of calcium to asymptomatic patients with mild to moderate hypocalcemia is contraindicated because doing so can cause severe cardiovascular, neuromuscular, or renal complications.

5. **Disposition**
   a. **Admission.** Patients with symptomatic hypocalcemia who require intravenous replacement therapy must be admitted to the hospital. These patients should be placed on continuous cardiac monitoring, and serial serum calcium levels should be obtained.
   b. **Discharge.** Asymptomatic patients may be discharged with appropriate follow-up.

B. **Hypercalcemia**
   1. **Discussion**
      a. **Definition.** Total calcium level exceeding 10.5 mg/dL or an ionized calcium level exceeding 2.7 mEq/L
      b. **Causes**
         i. **Endocrine causes.** Primary hyperparathyroidism, hyperthyroidism, pheochromocytoma, adrenal insufficiency, and acromegaly
         ii. **Malignancies.** Squamous cell carcinoma of the lung, breast cancer, kidney cancer, myeloma, and leukemia
         iii. **Granulomatous disorders.** Sarcoidosis, tuberculosis, histoplasmosis, and coccidioidomycosis
         iv. **Medications.** Excessive vitamin D or A intake, thiazides, lithium, and hormonal therapy for breast cancer can cause hypercalcemia.
         v. **Miscellaneous.** Immobilization, Paget disease, dehydration, excess calcium ingestion, and milk-alkali syndrome
   2. **Clinical features**
      a. **Signs and symptoms.** Weakness, depression, confusion, lethargy, personality changes, nausea, vomiting, anorexia, constipation, headache, and abdominal pain
      b. **Physical examination findings.** Dehydration, decreased motor strength, decreased mental status, ataxia, hyporeflexia, fractures, hypertension, weight loss, renal insufficiency, and cardiac arrest
   3. **Evaluation**
      a. **Laboratory studies** should include ionized calcium levels; serum calcium, protein, phosphate, magnesium, BUN, creatinine, glucose, amylase, and lipase levels; a serum electrolyte panel; and a CBC.
      b. **Electrocardiography.** ECG abnormalities include shortening of the QT interval, widening of T waves, bradyarrhythmias, bundle branch blocks, and second-degree and complete heart block.
   4. **Therapy.** Treatment is required for symptomatic patients with calcium levels greater than 12 mg/dL who are unable to maintain a good fluid intake or have abnormal renal function.
      a. **Fluid replacement.** Because patients with hypercalcemia are usually dehydrated, the initial and safest treatment is restoration of volume with large amounts of saline (5 to 10 L of normal saline in the first 24 hours).
      b. **Pharmacologic therapy**
         i. **Furosemide** (1 to 3 mg/kg) can be administered intravenously to enhance urinary output and increase renal excretion of calcium.
         ii. **Calcitonin** (2 to 4 IU/kg intramuscularly every 12 hours) diminishes calcium levels, usually within 12 hours. Calcitonin is useful for the initial treatment of symptomatic hypercalcemia greater than 14 mg/dL.

  iii. **Bisphosphonates** are used for longer term management of hypercalcemia related to bone resorption.

 c. **Dialysis.** Patients with severe symptoms and for patients with cardiac or renal disease

5. **Disposition.** Patients with a calcium level greater than 12 mg/dL, symptoms, or abnormal renal function require admission for continuous cardiac monitoring and serial calcium levels.

IV. MAGNESIUM IMBALANCE

A. Hypomagnesemia

 1. **Discussion.** Hypomagnesemia occurs when the serum magnesium concentration falls below 1.0 mEq/L.

 2. **Clinical features**

  a. **Symptoms.** Malaise, diffuse weakness, anorexia, nausea, vomiting, and seizures

  b. **Physical examination findings.** Mimic those of hypocalcemia, with nervous system complaints dominating the clinical picture. Chvostek sign, Trousseau sign, tremors, twitching, clonus, increased deep tendon reflexes, carpopedal spasm, frank tetany, delirium, movement disorders, and dysarthria

 3. **Evaluation**

  a. **Laboratory studies** include serum magnesium, calcium, BUN, creatinine, and glucose levels and a serum electrolyte panel.

  b. **Electrocardiography.** ECG findings include atrial and ventricular tachyarrhythmias, torsades de pointes, and a prolonged QT interval. Arrhythmias caused by hypomagnesemia may not respond to the usual antiarrhythmic therapy, but they may respond well to intravenous magnesium. Magnesium (2 g) should be administered rapidly over 2 minutes via an intravenous line to patients in pulseless ventricular tachycardia suspected of being hypomagnesemic (e.g., a patient with myocardial infarction who is taking diuretics).

  c. **Ancillary tests** (e.g., radiographs) may be required to diagnose the underlying cause.

 4. **Therapy**

  a. **Mild hypomagnesemia.** Oral supplementation. Magnesium hydroxide (200 to 600 mg, four times daily) is usually used.

  b. **Severe hypomagnesemia.** Marked neurologic manifestations or malignant ventricular arrhythmias is treated with 2 to 4 g of magnesium sulfate administered in 100 to 200 mL of 5% dextrose in water over 20 minutes. Additional treatment should be directed toward correcting the underlying cause of the hypomagnesemia.

 5. **Disposition.** Indications for admission include a serum magnesium level below 1 mEq/L, severe central neurologic manifestations, cardiac arrhythmias, and severe underlying disorders.

B. Hypermagnesemia

 1. **Discussion**

  a. **Definition.** Serum magnesium level greater than 2.5 mEq/L

  b. **Causes.** Because the kidney is efficient in excreting excess magnesium, hypermagnesemia is uncommon except in the presence of **renal failure or an iatrogenic cause.** Other causes of hypermagnesemia include rhabdomyolysis, tumor lysis, burns, tissue trauma, diabetic ketoacidosis, hypothyroidism, cathartic abuse, antacids, preeclampsia or eclampsia treatment, and adrenal insufficiency.

 2. **Clinical features**

  a. **Symptoms.** Nausea, vomiting, lethargy, mental confusion, and coma

  b. **Physical examination findings.** When magnesium level exceeds 4 mEq/L. Depression of the deep tendon reflexes, marked muscle weakness, bulbar paralysis, and respiratory insufficiency.

 3. **Evaluation**

  a. **Laboratory studies** include serum calcium, ionized calcium, BUN, and creatinine levels and a serum electrolyte panel.

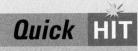

Quick HIT

Because only approximately 1% of the total body magnesium is sampled with a serum laboratory test, **patients with symptomatic hypomagnesemia may have normal or only minimally decreased serum magnesium levels.**

Metabolic Emergencies

b. **Electrocardiography.** Dysrhythmias and cardiac arrest can occur at serum magnesium levels exceeding 8 mEq/L, but the ECG manifestations of hypermagnesemia are variable and nonspecific.

4. **Therapy**

a. **Exogenous sources of magnesium should be removed.**

b. **Pharmacologic therapy**

i. **Calcium gluconate or calcium chloride.** Because calcium transiently reverses the effects of hypermagnesemia by acting as a direct antagonist, 10 mL of 10% calcium gluconate or calcium chloride solution can be given intravenously in symptomatic patients.

ii. **Furosemide.** In patients with normal renal function, brisk diuresis with intravenous normal saline and furosemide will enhance urinary magnesium excretion.

c. **Dialysis.** In patients with very high magnesium levels or in patients with renal failure, emergency peritoneal dialysis or hemodialysis may be required.

5. **Disposition.** Patients with magnesium levels above 8 mEq/L require admission to a monitored bed and should be considered for early dialysis. For patients with lower magnesium levels, admission depends on the underlying cause, the patient's hemodynamic status, and the presence of any comorbid factors (e.g., renal failure, cancer, psychiatric problems).

V. ACID–BASE IMBALANCE

A. **Normal physiology.** Acid–base balance refers to the maintenance of blood hydrogen ion concentration (see Clinical Pearl 7-1). The negative logarithm of this concentration, pH, is usually closely maintained between 7.35 and 7.45. Three homeostatic mechanisms maintain this balance:

1. **Buffer systems.** Soluble buffers mediate an immediate response to changes in pH. Carbonic acid, phosphoric acid, hemoglobin, and plasma proteins account for one-third of the body's buffering capacity. Intracellular tissue proteins are responsible for the remaining two-thirds.

2. **Respiratory mechanisms.** Through a respiratory response, changes in alveolar ventilation can promptly cause hydrogen ions to be excreted or retained by changing the concentration of components of the carbonic acid buffer system.

3. **Renal mechanisms** mediate a slow response to change in the total body hydrogen ion load by causing net excretion or production of hydrogen ions.

B. **Respiratory acidosis**

1. **Discussion**

a. **Definition.** Blood carbon dioxide tension (PCO_2) greater than 40 mm Hg and a decreased blood pH. It is associated with inadequate elimination of carbon dioxide by the lungs.

i. **Acute respiratory acidosis** is characterized by acute carbon dioxide retention leading to an increased PCO_2 but a minimal change in plasma bicarbonate concentration. For each 10 mm Hg increase in PCO_2, the plasma bicarbonate level increases 1 mEq/L and the blood pH decreases by 0.08.

ii. **Chronic respiratory acidosis** becomes apparent after 2 to 5 days. Renal compensation (i.e., increased hydrogen ion secretion and bicarbonate production in the distal nephron) is seen. For every 10 mm Hg increase

---

CLINICAL PEARL 7-1

Acid–Base Disturbances

1. **Respiratory acidosis:** PCO_2 >40 mm Hg and blood pH <7.35
2. **Respiratory alkalosis:** decreased PCO_2 and blood pH >7.45
3. **Metabolic acidosis:** plasma bicarbonate <24 and blood pH <7.35
4. **Metabolic alkalosis:** plasma bicarbonate decreased and blood pH >7.45

in P_{CO_2}, the plasma bicarbonate level increases 3 to 4 mEq/L and the blood pH decreases by 0.03.

b. **Causes** of respiratory acidosis include all disorders that reduce pulmonary function and carbon dioxide clearance: CNS lesions, sedative therapy and overdose, neuromuscular disorders (e.g., kyphoscoliosis, scleroderma, flail chest, rib fractures), pleural disease, obstructive airway disease (e.g., asthma, chronic obstructive pulmonary disease).

2. **Clinical features.** Respiratory acidosis may lead to symptoms of generalized CNS depression, reduced cardiac output, and pulmonary hypertension.

3. **Evaluation**

a. **Laboratory studies** should include an arterial blood gas (ABG), a serum electrolyte panel, BUN, creatinine, and glucose levels. It might also be useful to obtain urine drug screen results and a serum ethanol level.

b. **Electrocardiography** and **radiography** may be useful.

c. **Ancillary tests** (e.g., muscle biopsy) should take place outside of the emergency department.

4. **Therapy**

a. **Correction of the underlying cause** should be attempted. For example, in the case of drug-induced hypoventilation, vigorous attempts should be made to clear the offending agent from the body.

b. **Assisted ventilation.** A P_{CO_2} of more than 60 mm Hg may be an indication for assisted ventilation if CNS or pulmonary muscular depression is severe. Care must be taken not to normalize the P_{CO_2} in patients with chronic respiratory disturbances. Because renal compensatory mechanisms have already normalized the blood pH in these patients, rapid correction of the respiratory parameters can lead to a dangerous elevation of the blood pH.

C. **Respiratory alkalosis**

1. **Discussion**

a. **Definition.** Decreased P_{CO_2} and an increased pH. It is associated with excessive elimination of carbon dioxide by the lungs.

   i. **Acute respiratory alkalosis.** For each 10 mm Hg decrease in P_{CO_2}, the plasma bicarbonate level decreases by 2 mEq/L and the blood pH increases by 0.08. The serum chloride level also increases.

   ii. **Chronic respiratory alkalosis.** For each 10 mm Hg decrease in P_{CO_2}, the plasma bicarbonate level decreases by 5 to 6 mEq/L and the blood pH increases by 0.02. The serum chloride level also increases.

b. **Causes**

   i. **Anxiety** is the most common cause of respiratory alkalosis.

   ii. **Hypoxia** results in an increased respiratory rate and, thus, respiratory alkalosis.

   iii. **Primary pulmonary disorders** (e.g., pneumonia, asthma, pulmonary fibrosis, pulmonary embolism) lead to stimulation of the ventilatory rate, resulting in a low P_{CO_2}.

   iv. **Salicylate toxicity** initially causes overstimulation of the respiratory center, resulting in respiratory alkalosis.

   v. **CNS disorders** (e.g., cerebrovascular accident, tumor, infection, trauma) may be associated with inappropriate stimulation of ventilation.

   vi. **Pregnancy** and **progesterone therapy** cause an increase in respiratory rate, thereby decreasing the P_{CO_2}.

2. **Clinical features.** Acute alkalemia results in a generalized feeling of anxiety, severe obtundation, a tetany-like syndrome, and depressed cardiac function at a blood pH exceeding 7.73.

3. **Evaluation.** The ordering of tests should be directed toward finding the underlying cause. Some basic tests include an ABG, a CBC, a serum electrolyte panel, serum BUN and creatinine levels, a urine pregnancy test, liver studies, a salicylate level, a blood culture, and a chest radiograph.

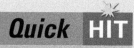

The anion gap is calculated from the electrolyte values: anion gap = $([Na^+] + [K^+]) - ([HCO_3^-] + [Cl^-])$. The normal range is 10 to 12 mEq/L.

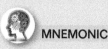

MNEMONIC

A Alcoholic Ketoacidosis
M Methanol
U Uremia
D DKA / starvation
P Paraldehyde / Propylene Glycol
I Iron / Isoniazid
L Lactic Acidosis
E Ethylene Glycol
C Cyanide, Carbon Monoxide
A Acetaminophen, Antiretrovirals (NRTI)
T Toluene

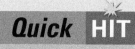

An anion gap greater than 35 mEq/L is usually caused by ethylene glycol, methanol, or lactic acidosis.

Quick HIT

The pH levels below 7.2 lead to decreased cardiac output, resistance to catecholamines, hypotension, and Kussmaul respiration (i.e., a rapid, regular, and deep respiratory rate).

4. **Therapy.** The primary goal of therapy is to correct the underlying cause. Most cases of respiratory alkalosis require no direct treatment.

D. **Metabolic acidosis**

1. **Discussion.** Decreased blood pH and a decreased plasma bicarbonate concentration (less than 24 mEq/L)

2. **Causes.** Metabolic acidosis is caused by the loss of bicarbonate or the accumulation of an acid other than carbonic acid (e.g., lactic acid). The causes of metabolic acidosis can be divided into those associated with a normal anion gap and those associated with an elevated anion gap. The gap represents anions that are present in the serum but are not routinely measured.

   a. **Anion gap metabolic acidosis.** The causes of an anion gap metabolic acidosis can be remembered using the mnemonic, "A MUDPILE CAT." The following are broad categories of disorders associated with anion gap metabolic acidosis:

      i. **Lactic acidosis** results from decreased oxygen delivery to tissues and is caused by conditions such as sepsis and shock. Lactic acidosis is the most common cause of anion gap metabolic acidosis.

      ii. **Ketoacidosis** is a condition characterized by increased ketone body formation that occurs as a complication of diabetes mellitus, prolonged starvation, and prolonged alcohol abuse.

      iii. **Renal failure** leads to an increased anion gap due to the accumulation of various organic and inorganic anions associated with a reduced glomerular filtration rate.

      iv. **Chemicals.** A variety of chemical substances (e.g., salicylates, methanol, ethylene glycol, paraldehyde, iron, isoniazid) can result in the accumulation of organic acids.

   b. **Nonanion gap metabolic acidosis** is caused by:

      i. **Conditions that lead to the renal loss of bicarbonate** (e.g., proximal tubular acidosis, distal tubular acidosis, acetazolamide therapy leading to carbonic anhydrase inhibition)

      ii. **Conditions that lead to the gastrointestinal loss of bicarbonate** (e.g., diarrhea, pancreatic fistula, ureterosigmoidostomy)

      iii. **Administration of hydrochloric acid, ammonium chloride, arginine hydrochloride, or oral calcium chloride**

3. **Clinical features.** The clinical features of metabolic acidosis are usually related to the underlying disorder.

4. **Evaluation**

   a. **Laboratory studies** should include an ABG; a CBC; a serum electrolyte panel; serum creatinine, BUN, and glucose levels; and urinalysis.

      i. The calculated osmolarity, which is used to calculate the osmolar gap, can be calculated as follows:

      Calculated osmolarity (mOsm/L) = 2 (Na) + (glucose / 18) + (BUN / 2.8) The osmolar gap (i.e., the difference between the measured osmolality and the calculated osmolarity) can aid in diagnosing the cause of an anion gap acidosis. Normally, the osmolar gap is 275 to 285 mOsm/L. Different substances increase the osmolar gap to varying degrees (Table 7-1).

      ii. Laboratory data may provide other clues as to the cause of the anion gap metabolic acidosis. For example:

         a) Hyperglycemia and glucosuria are characteristic of diabetic ketoacidosis, whereas the blood glucose level is lower and glucosuria is mild or absent in alcoholic ketoacidosis.

         b) Serum lactic acid levels are elevated in lactic acidosis, although the differential for an elevated serum lactic acid level is broad.

         c) Calcium oxalate or hippurate crystals may be evident in the urine of patients with anion gap metabolic acidosis as a result of ethylene glycol intoxication.

   b. **Ancillary tests** may be necessary to determine the specific cause of the metabolic acidosis.

Metabolic Emergencies

TABLE 7-1	Effect of Various Chemicals on the Osmolar Gap in Anion Gap Metabolic Acidosis	
Substance	**Amount Needed to Increase the Serum Osmolarity 1 mOsm/L (in mg/dL)**	**Increase in mOsm/L as a Result of Each mg/dL of Substance**
Methanol	2.6	0.38
Ethanol	4.3	0.23
Ethylene glycol	5.0	0.20
Acetone	5.5	0.18
Isopropyl alcohol	5.9	0.17
Salicylate	14.0	0.07

5. **Therapy.** Metabolic acidosis is no longer treated with **sodium bicarbonate** when the blood pH is less than 7.2. Complications of bicarbonate administration include hypernatremia, paradoxic cerebrospinal fluid acidosis, hypokalemia, hyperosmolality, and the induction of dysrhythmias.

E. **Metabolic alkalosis**
   1. **Discussion**
      a. **Definition.** Increased pH and an increased plasma bicarbonate concentration
      b. **Causes.** Increased bicarbonate results from either increased endogenous production with reduced renal excretion or exogenous administration of bicarbonate or another alkali.
         i. **Vomiting** or **nasogastric suction** causes a loss of gastric hydrochloric acid that leads to an increase in plasma bicarbonate. The decreased extracellular volume due to vomiting plus the chloride deficits reduce the glomerular filtration rate and increase the rate of bicarbonate and sodium reabsorption, helping to maintain the alkalosis.
         ii. **Diuretics** that increase sodium chloride loss lead to hydrogen ion loss, resulting in decreased bicarbonate production. Volume depletion by the sodium deficit reduces the glomerular filtration rate, stimulates proximal tubular reabsorption of bicarbonate, and maintains the metabolic alkalosis.
         iii. **Conditions characterized by excessive mineralocorticoid action** (e.g., Cushing disease, hyperaldosteronism, Bartter syndrome) stimulate hydrogen ion secretion, thereby raising the plasma bicarbonate level. Potassium depletion by a similar mechanism is also noted.
         iv. **Administration of alkali**, either as sodium bicarbonate or as organic ions (e.g., lactate, citrate, acetate), results in an increased plasma bicarbonate level.
         v. **Rapid correction of hypercapnia** in patients with a chronic state of respiratory acidosis leads to a transient state of hyperbicarbonatemia and an elevated pH.
   2. **Clinical features.** Signs and symptoms of metabolic alkalosis are usually dominated by the underlying disease state.
   3. **Evaluation**
      a. **Laboratory tests** should include an ABG report, a serum electrolyte panel, and serum glucose, BUN, and creatinine levels.
      b. **Ancillary tests** may be necessary to identify the underlying cause of the metabolic alkalosis.
   4. **Therapy.** The primary goal of therapy is to correct the underlying cause. Frequently, volume expansion is required.

I. HYPOGLYCEMIA

A. **Discussion**

1. **Definition.** Serum glucose level is **less than 50 mg/dL**.

2. **Etiology.** Glucose homeostasis is the result of a complex interaction between insulin (secreted by the pancreas), counterregulatory hormones (e.g., glucagon, catecholamine, glucocorticoids), and growth hormone. Traditionally, hypoglycemia is classified as either postprandial (reactive) or fasting.

   a. **Spontaneous hypoglycemia**

      i. **Postprandial (reactive) hypoglycemia** is characterized by declining glucose levels after a glucose load.

      ii. **Alimentary hypoglycemia** occurs in patients who have recently undergone gastrointestinal surgery.

      iii. **Prediabetic glucose intolerance.** Hypoglycemia may be an early manifestation of non–insulin-dependent diabetes mellitus.

      iv. **Functional (idiopathic) hypoglycemia.** Hypoglycemia occurs between the fed and fasting state.

      v. **Fasting hypoglycemia** occurs in patients with significant underlying pathologic conditions.

      vi. **Endogenous insulin excess** may result from **insulinomas** (nonmalignant pancreatic tumors) or **extrapancreatic neoplasms**.

      vii. **Regulatory hormone deficiencies.** Acquired or congenital deficiencies of glucagon, glucocorticoids, or growth hormone can lead to hypoglycemia.

      viii. **Organ failure.** Impaired liver or kidney function can lead to hypoglycemia.

      ix. **Systemic disease.** Shock, sepsis, and starvation can cause hypoglycemia.

   b. **Induced hypoglycemia**

      i. **Insulin-induced hypoglycemia**, seen in patients with diabetes, is the most common cause of hypoglycemia seen in the emergency department.

      ii. **Factitious hypoglycemia** may be seen in psychiatric patients (e.g., as a result of the ingestion of oral hypoglycemic agents by a patient with Munchausen syndrome).

      iii. **Chemical-induced.** Alcohol-induced hypoglycemia is found in malnourished, alcoholic patients. Other chemicals and medications can also induce hypoglycemia.

3. **Risk factors.** Young children and elderly patients are at high risk for the development of hypoglycemia.

B. **Clinical features** are caused by the direct effects of hypoglycemia on the central nervous system as well as its indirect effects on the sympathetic nervous system. Patients may be asymptomatic, or they may present with a wide variety of symptoms.

1. **Nonspecific systemic symptoms** include sweating, palpitations, hypertension, peripheral vasodilation, hyperventilation, tachycardia, dyspnea, pallor, and tremulousness.

2. **Neurologic symptoms** include paresthesia, neurologic deficit, diplopia, clonus, and transient hemiplegia.

3. **Psychiatric manifestations** include impairment of memory, change of personality, combative behavior, fatigue, headache, insomnia, nightmares, visual problems, catatonia, convulsions, and general sluggishness.

C. **Differential diagnoses.** Hypoglycemia may masquerade as neurologic, psychiatric, or cardiovascular disease. Stroke, diabetic ketoacidosis, nonketotic hyperosmolar coma, alcohol intoxication, alcohol withdrawal, and other causes of coma must all be ruled out.

D. **Evaluation.** Bedside glucose testing is a reliable test for ruling out hypoglycemia.

E. **Therapy**

1. Prehospital providers commonly administer one ampule (25 g) of 50% dextrose intravenously. Alcoholic patients should receive thiamine (100 mg administered intravenously) prior to receiving dextrose to prevent Wernicke-Korsakoff syndrome (see VIII). If intravenous access is unavailable, glucagon (0.5 to 2.0 mg) is administered intramuscularly or subcutaneously. The glucagon dose can be repeated twice.

2. A **meal high in complex carbohydrates** should be provided following initial treatment. If the patient is unable to swallow, a continuous intravenous infusion of 5% dextrose in water should be initiated.

F. **Disposition**

1. **Admission** is indicated for patients who have taken an oral hypoglycemic agent or long-acting insulin. Patients in whom no obvious cause for the hypoglycemia can be identified and patients with persistent neurologic deficits or cardiac complications (e.g., coronary or cerebrovascular insufficiency) should also be admitted.

2. **Discharge.** Patients whose symptoms are rapidly reversed without complications and in whom a clear cause for the hypoglycemia has been identified may go home. Patients with diabetes who experience a hypoglycemic episode should be taught how to adjust their insulin dose, food intake, or both based on their level of physical activity.

II. DIABETIC KETOACIDOSIS

A. **Discussion**

1. **Definition.** In insulin-dependent patients, diabetic ketoacidosis is characterized by hyperglycemia, ketonemia, and acidosis.

2. **Etiology.** Diabetic ketoacidosis is caused by a relative or absolute deficiency of insulin and increased levels of stress hormones (e.g., catecholamines, cortisol, growth hormone). Insulin deficiency leads to lipolysis, which in turn leads to the production of ketone bodies, resulting in an acidosis.

3. **Precipitating factors** include lack of insulin, infection, injuries, emotional stress, alcohol use, myocardial infarction, and cerebrovascular accident.

B. **Clinical features**

1. **Symptoms.** Nausea, vomiting, abdominal pain, polyuria and polydipsia, and altered mental status

2. **Physical examination findings**

   a. **Kussmaul respirations** (i.e., rapid, deep breathing) may be noted, and the breath often smells like **acetone.**

   b. **Dehydration** may be reflected by hypotension, reflex tachycardia, dry skin, and dry mucous membranes.

C. **Differential diagnoses.** Hypoglycemia, nonketotic hyperosmolar coma, isopropyl alcohol ingestion, alcoholic ketoacidosis, lactic acidosis, uremia, toxin ingestion, and starvation ketosis must be ruled out.

D. **Evaluation**

1. **Laboratory studies**

   a. A provisional diagnosis can be obtained via **blood gas** and **bedside glucose determinations.**

      i. **Hyperglycemia** (defined as a serum glucose level of at least 300 mg/dL) will be evident.

      ii. **Metabolic acidosis** is demonstrated by a serum bicarbonate concentration of less than 15 mEq/L and a pH of less than 7.3.

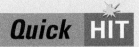

Quick HIT

Repeat laboratory measurements are required to confirm the diagnosis in patients who do not respond to glucose administration or who experience the recurrence of symptoms after treatment.

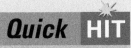

Quick HIT

Patients who are malnourished (i.e., have little glycogen reserve) may not have a measurable increase in serum glucose with administration of glucagon.

Endocrine Emergencies

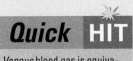

Quick HIT

Venous blood gas is equivalent to *arterial* in this circumstance and much less painful for the patient.

Endocrine Emergencies

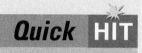

Be careful to correct fluid deficits over several hours as rapid fluid administration may result in cerebral edema, especially in children.

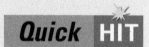

Potassium levels must be closely monitored throughout therapy.

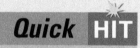

Occasionally, both nonketotic hyperosmolar coma and diabetic ketoacidosis are seen in the same patient.

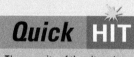

The severity of the altered mental status depends on the glucose level.

   b. A **serum biochemical profile** (**including** electrolytes, blood urea nitrogen [BUN], and creatinine levels), urinalysis, and ketone levels confirm the diagnosis.
      i. **Ketonemia** results from β-hydroxybutyrate and acetoacetate. Qualitative tests (e.g., the nitroprusside test) detect acetoacetate but not β-hydroxybutyrate.
      ii. **Electrolyte derangements** may be present, depending on the patient's hydration status.
   c. **Other studies,** such as a complete blood count (CBC), a chest radiograph, or an electrocardiogram (ECG), may be indicated to identify precipitating causes.

E. **Therapy**
   1. **Normal saline** should be administered at an initial rate of 1 L/hour for the first 2 to 3 hours. The average fluid deficit is 5 to 10 L. Clinical response and urine output are the best indicators of fluid status.
   2. **Insulin** is administered intravenously as a continuous infusion using a low-dose technique (i.e., 5 to 10 U/hour) until the ketonemia and acidosis have resolved.
   3. **Potassium** (20 mEq/L) should be added to the intravenous fluids early in therapy to correct the profound potassium deficiency associated with diabetic ketoacidosis. During the first day of treatment, the patient usually requires 100 to 200 mEq of potassium.
   4. **Phosphate.** It is unclear whether phosphate replacement is necessary. Phosphate is given either orally or intravenously if the patient's serum phosphate level decreases to below 1 mg/dL.

F. **Disposition.** Most patients with diabetic ketoacidosis need to be admitted, often to an intensive care unit (ICU). In patients with mild diabetic ketoacidosis, the ketoacidosis may resolve in the emergency department. These patients should be placed under observation until any underlying precipitating causes can be ruled out.

III. NONKETOTIC HYPEROSMOLAR COMA

A. **Discussion**
   1. **Definition.** Syndrome characterized by severe hyperglycemia, hyperosmolarity, and dehydration. Nonketotic hyperosmolar coma is less common than diabetic ketoacidosis and commonly occurs as an early manifestation of non–insulin-dependent diabetes.
   2. **Etiology**
      a. **Patients with diabetes** who have been subjected to a stressor (e.g., infection, stroke, gastrointestinal bleeding, pancreatitis) or who are taking thiazide diuretics, corticosteroids, phenytoin, cimetidine, propranolol, or calcium channel blockers may develop nonketotic hyperosmolar coma.
      b. **Nondiabetic patients.** Situations that cause severe dehydration or excessive glucose load (e.g., burns, heat stroke, peritoneal dialysis, hemodialysis, the ingestion of enormous amounts of sugar-containing foods) may cause this disorder in patients without diabetes.
   3. **Pathogenesis.** Nonketotic hyperosmolar coma and diabetic ketoacidosis represent different ends of a spectrum of lipid mobilization. Nonketotic hyperosmolar coma is precipitated by stress that increases glucose levels over days or weeks. The presence of a small amount of insulin is thought to suppress ketogenesis. Significant osmotic diureses leads to severe dehydration and altered mental status.

B. **Clinical features**
   1. **Patient history.** Most patients are elderly with either non–insulin-dependent diabetes (67% of patients) or insulin-dependent diabetes (33% of patients).
   2. **Symptoms.** Patients develop polydipsia and polyuria initially, followed by alterations in mental status. The disorder may go unrecognized until stupor and coma develop.
   3. **Physical examination findings.** Principal findings include dehydration, fever, hypotension, tachycardia, and variable respiratory patterns. A variety of neurologic signs, such as tremors, fasciculations, hemisensory deficits, and hemiparesis, may occur.

C. **Differential diagnoses.** Any disorder that can cause altered mental status (e.g., hepatic failure, uremia, sepsis, stroke, drug ingestion, lactic acidosis) must be considered.

D. **Evaluation**
1. **Glucose, ketones,** and calculated and measured **serum osmolarity values** are essential.
   a. The glucose level is typically 1,000 mg/dL or more.
   b. Although ketones may be present in small amounts, there is usually an absence of ketonemia and ketonuria.
   c. The serum osmolarity is greater than 350 mOsm/kg.
2. **Serum electrolyte, BUN,** and **creatinine levels; urinalysis;** and **venous blood gas determinations** are indicated.
   a. Serum sodium ranges from 120 to 160 mEq/L, and potassium depletion is usually severe.
   b. The BUN is usually elevated; the BUN:creatinine ratio usually exceeds 30:1.
3. **Other studies.** It is important to search for the underlying cause. A chest radiograph, ECG, computed tomography head scan, lumbar puncture, or cultures may be appropriate.

E. **Therapy**
1. **Fluid resuscitation.** The average fluid deficit is 8 to 12 L; therefore, administration of half-normal saline (or normal saline for hypotensive patients) is indicated. One-half of the patient's fluid deficit should be administered in the first 12 hours, and the remainder administered over the next 24 hours.
2. **Potassium** should be replaced early in the course of therapy. Usually, an infusion at a rate of 10 to 20 mEq/L for the first 24 to 36 hours is initiated if the patient's fluid status is such that he or she is able to produce urine.
3. **Insulin** is administered by continuous infusion (0.1 U/kg/hour). The insulin should be stopped when the blood glucose level reaches 300 mg/dL.
4. **Glucose** is indicated if the glucose level is below 250 mg/dL.
5. **Phosphate.** Administration of phosphate is controversial.
6. **Low-dose heparin** may be used to prevent arterial and venous thrombosis.

F. **Disposition.** Nonketotic hyperosmolar coma is associated with a high mortality rate. Patients are very ill and should be admitted to an intensive care service. Until the patient has been stabilized and other etiologies ruled out, transfer to other institutions is not advised.

IV. ALCOHOLIC KETOACIDOSIS

A. **Discussion**
1. **Definition.** Alcoholic ketoacidosis is usually seen in alcoholic patients who are forced to abruptly cease drinking alcohol after a drinking binge, but it may also be seen in first-time drinkers. These patients do not have diabetes mellitus.
2. **Pathogenesis.** The pathogenesis is uncertain. It is related to low insulin levels, reduction of available nicotinamide adenine dinucleotide, and increased ketone formation.

B. **Clinical features**
1. **Patient history.** The patient has recently stopped or limited alcohol consumption because of abdominal pain, nausea, and vomiting, not from a desire to stop drinking.
2. **Symptoms**
   a. **Diffuse abdominal pain** is typically present. Abdominal pain may be caused by alcohol-related diseases (e.g., pancreatitis, gastritis, hepatitis), or it may be caused by disorders unrelated to alcoholism (e.g., sepsis, pneumonia, pyelonephritis).
   b. **Symptoms of alcohol withdrawal** or **delirium tremens** may be noted.
3. **Physical examination findings**
   a. **Hydration status.** Dehydration occurs secondary to vomiting, diaphoresis, and decreased oral intake. The patient is acutely ill with hypotension and tachycardia.

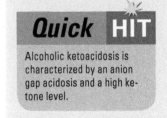

Quick **HIT**

Alcoholic ketoacidosis is characterized by an anion gap acidosis and a high ketone level.

b. **Vital signs.** Kussmaul respirations may be present, and the temperature may be elevated or normal.

c. **Mental status** varies from normal to comatose.

d. **Stigmata of alcoholism** (e.g., spider angiomata) may be noted.

C. **Differential diagnoses.** Any disorder that causes an anion gap acidosis must be ruled out. The most significant disorders to consider are diabetic ketoacidosis, hyperemesis gravidarum, starvation, cyanide poisoning, and isopropyl alcohol intoxication.

D. **Evaluation**

1. **Serum biochemical profile** will establish the presence of an anion gap acidosis. A mixed disorder may also be found (e.g., metabolic ketoacidosis may occur from vomiting and respiratory alkalosis may occur from fever, sepsis, or alcohol withdrawal).

2. **Ketone studies.** β-hydroxybutyric acid is the predominant ketone formed in alcoholic ketoacidosis. Because the nitroprusside test detects acetoacetate but not β-hydroxybutyrate, this test is of limited usefulness in patients with alcoholic ketoacidosis. As the patient undergoes treatment, acetoacetate levels increase, suggesting a false appearance of worsening of the ketoacidosis.

3. **Bedside glucose determination.** The blood glucose level may be low, normal, or minimally elevated. Most patients have normal to increased glucose levels.

E. **Therapy.** The reversal of ketoacidosis can take 12 to 18 hours.

1. **Saline solutions containing glucose** and **thiamine** are administered to treat dehydration. Glucose appears to improve the clinical response. Magnesium and vitamin supplements should be given if poor oral intake is suspected.

2. **Insulin.** Administration of insulin is not indicated unless the patient has concomitant diabetes mellitus.

3. **Bicarbonate.** Administration of bicarbonate is controversial. Most advocate administering bicarbonate only in the cardiac arrest situation with known severe acidosis.

F. **Disposition**

1. **Admission.** Patients who cannot tolerate oral fluids or who have a significant metabolic acidosis should be admitted. Underlying or precipitating illnesses and abdominal pain must be evaluated prior to discharge. Patients usually respond to therapy in 12 to 24 hours and may be discharged at that time.

2. **Discharge.** If the patient responds well to therapy in the emergency department, he or she may be discharged. Close follow-up and referral for alcoholism treatment are essential.

V. LACTIC ACIDOSIS

A. **Discussion**

1. **Etiology**

a. **Type A lactic acidosis** is caused by tissue hypoxia and is associated with a high mortality rate. The hypoxia may be related to hemorrhage or hypovolemic, cardiogenic, or septic shock.

b. **Type B lactic acidosis** is not associated with tissue hypoxia (see Clinical Pearl 8-1). This type of acidosis may occur abruptly or over a few hours. The mechanism predisposing a patient to type B lactic acidosis is not well understood.

CLINICAL PEARL 8-1

Types of B Lactic Acidosis

1. **Type B$_1$ lactic acidosis** is found in patients with diabetes, liver disease, sepsis, seizures, renal disease, and neoplasia.

2. **Type B$_2$ lactic acidosis** is associated with drugs, toxins, and chemicals. Ethanol is most commonly associated with this type of lactic acidosis; phenformin, fructose, and salicylate ingestion are also associated with type B$_2$ lactic acidosis.

3. **Type B$_3$ lactic acidosis** is associated with inborn errors of metabolism and is rare. Type I glycogen storage diseases and hepatic fructose biphosphate deficiency also cause type B$_3$ acidosis.

2. **Pathogenesis.** Lactic acidosis is caused by a buildup of lactic acid, which produces an anion gap acidosis. Lactate is a byproduct of glycolysis. The acidosis develops because the rate of production of lactate is greater than the rate of lactate utilization by the liver and kidneys.

B. **Clinical features** are nonspecific. The onset of illness is usually abrupt. The patient appears ill, and hypoventilation or Kussmaul respiration may be observed. Alterations in mental status range from lethargy to coma. Vomiting and abdominal pain may be present.

C. **Differential diagnoses** include those disorders that produce an anion gap acidosis (e.g., diabetic ketoacidosis, alcoholic ketoacidosis, renal failure, salicylate toxicity, methanol toxicity, ethylene glycol toxicity, paraldehyde toxicity, cyanide poisoning).

D. **Evaluation**
1. Blood gas; serum electrolyte, glucose, BUN, and creatinine levels; liver function studies; and a drug screen are necessary to make the diagnosis.
2. Measurement of lactate levels is indicative but not diagnostic of lactic acidosis. The normal lactate level (0.5 to 1.5 mEq/L) is increased to 5 to 6 mEq/L or more in patients with lactic acidosis. However, clinically insignificant factors that can increase the lactate level include exercise; hyperventilation; infusion of glucose, saline, and bicarbonate; and injections of insulin or epinephrine.

E. **Therapy**
1. If it can be identified, the underlying cause of the lactic acidosis should be treated.
2. **Adequate ventilation** and **volume replacement** are essential. Vasopressors are not indicated because they may actually decrease tissue perfusion.

F. **Disposition.** Patients with lactic acidosis are seriously ill and usually need to be admitted to the ICU.

VI. THYROID DISORDERS

A. **Thyroid storm**
1. **Discussion**
   a. **Definition.** Thyroid storm is a rare, life-threatening manifestation of hyperthyroidism that affects 1% to 27% of hyperthyroid patients.
   b. **Patient profile.** It is not possible to predict which hyperthyroid patients will develop thyroid storm. Patients commonly have hyperthyroidism for up to 2 years prior to the onset of thyroid storm, and most have antecedent Graves disease.
   c. **Etiology.** Thyroid storm is thought to be caused by changes in thyroid production or secretion, alteration of the body's response to thyroid hormone, and adrenergic hyperactivity.
   d. **Precipitating factors.** There are many nonspecific stressors that can precipitate a thyroid storm. Infection, pulmonary emboli, nonketotic hyperosmolar coma, diabetic ketoacidosis, surgery, burns, emotional stress, and trauma can cause thyroid storm. Iodine-131 therapy, thyroid hormone ingestion, premature withdrawal of antithyroid therapy, and contrast radiographic material can also precipitate thyroid storm.
2. **Clinical features**
   a. **Thyroid storm** is difficult to diagnose because the manifestations are protean. The clues to diagnosis include a history of hyperthyroidism, ocular signs of Graves disease, a widened pulse pressure, and a palpable goiter.
      i. **Systemic manifestations.** Heat intolerance and fever are commonly present. The pulse rate ranges from 120 to 200 beats/min but is out of proportion to the fever. Sweating is profuse and leads to dehydration.
      ii. **Cardiovascular manifestations** include increased systolic blood pressure, an elevated pulse pressure, a systolic flow murmur, sinus tachycardia, and atrial fibrillation. Cardiac arrhythmia, congestive heart failure (CHF), and pulmonary edema are also found.

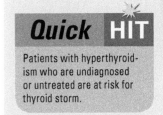

Quick HIT

Patients with hyperthyroidism who are undiagnosed or untreated are at risk for thyroid storm.

       iii. **Central nervous system manifestations** are common and vary from agitation and restlessness to psychosis and mental confusion to obtundation and coma. Proximal muscle weakness and myopathy may also be seen.

       iv. **Gastrointestinal disturbances** are variable, and weight loss is common. Nausea, vomiting, anorexia, abdominal pain, and hepatic dysfunction with jaundice may occur.

   b. **Apathetic thyrotoxicosis** is a rare form of thyroid storm found in older patients. In patients with apathetic thyrotoxicosis, the usual hyperkinetic manifestations of thyroid storm are absent. Patients present with lethargy, slow mentation, placid apathetic facies, and proximal muscle weakness. Atrial fibrillation and CHF may obscure the underlying thyrotoxicosis.

3. **Differential diagnoses.** Conditions that cause hypermetabolic states (e.g., cocaine intoxication, sympathomimetic excess, pheochromocytoma) should be considered in the differential diagnosis.

4. **Evaluation**

   a. **Thyroid function tests.** An elevated free thyroxine (T_4) level and a suppressed, unmeasurable thyroid-stimulating hormone (TSH) level confirm the diagnosis. In the rare condition of triiodothyronine (T_3) thyrotoxicosis, elevated T_3 levels are found in the presence of normal T_4 and TSH levels.

   b. **Other laboratory tests** that are frequently obtained include a serum electrolyte panel, cortisol levels, calcium levels, glucose levels, a CBC, and liver function tests.

      i. Elevated glucose and calcium levels are a common finding.

      ii. Normochromic, normocytic anemia, depressed cholesterol levels, and elevations in liver enzyme activity are fairly common.

5. **Therapy.** The underlying causes or precipitating events need to be evaluated and treated. No precipitating event is found in up to 50% of cases.

   a. **General supportive measures** include:

      i. Intravenous fluids to replace losses

      ii. Supplemental oxygen to compensate for increased consumption

      iii. Acetaminophen and cooling blankets to reduce fever

      iv. Digitalis and diuretics to treat CHF

      v. Antiarrhythmics (except atropine) to treat cardiac arrhythmias

      vi. Hydrocortisone

   b. **Minimization of thyroid hormone synthesis and release**

      i. **Propylthiouracil** (900 to 1,200 mg) or **methimazole** (90 to 120 mg) can be administered orally or via a nasogastric tube to inhibit thyroid hormone synthesis.

      ii. **Iodine** (in the form of **strong iodine solution** [1 mL three times daily], **potassium iodine** [10 drops of a solution containing 1 g/mL every 4 to 6 hours], or **sodium iodine** [1 g every 8 to 12 hours by slow intravenous infusion]) will prevent thyroid hormone release. Iodine preparations should be **administered 1 hour after the administration of propylthiouracil or methimazole** to prevent the synthesis of new hormone. Potassium-sparing diuretics and potassium-containing drugs should be used with caution in patients receiving potassium iodine because they can increase potassium load.

   c. **Beta blockade.** Administering **propranolol or esmolol** blocks the peripheral thyroid effects and inhibits peripheral conversion of T_4 and T_3. Pregnant patients and those with reactive airway disease, diabetes mellitus, or CHF should not receive propranolol.

6. **Disposition.** Patients diagnosed as having thyroid storm must be admitted to the ICU.

B. **Hypothyroidism and myxedema coma**

  1. **Discussion**

   a. **Hypothyroidism** is a slow, progressive disorder usually caused by subtotal thyroidectomy or radioactive iodine treatment. The prevalence

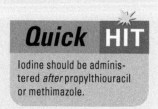

***Quick* HIT**

Iodine should be administered *after* propylthiouracil or methimazole.

of hypothyroidism varies from 0.1% to 1% and increases with age. Hypothyroidism is more prevalent in women.

   i. **Primary hypothyroidism** is failure of the thyroid gland to respond to TSH. It may be caused by therapy for Graves disease, subtotal thyroidectomy, autoimmune thyroiditis, iodine deficiency, or antithyroid drugs, or it may be congenital.

   ii. **Secondary hypothyroidism** is caused by failure of the anterior pituitary gland to release TSH. Causes include pituitary tumors, postpartum hemorrhage, and infiltrative disorders.

   b. **Myxedema coma** is a rare but life-threatening expression of hypothyroidism. It is most common during the winter months in elderly women with longstanding hypothyroidism. There are many precipitating factors, including infection, cardiovascular events, hemorrhage, and trauma.

2. **Clinical features**

   a. **Hypothyroidism**

      i. **Symptoms.** Fatigue, weakness, cold intolerance, constipation, weight gain, muscle cramps, diminished hearing, and mental disturbances. The voice may deepen. Neurologic manifestations include paresthesia, ataxia, delusions, hallucinations, and psychosis.

      ii. **Physical examination findings.** The skin feels dry and waxy, and nonpitting edema is present. Bradycardia, mild hypertension, and cardiac enlargement are also found.

   b. **Myxedema coma.** Patients present with the symptoms of hypothyroidism and are comatose.

      i. **Vital signs.** Eighty percent of patients with myxedema coma are hypothermic.

      ii. **Pulmonary signs.** Patients have respiratory distress characterized by hypoventilation, hypercapnia, and hypoxia.

      iii. **Cardiovascular manifestations** include cardiomegaly, ventricular arrhythmias, hypotension, and bradycardia.

      iv. **Neuropsychiatric manifestations** include seizures, ataxia, tremors, slow mentation, delusions, and psychosis.

      v. **Gastrointestinal and renal manifestations.** Patients frequently present with or have symptoms of megacolon, urinary retention, and abdominal distention.

3. **Differential diagnoses.** The differential diagnoses for myxedema coma include:

   a. **All causes of coma** (e.g., hypothermia, respiratory failure, electrolyte imbalance, hypoglycemia, stroke, drug overdose)

   b. **Chronic renal failure**

   c. **Nephrotic syndrome**

4. **Evaluation.** The diagnosis of myxedema coma is made on the basis of signs and symptoms of coma in a patient with hypothyroidism.

   a. Thyroid function tests and serum TSH levels can usually confirm the diagnosis.

   b. Laboratory studies and radiologic evaluation should be tailored to the presenting complaint.

      i. Patients may need a CBC, blood cultures, liver function tests, a serum electrolyte panel, renal function tests, arterial blood gas determinations, and/or serum calcium levels.

         a) Classic findings include hyponatremia, hypochloremia, hypoxia, and hypercapnia. Elevated serum creatinine kinase, aspartate aminotransferase, and lactate dehydrogenase are found.

         b) Variable potassium, calcium, and glucose levels are found.

      ii. A chest radiograph and ECG are usually necessary. A computed tomography head and obstructive gastrointestinal series may also be necessary. The chest radiograph demonstrates an enlarged cardiac silhouette, and the ECG usually shows bradycardia, T-wave inversion, prolongation of the PR interval, and low voltage.

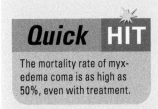

Quick HIT

The mortality rate of myxedema coma is as high as 50%, even with treatment.

Endocrine Emergencies

5. **Therapy.** Administration of medications, even in a normal dose, should be performed with caution.
   a. **General supportive measures**
      i. Oxygen and ventilatory support
      ii. Correction of hypothermia
      iii. Correction of electrolyte and glucose abnormalities
      iv. Administration of vasopressors
      v. Administration of antibiotics if the possibility of infection exists
      vi. Administration of hydrocortisone (300 mg/day) to ensure an adequate cortisol level
   b. **Specific therapy** is the administration of **intravenous thyroxine** (400 to 500 mg infused slowly, followed by 50 to 100 mg daily). **Triiodothyronine** can be given instead at a dose of 25 to 50 mg intravenously.
6. **Disposition.** All patients with myxedema coma need to be admitted to an ICU. Patients with uncomplicated hypothyroidism can be treated at home.

VII. ADRENAL INSUFFICIENCY AND ADRENAL CRISIS

A. **Discussion**
   1. **Normal physiology**
      a. The **adrenal medulla** secretes **catecholamines**.
      b. The **adrenal cortex** secretes **cortisol**, **aldosterone**, and **androgens**. Androgen production is significant in women but not in men.
         i. **Cortisol** is a potent hormone affecting glucose metabolism and water distribution. It also influences the pressor effects of catecholamines.
         ii. **Aldosterone** increases sodium reabsorption and potassium excretion.
   2. **Adrenal insufficiency** is a chronic disorder characterized by a lack of cortisol and aldosterone.
      a. **Primary adrenal insufficiency** results from the failure of the adrenal gland to produce cortical hormones. Primary insufficiency is uncommon and is most frequently caused by idiopathic autoimmune adrenalitis.
      b. **Secondary adrenal insufficiency** results from failure of the pituitary gland to secrete adrenocorticotropic hormone (ACTH). Secondary insufficiency is frequently caused by steroid suppression of the hypothalamic-pituitary-adrenal axis.
   3. **Adrenal crisis** is a medical emergency that can affect patients with chronic adrenal insufficiency who experience an acute stressful event (e.g., surgery, trauma, infection) or have abrupt cessation of corticosteroid therapy.
B. **Clinical features**
   1. Patients present with nonspecific complaints of weakness, fatigue, lethargy, anorexia, nausea, vomiting, abdominal pain, diarrhea, dizziness, and weight loss. Dehydration, hypotension, postural orthostasis, tachycardia, decreased heart size, lowered cardiac output, and decreased urine output are seen. The skin is cold and dry with increased brownish pigmentation over the exposed areas of the body. Mentation may be slowed, but coma is unlikely.
   2. In patients with secondary adrenal insufficiency, signs and symptoms of hypothalamic or pituitary disease (e.g., loss of sexual performance, menstrual irregularities, headache, galactorrhea, visual disturbances, features of acromegaly, and signs of hypothyroidism) may be noted as well.
C. **Differential diagnoses**
   1. The signs and symptoms of **adrenal insufficiency** are nonspecific and similar to those caused by many viral illnesses.
   2. In patients with **adrenal crisis**, any illness that causes cardiovascular compromise (e.g., acute myocardial infarction, sepsis, pulmonary embolism, heart failure, hypovolemia) should be considered.
D. **Evaluation**
   1. **Laboratory studies**
      a. **Serum biochemical profile.** Findings include mild to moderate hyponatremia, mild hypokalemia, hypoglycemia, hypercalcemia, moderate increases in BUN levels, and a mild metabolic acidosis.

b. **CBC.** Findings include lymphocytosis and mild eosinophilia.

c. **Corticotropin stimulation test.** This test can be used to differentiate primary from secondary causes of adrenal insufficiency. Baseline ACTH and cortisol levels should be drawn. Thirty minutes following the intravenous administration of 250 mg ACTH, a cortisol level is obtained. The administration of ACTH may be therapeutic as well as diagnostic. Dexamethasone will not interfere with this test.

2. **Electrocardiography.** An ECG shows flattened T waves, a prolonged QT interval, low voltage, prolongation of the PR or QRS intervals, ST-segment depression, and signs of hyperkalemia.

3. **Radiography.** A chest radiograph demonstrates a small, narrow heart. An abdominal radiograph may show calcification of the adrenal glands.

E. **Therapy**

1. **General supportive measures.** Fluids and vasopressors are administered to counteract dehydration and shock. Cardiac monitoring and determination of the central venous pressure can be used to monitor the response. It may be necessary to administer as many as 2 to 3 L of fluid over the first 8 hours.

2. **Therapy for adrenal crisis.** Patients suspected of having adrenal crisis should be treated before the confirmatory laboratory studies are returned.

a. **Hydrocortisone.** An intravenous push of 100 mg should be given and may be dose every 8 hours.

b. **Fludrocortisone** (0.05 to 0.1 mg) daily may be needed if hypotension and volume depletion persist.

F. **Disposition.** All patients with adrenal crisis must be admitted to the ICU.

9 NEUROLOGIC EMERGENCIES

Steve Pahner

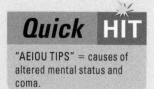

Neurologic Emergencies

I. ALTERED MENTAL STATUS AND COMA

A. Discussion

1. **Pathogenesis.** Coma or a change in mental status implies bilateral cortical disease or suppression of the reticular activating system.

2. **Causes.** The potential causes of altered mental status and coma are innumerable. The mnemonic "**AEIOU TIPS**" is an organized way of remembering the various potential causes of altered mental status and coma.

   a. *A* stands for **alcohol** (and **drugs** and **toxins**). Pharmacologic agents alter mental status through bilateral cortical suppression.

   b. *E* stands for **endocrine** and **environmental** causes.

      i. **Endocrine causes** include **hyperammonemia** (e.g., secondary to liver disease), **electrolyte abnormalities** (e.g., hyponatremia), and **hypo- and hyperthyroidism.**

      ii. **Environmental causes** include **hypo- and hyperthermia.**

   c. *I* designates **insulin poisoning** and **impaired glucose utilization**.

      i. **Hypoglycemia** is the most common cause of altered mental status seen in the emergency department (ED). Hypoglycemia may occur in any patient but is more commonly seen in patients with diabetes, alcoholics, neonates, patients with toxic ingestions, patients with poor nutrition states, and patients with pancreatic tumors or retroperitoneal sarcomas.

      ii. **Hyperglycemia** leading to diabetic ketoacidosis or nonketotic hyperosmolar syndrome may cause altered mental status.

   d. *O* signifies **oxygen deprivation** and **opiate poisoning**.

      i. **Oxygen deprivation (hypoxemia)** has multiple causes (e.g., pneumonia, cerebral hypoperfusion secondary to shock or cardiac arrhythmias, pulmonary embolism, bronchospasm).

      ii. **Opiate poisoning** depresses central respiratory centers, leading to acute hypoxia.

   e. *U* signifies **uremia**. Coma may occur secondary to rapid changes in the blood urea nitrogen level.

   f. *T* stands for **trauma**. Hypoperfusion and cerebral trauma may induce a change in mental status.

   g. *I* signifies **infection**. Both systemic and neurologic infection (e.g., meningitis, encephalitis) may induce a change in mental status. Infections and fever are a common cause in the elderly.

   h. *P* designates **psychiatric causes** and **porphyria**. Attributing a change in mental status to a psychiatric cause is a diagnosis of exclusion.

   i. *S* stands for **space-occupying lesions**, which induce an altered state of consciousness or coma by involving the bilateral cortical hemispheres or suppressing the reticular activating system.

      i. Bilateral cortical disease is generally secondary to metabolic or toxic causes.

      ii. Space-occupying lesions induce coma by increasing pressure on the reticular activating system, not by causing local neuronal destruction.

B. Evaluation. The patient presenting with an altered mental status requires a thorough physical examination, appropriate laboratory and diagnostic evaluation, and immediate treatment. The goal of the ED physician is to determine whether the etiology is metabolic or toxic in nature (as opposed to a structural defect). The former disease process is managed medically, whereas the latter is a potential surgical emergency.

1. **Stabilization**
   a. **Airway, breathing, and circulations (ABCs) and vital signs.** The airway, breathing, and circulatory status of the patient must be evaluated initially, and a full set of vital signs is essential.
   b. **Intravenous access, cardiac monitoring,** and **supplemental oxygen** should be established.
   c. **Oxygen and glucose levels** should be evaluated.
      i. **Hypoxemia** is corrected by administering **supplemental oxygen. Naloxone** should be administered intravenously in an adult to reverse opiate-induced respiratory depression. There are no case reports of adverse effects secondary to naloxone dosing; however, the patient may experience an acute opiate withdrawal syndrome.
      ii. **Hypoglycemia** is rapidly corrected by administering glucose. **Thiamine** should be administered prior to administering **glucose** in an adult to avoid precipitating Wernicke encephalopathy.

2. **Physical examination.** A thorough physical examination is essential.
   a. **General examination.** The patient should be undressed and the entire body examined. Clues to the cause of the altered mental status may include evidence of trauma, needle marks, perspiration, skin discoloration (e.g., jaundice), odors (e.g., alcohol, acetone), and rashes.
   b. **Head, ears, eyes, nose, and throat**
      i. **Head.** The head should be inspected for evidence of trauma. **Bilateral periorbital ecchymosis ("raccoon's eyes") or ecchymosis around the mastoid area (Battle sign)** suggests a basilar skull fracture.
      ii. **Eyes**
         a) **Pupils.** Pupillary size and reactivity should be assessed.
            1) **Miosis** results from multiple causes, which can be remembered using the mnemonic "COPS2":
               Clonidine and imidazoles
               Opiates
               Phenothiazines
               Sedative-hypnotic agents
               Cholinergics (e.g., pilocarpine, physostigmine)
               Organophosphates and carbamates
               Pontine hemorrhage
               Sleep
            2) **Mydriasis** may result from anticholinergic agents or sympathomimetic agents. A fixed and dilated pupil suggests uncal herniation of the temporal lobe on the ipsilateral side with resultant compression of cranial nerve III. However, in an alert patient, a fixed and dilated pupil may be secondary to local trauma, therapy with a cycloplegic agent, or aneurysmal compression of cranial nerve III.
         b) **Fundi.** The fundi should be inspected to rule out increased intracranial pressure (ICP). Check for papilledema, exudates, or hemorrhage.
      iii. **Ears.** The tympanic membranes should be inspected to rule out blood behind the membrane, which would indicate a basilar skull fracture. Signs of otitis media may suggest coexistence of central nervous system infection.
      iv. **Nose.** The nares are inspected to rule out a cerebrospinal fluid (CSF) leak.
      v. **Throat.** The pharynx should be inspected and a gag reflex elicited.
   c. **Neck.** Palpation of the cervical spine in a comatose patient is unnecessary. A cervical injury should be assumed and the neck immobilized. If the

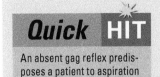

Quick **HIT**

An absent gag reflex predisposes a patient to aspiration and may be an indication for intubation.

Neurologic Emergencies

history and physical examination are not consistent with a traumatic injury, then the neck should be evaluated for signs of meningismus.

d. **Heart.** The heart should be examined for arrhythmias, murmurs (suggesting endocarditis), and rubs (suggesting uremic pericarditis). Blood pressure must be serially evaluated to rule out hypo- or hypertension.

e. **Lungs.** The respiratory rate and pattern must be evaluated.

   i. **Hypoventilation** may occur secondary to metabolic abnormalities or toxicity. An acute opiate overdose may present as a depressed level of consciousness and a decreased respiratory rate.

   ii. **Hyperventilation** may be seen in numerous disease states (e.g., metabolic acidosis, salicylate poisoning, hypoxia, hypercarbia).

   iii. **Cheyne-Stokes respiration** is a crescendo–decrescendo pattern of breathing that implies bilateral hemispheric dysfunction with an intact brain stem. This type of breathing accompanies metabolic disorders and may be the first sign of transtentorial herniation.

   iv. **Apneustic breathing** is characterized by a prolonged pause after inspiration (similar to breath holding) and is seen in patients with pontine infarction.

   v. **Ataxic breathing** is irregular breathing without a pattern; this type of breathing is preterminal.

f. **Abdomen and rectum.** A thorough abdominal examination, including a rectal examination, may aid in the diagnosis of an altered state of consciousness.

   i. The abdomen should be inspected for signs of trauma.

   ii. **Organomegaly** (e.g., hepatomegaly, splenomegaly, distended bladder), **ascites, bruits, masses, heme-positive stools,** and the presence or absence of **bowel sounds** may aid in determining the cause of the altered mental status. For example, a patient with an altered mental status who has no bowel sounds and a distended bladder may have ingested an anticholinergic medication. A patient with hepatomegaly and ascites may be suffering from hepatic encephalopathy.

3. **Neurologic examination.** The neurologic examination evaluates mental status, cranial nerve involvement, motor responses, cerebellar integrity, and reflexes.

a. **Glasgow Coma Scale** (Table 9-1). The Glasgow Coma Scale uses a point score (from 3 to 15) to categorize eye, verbal, and motor responses according to the severity of impairment.

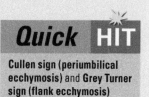

***Quick* HIT**

Cullen sign (periumbilical ecchymosis) and **Grey Turner sign (flank ecchymosis)** suggest retroperitoneal hemorrhage.

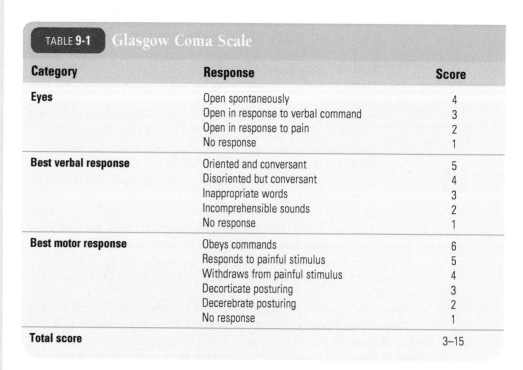

TABLE 9-1	Glasgow Coma Scale	
Category	**Response**	**Score**
Eyes	Open spontaneously	4
	Open in response to verbal command	3
	Open in response to pain	2
	No response	1
Best verbal response	Oriented and conversant	5
	Disoriented but conversant	4
	Inappropriate words	3
	Incomprehensible sounds	2
	No response	1
Best motor response	Obeys commands	6
	Responds to painful stimulus	5
	Withdraws from painful stimulus	4
	Decorticate posturing	3
	Decerebrate posturing	2
	No response	1
Total score		3–15

TABLE 9-2	Cranial Nerve Examination	
Cranial Nerve	**Function**	**Assessment**
I Olfactory	Smell	Ask patient to identify odors.
II Optic	Vision	Ask patient to read or count fingers.
III Oculomotor	Eye movement, pupillary constriction, and pupillary accommodation	Test eye movement, pupillary constriction, and pupillary accommodation and ptosis. Controls most of ocular muscles and levator palpebrae superioris muscle. Palsy results in eye in down and out position with ptosis. May have incomplete lesions
IV Trochlear	Eye movement	Test eye movement; have patient follow object. Moves eye down and out. With palsy patient, will tilt head forward to decrease diplopia
V Trigeminal	Facial sensation, masseter muscle innervation	Test facial sensation; have patient bite while palpating masseter muscle.
VI Abducens	Abducts eye	Ask patient to look to the side.
VII Facial	Facial movement, taste (anterior two-thirds of tongue)	Ask patient to wrinkle forehead and close eyes.
VIII Vestibulocochlear	Hearing and balance	Test hearing and balance.
IX Glossopharyngeal	Taste (posterior one-third of tongue), gag reflex, salivation	Test patient's gag reflex with a tongue depressor.
X Vagus	Lifts palate	Ask patient to say "ah" and observe symmetric elevation of the palate with the uvula midline.
XI Accessory	Innervates sternocleidomastoid and trapezius muscles	Ask patient to shrug shoulders and move head from side to side.
XII Hypoglossal	Innervates tongue	Ask patient to move tongue from side to side.

b. **Mental status exam.** The mental status exam primarily addresses the patient's orientation to person, place, and time. The ability to respond to voiced commands is then tested. If the patient does not respond to verbal stimuli, then response to noxious stimuli should be attempted.

c. **Cranial nerve assessment** is described in Table 9-2.

d. **Muscle strength assessment.** If the patient is able to follow simple commands, then the motor strength in major muscle groups should be documented on a point scale of 0 to 5 (Table 9-3).

TABLE 9-3	Evaluation of Muscle Strength
Grade	**Equivalent Patient Ability**
0/5	No detectable contraction
1/5	Palpable contraction, trace movement
2/5	Able to move when gravity is eliminated
3/5	Able to move fully against gravity but not resistance
4/5	Able to oppose gravity and resistance
5/5	Normal

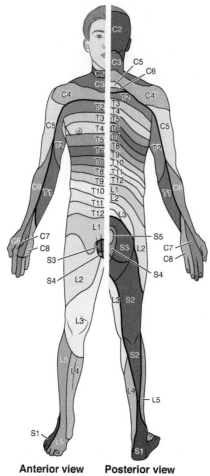

Anterior view   **Posterior view**

FIGURE

9-1   Pattern of dermatomal distributions and their innervation by the spinal roots.

e. **Sensory examination.** Responses to light touch, pain, proprioception, and a sensory level (in patients with spinal injuries) should be evaluated. Figure 9-1 shows the sensory dermatomes.

f. **Reflexes** should be assessed and graded on a scale from 0 to 4: 0 = no response, 1 = hypoactive, 2 = normal, 3 = brisk but not pathologic, and 4 = abnormally brisk with or without clonus (see Clinical Pearl 9-1).

g. **Cerebellar function** is assessed by gait, finger-to-nose testing, and heel-to-shin testing.

4. **Laboratory studies**

a. **Complete blood count.** A complete blood count should be performed to detect abnormalities (e.g., anemia, leukemia) or to confirm suspicions of an infectious process.

b. **Electrolyte status.** The discovery of electrolyte disturbances (e.g., hypo- or hypernatremia), a rapid change in blood urea nitrogen level, or detection of

CLINICAL PEARL   **9-1**

Reflexes and corresponding nerve roots: biceps (C5–C6), triceps (C7–C8), brachioradialis (C5–C6), quadriceps (L3–L4), ankle (S1–S2), and Babinski (pathologic extension of the toes on lateral stroking of the plantar surface of the foot).

an osmolar gap (typical in patients with toxic alcohol ingestions) may aid in diagnosis.

c. **Arterial blood gas analysis.** All patients with an altered mental status should be considered for arterial blood gas analysis to determine the acid–base status and to detect hypoxia and hypercarbia.

d. **Urine drug screen.** A urine drug screen may reveal the cause of the change in mental status.

e. **Specific or quantitative levels** (e.g., ammonia, calcium, thyroid hormone, salicylate, lithium, phenobarbital, carbamazepine, phenytoin, valproic acid, digoxin) may be ordered, depending on the patient's history and examination findings.

f. **CSF analysis.** A lumbar puncture may be necessary to rule out meningitis or encephalitis.

5. **Diagnostic studies**

a. **Electrocardiogram (ECG).** An ECG should be obtained to rule out a myocardial infarction, which may decrease cardiac output enough to elicit cerebral hypoperfusion. Brady- or tachyarrhythmias may also lead to cerebral hypoperfusion and a change in mental status.

b. **Computed tomography (CT) scan.** A brain CT scan may help to rule out mass lesions, hemorrhage, stroke, or trauma.

c. **Cervical spine imaging.** A patient with a change in mental status may have suffered trauma; if suspicious, a cervical spine CT should be performed to rule out injury.

d. **Electroencephalogram (EEG).** An EEG is a procedure designed to assess potential seizure activity and cortical functioning. This is usually an inpatient procedure.

C. **Disposition** of the patient with an altered level of consciousness depends entirely on the diagnosis. For example, a patient presenting with hypoglycemia secondary to inappropriate insulin dosing may be observed and subsequently discharged, a trauma patient with an acute intracranial bleed requires neurosurgical consultation, and a patient suffering acute salicylate poisoning may require urgent dialysis.

II. HEADACHE

A. **Migraine**

1. **Discussion.** Migraine headaches are generally recurrent attacks that vary widely in intensity, duration, and frequency.

a. **Onset.** They usually begin in adolescence or early adult life, although onset may occur in childhood. The development and persistence of migraines in later life is unusual.

b. **Predisposing factors.** Women are afflicted three times more often than men. There is a relationship to the menstrual cycle, with more attacks occurring during menses. During pregnancy, most women are symptom-free during the third trimester.

c. **Pathophysiology. Vascular hypothesis and neuronal hypothesis** have been considered.

2. **Clinical features.** Migraines are usually unilateral, throbbing, and associated with anorexia, nausea, and vomiting.

a. **Classic migraine** occurs in only 12% of patients with migraine and is often familial.

i. The prodromal phase is sharply defined, with the aura beginning up to 1 hour prior to the start of head pain. Contralateral manifestations include scotomas, fortification spectra, visual field defects, and transient amblyopia. Occasionally, the prodromal symptoms are motor or sensory.

ii. The aura is followed by a unilateral throbbing headache associated with nausea, vomiting, photophobia, and sonophobia.

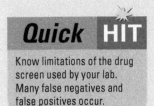

Quick **HIT**

Know limitations of the drug screen used by your lab. Many false negatives and false positives occur.

Neurologic Emergencies

    b. **Common migraine** is the most common migraine syndrome, occurring in over 80% of patients with migraine.
       i. The prodromal symptoms are not sharply defined and may consist of mood disturbances, fatigue, nausea, and vomiting. Visual disturbances are not present. The prodromal phase may precede the headache by hours or days.
      ii. The headache is unilateral, throbbing, and associated with photophobia, sonophobia, anorexia, nausea, vomiting, and general malaise.
    c. **Complex migraine** occurs when the neurologic symptoms persist beyond the headache phase of a classic migraine. These patients often present with disorders of speech including dysarthria, aphasia, dyslexia, and dysgraphia. Cranial nerve palsy can also be seen. Permanent sequelae may result from major or minor strokes secondary to ischemic or hemorrhagic infarcts.
    d. **Basilar artery migraine** primarily affects young, menstruating women.
       i. The prodromal symptoms are typically visual and include visual scintillations and visual loss throughout both visual fields. The visual disturbances are quickly followed by vertigo, ataxia, dysarthria, or tinnitus and peripheral paresthesias. Loss of consciousness may occur.
      ii. The prodrome lasts from a few minutes to up to an hour and is followed by a severe throbbing occipital headache and vomiting.

3. **Differential diagnoses.** There are numerous causes of headache. Some of the more common causes include temporomandibular joint syndrome, head injury, anemia, uremia, toxic effects from drugs or fumes, carbon monoxide poisoning, dental disease, Paget disease, sinusitis, refractive error, hypertension, hypoxia, temporal arteritis, and tumors.

4. **Therapy**
    a. **Acute therapy**
       i. **Sumatriptan** is a serotonin agonist that induces vasoconstriction. Contraindications to sumatriptan include ischemic heart disease, hypertension, headache with neurologic symptoms, concurrent ergotamine administration, and intravenous drug use. Several other triptan (e.g., naratriptan, zolmitriptan) medications, all of which have similar mechanisms of action, are also available for use. It is important to note that these headache patients may respond to one triptan but not another. Thus, multiple trials of the different triptans are appropriate before declaring the patient "triptan-unresponsive."
      ii. **Ergotamines** are potent vasoconstrictors. Contraindications are similar to those for sumatriptan.
     iii. **Antiemetics** (e.g., metoclopramide, prochlorperazine, droperidol) are often used successfully as first-line treatment for migraine; often, the headache will resolve with this treatment alone. Many physicians will give diphenhydramine prophylactically in an attempt to decrease adverse reactions. If the headache persists, either sumatriptan or dihydroergotamine may be given (in the absence of contraindications).
     iv. **Analgesics** and **nonsteroidal anti-inflammatory drugs** are also part of the treatment armamentarium. Narcotic analgesics are sporadically used but are usually avoided because of the potential for addiction and respiratory depression.
    b. **Prophylactic treatment.** ED physicians generally do not prescribe prophylactic treatment for migraines; however, the ED physician should be familiar with these medications because the patient may be taking them at the time he or she presents to the ED. Prophylactic agents include β-adrenergic blocking agents, anticonvulsants, ergotamine preparations, methysergide, cyproheptadine, monoamine oxidase inhibitors, nonsteroidal anti-inflammatory drugs, tricyclic antidepressants, and calcium channel blockers.

B. **Cluster headache**
   1. **Discussion.** Cluster headaches occur several times daily for weeks or months and are followed by long periods of pain-free intervals. The headaches are more common in the spring and fall.
      a. **Incidence.** Cluster headaches occur in 2% to 9% of patients who complain of headaches.
      b. **Predisposing factors.** Men are affected four to five times more frequently than women. Cluster headaches are often precipitated by ingestion of alcohol, use of nitroglycerin- or histamine-containing products, stress, changes in climate, and allergens.
   2. **Clinical features.** Cluster headaches are characterized by unilateral excruciating facial pain that is often accompanied by ipsilateral nasal congestion, lacrimation, and conjunctival injection. Horner syndrome (i.e., ptosis, miosis, and anhidrosis) may be seen; the ptosis and miosis are ipsilateral.
   3. **Therapy. One hundred percent oxygen** (8 to 10 L/min for 10 to 15 minutes) has been found to be helpful in treating cluster headaches. **Ergotamines, triptans** (e.g., sumatriptan, naratriptan), and **analgesics** are also used.
C. **Post–lumbar puncture headache**
   1. **Discussion.** Five percent to 30% of patients who undergo lumbar puncture develop a headache within hours or a few days of the procedure. The headache is thought to be secondary to low CSF pressure and a continuous CSF leak (see Clinical Pearl 9-2).
   2. **Clinical features.** Patients present with a bilateral pulsatile headache associated with nausea and vomiting, usually exacerbated by sitting upright and relieved by lying flat.
   3. **Therapy**
      a. Mildly symptomatic patients should receive **antiemetics, intravenous fluids,** and **analgesics.**
      b. Patients with persistent symptoms may require a trial of intravenous **caffeine** to increase the CSF pressure via cerebral vasoconstriction. Caffeine administration is generally reserved for younger patients and is contraindicated in patients with coronary artery disease or hypertension, patients taking theophylline, patients with a history of arrhythmias, and patients at risk for a vasospastic event.
      c. Severely symptomatic patients may require a "**blood patch**" (i.e., autologous transfer of blood to the epidural space at the site of the previous lumbar puncture). This procedure, performed by an anesthesiologist, is thought to stop leakage of CSF, thus restoring cerebral pressure.
   4. **Disposition.** Most patients with post–lumbar puncture headaches are discharged. Patients with complicating features require admission.
D. **Hypertensive headaches** are rare and overly diagnosed in the ED. An acute hypertensive headache requires a diastolic blood pressure elevation of approximately 25% or a sustained diastolic blood pressure greater than 130 mm Hg. Patients present with hypertension and a throbbing occipital headache. Treatment with antihypertensive agents relieves the headache, and most patients can be discharged. Patients with hypertensive urgency or crisis require admission (see Chapter 2.VI).
E. **Benign intracranial hypertension** occurs in young, obese females with irregular menses or amenorrhea. The patient presents with a severe headache, nausea, vomiting, and visual complaints. Papilledema is evident on physical examination. A CT scan will demonstrate signs of increased ICP without mass effect; the ventricles are slit-like. Lumbar puncture reveals CSF pressures greater than 250 mm Hg.

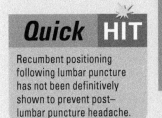

Quick HIT

Recumbent positioning following lumbar puncture has not been definitively shown to prevent post–lumbar puncture headache.

Neurologic Emergencies

CLINICAL PEARL 9-2

Prevent post–lumbar puncture headaches by using a small lumbar puncture needle, a nontraumatic lumbar puncture needle, entering dural space with bevel oriented laterally, and ensuring adequate hydration.

Therapy consists of repeated lumbar punctures to relieve pressure. Steroids may also be administered. Most patients are discharged, but patients with severe symptoms that fail to resolve with lumbar puncture require admission.

F. **Temporal arteritis**

1. **Discussion.** Temporal arteritis is a vasculitis of large and medium-sized arteries that includes the temporal artery. The disease occurs in elderly patients (the average age at the time of onset is 70 years). Left untreated, temporal arteritis may result in bilateral blindness.

2. **Clinical features.** Patients may present with unilateral, excruciating, burning pain over the affected artery. The disease is often associated with polymyalgia rheumatica and may present with systemic involvement including fever, polymyalgia, malaise, weight loss, and anorexia. Patients may have decreased visual acuity. Physical examination may reveal a tender, inflamed temporal artery. An afferent pupillary defect may be present.

3. **Evaluation.** Diagnosis is made by history, physical examination, and the demonstration of an erythrocyte sedimentation rate greater than 50 mm/h. Definitive diagnosis is established through arterial biopsy, although a negative biopsy does not exclude disease.

4. **Therapy** consists of the administration of high-dose steroids.

5. **Disposition.** Patients should be admitted to the hospital for the administration of systemic steroids and close observation. Consultation is recommended.

G. **Trigeminal neuralgia** affects older patients, especially women. The pain is secondary to trigeminal nerve hyperactivity. Clinically, patients present with unilateral facial pain (most commonly in the V2 distribution, although the V1 and V3 distributions may be affected). The pain is generally brief, intermittent, and described as "electric." The pain is triggered by eating, talking, or touching the face. Physical examination is unremarkable, and there are no neurologic deficits. Carbamazepine and gabapentin have shown benefit in treatment.

H. **Other causes of headache**

1. **Subarachnoid hemorrhage (SAH)**

a. **Discussion**

i. **Etiology.** SAH most commonly results from rupture of an **intracranial aneurysm.** The second most common cause is rupture of an **arteriovenous malformation.** Twenty-five percent of patients with a ruptured aneurysm will die the same day. Of the patients who survive, many are left with severe neurologic deficits. SAH is found in 1% of all ED patients with a headache.

ii. **Pathophysiology.** Saccular aneurysms occur most commonly at the bifurcations of the large arteries and subsequently rupture into the subarachnoid space.

b. **Clinical features**

i. **Headache.** Patients complain of the sudden onset of a headache that they may describe as "the worst headache of my life." The headache may be nonlocalized or may be localized to the occipital area and neck.

ii. **Loss of consciousness** occurs in 45% of patients secondary to decreased cerebral perfusion.

iii. **Vomiting** occurs secondary to increased ICP.

iv. **Focal neurologic deficits.** SAH is not usually associated with focal neurologic deficits. However, the presence of a focal neurologic deficit may aid in localization of the aneurysm. For example, an aneurysm at the junction of the posterior communicating artery and the internal carotid artery may result in a third nerve palsy associated with pupillary dilation, loss of light reflex, and retro-orbital pain.

v. **Meningismus** may be evident on physical examination secondary to irritation of the meninges.

c. **Evaluation**

i. **CT scan.** An unenhanced brain CT scan will detect an SAH in approximately 95% of affected patients within the first 24 hours. However,

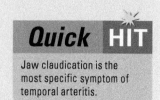

Quick HIT

Jaw claudication is the most specific symptom of temporal arteritis.

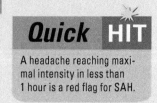

Quick HIT

A headache reaching maximal intensity in less than 1 hour is a red flag for SAH.

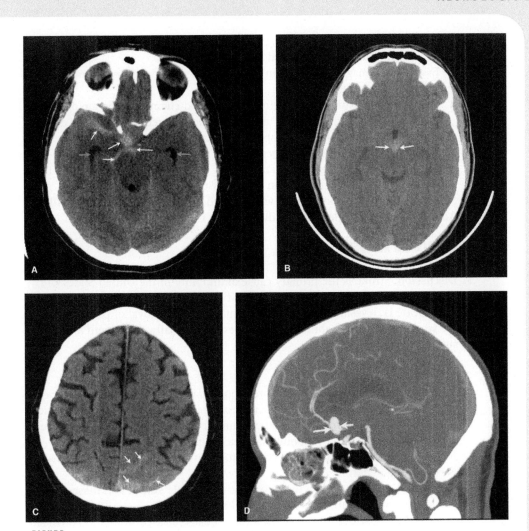

FIGURE 9-2 A to D: Computed tomography of subarachnoid hemorrhage.

the sensitivity of CT for detecting SAH drops significantly if the SAH occurred more than 36 to 48 hours prior to the scan (Figure 9-2).
  ii. **Lumbar puncture.** If the CT scan is unrevealing, then a lumbar puncture must be considered to rule out SAH.
 iii. **Cerebral angiography** will localize the site of aneurysm or rupture prior to neurosurgical intervention.
  iv. **ECG.** The ECG will frequently show ST-segment changes consistent with an ischemic process. Other abnormalities may include a widened QRS complex, an increased QT interval, and inverted T waves. Deeply inverted T waves are suggestive of an intracerebral hemorrhage (ICH; see III.A.1.b.i).
  d. **Therapy.** Urgent neurosurgical consultation is required. Intubate if coma is present. Elevate head of bed to promote venous drainage. Nimodipine should be administered to reduce vasospasm, which can lead to ischemic stroke. Goal blood pressure is systolic of 160 mm Hg.
  e. **Disposition.** Following neurosurgical correction of the bleed, patients are monitored in the intensive care unit (ICU).
 2. **Primary central nervous system tumors**
  a. **Discussion.** The principal primary tumors affecting the brain include **astrocytomas (glioblastoma multiforme** is the most devastating), **oligodendrogliomas, meningiomas, schwannomas,** and **lymphomas.**
  b. **Clinical features**
   i. **Headache** is insidious in onset. The pain is most severe on awakening. A new or unfamiliar headache should increase suspicion of a brain tumor.

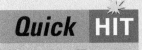

Quick HIT

Sixty-four-slice CT scanners approach 100% sensitivity for SAH if performed within 6 hours of onset of headache.

Neurologic Emergencies

ii. **Signs of increased ICP** (e.g., nausea, vomiting) may be present.

iii. **Focal neurologic signs** and **seizures** may occur.

c. **Evaluation.** Imaging studies (an enhanced CT scan or magnetic resonance imaging) aid in diagnosis.

d. **Therapy.** Neurosurgery, **radiation therapy**, and **chemotherapy** are often necessary. **Corticosteroid therapy** may be beneficial to reduce vasogenic edema.

e. **Disposition.** Outpatient workup is often acceptable; however, patients with a change in mental status or focal deficits need inpatient evaluation.

3. **Infections,** such as **meningitis**, **brain abscess**, and **sinusitis** (see Chapter 6.III.A, 6.III.C, and 6.V.A, respectively) can present with headache.

4. **Subdural** and **epidural hematomas** are discussed in Chapter 17.III.B.2 and 17.III.B.3.

5. **Acute angle closure glaucoma** is discussed in Chapter 12.

III. CEREBROVASCULAR ACCIDENT

A. **Stroke**

1. **Discussion.** Stroke is the primary cause of disability in the United States and the third leading cause of death after heart disease and cancer. Economically, this disease is devastating in terms of hospital costs, removal of patients from the work force, and rehabilitation expenses. Emotionally, the patient and family suffer immensely.

a. **Ischemic strokes**

i. **Thrombotic strokes**

a) **Atherosclerotic disease** predisposes patients to thrombotic strokes and is responsible for the majority of all strokes. The atherosclerotic vessel is hyperplastic and contains fibrous deposits that cause plaque formation in the subintimal area. Plaque formation leads to vessel narrowing and platelet adhesion, eventually leading to occlusion and infarction.

b) **Vasculitis, polycythemia, hypercoagulable states**, and **dissection** can also cause thrombotic stroke.

ii. **Embolic strokes** occur when a thrombus is released from a proximal site and lodges in a distal vessel, occluding the blood supply. The most common sources of emboli are the heart and major vessels (i.e., the carotid and vertebral arteries).

a) **Cardiac sources of emboli** include mural thrombi (secondary to myocardial infarction and arrhythmias, especially atrial fibrillation), valvular heart disease with resultant thrombus formation, ventricular septal defects with thrombus formation, and cardiac tumors.

b) **Rare causes of emboli** include septic emboli secondary to endocarditis, fat emboli secondary to long bone fractures, and particulate emboli seen in intravenous drug abusers.

iii. **Hypoperfusion strokes** generally result from decreased cardiac output. The areas of the brain most susceptible to hypoperfusion injury are the "watershed" areas, located at the periphery of the major vessels. Ischemic hypoperfusion strokes do not present with a discrete syndrome because a diverse population of neurons is affected.

b. **Hemorrhagic strokes** may be intracerebral or subarachnoid.

i. **ICH.** Intracerebral/intracranial hemorrhage. Bleeding occurs directly into the cerebral parenchyma.

a) **Etiology.** The majority of ICHs are associated with **chronic hypertension**.

b) **Pathophysiology.** Small intracerebral vessels are damaged by longstanding hypertension and eventually rupture and bleed. Hypertensive bleeds most commonly occur in the putamen and internal capsule, thalamus, pons, and cerebellum. The hemorrhage enlarges, leading to compression of local neurons. Increased ICP may lead to neuronal dysfunction in adjacent brain tissue. A large hematoma may gain access to the ventricular system and displace midline structures, leading to coma and death.

ii. **SAH** is discussed in II.H.1.

2. **Clinical features.** Only the clinical features of the major syndromes are discussed here (see Clinical Pearl 9-3). The easiest method of approaching stroke is to think about the vascular distribution of the brain (Figure 9-3).

   a. **Small artery disease.** Lacunar infarcts elicit several distinct syndromes and are commonly associated with hypertension. The structures involved include the basal ganglia, internal capsule, thalamus, and brain stem.

      i. Most frequently, a purely motor deficit leading to contralateral motor weakness of the face, arm, and leg results. There is no associated sensory loss. This infarct is localized to the internal capsule or pons.

      ii. A pure sensory stroke is secondary to infarction of the ventral posterior nuclei of the thalamus and results in contralateral sensory loss of the face, arm, and leg.

      iii. Patients with clumsy hand–dysarthria syndrome present with slurred speech and weakness and ataxia of the upper limb. Lesions of the anterior limb of the internal capsule give rise to this syndrome.

3. **Evaluation**

   a. **ABCs.** ABCs should be evaluated in all patients who are experiencing a cerebrovascular accident. These patients are potentially critical and should therefore have a safety net of intravenous access, cardiac monitoring, and supplemental oxygen.

CLINICAL PEARL 9-3

Clinical Presentation of Major Vessel Ischemic Stroke

Middle cerebral artery. Patients present with contralateral hemiplegia, hemianesthesia, and homonymous hemianopsia (blindness affecting either the right or left half of the visual fields of both eyes). Aphasia occurs when the hemisphere dominant for language is affected. Patients may display conjugate eye deviation toward the side of the lesion (away from the deficit).

Anterior cerebral artery. Patients display contralateral paralysis and sensory loss of the lower extremity, urinary incontinence, infantile reflexes such as suck and grasp, and slowness in mentation with perseveration.

Internal carotid artery. A patient with a stroke localized to the internal carotid artery shows signs of middle and anterior cerebral artery stroke because both vessels originate from the internal carotid. The internal carotid also supplies the optic nerve; therefore, monocular blindness may occur. Patients with internal carotid lesions will often have an audible bruit over the carotid. Collateral blood flow from the circle of Willis and between the internal and external carotid systems varies from person to person; therefore, complete occlusion of the internal carotid artery may leave a patient with little deficit, or the patient may be semicomatose secondary to the large area of infarction involved.

Posterior cerebral artery. Occlusion of the posterior cerebral artery induces a homonymous hemianopsia secondary to visual cortex infarction.

Vertebrobasilar system (Figure 9-3). To appreciate strokes involving the vertebrobasilar artery system, the blood supply must be reviewed. The vertebral arteries ascend along the anterior surface of the medulla and enter the posterior fossa via the foramen magnum. The two vertebral arteries then merge to form the basilar artery. Branches of the basilar artery supply the pons and the cerebellum. The basilar artery then branches into the two posterior cerebral arteries, which supply the occipital lobes, temporal lobes, the thalamus, and the upper brain stem.

1. Neurologic deficits involving the vertebrobasilar system are often subtle and include vertigo, diplopia, dysphasia, ataxia, cranial nerve palsies, and bilateral limb weakness. Crossed neurologic deficits (e.g., an ipsilateral cranial nerve deficit coupled with contralateral motor weakness) are the hallmarks of vertebrobasilar stroke.

2. The **lateral medullary (Wallenberg) syndrome** involves the vertebrobasilar system and affects the brain stem and cerebellum (Figure 9-4).

   a. The affected area of the brain stem includes the cranial nerves or nerve tracts that supply cranial nerves V, IV, and X; therefore, the patient experiences hoarseness, dysphasia, and decreased ipsilateral facial sensations.

   b. The vestibular nuclei are affected, leading to nausea, vomiting, and vertigo.

   c. The spinothalamic tract is affected, leading to contralateral loss of pain and heat sensation.

   d. Disruption of the sympathetic tract leads to Horner syndrome.

   e. Cerebellar dysfunction produces ataxia. Patients experiencing a cerebellar stroke may initially present with the inability to ambulate or a "drop attack," which may be followed by nausea, vomiting, and vertigo. Cranial nerve deficits may also occur.

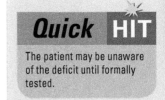

Quick HIT

The patient may be unaware of the deficit until formally tested.

Neurologic Emergencies

Neurologic Emergencies

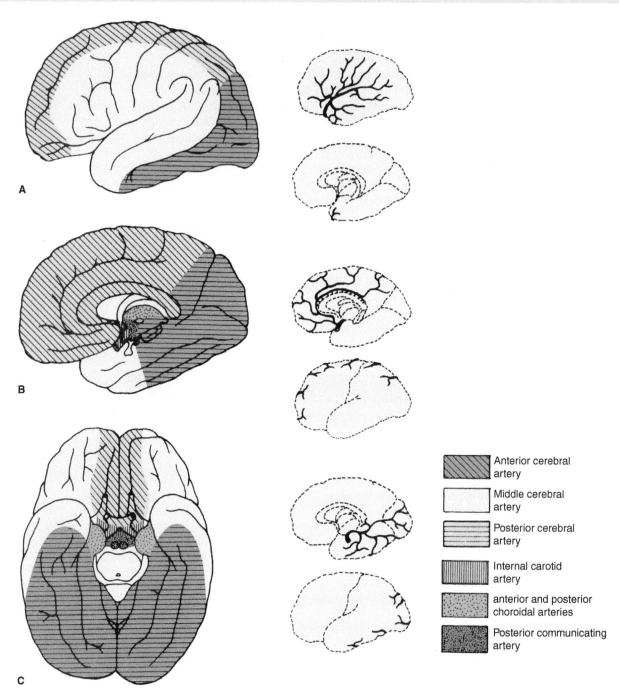

Anterior cerebral
artery

Middle cerebral
artery

Posterior cerebral
artery

Internal carotid
artery

anterior and posterior
choroidal arteries

Posterior communicating
artery

FIGURE 9-3 Surface distribution of the anterior, middle, and posterior cerebral arteries. **(A)** Lateral view of the left cerebral hemisphere. **(B)** Medial view of the left cerebral hemisphere. **(C)** Ventral view of the cerebrum. The figures to the *right* show the branches of the arteries.

(Reprinted with permission from DeMyer. *NMS Neuroanatomy*. 2nd ed. Baltimore: Williams & Wilkins; 1997:403.)

b. **Physical examination.** A complete examination should be performed to elucidate clues regarding the cause of the stroke. Major arteries should be auscultated for bruits, and arrhythmias and murmurs should be ruled out. The skin should be assessed for signs of peripheral vascular disease, needle marks suggesting intravenous drug abuse, and petechiae or ecchymosis suggesting endocarditis, sepsis, or coagulopathy.

c. **Neurologic examination.** A complete neurologic examination must be performed.

d. **Laboratory studies.** A complete blood count should be performed to evaluate for anemia, an infective process, or a hyperviscosity state. Electrolytes

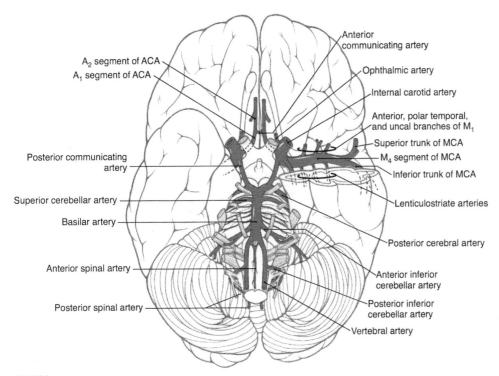

FIGURE 9-4 **Vertebrobasilar artery system.** *CN*, cranial nerve.

(From Haines DE. *Neuroanatomy in Clinical Context: An Atlas of Structures, Sections, Systems, and Syndromes.* 9th ed. Baltimore: Wolters Kluwer Health; 2015.)

should be corrected, and baseline coagulation studies should be performed to rule out a coagulopathy and to guide therapy for those patients requiring anticoagulation.

  e. **Diagnostic studies**
   i. A **12-lead ECG** should be used to detect arrhythmias and rule out myocardial infarction.
   ii. An **unenhanced CT scan** should be obtained in all patients to rule out ICH. An infarct is treated medically, whereas an intracerebral bleed may need urgent neurosurgical intervention.
   iii. **Ancillary tests** generally reserved for inpatients include an echocardiogram to rule out cardiac thrombosis and carotid duplex scanning to detect carotid stenosis.

4. **Therapy**
  a. **Ischemic stroke**
   i. **Management of hypertension.** The management of hypertension during a cerebrovascular accident is controversial. Only severe hypertension (defined by a systolic blood pressure greater than 220 mm Hg or a diastolic pressure greater than 120 mm Hg) should be treated because a sudden decrease in blood pressure may increase the infarct size. The goal of antihypertensive therapy should be to lower the systolic blood pressure to less than 180 mm Hg. Pharmacologic agents used include nitroprusside, nicardipine, and labetalol.
   ii. **Anticoagulation therapy.** The use of anticoagulation in the ED for a stroke victim should be initiated only in consultation with a neurologist. Immediate heparinization may be considered in those patients with progression of the stroke syndrome in whom an ICH has been ruled out.
    a) An embolic stroke may be treated with anticoagulation; however, anticoagulation is generally withheld for 3 to 4 days to prevent a hemorrhagic stroke.
    b) Anticoagulation has not proved beneficial in thrombotic strokes.

Quick HIT

Noncontrast CT scan may not detect an ischemic stroke until 6 to 72 hours after the initial infarct.

Quick HIT

Magnetic resonance imaging (to visualize deficits not seen on the CT scan) and CT angiogram and CT perfusion (to evaluate cerebral vessel patency and tissue perfusion) are being performed more frequently in the ED.

Quick HIT

All patients should have frequent blood pressure monitoring. Overcorrection of blood pressure may lead to a worse outcome.

Neurologic Emergencies

      iii. **Antiplatelet agents** (e.g., **aspirin**). The use of antiplatelet agents is probably not immediately beneficial to the patient; however, a patient with a transient ischemic attack (TIA; see III.B) or a small stroke may benefit from chronic treatment with these agents.

      iv. **Surgery.** Early neurosurgical consultation is needed for all patients with a cerebellar infarct to determine the need for posterior fossa decompression. Cerebellar swelling can lead to rapid deterioration with herniation.

      v. **Thrombolytic therapy.** Thrombolytic therapy (e.g., with **tissue plasminogen activator**) should be administered with neurologic consultation for eligible candidates (see Clinical Pearl 9-4).

    b. **Hemorrhagic stroke** may require neurosurgical treatment. Supportive measures include actions to decrease the ICP (e.g., hyperventilation, mannitol, diuretics).

  5. **Disposition.** All patients suffering a new stroke should be admitted to the hospital for further workup, education, and rehabilitation. Patients with large infarcts, an impaired gag reflex, mental status changes, cerebellar strokes, or cerebral hemorrhage should be admitted to the ICU for close monitoring because deterioration of the patient's condition can be devastating.

B. TIA

  1. **Discussion.** A TIA is a cerebrovascular accident that resolves within 24 hours. Thrombotic strokes are frequently preceded by a TIA affecting the same region as the ensuing stroke, although the exact incidence of TIAs progressing to full strokes is unknown. TIAs can result from plaque ulceration or embolism of platelet aggregates from atherosclerotic vessels. Alternatively, embolism from heart valves may result in a TIA. Any hemodynamic insult that results in cerebral hypoperfusion may lead to a TIA.

  2. **Clinical features.** Clinically, TIAs present as a stroke syndrome; however, the symptoms may have resolved at the time of presentation.

  3. **Evaluation.** Workup in the ED would include a prothrombin time and partial thromboplastin time, an ECG, and a CT scan of the head to rule out hemorrhage. Serial examination should follow neurologic symptoms to document progression or resolution.

  4. **Therapy** in the ED entails antiplatelet therapy.

  5. **Disposition.** All patients with new-onset TIAs or increasingly severe TIAs should be hospitalized for further evaluation and treatment. Cerebral circulation and the feasibility of surgery can be evaluated on an inpatient basis using cerebral artery angiography or carotid duplex ultrasonography. Patients with documented vertebrobasilar lesions should be considered potential candidates for anticoagulation.

CLINICAL PEARL 9-4

Tissue Plasminogen Activator Guidelines

1. **Eligibility.** Candidates should be older than 18 years and have clinical evidence of an ischemic stroke, and the onset of symptoms must have occurred within the last 3 hours.
2. **Contraindications** (absolute and relative) include:
   a. Radiologic evidence or high clinical suspicion of ICH
   b. A history of ICH, neoplasia, arteriovenous malformation, or aneurysm
   c. Coagulation disorders
   d. Seizure at the onset of stroke
   e. Severe neurologic deficit
   f. Uncontrolled hypertension (i.e., a systolic blood pressure greater than 185 mm Hg or a diastolic blood pressure greater than 110 mm Hg)
   g. A history of surgery, head trauma, or a previous stroke within the previous 3 months
   h. Active internal bleeding
3. **Dosage.** In eligible patients, tissue plasminogen activator is given at a dose of 0.9 mg/kg intravenously, up to a total dose of 90 mg. No anticoagulants or antiplatelet agents should be administered until 24 hours after the tissue plasminogen activator infusion is complete.

IV. VERTIGO

A. **Discussion.** In patients complaining of "dizziness," the primary challenge to the ED physician is to determine what the patient means by that term. Vertigo, the illusion of motion, must be distinguished from light-headedness or near-syncope.

1. **Etiology.** The end organs of the vestibular system are situated in the bony labyrinths of the inner ear and consist of the semicircular canals and the otolithic apparatus, the utricle and saccule. The neural output of these end organs is conveyed to the vestibular nuclei in the brain stem via cranial nerve VIII. Projections from the vestibular nuclei include cranial nerves III, IV, and VI; the spinal cord; the cerebral cortex; and the cerebellum. Vertigo may occur with disruption of any of these structures.

   a. **Peripheral vertigo** is caused by dysfunction of structures peripheral to the brain stem.

      i. **Vestibular neuritis** is thought to be of viral origin and affects the vestibular nerve. Patients generally present with acute onset of vertigo with associated nausea and vomiting but no hearing loss. Head positioning worsens the symptoms. History may disclose an upper respiratory tract infection in the weeks preceding the disease. The vertigo may last for days or weeks.

      ii. **Labyrinthitis** is characterized by vertigo with associated hearing loss. This disease is presumed to be viral in origin. Bacterial labyrinthitis is extremely rare but may occur secondary to otitis media, mastoiditis, meningitis, or surgery. Labyrinthitis may also occur secondary to trauma as a result of disruption of the otoconia.

      iii. **Ménière disease** classically presents as a triad of hearing loss, tinnitus, and vertigo. The pathophysiology of Ménière disease is unknown; however, all forms lead to dilation of the endolymphatic systems of the middle ear. The typical patient is older than 50 years and has progressive tinnitus and deafness in the affected ear with acute onset of vertigo. Attacks range from several per week to every few years.

      iv. **Benign paroxysmal positional vertigo** occurs when the patient moves his or her head and is the most common cause of vertigo in the elderly. There is no associated hearing loss or tinnitus. The disease is thought to result from calcium carbonate crystal deposition in the inner ear.

      v. **Drug-induced vertigo.** Vertigo may be caused by aminoglycosides, furosemide, nonsteroidal anti-inflammatory drugs (especially indomethacin), cytotoxic agents (e.g., cisplatin), and anticonvulsants (e.g., phenytoin, carbamazepine).

   b. **Central vertigo** involves disease processes affecting the brain stem or cerebellum.

      i. **Acoustic schwannomas** or **meningiomas** affect cranial nerve VIII. These tumors have the highest incidence in the fifth decade of life. The vertigo, which is of gradual onset, is generally preceded by hearing loss.

      ii. **Cerebellar pontine angle tumors** are characterized by vertigo, hearing loss, and nystagmus. Symptoms are gradual in onset. Cranial nerves V, VII, IX, and XII may be affected. Ipsilateral cerebellar abnormalities may also be noted.

      iii. **Cerebellar infarction** may cause the sudden onset of vertigo. Cerebellar signs are present along with cranial nerve deficits.

      iv. **Cerebellar hemorrhage** is characterized by vertigo and an occipital headache. Gaze is affected secondary to sixth nerve involvement, and the patient cannot look toward the side of the lesion. Other cranial nerves are often affected.

      v. **Vertebrobasilar insufficiency** may lead to vertigo. In these patients, cranial nerve function and cerebellar function are disrupted.

B. **Clinical features** (Table 9-4)

1. **Peripheral vertigo.** Vertigo of peripheral origin usually is an intense spinning sensation accompanied by nausea and vomiting. The onset is generally acute and the vertigo is aggravated by positional changes. Tinnitus and hearing loss may accompany the vertigo. The nystagmus is fatigable and inhibited by ocular fixation.

Quick HIT

The primary consideration in patients with true vertigo is determining whether the vertigo is of peripheral or central origin.

Neurologic Emergencies

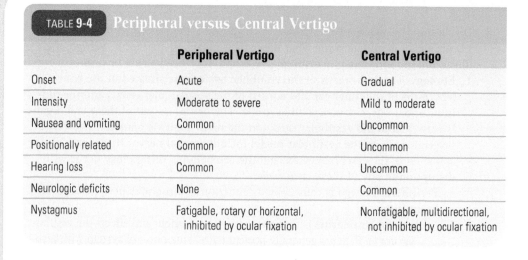

TABLE 9-4 Peripheral versus Central Vertigo	Peripheral Vertigo	Central Vertigo
Onset	Acute	Gradual
Intensity	Moderate to severe	Mild to moderate
Nausea and vomiting	Common	Uncommon
Positionally related	Common	Uncommon
Hearing loss	Common	Uncommon
Neurologic deficits	None	Common
Nystagmus	Fatigable, rotary or horizontal, inhibited by ocular fixation	Nonfatigable, multidirectional, not inhibited by ocular fixation

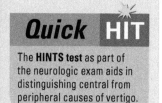

2. **Central vertigo.** Vertigo of central origin is generally less intense and not positionally related. Central vertigo is accompanied by brain stem or cerebellar signs (e.g., cranial nerve dysfunction). Nystagmus is not fatigable and is not inhibited by ocular fixation.

C. **Evaluation**
   1. **Patient history.** The history is most important in diagnosis.
   2. **Physical examination**
      a. **Ears.** The ears should be inspected.
      b. **Eye movements**, with emphasis on nystagmus, are tested.
   3. **Neurologic examination.** A complete neurologic examination is necessary to determine whether the condition is central or peripheral in origin. For example, any cranial nerve abnormality suggests a central process.
   4. **Diagnostic imaging studies.** Cerebral imaging studies are indicated in patients with central vertigo to rule out tumor, hemorrhage, or infarction. In many cases, a noncontrast CT scan is inadequate for diagnosing a tumor or infarct; thus, the patient may need to undergo magnetic resonance imaging.

D. **Therapy**
   1. **Peripheral vertigo.** Patients suffering from peripheral causes of vertigo benefit from hydration and time. Medications used in the treatment of vertigo include antihistamines, anticholinergics, antiemetics, and benzodiazepines. Most patients require reassurance that their symptoms are benign, and patients must also be advised that their symptoms may be protracted. Patients with BPPV may benefit from an otolith repositioning maneuver (e.g., Epley maneuver).
   2. **Central vertigo.** A patient with central vertigo will need to be seen by a neurologist and, possibly, a neurosurgeon.

E. **Disposition**
   1. **Peripheral vertigo.** Patients with peripheral vertigo are often discharged after arranging follow-up with an otolaryngologist. Admission is necessary for patients with the potential for self-injury, patients who are experiencing intractable vomiting, and any patient who lives alone.
   2. **Central vertigo.** Patients with central vertigo require admission, neurologic or neurosurgical consultation, and additional testing.

V. SEIZURES

A. **Discussion.** Seizures affect approximately 1% to 2% of the population. Ten percent of the population will experience at least one seizure in a lifetime.
   1. **Definitions**
      a. **Epilepsy** is a clinical condition in which patients are subject to recurrent seizures. The term "epileptic" is reserved for patients with fixed lesions or irreversible causes of seizures.

b. **Status epilepticus** is defined as continuous seizure activity for more than 30 minutes or two or more seizures without full recovery between seizures.

2. Etiology
   a. **Idiopathic (primary) seizures** have no discernible cause.
   b. **Symptomatic (secondary) seizures** occur in response to identifiable neurologic pathology. Some of the more common causes of seizures include:
      i. **Structural defects**
      ii. **Neoplastic disorders**
      iii. **Vascular disorders** (e.g., subdural or epidural hematoma, SAH, arteriovenous malformation, vasculitis)
      iv. **Degenerative disorders**
      v. **Toxins**
         a) **Substance withdrawal** (e.g., ethanol, benzodiazepines, barbiturates, clonidine, baclofen)
         b) **Overdose** (e.g., theophylline, isoniazid, cyclic antidepressants, anticonvulsants, lithium, sympathomimetics, antihistamines, nicotine, salicylates)
      vi. **Metabolic derangements**
         a) **Electrolyte imbalance** (e.g., hypoglycemia, hyponatremia, hypocalcemia, hypomagnesemia)
         b) **Hypoxia** or **anoxic-ischemic injury**
         c) **Uremia, hepatic failure,** or **pyridoxine deficiency**
      vii. **Infections** (e.g., meningitis, encephalitis, brain abscess)
      viii. **Eclampsia**
      ix. **Fever**

3. Classification
   a. **Generalized seizures**
      i. **Absence seizures**
      ii. **Generalized seizures** may be **tonic–clonic, clonic, tonic, myoclonic,** or **atonic.**
   b. **Partial seizures**
      i. **Simple partial seizures** may be **motor, somatosensory, autonomic,** or **psychic.**
      ii. **Partial seizures with secondary generalization**
      iii. **Complex partial seizures**
   c. **Status epilepticus** may be **tonic–clonic, absence,** or **focal.**

B. **Clinical features**
   1. **Generalized seizures** are initiated deep within the brain stem and involve both cerebral hemispheres. Consciousness is always lost.
      a. **Absence seizures,** brief periods of loss of consciousness that are not accompanied by motor activity, occur most frequently in children 5 to 10 years of age. The attack ends quickly, and the child resumes previous activity. Children with petit mal seizures are often thought to be daydreaming. The attacks may occur frequently, leading to poor academic performance. The frequency of episodes tends to lessen as the child matures.
      b. **Generalized tonic–clonic seizures** begin with a loss of consciousness.
         i. **Tonic phase.** The patient's torso and extremities are extended. The patient may become apneic, lose bowel or bladder control, and vomit.
         ii. **Clonic phase.** The clonic phase immediately follows; the patient exhibits clonic movements of the torso and extremities. The patient will often inadvertently bite his or her tongue. The attack is generally short-lived, lasting 1 to 2 minutes.
         iii. **Postictal phase.** During the postictal period, the patient is flaccid and unconscious. Consciousness then returns gradually; postictal confusion may last for several hours.
   2. **Partial seizures.** Loss of consciousness does not occur.
      a. **Simple partial seizures** begin in a localized area of the brain and may cause motor, sensory, or psychic symptoms. The occurrence of partial seizures

implies a structural brain lesion. Nearby cerebral areas may be affected, leading to localized spread of epileptiform discharges. For example, a patient may present with twitching of the right thumb that progresses to clonic movements of the entire right extremity and right side of the face. Progression of a partial seizure in this form is termed "**Jacksonian march.**"

    b. **Secondary generalization of partial seizures** may occur, resulting in loss of consciousness and convulsive motor activity. **Todd paralysis** is a postictal focal neurologic deficit that can provide a clue as to the seizure focus.

    c. **Complex partial seizures (temporal lobe or psychomotor seizures)** are initiated in the temporal lobe. Consciousness or mentation is affected. Clinically, patients may experience hallucinations, memory disturbances, visceral symptoms, and/or affective disorders. Patients with temporal lobe epilepsy are often mistakenly referred to a psychiatrist.

C. Evaluation

  1. **Patient history.** An adequate history is essential in all patients presenting with a seizure.

    a. Interviews with bystanders, paramedics, and family members will help to establish that the patient did indeed suffer a seizure.

    b. An attempt should be made to ascertain the cause of the seizure. A history of previous seizures, medical compliance with anticonvulsant medications, coincident illnesses, headaches, head trauma, toxin exposure, toxin withdrawal, pregnancy, or neurologic symptoms may offer a clue.

  2. **Physical examination,** including vital signs, may confirm that a seizure actually did occur (e.g., lacerations on the tongue, evidence of bowel or bladder incontinence) and alert the physician to a probable cause (e.g., trauma).

  3. **Neurologic examination.** A complete neurologic examination is essential.

  4. **Diagnostic imaging studies.** A noncontrast CT scan is generally performed on a patient with a new-onset seizure to rule out mass lesions.

  5. **Laboratory studies.** A patient with new-onset seizures must undergo a thorough evaluation to determine a cause. These patients should be monitored and intravenous access obtained. Essential diagnostic studies include pulse oximetry, an ACCU-CHEK, electrolyte levels (including calcium and magnesium), appropriate cultures if infection is suspected, toxicologic screening, and pregnancy testing.

D. **Therapy** depends on the cause of the seizure and the clinical presentation.

  1. **Patients with a seizure history who present to the ED following a seizure** should be questioned in an attempt to discern possible inciting factors.

    a. If the patient is on an antiepileptic drug that can have a level obtained, this should be drawn.

      i. If the level is found to be low, then the patient may be given a loading dose or started on the appropriate medication.

      ii. If the level is determined to be adequate and it is determined that the patient has experienced a single breakthrough seizure, or if the frequency of breakthrough seizures has increased, then the patient's neurologist should be consulted for continued management.

    b. Should the patient not recover fully from a simple seizure, the seizure should be considered a new-onset seizure and worked up appropriately.

  2. **Patients who are having a seizure** need to be protected from self-harm. The patient should be turned on his or her side to prevent aspiration if vomiting should occur. Side rails should be up and padded. Intravenous administration of anticonvulsant medications is not required for an uncomplicated seizure.

  3. **Status epilepticus** is treated aggressively. Stabilization, diagnostic evaluation, and pharmacologic intervention are performed simultaneously.

    a. **Stabilization**

      i. Airway compromise should be aggressively treated with intubation.

      ii. Cardiac monitoring, intravenous access, and supplemental oxygen are instituted. Continuous pulse oximetry and ACCU-CHEKs are performed throughout the resuscitation. Blood pressure should be closely monitored, and a rectal temperature should be obtained initially and followed. A Foley catheter is inserted to monitor urine output.

b. **Diagnostic evaluation**

i. **Laboratory studies.** Electrolyte levels (including calcium, magnesium, and phosphorus), liver function tests, prothrombin time and partial thromboplastin time, ethanol levels, anticonvulsant drug levels, drug levels of potentially convulsant medications, toxicologic screening, pregnancy testing, and creatinine phosphokinase levels (to assess rhabdomyolysis) should be ordered. Arterial blood gas analysis is ordered to assess acidemia and hypercarbia.

ii. **Diagnostic imaging studies**

a) An **ECG** is obtained to assess for toxicity.

b) A **head CT scan** is also performed during the course of treatment; a lumbar puncture should be performed if CT results are unremarkable.

c) **Continuous EEG recordings** are performed on paralyzed patients and those in a barbiturate coma.

c. **Pharmacologic treatment**

i. **Intravenous dextrose** is administered to counteract hypoglycemia.

ii. **Thiamine** (100 mg) and **magnesium sulfate** (2 g) are administered intravenously to alcoholic patients.

iii. **First-line agents.** Benzodiazepines (e.g., lorazepam, diazepam, midazolam) are first-line agents in the treatment of status epilepticus. Generally, lorazepam in 2-mg increments is administered intravenously (up to a maximum dose of 10 mg).

iv. **Coadministration agents.** In cases of status epilepticus, benzodiazepines act quickly to control the seizures, but they have a relatively short window of action (30 to 40 minutes at the most). During this window of opportunity, the patient should be loaded with fosphenytoin (or phenytoin), and if seizures are still not controlled, another intravenous antiseizure medication should be added (e.g., phenobarbital, valproic acid). **Pyridoxine** (6 g, to counteract potential isoniazid poisoning) should be considered.

a) **Fosphenytoin (or phenytoin).** If hypotension occurs, slow the infusion rate but still administer the entire dose.

b) **Phenobarbital.** The patient should be monitored for hypotension. The patient should be intubated for airway protection.

c) **Valproic acid.** Second line

d) **Levetiracetam.** Less evidence-based but possibly effective.

v. **Pentobarbital anesthesia.** If seizures continue despite therapy with benzodiazepines, fosphenytoin (phenytoin), and phenobarbital, an anesthesiologist should be consulted for pentobarbital anesthesia. Neurologic consultation must also be obtained for continuous EEG monitoring.

E. **Disposition.** All patients with status epilepticus are admitted to an ICU. Patients with a treatable underlying cause of seizure, patients with uncontrollable seizures, patients with an unclear etiology of the seizure, and patients who may not receive expedient outpatient follow-up should also be admitted to the hospital.

VI. PERIPHERAL NEUROPATHIES

A. **Chronic neuropathies** develop over months to years. Patients presenting to the ED with a history consistent with a chronic neuropathy may be referred to their primary care physicians. Chronic neuropathy has many causes:

1. **Diseases** (e.g., diabetes, uremia, alcoholism, liver disease, amyloidosis, hypothyroidism, porphyria, lupus, vasculitis, multiple myeloma, polycythemia, sarcoidosis, tuberculosis, scleroderma, hypoglycemia, biliary cirrhosis, acromegaly, malabsorption syndrome, carcinoma, lymphoma, genetic disorders)

2. **Vitamin deficiencies** (e.g., thiamine, pyridoxine, vitamin B_{12}, folic acid, riboflavin, pantothenic acid)

3. **Toxins** (e.g., heavy metals, acrylamide, carbon disulfide, organophosphates, nitrous oxide, hexacarbons, methyl bromide, ethylene oxide, methylbutylketone, pyraminyl, polychlorinated biphenyls)

4. **Drugs** (e.g., amiodarone, colchicine, dapsone, disulfiram, ethambutol, hydralazine, isoniazid, metronidazole, nitrofurantoin, phenytoin, Taxol)

B. **Acute neuropathies**

1. **Guillain-Barré syndrome** is an acute inflammatory demyelinating neuropathy.

a. **Clinical features.** Patients classically present with a prodromal illness, followed in 1 to 3 weeks by an ascending motor paralysis that peaks in 10 to 14 days. Diagnosis is based on the history and physical findings consistent with an acute motor neuropathy (e.g., absent reflexes, cranial nerve palsies, autonomic dysfunction).

b. **Differential diagnoses. Tick paralysis** (see Chapter 6.VIII.B.3) has a similar presentation to that of Guillain-Barré syndrome.

c. **Evaluation.** CSF analysis demonstrates an elevated protein level.

d. **Therapy** is primarily supportive. They should be admitted to a unit where their respiratory status can be closely monitored. Patients may progress to respiratory failure requiring mechanical ventilation. Patients with Guillain-Barré syndrome may benefit from intravenous immunoglobulin.

2. **Botulism** is caused by a preformed toxin elaborated by *Clostridium botulinum*. The toxin acts at the presynaptic terminal to prevent acetylcholine release, leading to paralysis. Sources of infection include improperly prepared food and raw honey.

a. **Clinical features.** Initial symptoms include nausea, vomiting, and xerostomia. Neurologic findings include cranial nerve palsies (especially affecting the ocular muscles), followed by a descending motor paralysis. Sensation and mental status are not affected.

b. **Therapy** includes supportive care and, possibly, mechanical ventilation. Decontamination can be attempted with activated charcoal. Botulinum antitoxin may be administered in consultation with an infectious disease specialist.

3. **Bell's palsy** is an idiopathic mononeuritis of cranial nerve VII.

a. **Clinical features.** The patient presents with paresis of the facial musculature on the affected side. The patient is unable to wrinkle the forehead and close the eye on the affected side. The nasolabial fold is lost, and the mouth sags on the affected side.

b. **Differential diagnoses** include trauma, otitis media, herpes zoster oticus (Ramsay Hunt syndrome), and tumors.

c. **Therapy** for idiopathic Bell's palsy consists of patience and the administration of eye lubricants. Oral steroids should be prescribed if no contraindications. An otolaryngologist or neurologist performs the follow-up. Acyclovir has shown improvement in severe cases.

VII. MUSCLE DISORDERS

A. Myopathies

1. **Discussion**

a. Most patients with myopathies present to the ED because of complications of the disease. A patient with a myopathy will eventually not be able to adequately clear secretions and swallow properly; therefore, these patients are susceptible to respiratory tract infections.

b. The weakness characteristically seen in any myopathy is secondary to **degeneration of muscle fibers**. Initially, the dying fibers are replaced by regeneration. Ultimately, renewal cannot keep pace and progressive fiber loss ensues.

2. **Differential diagnoses.** Myopathies must be differentiated from **neuropathies** and **diseases of neuromuscular transmission** (e.g., myasthenia gravis).

a. Myopathies generally affect large proximal musculature groups and then progress distally. Neuropathies, on the other hand, usually present with distal symptoms that progress proximally. Diseases of neuromuscular transmission initially affect the extraocular and bulbar musculature.

b. Neurologic examination of a patient with a myopathy will reveal preservation of sensation and reflexes (as opposed to the findings in a patient with a neuropathy).

3. **Evaluation.** Finding an elevated creatine phosphokinase level, an increased erythrocyte sedimentation rate, and leukocytosis may aid in the diagnosis of a myopathy.

4. **Clinical entities**

a. **Muscular dystrophy.** The muscular dystrophies (Table 9-5) are a group of inherited disorders that lead to muscular degeneration.

   i. **Duchenne muscular dystrophy** is an X-linked trait that develops in boys before the age of 5 years, leaving them wheelchair-bound by age 12 years.

   ii. **Fascioscapulohumeral muscular dystrophy** is autosomal dominant, affecting both sexes equally, and beginning in adolescence. The face, shoulder, and pelvic girdle are affected early.

   iii. **Limb–girdle muscular dystrophy** is autosomal dominant and characterized by weakness in the shoulder girdle or the pelvic girdle.

   iv. **Myotonic muscular dystrophy** is an autosomal dominant disease that is characterized by myotonia (i.e., delayed relaxation of muscle after voluntary contraction) as well as weakness.

b. **Glycogen storage diseases** are inherited myopathies in which the muscle enzymes, phosphorylase or phosphofructokinase, are limited, leading to impairment of glycogen breakdown with subsequent intracellular glycogen accumulation and myofilament distortion. The disorder generally affects men in their late teens. After vigorous exercise, the patient complains of muscle pain, stiffness, and weakness. Rhabdomyolysis (see VIII.B) may ensue and requires treatment.

c. **Acute periodic paralysis** is another inherited disorder that occurs primarily in men during the first two decades of life. The disease may be hypokalemic, hyperkalemic, or normokalemic. History will reveal a period of intense physical exertion, trauma, surgery, or cold weather preceding the attack. Attacks generally last for a few hours and resolve. Laboratory determinations of potassium and creatine phosphokinase should be performed; patients suspected of having the disorder should be referred to a neurologist.

d. **Polymyositis** is an inflammatory disorder of skeletal muscle that affects the proximal musculature. **Dermatomyositis** is a form of polymyositis

Neurologic Emergencies

TABLE 9-5	Muscular Dystrophies			
	Duchenne	**Fascioscapulohumeral**	**Limb–Girdle**	**Myotonic**
Inheritance	X-linked recessive	Autosomal dominant	Autosomal recessive	Autosomal dominant
Sex	Male	Both	Both	Both
Onset	Younger than 5 years	Adolescence	Adolescence	Infancy to adolescence
Initial symptoms	Pelvic girdle	Shoulder girdle	Pelvic girdle or shoulder girdle	Extremities
Progression	Rapid	Slow	Slow	Slow
Serum creatinine phosphokinase	High	Normal	Slightly increased	Normal
Myotonia	Absent	Absent	Absent	Present

accompanied by a rash that has a predilection for the face and chest and extensor surfaces of the joints.

    i. **Etiology**

      a) **Infectious causes** of polymyositis include trichinosis, toxoplasmosis, malaria, viral diseases, and Lyme disease.

      b) **Metabolic and endocrine causes** of polymyositis include hyper- and hypothyroidism, adrenocortical excess, and hyperparathyroidism.

      c) **Pharmaceutical causes** include steroids, aminocaproic acid, clofibrate, colchicine, amiodarone, L-tryptophan, β blockers, chloroquine, D-penicillamine, vincristine, and opiates.

    ii. **Predisposing factors.** Ten percent of patients diagnosed with polymyositis have an occult malignancy; 20% have a connective tissue disorder (e.g., systemic lupus erythematosus, rheumatoid arthritis, scleroderma). Microscopically, the muscle is infiltrated by lymphocytes, suggesting a cell-mediated autoimmune disorder.

    iii. **Therapy** is with **steroids**.

B. **Rhabdomyolysis** is skeletal muscle injury that leads to the release of myocellular contents into the plasma.

  1. **Etiology.** Rhabdomyolysis is caused by:

    a. **Myopathies**

    b. **Excessive physical exertion** (e.g., seizures)

    c. **Muscular ischemia** (e.g., compartment syndrome; see Chapter 18.VII.A)

    d. **Temperature extremes**

    e. **Direct muscle injury** (e.g., burns, trauma)

    f. **Toxins** (e.g., ethanol, sympathomimetics, seizure-inducing agents)

  2. **Evaluation.** The diagnosis of rhabdomyolysis rests on the laboratory workup. Serum creatine phosphokinase levels are elevated. Although a urine dipstick will show "large" blood, few or no red blood cells are seen because myoglobin and hemoglobin cross-react on the urine dipstick.

  3. **Therapy**

    a. The primary goal is to halt further muscular destruction. The underlying cause must be treated. Induction of paralysis with a nondepolarizing neuromuscular blocker and subsequent endotracheal intubation may be required to halt muscular activity.

    b. Prevention of complications is also important. The toxic ferrihemate molecule released from myoglobin in patients with rhabdomyolysis produces acute renal tubular necrosis leading to renal failure. Hydration (to the point of a good urine output) and alkalinization of the urine (to prevent the release of ferrihemate from myoglobin) are necessary. A urine pH of greater than 6 and a urine output of 2 mL/kg/hour are desirable.

VIII. NEUROLEPTIC MALIGNANT SYNDROME

A. **Discussion.** Neuroleptic malignant syndrome (NMS) is a clinical syndrome composed of the triad of **hyperthermia**, **rigidity**, and **altered mental status**.

  1. **Etiology.** NMS occurs secondary to dopamine antagonism, dopamine agonist withdrawal, and dopamine depletion.

    a. **Dopamine antagonism**

      i. **Therapy with antipsychotic agents** (most commonly the depot form of fluphenazine and haloperidol) is the most common cause of NMS.

      ii. **Therapy with dopamine antagonists** (e.g., metoclopramide) may induce NMS.

    b. **Withdrawal of dopamine agonists** (e.g., L-dopa, bromocriptine, amantadine) may precipitate NMS.

    c. **Dopamine depletion. Catecholamine-depleting agents** (e.g., tetrabenazine) have been implicated in the development of NMS.

  2. **Incidence.** NMS occurs in 0.5% to 1.4% of patients taking neuroleptics.

  3. **Risk factors**

    a. A patient restarted on neuroleptics after a prior episode of NMS suffers a recurrence rate of approximately 33%.

    b. Men are affected five times as often as women, and the peak incidence occurs at 20 to 40 years of age.

    c. Other risk factors include antecedent psychomotor agitation, rate-of-dosage increases, maximum dosages, dehydration, heat, and withdrawal of dopamine agonists.

  4. Complications of NMS include rhabdomyolysis with renal failure, metabolic acidosis, dehydration, respiratory failure due to inadequate ventilation, acute respiratory distress syndrome, disseminated intravascular coagulation, hepatitis, and multisystem organ failure.

B. Clinical features

  1. Fever occurs in 98% of patients. Of these patients, 87% have temperatures greater than 38°C, and 40% have temperatures greater than 40°C.

  2. Altered mental status occurs in 97% of patients and varies from stupor to coma.

  3. Rigidity occurs in 97% of patients and may manifest as generalized or "lead pipe" rigidity. Trismus, opisthotonus, myoclonus, and hyperreflexia may occur.

  4. Signs of autonomic instability are evident in 95% of patients and include sinus tachycardia, hyper- or hypotension, diaphoresis out of proportion to temperature, and tachypnea.

C. Differential diagnoses

  1. Malignant hyperthermia can occur 1 to 2 hours after administration of an anesthetic or paralytic agent. The rigidity associated with NMS is blocked by paralytic agents, whereas that associated with malignant hyperthermia is not. Malignant hyperthermia occurs secondary to abnormal sarcoplasmic reticulum function; therefore, a paralytic agent will not yield any effect.

  2. Serotonin syndrome results from increased serotoninergic activity. A medication search will differentiate the two syndromes.

  3. Lethal catatonia occurs in psychiatric patients. This syndrome is not characterized by muscular rigidity.

  4. Central nervous system infections (e.g., meningitis, encephalitis, sepsis) present with fever and altered mental status, but rigidity is generally not present.

  5. Parkinsonism may be confused with NMS.

D. Evaluation

  1. Laboratory studies. Elevated serum creatine phosphokinase, a sign of rhabdomyolysis, is seen in 95% of patients. Leukocytosis occurs in 98% of patients.

  2. CT and **lumbar puncture** are negative in 95% of patients.

E. Therapy. Supportive care is the mainstay of treatment.

  1. ABCs. Patients with NMS are in critical condition, and primary attention to airway, breathing, and circulation should be maintained.

  2. Cooling measures should be used to reduce the fever, such as ice packs to the axilla and groin, a cooling fan, or a cooling blanket.

  3. Fluid administration and **alkaline diuresis** are used to treat rhabdomyolysis. Creatine phosphokinase levels and renal function must be monitored.

  4. Pharmacologic therapy

    a. Bromocriptine, a dopamine agonist, is administered orally in dosages of 2.5 to 7.5 mg every 8 hours.

    b. Dantrolene inhibits calcium release from the sarcoplasmic reticulum, thereby preventing muscular contraction. Dantrolene is administered intravenously in 1- to 2-mg/kg increments every 6 hours.

    c. Nondepolarizing neuromuscular junction blocking agents may be used to induce paralysis in patients with severe rigidity and hyperthermia. The patient will require mechanical ventilation. Prior to paralysis, patients with severe rigidity may not be able to be ventilated.

    d. Nicardipine may be used to treat hypertension.

F. Disposition. Any patient with a tentative diagnosis of NMS is admitted to the ICU for monitoring and therapy.

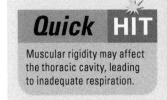

Quick HIT

Muscular rigidity may affect the thoracic cavity, leading to inadequate respiration.

Neurologic Emergencies

RHEUMATOLOGIC AND ALLERGIC EMERGENCIES

Joseph Bales • Salvator Vicario

I. ANAPHYLAXIS

A. **Discussion**

1. **Anaphylaxis is an acute, life-threatening syndrome** initiated by the release of chemical mediators from mast cells and basophils. **Histamine** is the major preformed chemical mediator. Others are Hageman factor pathway enzymes, proteoglycans, neutrophil chemotactic factor, and eosinophil chemotactic factor.

2. **Anaphylactic versus anaphylactoid reactions**

   a. Anaphylactic reactions involve antibody–antigen interactions mediated by immunoglobulin E (IgE), whereas anaphylactoid reactions occur via diverse mechanisms directly degrade mast cells.

      i. **Anaphylaxis**

         a) In IgE-mediated reactions, there has been prior exposure to the antigen, production of specific IgE by plasma cells, and binding of the IgE to receptor sites on mast cells and basophils. This causes the release of preformed mediators, especially histamine, which leads to a series of secondary effects, culminating in anaphylaxis.

         b) Causes of anaphylaxis include foods accounting for one-third of all cases, antibiotics, foreign proteins (e.g., streptokinase), *Hymenoptera* venom, and preservatives. Approximately one-third of all cases are idiopathic.

      ii. **Anaphylactoid reactions**

         a) Anaphylactoid reactions occur via mechanisms that do not involve IgE. The sequence of events involves the direct release of mediators from mast cells and basophils.

         b) Causes of anaphylactoid reactions include human plasma and blood products, direct histamine releasers (e.g., opiates, curare, dextran, radiocontrast media), and miscellaneous agents and processes, such as exercise, physical factors, vibration, nonsteroidal anti-inflammatory drugs (NSAIDs), and mastocytosis.

   b. Anaphylactic and anaphylactoid reactions are clinically the same because comparable mediators produce similar target organ sequelae. Treatment for both reactions is directed at the end-organ signs and is the same. Because of these similarities, the term anaphylaxis will be used to encompass both IgE and non-IgE reactions.

B. **Clinical features** (see Table 10-1)

1. Symptoms are most likely to occur minutes after exposure to the triggering agent but may occur in seconds to a few hours. Early or subtle signs and symptoms of anaphylaxis include cutaneous flushing, pruritus, voice change, and sense of impending doom. Usually, the later the symptoms occur, the less severe the reaction.

2. Clinical findings prominently involve the skin (urticaria), the upper airways (laryngeal edema, hoarseness, stridor), the lower airways (bronchospasm), the cardiovascular system (hypotension, vasodilation, dysrhythmia, myocardial infarction [MI]), and the gastrointestinal system (abdominal cramps).

TABLE 10-1	Clinical Manifestations of Anaphylaxis
Organ System	**Reaction**
Cutaneous	Diaphoresis Flushing Pruritus Piloerection Urticaria Angioedema
Head, ears, eyes, nose, and throat	Conjunctivitis Rhinorrhea/nasal congestion Metallic taste Hoarseness Stridor
Pulmonary	Tachypnea Dyspnea Cough Wheezing
Cardiovascular	Tachycardia Dysrhythmia Hypotension
Gastrointestinal	Abdominal cramps Nausea and vomiting Diarrhea
Neurologic	Altered mental status Dizziness Seizure

3. Death may occur from respiratory causes (70%) or from cardiovascular causes (25%). (Autopsy findings include acute pulmonary hyperinflation, laryngeal edema, visceral congestion, pulmonary edema, intra-alveolar hemorrhage, urticaria/angioedema, and MI.)

C. **Differential diagnoses.** The diagnosis of anaphylaxis is generally readily apparent based on history and clinical findings but may sometimes be confused with overlapping or other distinct entities (see Clinical Pearl 10-1).

D. **Evaluation.** History and physical examination are key for making the diagnosis and for assessing the severity of the reaction in order to plan the management strategy.

   1. **Patient history**

      a. The cause for the anaphylaxis should be determined.

         i. Penicillin antibiotics are a leading cause of adverse drug reactions. Most reactions occur after parenteral administration rather than the oral route.

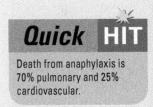

Death from anaphylaxis is 70% pulmonary and 25% cardiovascular.

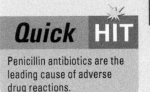

Penicillin antibiotics are the leading cause of adverse drug reactions.

CLINICAL PEARL 10-1

Differential diagnosis involves the following:

1. Judging whether the symptoms and signs represent a simple allergic or pseudoallergic reaction (e.g., asthma exacerbation, urticaria), as opposed to anaphylaxis
2. Considering whether some of the symptoms and signs represent a secondary process (e.g., MI)
3. Determining if a completely different type of problem could be occurring (e.g., drug intoxication, hypovolemic shock)

Rheumatologic and Allergic Emergencies

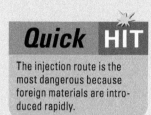

The injection route is the most dangerous because foreign materials are introduced rapidly.

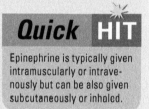

Epinephrine is typically given intramuscularly or intravenously but can be also given subcutaneously or inhaled.

    ii. Radiocontrast media cause anaphylactoid reactions at a rate of 0.22% for ionic (high osmolar) agents. The risk of death has been estimated to be 1 in 10,000 (0.01%). Nonionic (low osmolar) agents cause anaphylactoid reactions at a rate of 0.04%.

    iii. Lidocaine and other local anesthetics rarely cause true allergic reactions, but many patients report "allergy to 'caines'" because a variety of nonallergic reactions are associated with its administration.

  b. The route and timing of exposure should be ascertained. The route may be by injection, ingestion, inhalation, or cutaneous absorption.

  c. Additional information that may be important for the assessment and management of the case should include prior reaction to the same substance and severity of that reaction; underlying medical problems, such as cardiovascular disease or pulmonary disease; current medications, including β blockers, antihistamines, and corticosteroids; and medication allergies.

  2. Laboratory testing (see Table 10-2)

  3. Radiography. A chest radiograph may reveal hyperinflation or atelectasis.

E. Therapy

  1. Prompt intervention is vital

    a. Exposure to antigen must be terminated, and vital signs monitored. Any intravenous infusion of antigen should have been stopped at onset of the reaction and any topical preparations removed. If the agent was recently ingested, gastric lavage should be considered.

    b. **Epinephrine** is administered to prevent mediator release. It relaxes laryngeal and bronchial smooth muscle and supports blood pressure.

      i. **Side effects.** Epinephrine may cause vomiting, hypertension, tremor, and tachydysrhythmia.

      ii. **Possible contraindications** include cardiac ischemia, severe hypertension, and pregnancy. Glucagon can be substituted if epinephrine is contraindicated.

      iii. **Dosage and administration**

        a) Epinephrine 0.1% (1:1,000 preparation). In patients with stable vital signs, epinephrine 0.1% is given subcutaneously or intramuscularly every 15 minutes as required. The dosage is 0.3 to 0.5 mL for adults and 0.01 mg/kg for children.

        b) Epinephrine 0.01% (1:10,000 preparation) is administered intravenously when there is significant airway compromise or shock. For adults, the dosage is 1 to 3 mL, administered slowly intravenously (or diluted in normal saline to 10 mL and administered via an endotracheal tube). Children receive 0.1 mg/kg by slow intravenous infusion.

TABLE 10-2 Differential Diagnoses of Anaphylaxis	
Asthma exacerbation	Hypovolemic shock or sepsis
Carcinoid syndrome	Mastocytosis
Cerebrovascular accident	Myocardial infarction
Drug intoxication	Pulmonary embolus
Hereditary angioedema	Seizure disorder
Hyperventilation	Urticarial syndrome
Hypoglycemia	Vasovagal syncope
Laryngeal foreign body	Trauma to larynx

   c. **Stabilization of airway, breathing, and circulation (ABCs)**
      i. The airway should be observed closely and supported as needed with endotracheal intubation or cricothyrotomy.
      ii. High-flow oxygen should be administered.
      iii. Blood pressure should be supported by placing the patient in a recumbent position, by infusing intravenous fluids, and, if necessary, by administering a continuous infusion of epinephrine.
   d. **Treatment of bronchospasm** is with β agonists or nebulized epinephrine.
   e. **Histamine receptor blockade**
      i. Histamine-1 receptors should be blocked with an antihistamine such as diphenhydramine (1 to 2 mg/kg intravenously, up to a total dose of 50 mg, initially and every 6 to 8 hours as needed, for adults and children).
      ii. Histamine-2 receptors. Blocking of the histamine-2 receptors with an agent such as cimetidine or ranitidine may also be advantageous.
   f. **Prevention of late-phase reactions.** A corticosteroid (e.g., prednisolone, 1 to 2 mg/kg intravenously every 6 hours until conversion to oral medication) should be administered intravenously in an attempt to abort late-phase reactions.
   g. **Treatment of refractory anaphylaxis.** In the presence of β blockade, anaphylaxis may be particularly refractory to treatment, and glucagon (0.05 mg/kg administered as an intravenous bolus, followed by an infusion at a rate of 0.07 mg/kg/hour) may need to be employed.
  2. **Late-phase reactions** may occur in the ensuing 6 to 48 hours. The treatment strategy for a late-phase reaction is the same as that for an initial reaction.

F. **Disposition**
  1. **Discharge.** Patients who present with a mild reaction, respond well to treatment, remain asymptomatic for 4 to 6 hours after initial treatment, and are reliable with good support systems may be considered for discharge home.
   a. These patients should be instructed to use oral antihistamines and steroid medication for several days and to return to the emergency department (ED) if there is any return of symptoms. They should be advised to avoid the suspected agent or agents and to follow up with their primary care physician.
   b. Patients with conditions such as *Hymenoptera*-sting anaphylaxis need instructions regarding acquisition of a medical alert bracelet, tag, or card; provision of epinephrine autoinjector (e.g., EpiPen [Mylan]) so that early treatment may be self-initiated in the event of another episode of anaphylaxis; and referral to an allergist.
  2. **Admission.** Patients with persistent or recurring airway edema, bronchospasm, hypotension, cardiovascular complications, or altered mental status require hospital admission to an intensive care unit. Patients who receive treatment for an initially severe anaphylactic reaction but who rapidly become asymptomatic can be admitted to the hospital in case a late-phase reaction occurs, although this is becoming less common.

G. **Prevention of anaphylaxis**
  1. Allergic reactions should be clearly documented in the medical record.
  2. Inquiries regarding history of allergy should be made before administering a medication, and any worrisome report should be heeded.
  3. When possible, drugs that are highly allergenic should be given orally rather than parenterally. If an injection is given, the patient should be observed for 20 to 30 minutes.
  4. Desensitization may be feasible and indicated for certain agents such as penicillin, *Hymenoptera* venom, and aspirin (Table 10-3).

II. URTICARIA AND ANGIOEDEMA

A. **Discussion.** Urticaria and angioedema are associated conditions. Reports indicate 15% to 23% of the population of the United States may have had urticaria, and

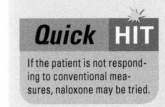

Quick **HIT**

If the patient is not responding to conventional measures, naloxone may be tried.

Rheumatologic and Allergic Emergencies

TABLE 10-3 Local Anesthetic Chemical Groups		
Group I: Esters[a]	**Group II: Amides**[b]	**Others**[c]
Benzocaine	Bupivacaine	Dibucaine
Procaine	Lidocaine	Dyclonine
Proparacaine	Mepivacaine	Pramoxine
Tetracaine	Prilocaine	

[a]May cross-react.
[b]Unlikely to cross-react.
[c]For mucous membrane administration.

half of the cases are accompanied by angioedema. Occasionally, angioedema occurs alone.

1. **Definitions**
   a. **Urticaria** is characterized by pruritic, erythematous, cutaneous elevations that blanch with pressure and clear or migrate within 12 to 24 hours.
      i. Acute urticaria usually lasts for 2 to 3 days but may persist for 4 to 6 weeks. It occurs in younger patients and is more prevalent in those who are atopic. Commonly identified causes include drugs, foods, and infections; however, in over 50% of patients, the cause is not determined.
      ii. Chronic urticaria persists for more than 6 weeks. It affects predominantly young adults and is approximately twice as common in women as in men. Occasionally, the cause is one of the physical urticarias (see II.A.3), but more than 75% of cases are classified as idiopathic.
   b. **Angioedema** is characterized by swelling originating subcutaneously or submucosally. Symptoms typically last longer but are less pruritic than the wheals of urticaria.

B. **Differential diagnoses**
   1. Early maculopapular rashes or local reactions to insect bites may initially resemble urticaria, but over time, urticaria can be diagnosed by its characteristic appearance together with its transient pattern.
   2. Distinguishing features of some forms of urticaria that have more serious prognostic significance and special therapeutic implications are as follows:
      a. Urticarial vasculitis is characterized by wheals that last more than 24 hours and a biopsy that shows evidence of vascular damage.
      b. Urticaria pigmentosa occurs in systemic mastocytosis.
      c. Hereditary angioedema, or C1q esterase deficiency, has a predilection for the upper airways. Patients typically have a low level of C4 during and between attacks.

C. **Evaluation**
   1. **History and physical examination.** Preliminary visual survey usually identifies a patient as having an urticaria/angioedema syndrome (Figure 10-1). As long as the airway is not compromised and there is no concomitant hypotension or wheezing (which would suggest that the cutaneous findings are actually part of an anaphylactic reaction), evaluation proceeds with detailed history. In cases of acute urticaria, history of exposure to agents that may cause an IgE reaction or other type of reaction is sought, plus information that might suggest that this is the first presentation of a systemic illness or physical urticaria.
   2. **Laboratory studies.** Laboratory testing in the ED is generally not indicated for acute urticaria and is rarely indicated for chronic urticaria. Clinic evaluation of chronic urticaria may include screening for collagen vascular disease (e.g., erythrocyte sedimentation rate [ESR], antinuclear antibodies, rheumatoid factor), thyroid disease (e.g., thyroid function tests), infections (e.g., stool analysis for ova and parasites if there is eosinophilia, hepatitis panel, Epstein-Barr virus

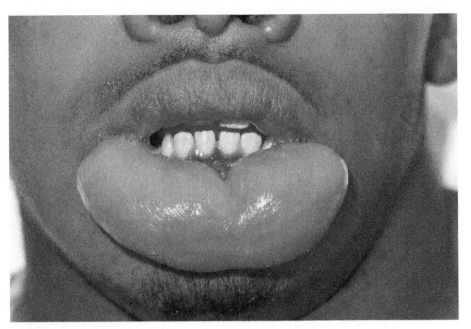

FIGURE 10-1 Patient with angioedema.
(Courtesy of Lawrence B. Stack, MD.)

detection), neoplastic disease (e.g., complete blood count [CBC], chest radiograph), and complement pathway disorders (e.g., complement levels).

D. **Therapy.** General measures include avoidance of any identified causative agent and treatment of underlying contributing conditions. In addition:

1. Antihistamines are the mainstay of symptomatic management for urticaria and angioedema.

    a. The most widely used antihistamines are the traditional histamine-1–receptor blockers hydroxyzine and diphenhydramine. Newer agents, such as loratadine, are less sedating and more convenient in terms of dosing.

    b. Adjunctive treatment with histamine-2–receptor antagonist (e.g., cimetidine) may be helpful.

2. Corticosteroids are used when antihistamines do not adequately control the signs and symptoms. Because of the potential for adverse long-term effects, the medication is stopped after 1 to 3 weeks, or is tapered or stopped once symptoms are controlled.

3. Epinephrine 0.1% (0.3 mL of 1:1,000 preparation intramuscularly or subcutaneously) is occasionally necessary for patients with acute, severely symptomatic urticaria or when angioedema may be beginning to compromise the upper airway.

4. Hereditary angioedema may require a recombinant C1-inhibitor or long-term control with certain androgens. Fresh frozen plasma, which contains C1-inhibitor and angiotensin-converting enzyme, has been shown to have some benefit in angiotensin-converting enzyme inhibitor induced angioedema.

5. Intubation may be needed for airway management, especially in patients with a reaction to angiotensin-converting enzyme inhibitors or in patients with hereditary angioedema.

E. **Disposition**

1. **Discharge**

    a. Patients with acute urticaria/angioedema may be discharged with instructions to follow up in clinic if medications are ineffective or if the problem persists for more than 6 weeks.

    b. Patients with chronic urticaria/angioedema who have not had a diagnostic workup should be referred to a primary care physician or allergy specialist for evaluation.

2. **Admission.** Only patients with airway compromise need to be admitted to the hospital. Airway management should be a top priority.

CLINICAL PEARL | **10-2**

Spinal Cord Anatomy

1. The corticospinal tract provides motor innervation to muscles on the same side.
2. The spinothalamic tract, or lateral column, carries superficial pain, deep pain, light touch, and temperature sensation from the opposite side of the body (decussation occurs two dermatome levels above the point of nerve root entry).
3. The posterior column carries proprioception, light touch, and vibration from the same side of the body.

III. NECK PAIN

A. Discussion

  1. Anatomy

    a. The musculoskeletal structures of the neck include the cervical vertebrae, intervertebral disks, supporting muscles, and ligaments (see Clinical Pearl 10-2).

      i. The seven cervical vertebrae are connected by the anterior and posterior longitudinal ligaments.

      ii. Intervertebral disks consist of a shock-absorbing central nucleus pulposus surrounded by an annulus fibrosis.

      iii. Facet joints, one on each side of the spine, connect the vertebral elements posteriorly.

    b. **Neuroanatomy.** The individual nerve roots emerge from the spinal canal through the intervertebral neural foramina, located on the right and left sides of the vertebral bodies.

  2. Causes of neck pain include:

    a. **Musculoskeletal disorders**

      i. **Mechanical disorders**

        a) Disk disease. The nucleus pulposus and annulus fibrosis tend to undergo progressive degeneration after the fourth decade of life, decreasing the ability of the intervertebral disk to absorb shocks and stimulating local nerve endings, causing pain that can be perceived along the neck at any level.

        b) Arthritis, particularly osteoarthritis, may involve the facet joints and may also produce pain along the neck at any level.

        c) Muscle spasm or torticollis (congenital, spasmodic, drug-induced, hysterical)

        d) Muscle strain or ligament strain (e.g., acute posterior cervical strain)

        e) Tendinitis (occipital, sternocleidomastoid)

        f) Cervical spondylosis

        g) Thoracic outlet syndrome, which may be confused with cervical disk disease associated with nerve root compression

        h) Skeletal congenital causes, including fused vertebrae, hemivertebrae, instability of the atlantoaxial joint, and spinal stenosis

      ii. **Medical disorders** or processes in the bone of the cervical column may cause neck pain and associated symptoms of systemic disease. Specific disorders include:

        a) Inflammatory arthritis (rheumatoid arthritis, juvenile rheumatoid arthritis, ankylosing spondylitis, Reiter syndrome, psoriatic arthritis, the enteropathic arthritides)

        b) Osteomyelitis (e.g., staphylococcal, tubercular)

        c) Discitis

        d) Abscess

        e) Primary or metastatic neoplasms (e.g., multiple myeloma)

        f) Paget disease

        g) Diffuse idiopathic skeletal hyperostosis

     b. Soft tissue disorders of structures such as the blood vessels, endocrine glands, exocrine glands, respiratory structures, and alimentary structures can also cause neck pain. Meningeal irritation may cause symptoms in patients with meningitis or subarachnoid hemorrhage.

        i. Thyroiditis

        ii. Cervical lymphadenitis

        iii. Pharyngeal infections

        iv. Sialoadenitis

        v. Carotodynia

        vi. Thyroglossal duct cyst

        vii. Meningitis

        viii. Epidural abscess

        ix. Carotid dissection

        x. Subarachnoid hemorrhage

     c. Referred pain. The symptom of neck pain may be a referred symptom from a remote somatic or visceral structure that has cervical nerve root innervation based on a common embryologic origin. Pain referred from other sites but perceived in the neck includes pain secondary to tumor or other process in the apex of the lung, pain secondary to gastrointestinal conditions (e.g., gallbladder disease, pancreatic disease, hiatal hernia, gastric ulcer), or cardiovascular causes including infarction and thoracic aneurysm.

  3. Pathogenesis

     a. Neck pain as a result of muscle spasm and ligamentous strain

        i. Trauma may cause muscle spasm or ligamentous strain of the neck. "Whiplash" (cervical strain syndrome) describes an injury to muscles and ligaments that have been forcibly extended and flexed.

        ii. "Neck stiffness" exists as a common disorder in the working population. Sustained position, such as extension of the neck while doing overhead work or flexion of the neck while sitting at a typewriter or computer, causes spasm of the neck muscles and neck pain that may be associated with headache or shoulder-arm-hand pain.

     b. Neck pain as a result of arthritis. Osteoarthritis, ankylosing spondylitis and the other spondyloarthritides, rheumatoid arthritis, and juvenile rheumatoid arthritis may cause neck pain. Rarely, neck pain is associated with gout and calcium pyrophosphate deposition disease.

        i. In patients with rheumatoid arthritis, cervical spine disease may progress, placing the patient at risk for neurologic injury.

        ii. Atlantoaxial subluxation may be present.

        iii. Cord compression may follow minor trauma or be insidious. In patients with spondyloarthropathy, the inflexible cervical spine is susceptible to fracture with minor trauma.

     c. Neck pain as a result of intervertebral disk disease. Cervical disks may rupture after minor or major trauma. In most patients, hyperextension aggravates the pain, and rotation and lateral movements are moderately restricted. If the cervical herniation is large and centrally located, spinal cord compression may result. More commonly, however, the disk protrusion impinges on a nerve root and causes radicular symptoms and signs.

     d. Neck pain as a result of cervical spondylosis. Cervical spondylosis is characterized by degenerative and arthritic changes in the cervical spine that affect nerve roots and the spinal cord. The constellation of pathologic changes includes bone formation in the bony canal (spondylosis), narrowing of the intervertebral disk spaces (by herniation of the nucleus pulposus or by degeneration and desiccation of the disk with aging), formation of osteophytes on the vertebrae, and partial subluxation of one or more vertebrae. Cervical spondylosis is most common at the C5–C6 interspace.

B. Clinical features

  1. Neurologic signs and symptoms may result from mechanical or medical musculoskeletal disorders of the neck that involve the nerve roots or spinal cord.

Rheumatologic and Allergic Emergencies

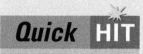

Quick HIT

Objective signs of nerve root compression are muscle weakness, decreased sensation in a dermatomal distribution, and decreased associated deep tendon reflex.

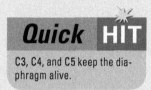

Quick HIT

C3, C4, and C5 keep the diaphragm alive.

The neural foramina and the spinal cord can be encroached on by a bulging intervertebral disk or an osseous proliferation from the vertebral body, facet joints, or neural foramina. They may also be encroached on by masses related to infection, tumor, or bleeding.

   a. **Radicular symptoms and signs.** When the encroachment involves a nerve root, irritation of the dorsal sensory root produces neuralgic pain, which is dermatomal and "electric" in nature, and irritation of the ventral motor root produces myalgic pain, which is sclerotomal and "achy" in nature.

      i. The first through the seventh cervical nerves exit above the cervical vertebrae of the same number, whereas the eighth cervical nerve exits below the seventh cervical vertebra. Because the cervical spinal nerves may consist of separate ventral motor and dorsal sensory bundles at the point of the neural foramina, production of isolated motor or sensory symptoms rather than as combined deficits is common.

      ii. Cervical roots 3, 4, and 5 supply innervation to the diaphragm via the phrenic nerves. Innervation in the upper extremity attributable to nerve roots C5–T1 is summarized in Table 10-5. Dermatomes (regions of skin from which afferent fibers converge at a single nerve root) are shown in Chapter 9, Figure 9-1.

   b. **Spinal cord compression symptoms and signs.** When the encroachment involves the spinal cord, patients may present with numb or spastic paraparesis. The degree of neck pain is variable. When there is extensive spinal cord injury, there can be initial loss of function below the level of the injury, known as spinal shock (see Chapter 17.IV.B.3). Specific cord syndromes are discussed in Chapter 17.IV.B.2.

  2. **Systemic signs.** Fever or weight loss may be present in patients with infectious, inflammatory, or neoplastic processes.

C. Differential diagnoses. Although many of the causes of neck pain do not represent an emergency, the life- or limb-threatening causes of neck pain must be systematically excluded. These include:

  1. Spinal instability resulting from mechanical injury, osteomyelitis, or tumor
  2. Cord vulnerability as a result of spinal instability, abscess, hematoma, or tumor
  3. Meningitis
  4. Subarachnoid hemorrhage
  5. MI
  6. Thoracic aneurysm

D. Evaluation. A directed history and focused musculoskeletal and neurologic examination are required to develop a preliminary differential diagnosis.

  1. **Patient history**

   a. The time and circumstances of onset, the location, and the quality of the pain should be determined, as well as constancy versus intermittency, and exacerbating or relieving factors (Table 10-4).

   b. The presence or absence of associated neurologic symptoms needs to be established. Neurologic complaints may reflect nerve root irritation or cord compression. Symptoms of dizziness, visual changes, and ataxia may be related to vertebral artery compression.

   c. The past medical history is important, especially in regard to a possible underlying anatomic abnormality, rheumatologic disorder, or immunosuppressive condition. Congenital abnormalities should be considered in children who present with neck pain.

  2. **Physical examination.** In the setting of trauma or suspected neck instability from other causes, prompt and continued immobilization is necessary throughout the evaluation process to minimize the risk of cord injury.

   a. **Evaluation of the musculoskeletal structures of the neck**

      i. The neck should be examined with respect to possible bony injury or abnormality. The neck muscles are examined for tenderness or spasm.

      ii. If spine instability is not suspected, active range of motion should be tested (i.e., flexion, extension, rotation to the left and right, and lateral bending to the left and right).

TABLE 10-4	Innervation of the Upper Extremity			
Root	**Reflex**	**Muscles**	**Action**	**Sensation**
C5	Biceps reflex	Deltoid Biceps	Shoulder abduction Flexion of the supinated forearm	Lateral upper arm
C6	Brachioradialis reflex (biceps reflex)	Extensor carpi radialis, extensor carpi ulnaris Biceps	Wrist extension Flexion of the supinated forearm	Lateral forearm and thumb
C7	Triceps reflex	Flexor carpi radialis, flexor carpi ulnaris Extensor digitorum Triceps	Wrist flexors Finger extension Forearm extension at elbow	Middle finger
C8	None	Flexor digitorum superficialis, flexor digitorum profundus Hand intrinsics	Finger flexion Digit abduction and adduction	Medial forearm and fourth digit
T1	None	Hand intrinsics	Digit abduction and adduction	Median midarm

b. **The soft tissues** of the neck should be inspected for swelling or asymmetry, and the midline tracheal position should be verified. The patient's neck should be palpated for thyroid abnormalities, lymphadenopathy, enlargements consistent with cysts or other tumors, and areas of induration or fluctuance consistent with abscess. Carotid artery pulsations should be checked.

c. **General physical examination.** A general physical examination is performed, paying special attention to the area of concern if a type of referred pain is suspected.

d. **Neurologic examination**

i. Motor and sensory function and sphincter tone should be tested as well as reflexes.

a) Muscle strength testing in the upper extremities should include the biceps (flexion of the elbow), triceps (extension of the elbow), wrist extensors and flexors, hand and finger flexors, and intrinsic muscles of the hand.

b) Sensory testing should include pain and vibration and an attempt to delineate an anatomic deficit.

3. **Laboratory and diagnostic imaging studies**

a. If there is localized spinal tenderness or if the neurologic examination is abnormal, cervical spine computed tomography (CT) should be obtained. If abnormality is present or there are neurologic deficits, magnetic resonance imaging or myelography should be ordered.

b. If underlying disease is suspected, workup may include a CBC, ESR, a CT head, a magnetic resonance imaging or CT of the neck, and/or cerebrospinal fluid analysis for evaluation for meningitis or hemorrhage.

c. In patients with neurologic deficits associated with the pain, neurologic or neurosurgical consultation is usually necessary, often before specialized imaging tests are ordered.

E. **Therapy**

1. **Spasm, strain, or sprain.** Cervical symptoms caused by simple spasm, strain, or sprain are managed with anti-inflammatory medications, and mobilization as guided by pain control. Improvement should occur within 1 to 2 weeks. For patients with more severe pain or spasm, narcotic analgesics or muscle relaxants may also be prescribed. Local injection of an anesthetic agent at key anatomic points may be considered for selected patients.

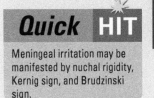

Quick **HIT**

Meningeal irritation may be manifested by nuchal rigidity, Kernig sign, and Brudzinski sign.

Rheumatologic and Allergic Emergencies

2. **Disk disease and cervical spondylosis** includes rest and anti-inflammatory and analgesic medications.

F. **Disposition**

1. **Discharge.** Most patients with musculoskeletal neck pain, including patients with stable cervical disk disease, may be discharged home with arrangements for outpatient follow-up.

2. **Admission.** Patients with unstable or rapidly progressive neurologic symptoms or findings consistent with cord compression as well as patients in whom a serious medical condition (e.g., meningitis, osteomyelitis, abscess, MI, hemorrhage) is suspected require inpatient hospital management.

IV. THORACIC AND LUMBAR BACK PAIN

A. **Discussion**

1. **Anatomy**

a. **Musculoskeletal structures.** The thoracic spine consists of 12 vertebrae and the lumbar spine consists of 5 vertebrae, with intervertebral disks. The column is supported by ligaments and paraspinous muscles. The posterior aspects of the vertebrae form the spinal canal, neural foramina, and facet or apophyseal joints. The sacrum connects with the iliac bones of the pelvis.

b. **Neuroanatomy.** The pattern of innervation is a complex anastomosis that serves multiple structures and levels, explaining the diffuse and nonspecific nature of pain associated with back disorders of varying causes.

2. **Causes of back pain.** Like neck pain, back pain may be caused by mechanical and medical disorders of the musculoskeletal structures of the spine. The precise cause of back pain can be identified in less than 25% of patients. Herniated disk, spinal stenosis, and compression fracture are identified most often.

a. **Mechanical causes** of back pain include:

   i. **Degenerative disk disease**

   ii. **Osteoarthritis** of the facet joints

   iii. **Muscle spasm**

   iv. **Ligament or muscle strain**

   v. **Intervertebral disk disease**

   vi. **Spinal stenosis**

   vii. **Epidural** or **intradural tumors** in the spinal canal may produce a syndrome similar to that of a ruptured disk.

   viii. **Spondylolysis** and **spondylolisthesis**

   ix. **Spina bifida** (rare)

b. **Medical causes** of thoracic and lumbar pain include **inflammatory arthritis** (ankylosing spondylitis and the other spondyloarthritides), **infection, neoplasm**, and other underlying diseases and processes (e.g., **spinal osteomyelitis, epidural abscess**).

c. **Referred pain.** Disorders of the abdominal, retroperitoneal, and pelvic viscera can cause pain that is perceived in the region of the spine. However, back pain is rarely the only symptom, and it is not aggravated by activity or relieved by rest, as is most pain of spinal origin. From an emergency standpoint, it is important to realize that **abdominal aortic aneurysm** and **aortic dissection** may give rise to back pain (see Clinical Pearl 10-3).

3. **Differential diagnoses**

a. **Life-threatening causes of back pain**, such as abdominal aortic aneurysm or abdominal dissection, must be ruled out.

b. **Nonanatomic, nonorganic presentations** such as whole leg pain, numbness, and/or weakness are associated with psychological stressors.

4. **Clinical findings. Neurologic symptoms** may result from mechanical or medical musculoskeletal disorders of the back that involve the nerve roots or spinal cord, such as intervertebral disk protrusion, osseous proliferation, or masses due to infection, tumor, or bleeding.

a. **Radicular symptoms and signs** are produced when there is nerve root irritation or impingement at the neural foramina. The lumbar and sacral nerve

1. In general, upper abdominal diseases (peptic ulcer disease, tumors of the stomach, duodenum, and pancreas) are referred to the lower thoracic spine, lower abdominal diseases (colon tumors, colon inflammatory disease) are referred to the lumbar spine, and pelvic diseases (endometriosis; invasive carcinoma of the uterus, cervix, or bladder; uterine malposition; dysmenorrhea; chronic prostatitis; carcinoma of the prostate) are referred to the sacral region.
2. Renal pain is perceived in the costovertebral angle.
3. Diseases of retroperitoneal structures (e.g., lymphomas, sarcomas) may evoke pain in the adjacent part of the spine. Retroperitoneal bleeding, especially in an anticoagulated patient, can cause back pain.

root motor and sensory innervation patterns are summarized in Table 10-5 and Chapter 9, Figure 9-1.

  b. **Spinal cord compression symptoms and signs.** Specific spinal cord syndromes are discussed in Chapter 17.IV.B.2.
    i. **Compression of the spinal cord above T12** results in a constellation of possible **upper motor neuron** or **long tract signs**: spasticity, hyperactive deep tendon reflexes, suppressed superficial skin reflexes, positive Babinski sign, acute urinary retention with overflow incontinence, and fecal retention. Acutely, however, these signs may not be apparent because of transient spinal shock producing flaccid paralysis, areflexia, and hypotension.
    ii. **Compression in the spinal canal below T12**, and specifically below the level of the conus medullaris, results in a constellation of **lower motor neuron** or **nerve root signs**.
5. **Evaluation.** The history and physical examination provide the diagnosis in most cases.
  a. **Patient history**
    i. **Possible precipitating factors.** In the approach to the patient with back pain, the **patient's age** and the **circumstances of the onset of the pain** are important. There may be **antecedent trauma**, minor to major, or a **history of lifting or strain**. There may be a **history of prior episodes**. **Occupational history** may be relevant.
    ii. **Symptoms**
       a) **Neurologic symptoms.** Information pertaining to possible nerve root irritation, spinal cord compression, or cauda equina syndrome should be elicited. Patients may complain of motor weakness; numbness; paresthesias; or bowel, bladder, or sexual dysfunction.
       b) **Associated symptoms** (e.g., fever, weight loss) may be present, or there may be pertinent risk factors for infection, such as chronic steroid use or intravenous drug abuse.

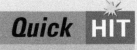

Quick HIT

In the **cauda equina syndrome**, flaccid paralysis, areflexia, a negative Babinski sign, and urinary and fecal incontinence due to loss of sphincter tone may be seen.

Rheumatologic and Allergic Emergencies

TABLE **10-5**	Innervation of the Lower Extremity			
Root	**Reflex**	**Muscles**	**Action**	**Sensation**
L4	Patellar reflex	Anterior tibialis	Dorsiflexion and inversion of foot	Medial regions of lower leg and foot
L5	None	Extensor hallucis longus	Dorsiflexion of great toe	Lateral region of midleg, dorsum of foot
S1	Achilles reflex	Peroneus longus and brevis	Plantar flexion and eversion of foot	Lateral region of foot
S2, S3, S4	Superficial anal reflex	Bladder, foot intrinsics	Toe abduction and adduction	Perineal region

iii. **Past medical history** is important in general and for any prior back pain evaluation and treatment in particular.

iv. **Psychosocial issues** (e.g., current work status, disability, compensation, litigation) should be discussed because they may influence the assessment, management, and outcome of treatment for back pain.

b. **Physical examination.** The back should be examined, and a neurologic examination should be performed. The general examination is important to evaluate the patient for a medical disorder as a cause of back pain.

   i. **Examination of the back**

      a) **Inspection**

         1) The back should be inspected for **signs of infection and trauma.**

         2) **Unusual skin markings**, which may denote underlying neurologic or bone pathology, should be noted.

         3) The **posture** should be analyzed. The lumbar curve may be straightened by paravertebral muscle spasm.

      b) **Bony palpation** of the posterior aspect of the back should be performed. The spinous processes are palpated. Evaluation of the coccyx is accomplished through rectal examination. The sacroiliac joints should be palpated for tenderness.

      c) **Soft tissue palpation** of the posterior aspect of the back is also performed.

         1) The interspinous ligaments connect the adjoining processes, and the supraspinous ligament connects the spinous processes from the seventh cervical vertebra to the sacrum. If either is ruptured, there may be localized pain and a palpable defect between the spinous processes.

         2) The paraspinal muscles are palpated for tenderness, spasm, or defects.

         3) The sciatic nerve exits the pelvis midway between the greater trochanter and the ischial tuberosity, runs vertically down the midline of the posterior thigh, and divides into the tibial and peroneal nerves. The sciatic nerve is most likely to be palpable with the hip flexed. Tenderness can be caused by a herniated disk or a space-occupying lesion compressing the contributing nerve roots.

      d) **Range-of-motion testing** (flexion, extension, lateral bending, and rotation) should be performed to detect restrictions in movement and patterns of exacerbation of pain.

   ii. **Selected special tests** may be performed.

      a) **Straight leg raising** is conducted to reproduce the back or leg pain. The patient may complain of pain in the posterior thigh (hamstring or sciatic), pain all the way down the leg (sciatic), pain in the low back, or pain in the opposite leg. With the leg lowered below the angle producing pain, the foot should be dorsiflexed to stretch the sciatic nerve, which would be expected to reproduce sciatic pain.

      b) **Crossed straight leg raising.** In this test, the uninvolved leg is raised. If this produces back and sciatic pain on the opposite side, a herniated disk or comparable condition is suggested.

      c) **Hoover test.** This test gives an estimate of the patient's effort during straight leg raising. The examiner cups one hand under each of the patient's heels. There should be downward pressure from the leg that is not being actively raised.

   iii. **Neurologic examination of the lower body** should be performed, including assessment of motor strength, sensation, reflexes, and sphincter tone.

   iv. **Evaluation for extraspinal causes of back and leg pain**

      a) **Examination of the abdomen and lower extremities.** Pulsatile abdominal masses and bruits, diminished pulses, and color or temperature changes in the distal extremities suggest vascular disease.

      b) **Pelvic examination** and **rectal examination** may also be indicated.

Quick HIT

Crossed straight leg raising is the most specific positive finding for radiculopathic lumbar disease.

CLINICAL PEARL 10-4

Plain films should be obtained for "red flags": patients younger than 18 or older than 50 years, pain greater than 6 weeks, history of malignancy, unrelenting or night pain, urinary or fecal incontinence, patients with systemic symptoms (fever or weight loss), patients with an acute injury and localized tenderness, intravenous drug abusers, and patients with neurologic deficits.

    c. **Diagnostic imaging studies (see Clinical Pearl 10-4)**
       i. Emergent magnetic resonance imaging and surgical consultation are necessary for patients with suspected cord impingement or cauda equina syndrome.
      ii. A bone scan or positron emission tomography scan may be obtained inpatient for patients with suspected infectious or malignant conditions.
    d. **Laboratory studies** should be considered for selected patients. An ESR may be helpful in those with systemic symptoms or with risk factors for inflammatory or infectious diseases. Appropriate arrays of other blood and urine tests specific to the suspected conditions should be conducted for patients being evaluated for medical causes of spinal column disease and for referred pain.

6. **Therapy**
    a. **NSAIDs** or **acetaminophen** is the first line of treatment for most patients with musculoskeletal back pain. Some patients (e.g., those with a compression fracture) require **short-term narcotic analgesics**.
    b. **Short-term muscle relaxants** may benefit patients with muscle spasm.
    c. **Gradual return to tolerated activities** is more beneficial than bed rest for most causes of back pain.

7. **Disposition**
    a. **Discharge.** Most patients can be discharged home with appropriate medications and instructions for outpatient follow-up.
    b. **Admission** is necessary for patients with cauda equina syndrome and for patients with syndromes thought to be infectious or rapidly progressive in terms of neurologic impairment.

B. **Specific disorders causing thoracic and lumbar back pain**
  1. **Low back strain.** The most common cause of back pain, low back strain may be related to muscle spasm and ligamentous strain from a specific traumatic episode or repeated stress. Typically occurring in patients between the ages of 20 and 40 years, the pain may be in the back, buttock, or one or both thighs, and the pain may be accentuated by standing and alleviated by lying. The back examination may show the nonspecific signs of muscle spasm and loss of lumbar lordosis, and the neurologic examination is normal.
  2. **Herniated intervertebral disk.** Tears in the annulus fibrosus allow the contents of the nucleus pulposus to herniate and compress neural elements. The lower lumbar region (L4, L5, S1) has the most mobility and has the highest incidence of herniated disks; only 1% of all disk herniations are thoracic.
    a. **Patient history.** Patients are typically between the ages of 30 and 50 years. The patient may give a history of acute pain following the sensation of sudden, but minor, pressure on the spine. The pain is often sharp or lancinating in character and may be associated with nerve root irritation, cord compression, or cauda equina syndrome.
    b. **Signs and symptoms**
       i. **Sciatic symptoms** are radicular in nature and tend to be exacerbated by maneuvers such as bending, which increase intradiscal pressure. A **positive straight leg raising test is 75% diagnostically accurate**, and a positive crossed straight leg raising test increases the accuracy.
      ii. **Neurologic symptoms** predict the actual anatomic lesion level approximately 50% of the time, and neurologic signs predict the correct level approximately 75% of the time. In the cauda equina syndrome, a central

midline herniation causes paralysis of the sacral roots, leading to bowel and bladder dysfunction and the inability to walk. Prompt recognition and surgical intervention are necessary to minimize permanent bladder and bowel dysfunction.

3. **Spondylolysis and spondylolisthesis.** Spondylolisthesis is forward slippage of one vertebra on another, most often L5 on S1, or L4 on L5. It is secondary to spondylolysis, a separation at the pars interarticularis (a segment near the junction of the pedicle with the lamina). In many cases, spondylolysis seems to be caused by trauma to a congenitally abnormal segment in the pars interarticularis.

   a. **Patient history.** Most often seen in teenagers, spondylolisthesis is associated with backache and is sometimes accompanied by pain that radiates down the legs as a result of stretching of a nerve root or herniation of a disk.

   b. **Physical examination findings.** A palpable "step-off" from one process to another may be an indication of this condition.

4. **Osteoarthritic spinal disease** occurs later in life and may involve any part of the spine; the lumbar area is more often involved than the thoracic area.

   a. The pain is exacerbated by motion and improved with rest; associated complaints include stiffness and limitation of motion.

   b. In osteoarthritis, the severity of the symptoms bears little relation to the radiologic findings. Pain may be present when there are minimal findings on radiographs; conversely, there may be marked spur formation, ridging, and bridging of vertebrae without symptoms.

5. **Ankylosing spondylitis** usually occurs in young adult men. Initial symptoms may be intermittent pain in the middle or low back; occasionally, there is radiation of pain to the back of the thighs. Limitation of movement becomes constant and progressive. Associated musculoskeletal examination findings may be tenderness of the sacroiliac joints, limitation of hip range of motion, and limitation of chest expansion. A similar back pain syndrome may be present in patients with Reiter syndrome, psoriatic arthritis, and chronic inflammatory bowel disease.

6. **Spinal stenosis** represents a continuum of disease: Disk degeneration is followed by posterior facet disease, which then develops into progressive articular facet, laminar, and vertebral encroachment with osteophytic formation and ultimately vertebral fusion.

7. **Vertebral compression fractures** are common, especially in elderly patients, and are usually the result of a flexion injury. The force required to cause the fracture is minimal when there is underlying bone disease (e.g., osteoporosis, multiple myeloma, metastatic cancer).

   a. The thoracic spine is most likely to be affected. In the T2 through T10 area, stable compression fractures with less than 25% anterior wedging tend to occur.

   b. Because of the relative immobility of the thoracic spine (as compared with the lumbar spine), more complicated and unstable fractures tend to occur when the thoracolumbar level of the spine is injured.

   c. Disruption of the posterior ligaments in the lumbar region also produces unstable fractures.

V. MONARTICULAR ARTHRITIS

A. **Discussion.** Monarticular arthritis is characterized by **pain** and **inflammation** in an isolated joint.

   1. **Septic arthritis** and the **crystal-induced arthropathies** (i.e., **gout, pseudogout**) are the key causes of acute monarticular arthritis that need to be addressed in the ED. Joint infection can coexist with gout or pseudogout: Infection in a joint with any microcrystalline deposition process can lead to crystal shedding and subsequent synovitis from both crystals and microorganisms.

      a. **Septic arthritis** may be **bacterial, tuberculous,** or **fungal** in etiology, and it has the potential for rapid disease progression. Cases are usually classified as those

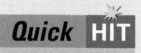

Quick HIT

Almost any joint disorder is capable of presenting initially as monarticular arthritis, but usually, the practitioner can identify patients who might have an acute inflammatory or infectious condition and appropriately proceed with vigorous evaluation and treatment in the ED.

Rheumatologic and Allergic Emergencies

that are caused by *Neisseria gonorrhoeae* (**disseminated gonococcal arthritis**) and those that are caused by all other organisms (**nongonococcal arthritis**).

  i. **Disseminated gonococcal arthritis.** *N. gonorrhoeae* is the most common cause of bacterial arthritis in urban centers. Disseminated gonococcal arthritis tends to be a disease of young, sexually active, healthy adults. Women, especially pregnant or menstruating women, are affected more often than men.

  ii. **Nongonococcal arthritis**

   a) **Causes.** *Staphylococcus aureus* is the bacterium most frequently cultured, followed by various species of streptococci. Other causative organisms are *Escherichia coli* and *Pseudomonas aeruginosa* in elderly patients and intravenous drug users and *Haemophilus influenzae* in young children and, rarely, in adults. When joint infection is present in patients with HIV, opportunistic and less common microorganisms, such as *Cryptococcus neoformans* and *Salmonella*, have been identified.

   b) **Pathogenesis**

    1) An ongoing illness or problem may allow hematogenous spread of bacteria to a joint. At-risk patients include those with impaired host defense mechanisms, those with indwelling venous catheters, those with chronic arthritis (especially rheumatoid arthritis), and intravenous drug users.

    2) Alternatively, microorganisms may be directly introduced into the joint through a deep penetrating wound (including human bite and animal bite wounds), contiguous osteomyelitis, intra-articular injection or aspiration, arthroscopy, or prosthetic joint surgery.

 b. **Gout.** In this condition, sodium urate crystals precipitate in and around the joints of the extremities when the concentration of urate exceeds its solubility.

  i. **Patient history.** Gout is more common in men than in women; when it occurs in women, it is most often seen in postmenopausal women. Patients may have a history of food overindulgence, heavy alcohol intake, use of medications (e.g., diuretics), or trauma. Obesity and hypertriglyceridemia are also associated with gout.

  ii. **Phases.** In primary hyperuricemia, the tendency toward acute gout increases with the serum urate level. In the natural history of gout, the phases include:

   a) **Asymptomatic hyperuricemia** (serum urate concentration greater than 7 mg/dL)

   b) **Acute monarticular arthritis with few constitutional symptoms**

   c) **Arthritis attacks** that are **polyarticular, associated with fever, and/or occurring at shorter intervals**

   d) **Tophi** and **chronic arthritis** with superimposed exacerbations

  iii. **Associated problems** can include renal disease and uric acid nephrolithiasis.

 c. **Pseudogout,** which clinically resembles acute gouty monarthritis, **is a form of calcium pyrophosphate deposition disease (CPPD).** (More chronic forms may resemble osteoarthritis, neuropathic arthropathy, rheumatoid arthritis, and ankylosing spondylitis.) Surveys have shown the radiographic incidence to be as high as 25% in some populations, but many of these patients are asymptomatic.

  i. **Pathogenesis.** Crystals of CPPD develop in cartilages and other connective tissue. The precise reasons for crystal deposition are not known.

  ii. **Patient history**

   a) CPPD increases in prevalence with age and is somewhat more prevalent in men. It is associated with hyperparathyroidism and hemochromatosis, and CPPD crystalline deposits have been identified in patients with hypothyroidism, urate gout, and Wilson disease, as well as in kindreds without an identified specific metabolic defect.

   b) An attack of pseudogout may be precipitated by trauma, surgical procedures, or serious medical illness.

2. **Other conditions.** Acute monarticular arthritis may be the atypical presentation of a number of other inflammatory conditions that usually cannot be definitively diagnosed in the ED.
   a. If the patient does not appear ill, the monarticular arthritis may be a presentation of **rheumatoid arthritis** or one of the **seronegative spondyloarthropathies**.
   b. If the patient shows signs of systemic illness, the patient may have **enteropathic arthritis** or **systemic autoimmune disease**.

B. **Clinical features**
   1. **General**
      a. **Symptoms.** The patient usually describes a short course of increasing pain, redness, swelling, and immobility of a single joint, sometimes associated with fever, skin lesions, or other symptoms and signs related to the specific disease process.
      b. **Physical examination findings.** Examination of the joint usually reveals swelling, warmth, and/or redness that is not present on the contralateral side. Effusion may be present.
   2. **Septic arthritis**
      a. **Disseminated gonococcal infection.** Twenty-five percent to 50% of patients present with a single hot, swollen joint, whereas the others usually have migratory polyarthralgia or polyarthritis. Fever, dermatitis, and tenosynovitis are the most common findings on the initial examination. The skin lesions are usually small papules located on the trunk or extremities.
      b. **Nongonococcal bacterial arthritis.** Patients may be febrile. The knee is most often affected in adults, and the hip is most often affected in children. Bacterial infection of the sternoclavicular and sacroiliac joints is associated with intravenous drug use.
   3. **Gout**
      a. The typical gout attack begins suddenly, often at night, and within a few hours the joint becomes visibly inflamed and exquisitely tender. The skin is often tense and shiny. Swelling is related to synovial effusion and to periarticular edema. The attacks usually subside within a few days to a few weeks, even if untreated.
      b. Gout typically occurs in the lower extremity, often confined to the **first metatarsophalangeal joint (podagra)**. Involvement of other joints of the foot may occur simultaneously or in rapid succession. In the chronically untreated hyperuricemic patient with recurrent attacks, there is involvement of an increasing number of joints in addition to those of the feet (e.g., the hands, wrists, ankles, knees, elbows). Tophi may be present if gout has been untreated for approximately 10 years.
   4. **Pseudogout** by far most commonly involves the **knee joint**. Attacks generally last up to 10 days but may persist for months. Findings consistent with acute synovitis are noted, and fever (as high as 40°C) may occur.

C. **Differential diagnoses**
   1. **Septic arthritis**, **gout**, and **pseudogout** are the prime diagnostic considerations when a patient presents to the ED with a clinical picture consistent with monarticular arthritis.
   2. **Periarticular problems.** Localized periarticular processes (e.g., bursitis, tendinitis, soft tissue infection, bone disease) may cause pain and swelling near a single joint. Bone pain may be caused by Paget disease or osteomyelitis, or it may be related to hemoglobinopathies, pulmonary hypertrophic osteoarthropathy, or malignancy.
   3. **Noninflammatory monarticular arthritis**
      a. **Structural joint problems** may be related to trauma or overuse, internal derangement, loose body, fracture, neuropathic joint, or osteonecrosis.
      b. **Hemarthrosis** is a consideration in patients with bleeding disorders or in those taking anticoagulants.
      c. **Congenital disorders.** Pediatric patients may present with congenital dysplasia of the hip, slipped capital femoral epiphysis, or osteochondritis dissecans.

    d. Osteoarthritis. Older patients with osteoarthritis fairly often present with monarthritis of the knee, hip, or other joints.

4. **Underlying inflammatory conditions.** Monarticular arthritis may be part of the pattern of exacerbation and remission of many of the rheumatologic diseases that are usually classified as polyarticular, such as rheumatoid arthritis, psoriatic arthritis, Reiter syndrome, and systemic lupus erythematosus (SLE). Similarly, enteropathic arthritis is more commonly polyarticular, but monarticular arthritis may be associated with Whipple disease, intestinal bypass, ulcerative colitis, and regional enteritis.

5. **Rare or less obvious causes of monarticular arthritis.** Hydroxyapatite deposition, crystal-induced arthropathies other than gout and pseudogout, sarcoid, Lyme disease, and myriad other conditions may present as acute monarticular arthritis. Furthermore, when a single joint is persistently inflamed, consideration must be given to the possibilities of indolent infection caused by slow-growing organisms, such as *Mycobacterium tuberculosis*, *Sporotrichum schenckii*, or *Candida*, and tumors, particularly pigmented villonodular synovitis.

D. Evaluation

1. **Laboratory studies**

    a. Rapid-turnaround blood tests that may contribute to the diagnosis include a **CBC, ESR,** and **uric acid and calcium levels.** However, a patient with gout may not have hyperuricemia at the time of the acute attack, and most patients with pseudogout do not have hypercalcemia.

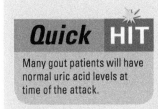

Many gout patients will have normal uric acid levels at time of the attack.

    b. If gonococcal arthritis is suspected, **testing for sexually transmitted infections** should be conducted. Genitourinary testing is positive in 80% of patients with disseminated gonococcal infection.

    c. Blood cultures are drawn in patients with suspected septic arthritis. In nongonococcal bacterial arthritis, blood cultures are positive approximately 50% of the time, although they are positive less than 20% of the time in patients with disseminated gonococcal infection.

2. **Imaging studies.** Radiographs of the involved joint are usually obtained to rule out fracture and bone disease and to assess for findings consistent with specific forms of arthritis.

    a. In septic arthritis, routine radiographs generally reveal only joint effusion. A CT scan may be helpful in diagnosing infection of the sternoclavicular or sacroiliac joints.

    b. In early gout, radiographs are expected to be negative, but in chronic gout, there may be erosions of bone of 5 mm or more in diameter.

    c. In pseudogout, there may be radiographic evidence of calcinosis in cartilage and other structures.

3. **Arthrocentesis** is performed to obtain a sample of the joint fluid for study. The joint fluid is analyzed for cell count, glucose and protein levels, viscosity or mucin clot, crystals, and Gram stain characteristics. It is cultured for bacteria (aerobic and anaerobic), acid-fast bacilli, and fungi. Table 10-6 lists findings typical of various conditions.

    a. Septic arthritis

        i. In **disseminated gonococcal arthritis,** *N. gonorrhoeae* is cultured in less than 50% of purulent joints. The mean white blood cell (WBC) count is over 50,000/mm^3.

        ii. In **nongonococcal bacterial arthritis,** the mean synovial fluid WBC count is approximately 100,000/mm^3, but initial counts may be in the same range as inflammatory arthritis. The causative organism is cultured approximately 90% of the time. Low levels of glucose are present in approximately 50% of patients with septic joints but can also occur in rheumatoid arthritis.

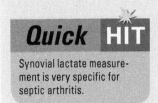

Synovial lactate measurement is very specific for septic arthritis.

    b. Gout. In patients with gout, synovial fluid aspirated early in the clinical course of joint inflammation contains negatively birefringent needle-like crystals in polymorphonuclear leukocytes (PMNs). The WBC count in the synovial fluid is usually approximately 15,000/mm^3 but occasionally is in the range of 70,000/mm^3.

Rheumatologic and Allergic Emergencies

TABLE **10-6** Synovial Fluid Characteristics				
Diagnosis	**Appearance**	**Mucin Clot**	**WBC/mm³**	**Sugar (% of Blood Level)**
Normal	Straw-colored clear	Good	<200	≅100
Degenerative joint disease	Slightly turbid	Good	<2,000	≅100
Traumatic arthritis	Straw-colored bloody, or yellow	Good	≅2,000	
Rheumatoid arthritis	Turbid	Fair to poor	5,000–50,000	<50–75
Spondyloarthropathies	Turbid	Fair to poor	5,000–50,000	<50–75
Acute gout, pseudogout	Turbid	Fair to poor	5,000–50,000	≅90
Septic arthritis	Very turbid or purulent	Poor	50,000–200,000	<50
Tuberculous arthritis	Turbid	Poor	≅25,000	<50

WBC, white blood cell.

    c. **Pseudogout.** The synovial fluid WBC count is usually less than 15,000/mm³, although the count may reach 70,000/mm³ or higher. In pseudogout, the crystals are weakly positively birefringent and rhomboid in shape.

  E. **Therapy**

    1. **Septic arthritis**

      a. **Antibiotics.** The selection of the initial antibiotic is based on the results of the Gram stain and the leading organisms in the differential diagnosis. Table 10-7 contains guidelines regarding empiric therapy.

TABLE **10-7** Suggested Empiric Therapy for Septic Arthritis and Bursitis			
Diagnosis	**Patient Profile**	**Likely Causative Organisms**	**Intravenous Antibiotics**
Septic arthritis	Infant (<3 months)	*Staphylococcus aureus* Enterobacteriaceae Group B streptococcus	PRSP + third-generation cephalosporin
	Child (3 mo to 6 y)	*S. aureus* *Haemophilus influenzae* Streptococci Enterobacteriaceae	PRSP + third-generation cephalosporin
	Adult	*S. aureus* Group A streptococcus Enterobacteriaceae	PRSP + aminoglycoside Ceftriaxone or cefotaxime
	Adult with possible sexually transmitted infection contact	Gonococci	Vancomycin + ciprofloxacin
	Prosthetic joint, post-operative, post–intra-articular injection	*Staphylococcus epidermidis* *S. aureus* Enterobacteriaceae *Pseudomonas* species	
Septic bursitis		*S. aureus*	PRSP (intravenously or orally)

PRSP, penicillinase-resistant synthetic penicillin.

Rheumatologic and Allergic Emergencies

  b. **Drainage.** Most rheumatologists recommend an initial trial of closed-needle aspiration (arthrocentesis), once or twice daily, in all joints except the hips, which should be managed with open drainage (arthrotomy).

  c. **Immobilization.** A splint or cast is used to immobilize the joint in a position of function. The patient should begin passive range-of-motion exercises as soon as possible.

 2. **Crystal-induced arthritis.** When a joint of the lower extremities is involved, a cane or crutches may facilitate limited ambulation.

  a. **Oral NSAIDs** are first-line therapy. **Narcotic analgesics** may be needed adjunctively. Low-dose salicylates (less than 3 g/day) should be avoided because they increase hyperuricemia through renal mechanisms.

   i. **Indomethacin** is the NSAID traditionally used to treat crystal-induced arthritis. The first dose is 75 to 150 mg, followed by 50 mg every 8 hours. Smaller doses are frequently effective (e.g., 50 mg initially and then 25 to 50 mg every 8 hours).

   ii. **Other NSAIDs,** such as **ibuprofen** and **naproxen,** are also effective and may have fewer side effects than indomethacin. In adults, **ketorolac** may be administered, intravenously or intramuscularly, to initiate treatment.

  b. **Colchicine** administration can abort acute gout attacks. However, colchicine does not affect the course of rheumatoid arthritis and does not have a predictable effect in pseudogout. The oral dose of colchicine is 0.6 mg every 1 to 2 hours for up to a maximum of 14 doses. Oral colchicine frequently causes nausea, vomiting, and diarrhea. Significant improvement in signs and symptoms is expected in 12 to 24 hours, at which point the dosage can be tapered to 0.6 mg two to three times daily.

  c. **Prednisone** may be employed for refractory cases of gout or pseudogout or when the standard treatment regimens are contraindicated. Glucocorticoids can be administered orally or parenterally.

  d. **Allopurinol** or **probenecid** is used to treat hyperuricemia in patients with gout after remission of the acute attack.

  e. **Joint aspiration** seems to be therapeutic in patients with pseudogout.

 F. **Disposition**

  1. **Discharge**

   a. Most patients with straightforward crystal-induced arthritis can be treated as outpatients. Prescriptions are usually written to cover the first week of therapy. Clinic follow-up is important to ensure resolution of the acute episode and also to address underlying health issues and any recurrent episodes. Possible indications for admission are intractable pain or uncertainty regarding the diagnosis.

   b. When a patient has an acutely inflamed joint but an evaluation not diagnostic and not suspicious for infection, discharge home with cultures pending is acceptable with close follow-up. Outpatient workup, such as serologic tests or special radiographs, may be appropriate to initiate from the ED if the institution is set up to do this.

  2. **Admission.** Patients who have been diagnosed as having septic arthritis, as well as those suspected of having septic arthritis, should be admitted to the hospital.

VI. POLYARTICULAR ARTHRITIS

 A. **Discussion.** Polyarticular arthritis is characterized by **pain in multiple joints**; it can be inflammatory or noninflammatory.

  1. **Noninflammatory polyarticular arthritis. Osteoarthritis** is the primary disorder in this category. Recognized forms are hereditary osteoarthritis of the hands, hereditary primary generalized osteoarthritis, traumatic osteoarthritis, and osteoarthritis secondary to metabolic disease.

  2. **Inflammatory polyarthritis.** Many types of disorders cause inflammatory polyarthritis. They are subdivided according to the location of the arthritis and the number of joints involved: **peripheral polyarticular** (involving five or more joints), **peripheral pauciarticular** (involving two to four joints), and

peripheral with axial involvement (involving one or both sacroiliac joints and/or the spine).

    a. **Peripheral polyarticular arthritis.** Rheumatoid arthritis is the prototypical inflammatory peripheral polyarthritis. SLE and some forms of viral arthritis, such as that caused by HIV, are also in this group. Psoriatic arthritis occasionally has a polyarticular presentation.

    b. **Peripheral pauciarticular arthritis.** Psoriatic arthritis, Reiter syndrome, and enteropathic arthritis most frequently present as peripheral pauciarticular disease. Other conditions that are members of this category are rheumatic fever, Behçet disease, bacterial endocarditis, Lyme disease, sarcoidosis, and polyarticular gout.

    c. **Peripheral polyarthritis with axial involvement** is seen in ankylosing spondylitis. In this condition, the peripheral arthritis may precede the back symptoms, particularly in the juvenile-onset form. A minority of patients with Reiter syndrome initially presents with polyarthritis and axial involvement, but most develop sacroiliitis or spine disease at some point during the course of the disease. Enteropathic arthritis may present as peripheral arthritis, axial arthritis, or a combination of the two.

B. **Clinical features.** Polyarticular arthritis may present to the ED practitioner as a recurrent symptom in a previously diagnosed disease, as a new symptom in a previously diagnosed disease, or as the first presentation of an as-yet undiagnosed disorder.

    1. **General**

        a. **Patient history.** Important history details include age, gender, acuteness of the illness, anatomic location and symmetry of the arthritis, and relevant exposures. Past medical history is important, including particulars of diagnostic evaluation and treatment.

        b. **Symptoms**

          i. The patient usually describes onset of pain in multiple joints, with individual joint involvement being simultaneous, additive, or migratory. The patient may describe evidence of inflammation (e.g., redness, warmth, swelling) or evidence of mechanical dysfunction (e.g., joint locking or giving way).

          ii. There may be nonspecific associated symptoms (e.g., fever, night sweats, weight loss), symptoms suggestive of other musculoskeletal involvement (e.g., back pain), or symptoms suggestive of other organ involvement (e.g., rash, oral or genital lesions, diarrhea, chest pain).

    2. **Specific clinical presentations.** Recognition of clinical presentations may assist in determining the diagnosis.

        a. **Osteoarthritis** is the most common cause of polyarthritis.

          i. **Patient history.** Rare in patients younger than 40 years, the incidence of osteoarthritis increases with age.

          ii. **Symptoms** usually develop gradually, but patients may present with the acute development of pain, redness, and swelling.

          iii. **Physical examination findings** include **Heberden nodes** (i.e., bony enlargements of the distal interphalangeal joints) and **Bouchard nodes** (i.e., bony enlargements of the proximal interphalangeal joints). The next most frequent area of involvement in osteoarthritis is the thumb base, and on examination there may be swelling, tenderness, and crepitus. Other frequently involved sites are the hips, knees, and spine.

        b. **Rheumatoid arthritis,** a systemic chronic inflammatory disorder, is characterized by joint involvement.

          i. The initial presentation of rheumatoid arthritis often is the **symmetric inflammation of the small joints of the hands and feet,** although large joints such as the knees and ankles are sometimes affected first. Associated **extra-articular manifestations** may involve the eyes (e.g., as part of Sjögren syndrome), the hematologic system (e.g., as part of Felty syndrome), the lungs, the heart, the blood vessels, and the neuromuscular system.

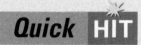

Quick HIT

In patients with inflammatory causes of polyarthritis, associated inflammatory involvement of other organ systems of the body may also be part of the presentation.

    ii. **Rheumatoid nodules** (i.e., subcutaneous nodules ranging from a few millimeters to over 20 mm in diameter occurring in areas exposed to pressure) may be found on physical examination in patients with chronic disease.

c. **Psoriatic arthritis** afflicts 5% to 8% of patients with psoriasis. In the asymmetric pauciarticular inflammatory type, the arthritis is typically preceded by psoriasis by many years, and the proximal interphalangeal and distal interphalangeal joints are most frequently involved. There are also syndromes of symmetric arthritis and psoriatic spondylitis. Physical examination may reveal sausage-shaped digits (dactylitis), onychodystrophy, and psoriatic skin lesions.

d. **Enteropathic arthritis** occurs in 10% to 20% of patients with ulcerative colitis and Crohn disease. The arthritis tends to be acute, in association with an initial flare of bowel disease, and does not result in bony destruction. In most patients, the knees, ankles, elbows, and wrists are affected.

e. **Spondylarthritides.** The spondylarthritides are characterized by involvement of the sacroiliac joints, by peripheral inflammatory arthropathy, by the absence of rheumatoid factor, and by the presence of human leukocyte antigen–B27. Ankylosing spondylitis and Reiter syndrome fall into this category, as well as the subtypes of psoriatic, juvenile, and inflammatory bowel disease associated with sacroiliitis.

    i. **Ankylosing spondylitis.** Predominant features are back discomfort and sacroiliitis.

        a) **Symptoms.** The back pain, which usually first manifests in patients younger than 40, is insidious in onset, persistent, and associated with morning stiffness and improvement with exercise.

        b) **Physical examination findings**

           1) **Signs of associated conditions** (e.g., anterior uveitis, aortic valve insufficiency) may be seen.

           2) **Local signs.** Patients with ankylosing spondylitis may have **loss of spinal lordosis**, **muscle spasm**, and **decrease in mobility** in both the anterior and lateral planes of the body.

           3) **Peripheral joint involvement** occurs in approximately 25% of cases, especially in the lower limbs, but also in the shoulder and hip. Other musculoskeletal features may be **plantar fasciitis**, **costochondritis**, and **Achilles tendinitis**.

    ii. **Reiter syndrome**

        a) **Patient history.** A reactive arthritis, triggered by a specific etiologic agent (e.g., *Shigella*, *Salmonella*, *Yersinia*, *Chlamydia trachomatis*, *Campylobacter*) in a genetically susceptible host

        b) **Signs and symptoms.** The **classic clinical triad** is **urethritis**, **conjunctivitis**, and **arthritis**. **Mucocutaneous lesions** may also be present.

           1) **Arthritis.** In Reiter syndrome, arthritis is usually asymmetric. It typically involves the joints of the lower extremities, such as the knee, ankle, subtalar, metatarsophalangeal, and toe interphalangeal joints. As in psoriatic arthritis, dactylitis may be a distinguishing feature.

           2) **Mucocutaneous lesions.** The characteristic skin lesions are keratoderma blennorrhagica and lesions of the glans penis (circinate balanitis).

f. **SLE** is an autoimmune disease with myriad clinical manifestations (see VII.B.1). The severity and activity of the disease are highly variable. Almost all patients experience arthralgias and myalgias, and most develop intermittent arthritis.

    i. Patients with SLE tend to develop fusiform swelling of the joints, diffuse puffiness of the hands and feet, and tenosynovitis. Frequently involved joints are the proximal interphalangeal and metacarpophalangeal joints of the hands, the wrists, and the knees, in a symmetric pattern.

  ii. Joint deformities develop in approximately 25% of patients (e.g., a swan-neck deformity or ulnar deviation, as in rheumatoid arthritis).

C. **Differential diagnosis**
   1. **Inflammatory polyarthritis**
      a. **Rheumatic conditions.** Inflammatory polyarthritis is caused by rheumatic conditions (e.g., rheumatoid arthritis, psoriatic arthropathy, enterohepatic arthropathy, SLE) as well as most variations of juvenile rheumatoid arthritis.
      b. **Infection.** Inflammatory polyarthritis may occur in conjunction with bacterial infections, such as endocarditis, acute rheumatic fever, and disseminated gonococcal infection.
      c. **Microcrystalline disease.** Inflammatory polyarthritis is a possible presentation of microcrystalline disease, such as gout and pseudogout.
   2. **Noninflammatory polyarticular arthritis** is generally caused by osteoarthritis. Contributing factors may be heredity, acute or repeated trauma, developmental defects, and metabolic abnormalities including hypothyroidism and the osteoarthritic form of CPPD as well as hemochromatosis, ochronosis, and acromegaly.
   3. **Polyarthralgia** must be distinguished from polyarthritis. Polyarthralgia can occur in serum sickness, drug-induced lupus, and Henoch-Schönlein purpura. It can occur in association with metabolic disorders (e.g., hypothyroidism, hyperthyroidism) or in association with viral infections.
   4. **Periarticular problems** must also be distinguished from polyarthritis.
      a. Joint pain may be related to trauma or inflammation of the ligaments, tendons, or bursae.
      b. Muscular causes of pain include viral infection, polymyalgia rheumatica, polymyositis, and dermatomyositis.
      c. Vasculitis and vaso-occlusive disease occasionally present with periarticular pain.
      d. Peripheral neuropathies and compression neuropathies (e.g., carpal tunnel syndrome) may present with periarticular pain.
      e. When axial symptoms are present, nonrheumatologic diseases of the spine (e.g., spinal stenosis, spondylolisthesis) should be considered.
      f. Myeloma, widely metastatic cancers, osteonecrosis, and bone disease associated with sickle cell crises and pulmonary disease may present with bone and joint pain.

D. **Evaluation**
   1. **Laboratory studies**
      a. **Osteoarthritis.** No laboratory studies are diagnostic of osteoarthritis, but special laboratory tests may identify one of the causes of metabolic osteoarthritis.
      b. **Inflammatory disorders.** The inflammatory disorders may be associated with abnormalities of the CBC and ESR. Other tests that may assist in classifying the disorders are rheumatoid factor, antinuclear antibodies, and complement levels; however, the results of these tests are generally not available at the time of the visit to assist in decision making.
         i. Human leukocyte antigen–B27 testing is generally not needed for the diagnosis of ankylosing spondylitis but may be helpful in classifying one of the variant spondyloarthropathies when radiographs are nondiagnostic.
         ii. Cultures or serologic tests are occasionally helpful in identifying the triggering agent of the reactive arthritis of Reiter syndrome.
         iii. When an underlying infection (e.g., HIV, gonococcal infection, hepatitis B, Lyme disease, rheumatic fever, endocarditis) is suspected as the basis for polyarthritis, conventional diagnostic testing should be conducted.
   2. **Diagnostic imaging studies.** Radiographs of selected involved joints may assist in diagnosis.
      a. **Osteoarthritis.** Characteristic changes include joint-space narrowing as articular cartilage is lost, subchondral bone sclerosis, subchondral cysts, and marginal osteophytes. Osteophytosis alone may be attributable to aging rather than osteoarthritis.

b. **Rheumatoid arthritis.** Characteristic changes include soft tissue swelling, loss of cartilage space, demineralization, erosions, bony ankylosis, subluxations, and subchondral cysts.

c. **Psoriatic arthritis.** Radiographic findings in psoriatic arthritis are similar to those in rheumatoid arthritis, but there may be more involvement of the distal interphalangeal joints, a "pencil-in-cup" appearance to the proximal and distal terminal phalanx, or an "opera-glass" deformity of one phalanx telescoping into its neighbor.

d. **Enteropathic arthritis.** In arthritis associated with gastrointestinal disease, peripheral joint radiographs show soft tissue swelling or effusion without erosion or destruction.

e. **Spondylarthritides**

   i. **Ankylosing spondylitis** is diagnosed by the presence of sacroiliitis, which may be based on the findings of juxta-articular sclerosis, blurring of the joint margin, and narrowing. In more advanced disease of the sacroiliac joint, there may be erosions, joint-space destruction, and total ankylosis. The lumbar spine initially shows squaring of the superior and inferior margins of the vertebral bodies; in some advanced cases, "bamboo spine" is seen.

   ii. **Reiter syndrome.** Early or mild findings consist of juxta-articular osteoporosis. In more serious disease, marginal erosions and loss of joint space can be seen. As in the other spondyloarthropathies, periostitis occurs. Spurs may occur at the insertion of the plantar fascia.

3. **Arthrocentesis** and synovial fluid analysis may be performed to determine if the fluid is more consistent with noninflammatory or inflammatory arthritis and to investigate the possibilities of crystal-induced arthritis and septic arthritis (see Table 10-6).

E. **Therapy**

1. **Osteoarthritis** is treated symptomatically with NSAIDs or acetaminophen. Narcotics and corticosteroids are rarely indicated. If steroids are used, intra-articular or periarticular injection is preferable to systemic administration, and steroid therapy should be limited to every 4 to 6 months. Activities and physical therapy should be tailored to the severity of the degenerative process. Orthopedic surgery may be needed in advanced cases.

2. **Acute polyarthritis secondary to rheumatologic conditions** is generally managed with NSAIDs as first-line agents, sometimes supplemented with narcotic analgesics. In more severe cases and flares, systemic corticosteroids are also given. Chronic rheumatoid arthritis is managed with suppressive therapy, such as methotrexate or monoclonal antibody disease modifying drugs. Ultimately, orthopedic surgery may be necessary. Prolonged administration of a long-acting tetracycline may ameliorate *Chlamydia*-induced Reiter syndrome.

3. **Acute diseases or underlying conditions causing acute polyarthritis** should be managed according to conventional measures, with symptomatic treatment of the joint pain.

F. **Disposition**

1. **Discharge**

   a. Patients with osteoarthritis are managed in the outpatient setting by the primary care physician.

   b. Most patients with rheumatologic disorders can be managed as outpatients by the patient's primary care or specialty physician.

   c. Patients with psoriasis and underlying conditions such as bowel disease are generally managed according to the severity of the underlying disease rather than the severity of the arthritis.

2. **Admission.** Criteria for admission include:

   a. An unclear diagnosis

   b. Painful and incapacitating arthritis

   c. Severe underlying conditions, such as rheumatic fever or endocarditis

11 DERMATOLOGIC EMERGENCIES

William B. Adams

I. APPROACH TO THE PATIENT WITH DERMATOLOGIC LESIONS

A. **Patient history.** Answers to the following questions should be sought:
1. **General questions:** Duration, changes over time, exacerbating/alleviating factors, travel?
2. **Questions about symptoms:** Itching, painful, associated symptoms?
3. **Questions about the past medical history:** New medications, occupational and social history, family history?

B. **Physical examination.** The patient's entire body should be examined, and the lesion should be palpated (see Clinical Pearl 11-1).
1. **Location of lesions**
   a. **Site.** The location of the lesions on the body may offer a clue to the diagnosis. For example, varicella spares the palms and soles, and scabies favors the finger web spaces.
   b. **Extent.** Are the lesions localized or generalized?
   c. **Arrangement.** Are the lesions grouped or solitary?
2. **Appearance of lesions**
   a. **Margins** can be raised (as in psoriasis) or more active peripherally (as in tinea).
   b. **Color.** Melanin and hemoglobin are responsible for the colors of lesions.
   c. **Shape.** Annular lesions have clear or contrasting centers (e.g., the target lesions of Stevens-Johnson syndrome).
   d. **Scale.** The epidermis is replaced every 28 days. In psoriasis, the basal cells are mitotically active and produce epidermis or scale.

C. **Differential diagnoses.** Many **systemic diseases** have cutaneous manifestations. For example:
1. Necrobiosis lipoidica diabeticorum, an oval, yellowish, shiny plaque with sharp borders, is a characteristic lesion usually located on the shins of patients with diabetes.
2. Erythema nodosum lesions may be seen in patients with ulcerative colitis.
3. Erythema multiforme can be associated with viral infections such as herpes simplex.

D. **Evaluation**
1. **Microscopic examination.** An ordinary microscope can be used to examine scrapings from skin lesions.
   a. A **potassium hydroxide (KOH) slide preparation** is used when dermatophyte infections are suspected. The slide is examined for long, thin, branching hyphae.
   b. A **Tzanck slide preparation** can confirm the diagnosis of herpes infections. Vesicle contents are smeared on a slide, and Wright's stain or methylene blue is used for staining. Alternatively, the slide can be sent for direct fluorescent assay or enzyme-linked immunosorbent assay.
2. **Wood's light examination.** A Wood's light is an ultraviolet lamp that emits radiation at a wavelength of 360 nm.
   a. In the presence of certain species of tinea capitis infection, the hair shaft will fluoresce bright green.
   b. Cutaneous corynebacterial infections fluoresce coral pink.

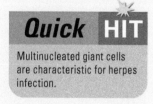

Quick **HIT**

Multinucleated giant cells are characteristic for herpes infection.

Dermatologic Emergencies

254

Types of Lesions

a. **Macules** are flat lesions, measuring less than 1 cm in diameter that are different in color from the normal skin tone (e.g., measles).

b. **Papules** are circumscribed, palpable elevations of the skin measuring less than 1 cm in diameter (e.g., scabies).

c. **Nodules** are circumscribed, palpable elevations of the skin measuring greater than 1 cm in diameter (e.g., erythema nodosum).

d. **Patches** are flat lesions greater than 1 cm in diameter (e.g., pityriasis rosea).

e. **Plaques** are raised lesions measuring greater than 1 cm in diameter (e.g., psoriasis).

f. **Pustules** are raised lesions greater than 0.5 cm in diameter that contain yellow fluid (e.g., abscesses).

g. **Vesicles** are raised lesions up to 0.5 cm in diameter that contain clear fluid (e.g., herpes simplex).

h. **Bullae** are vesicles that are greater than 0.5 cm in diameter (e.g., pemphigus).

i. **Crust** is a dried exudate (e.g., impetigo).

3. **Skin biopsy** can be performed with basic surgical tools (e.g., forceps, scalpel, curette, scissors, and a needle holder) and is best performed by a dermatologist. A specific section of the lesion must be biopsied to obtain a satisfactory specimen for pathology. In addition, the specimen may need to be sent for immunofluorescence studies, electron microscopic examination, or culture.

II. DISORDERS CHARACTERIZED BY VESICULAR LESIONS

A. **Herpes simplex**, an eruption of a painful group of vesicles usually occurring on the genitals or around the mouth, is discussed in Chapter 5.V.B and Chapter 6.IV.F.

B. **Varicella (chickenpox)**

1. **Discussion.** The disease is spread by airborne droplets or contact with vesicle fluid and is highly contagious; patients are no longer contagious when all of the lesions have crusted over. The incubation period is 14 to 21 days.

2. **Clinical features.** Papules progress to vesicles that crust over. Lesions of various stages are seen simultaneously. The rash starts on the trunk and spreads to the face and extremities, sparing the palms and soles.

3. **Differential diagnoses** include herpes simplex, bullous impetigo, and disseminated herpes zoster.

4. **Evaluation.** Diagnosis in the emergency department is usually made on the basis of the patient history and physical examination findings. However, a Tzanck smear of vesicle fluid or serologic titers can confirm the diagnosis.

5. **Therapy**

   a. **Diphenhydramine** (25 mg orally four times daily for adults; 5 mg/kg every 24 hours divided in four doses for children) can be administered to relieve itching. **Menthol lotion** can also provide relief from itching.

   b. **Intravenous acyclovir** (10 mg/kg every 8 hours for 7 to 10 days) is indicated for immunosuppressed patients.

   c. **Oral antibiotics** (e.g., cloxacillin) can be prescribed for patients with secondarily infected lesions.

6. **Disposition.** Hospital admission is warranted for patients with complications (e.g., pneumonia, cellulitis, encephalitis, Reye syndrome).

C. **Herpes zoster (shingles)**

1. **Discussion.** Herpes zoster is the reactivation of the varicella virus (chickenpox) along one or two contiguous dermatomes (Figure 11-1). This condition is most common in elderly patients and is associated with immunosuppression (which occurs with chemotherapy, leukemia, Hodgkin lymphoma, and other malignancies).

2. **Clinical features**

   a. Pain, burning, and hyperesthesia precedes the eruption of vesicles.

   b. Lesions occur on the face, neck, thorax, lumbosacral area, and tip of the nose. The eruption is limited to one side of the body in most cases.

      i. **Ramsay Hunt syndrome** involves cranial nerve VII; vesicles are seen in the ear canal or on the pinna. This syndrome can lead to hearing

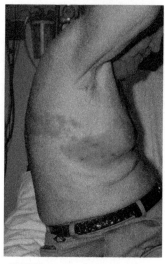

FIGURE 11-1 Herpes zoster intradermal distribution.
(Courtesy of Lawrence B. Stack, MD.)

loss, facial paralysis, and loss of taste in the anterior two-thirds of the tongue.

    ii. **Serious ocular complications** can result from involvement of the trigeminal nerve; lesions are seen on the tip of the nose. Fluorescein stain with slit-lamp eye examination may reveal a dendritic pattern consistent with a serious viral infection of the cornea.

3. **Differential diagnoses** include herpes simplex, poison ivy, contact dermatitis, and localized bacterial infection.

4. **Evaluation**

    a. For lesions involving the nose tip or periorbital area, the eye should be fluorescein-stained to evaluate for herpetic keratitis; consultation with an ophthalmologist is warranted.

    b. A positive Tzanck smear of vesicle fluid and rising viral titers are diagnostic but seldom needed.

5. **Therapy**

    a. **Acyclovir**

        i. **Oral acyclovir** (800 mg five times daily for 5 to 10 days) is effective if therapy is initiated within 48 hours of the appearance of lesions.

        ii. **Intravenous acyclovir** (10 mg/kg over 1 hour every 8 hours for 7 days) is indicated for patients with severe outbreaks, patients with herpes keratitis, and immunosuppressed patients.

        iii. **Topical acyclovir** can be applied four times daily for 10 days.

    b. **Prednisone** can be administered orally to shorten the duration of symptoms and is given as a tapered dose, starting at 30 mg.

    c. **Analgesics** may be needed; some patients will require opiate medications. **Capsaicin cream** can be applied topically five times daily and is useful for patients with postherpetic neuralgia.

6. **Disposition.** Admission is required for immunocompromised patients, patients with ophthalmologic herpes zoster, and patients with complications (e.g., meningitis, peripheral neuropathy, cutaneous dissemination).

III. DISORDERS CHARACTERIZED BY VESICULOBULLOUS LESIONS

    A. **Erythema multiforme**

        1. **Discussion**

            a. **Definitions**

Dermatologic Emergencies

      i. **Erythema multiforme minor** is characterized by a skin rash, which may be accompanied by involvement of one mucous membrane site.

     ii. **Erythema multiforme major (Stevens-Johnson syndrome)** is characterized by severe and extensive mucous membrane involvement and the involvement of multiple organ systems.

  b. **Etiology.** Erythema multiforme appears to be a **hypersensitivity reaction** to drugs, infectious organisms, and other unknown entities. Causes include:

      i. **Drugs** (especially aspirin, penicillins, sulfonamides, phenytoin, rifampin, and phenobarbital)

     ii. **Infectious diseases,** most commonly herpes simplex, *Mycoplasma* infection, Coxsackie and adenovirus infections, hepatitis B, and histoplasmosis

    iii. **Vaccines,** including bacille Calmette-Guérin and the poliomyelitis vaccine

    iv. **Idiopathic** (50% of cases)

2. **Clinical features.** The onset is sudden. Fever, malaise, and arthralgias are common. The lesions usually spare the trunk.

  a. **Dermal lesions.** The rash may present as erythematous macules, papules, wheals, vesicles, or bullae. It appears mostly on the palms, soles, and dorsa of the extremities. The dermal lesions ("target lesions") are papules or vesicles surrounded by a zone of normal skin and then a halo of erythema; they resemble a bull's eye target (Figure 11-2).

  b. **Mucosal lesions.** Hemorrhagic lesions can be found on the lips and oral mucosa.

  c. A **burning sensation** is present on the skin and mucous membranes. Pruritus is absent.

3. **Differential diagnoses**

  a. The **dermal lesions** must be differentiated from secondary syphilis, contact dermatitis, and meningococcemia.

  b. The **mucosal lesions** must be differentiated from pemphigus and herpetic stomatitis.

4. **Evaluation.** Diagnosis depends primarily on history and physical examination findings. Skin biopsy specimens show edema, extravasated erythrocytes, and necrolysis in the epidermis.

5. **Therapy**

  a. The cause should be treated (e.g., with antibiotics or termination of drug therapy) if it can be identified.

FIGURE 11-2 Target lesions of erythema multiforme.
(Courtesy of Lawrence B. Stack, MD.)

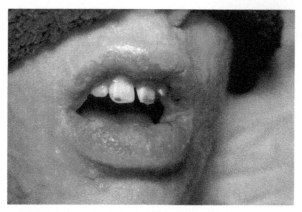

FIGURE

11-3 Sulfonamide-induced Stevens-Johnson syndrome.

(Courtesy of Lawrence B. Stack, MD.)

b. The use of systemic corticosteroids is controversial and has been associated with both remission of the disease and with secondary, fatal, respiratory infections. If steroid treatment is used, prednisone (2 mg/kg/day) is given with subsequent tapering.

6. **Disposition.** Patients with mild cases are treated as outpatients; patients with more severe mucous membrane involvement require hospitalization. Recurrent attacks lasting 2 to 4 weeks and usually occurring in the spring or autumn have been reported.

B. **Stevens-Johnson syndrome** (Figure 11-3)

1. **Discussion.** Stevens-Johnson syndrome is a severe form of erythema multiforme, associated with a mortality rate of 10%. The disease is most common in children and young adults. Complications include blindness, renal failure, meningitis, necrotizing tracheobronchitis, dehydration, secondary bacterial infection, arrhythmias, and congestive heart failure.

2. **Clinical features**

   a. **Upper respiratory tract infection, headache, fever, hematuria, diarrhea,** and **arthralgias** can precede the rash.

   b. **Rash.** Skin lesions are burning but not pruritic.

      i. **Bullae** appear in 1 to 14 days on the skin and the mucous membranes of the mouth, genitalia, and anus.

      ii. **Ulcers.** Corneal ulcers can lead to blindness. Ulcerative stomatitis leads to hemorrhagic crusting. Patients are unable to eat or drink and continuously drool.

      iii. **Vesicles** rupture and leave denuded bases and necrotic epithelium.

   c. **Signs of toxic epidermal necrolysis (TEN)** may develop (see XI.A). **Urinary retention** can result from urethral involvement.

3. **Differential diagnoses** include TEN and pemphigus.

4. **Evaluation.** Skin biopsy findings include necrolysis with edema and erythrocytes in the dermis.

5. **Therapy**

   a. **Definitive treatment** entails **treating the cause** if it can be identified (e.g., with antibiotics or termination of drug therapy). **Prednisone** (80 to 120 mg/day in divided doses) can be administered orally with subsequent tapering. **Intravenous immunoglobulin** has also been used successfully to halt progression of TEN. It is important to note that treatment with prednisone or intravenous immunoglobulin is controversial and varies from one institution to another.

  b. **Supportive treatment**
    i. **Cool, wet compresses**
      a) **Aluminum acetate** compresses are applied to blisters.
      b) Compresses soaked in **potassium permanganate solution** are applied to bullous lesions.
    ii. **Anesthetic troches, 2% viscous lidocaine, or 10% sodium bicarbonate mouthwashes** can be used to soothe mouth lesions. If the patient cannot tolerate a liquid diet, he or she will require **intravenous rehydration**.
    iii. **Antibiotic therapy** is indicated for patients with secondary bacterial infections.
    iv. **Ophthalmology consult.** An ophthalmologist should be consulted.
    v. **Urology consult.** Urology should be consulted if genitourinary involvement is suspected.
  6. **Disposition.** Patients with severe mucous membrane involvement require admission to a burn unit for reverse isolation and treatment of fluid and electrolyte imbalances.
C. **Pemphigus vulgaris**
  1. **Discussion.** Pemphigus vulgaris is a rare disease that affects elderly patients. The mortality rate is 10%; most deaths result from steroid complications, secondary infection, dehydration, or thromboembolism. Pemphigus vulgaris is caused by the attachment of immunoglobulin G autoantibodies to the epidermis. It has been associated with D-penicillamine and captopril administration.
  2. **Clinical features**
    a. **Mucosal** lesions and erosions are very common. Examination of all mucosal sites is warranted.
    b. **Nonpruritic, painful, flaccid bullae** appear that rupture easily. Blisters can be extended or new bullae formed by applying firm tangential pressure on intact epidermis.
    c. **Weakness, weight loss,** and **dysphagia** may be presenting complaints.
  3. **Differential diagnoses** include erythema multiforme, bullous impetigo, and herpes zoster.
  4. **Evaluation.** Biopsy of lesions shows eosinophils, intraepidermal bullae, and acantholysis. Indirect immunofluorescent staining shows immunoglobulin G antibodies. Serum titers can be followed to evaluate the effectiveness of therapy.
  5. **Therapy**
    a. **Prednisone** (200 to 350 mg/day) for 5 to 10 weeks is used until cessation of new blister formation occurs. The dosage is then reduced to 40 mg on alternative days and tapered over the course of 1 year.
    b. **Azathioprine** (100 mg/day) is added to the regimen and the dosage is reduced over a 4- to 6-month period. **Methotrexate** and **cyclophosphamide** can be used instead of azathioprine.
    c. **Topical analgesics** (e.g., viscous lidocaine) can be used to alleviate the pain associated with oral lesions.
  6. **Disposition.** Patients with severe cases and oral lesions may require hospital admission for intravenous hydration. Others can be treated as outpatients with close follow-up.

IV. DISORDERS CHARACTERIZED BY PAPULOSQUAMOUS ERUPTIONS

A. **Psoriasis**
  1. **Discussion.** Psoriasis, a hereditary disorder, is a chronic, recurrent disease that is worse in the winter and during periods of stress. Psoriasis is also exacerbated by drugs (especially lithium, β blockers, nonsteroidal anti-inflammatory drugs, angiotensin-converting enzyme (ACE) inhibitors, and withdrawal from systemic steroids) and repeated minor trauma to the skin. Complications include hypo- and hyperpigmented areas and psoriatic arthritis.
  2. **Clinical features.** The clinical presentation can be diverse. Patients have recurring remissions and exacerbations.
    a. Papules and well-defined white, scaly lesions are seen most often on the knees, elbows, scalp, gluteal cleft, and nails (Figure 11-4).

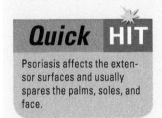

Quick HIT

Psoriasis affects the extensor surfaces and usually spares the palms, soles, and face.

Dermatologic Emergencies

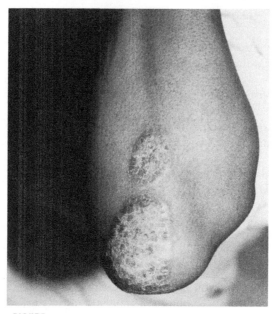

FIGURE
11-4 Psoriasis rash.

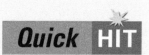

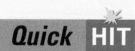

　　b. Removal of the scale results in the appearance of blood droplets (**Auspitz sign**).

3. **Differential diagnoses** include tinea corporis, eczema, pityriasis rosea, candidiasis, and seborrheic dermatitis.

4. **Therapy** may be initiated in the emergency department, but outpatient follow-up and treatment are necessary.

　　a. **Triamcinolone acetonide 0.1%**, a corticosteroid, can be applied twice daily for 2 weeks. To maximize effectiveness, following topical application, the area should be covered with plastic wrap if possible.

　　b. **Coal tar**, in the form of a 5% gel, can be applied twice daily to lesions. A tar shampoo can be used for scalp lesions.

　　c. **Anthralin 0.1%** can be used by patients with chronic plaques. The topical preparation is applied and washed off in 20 minutes.

　　d. **Ultraviolet light therapy**

　　　　i. **Ultraviolet B light therapy** (twice weekly) is combined with tar therapy for patients with severe psoriasis.

　　　　ii. **Ultraviolet A light therapy** is used in combination with **psoralens**, a chemotherapeutic agent. PUVA (Psoralens + ultraviolet A) is reserved for patients who do not respond to conventional treatments.

　　e. **Methotrexate** is prescribed by dermatologists in resistant cases.

5. **Disposition.** Most patients are treated as outpatients.

B. **Pityriasis rosea**

1. **Discussion.** This skin eruption is seen in patients between 10 and 35 years of age.

2. **Clinical features.** A **herald patch**, a single, oval lesion on the trunk or an extremity, is followed by erythematous scaly plaques in 1 to 2 weeks (Figure 11-5).

3. **Differential diagnoses** include tinea corporis, psoriasis, eczema, a drug eruption resulting from captopril therapy, and secondary syphilis.

4. **Therapy.** Most cases resolve spontaneously in 4 to 7 weeks.

　　a. **Diphenhydramine** (25 mg every 6 hours for adults, 5 mg/kg/24 hours in four divided doses for children) can be used to relieve pruritus.

　　b. **Triamcinolone acetonide 0.1% cream** can be applied twice daily.

　　c. **Ultraviolet B light** treatments hasten resolution.

5. **Disposition.** Patients are treated on an outpatient basis.

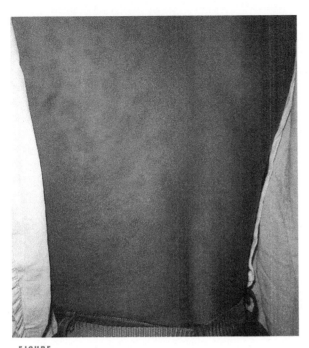

11-5 Christmas tree rash of pityriasis rosea.

V. DERMATITIS

A. **Contact dermatitis**

1. **Discussion.** Inflammation of the skin is caused by a primary irritant or allergen.
   a. **Irritant dermatitis** is caused by caustic industrial solvents and detergents.
   b. **Allergic contact dermatitis** involves a delayed hypersensitivity reaction mediated by lymphocytes.

2. **Clinical features.** Skin lesions appear as red macules and papules. Vesicles or bullae may be present. The lesions are pruritic.

3. **Differential diagnoses** include drug reaction, scabies, syphilis, and herpes.

4. **Evaluation.** Diagnosis is largely on the basis of patient history and physical examination findings. Patch skin testing with allergens can be performed by a dermatologist.

5. **Therapy.** Mild dermatitis resolves in 7 to 10 days.
   a. **Minimization of contact.** An effort should be made to eliminate contact with irritants or allergens.
   b. **Supportive therapy** entails relief of pruritus. Measures include:
      i. **Diphenhydramine** (25 mg every 6 hours for adults, 5 mg/kg/24 hours in four divided doses for children)
      ii. **Colloidal oatmeal baths**
      iii. **Hydrocortisone 1% cream** (applied twice daily)
      iv. **Oral prednisone** (30 to 80 mg daily tapered over a few weeks; shorter courses result in rebound) for patients with severe cases of contact dermatitis

6. **Disposition.** Patients are treated on an outpatient basis. Complications include hyperpigmentation of skin.

B. *Toxicodendron (Rhus)* **dermatitis**

1. **Discussion**
   a. **Etiology. Poison ivy, poison oak,** and **poison sumac** belong to the genus *Toxicodendron (Rhus)* and produce a sensitizing oleoresin, **urushiol.** Cross-sensitivity exists among poison ivy, poison oak, and poison sumac.
   b. **Transmission.** Eruptions can occur 8 hours to 1 week after exposure but usually develop within 2 days. The rash is not spread by contact with the blister fluid; rather, scratching with antigen-contaminated fingernails disseminates the dermatitis. A soap and water bath or shower will remove these oils and decrease the contact spread.

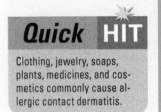

Quick **HIT**

Clothing, jewelry, soaps, plants, medicines, and cosmetics commonly cause allergic contact dermatitis.

Dermatologic Emergencies

2. **Clinical features.** Vesicles and blisters can be linear if the leaf or stem was drawn across the skin. The rash may seem to "spread," but it is due to a variable immune reaction that resolves over several days.

3. **Differential diagnoses** include drug reaction, scabies, syphilis, and herpes.

4. **Therapy.** Mild cases of *Toxicodendron* dermatitis resolve in 7 to 10 days.
   a. **Minimizing contact.** Washing the skin, hands, and fingernails with soap inactivates the oleoresin and is most effective within 30 minutes of exposure.
   b. **Supportive therapy** is the same as for contact dermatitis (see V.A.5.b).
   c. **Education.** Patients should be shown the appearance of poison ivy so that it can be avoided.

5. **Disposition.** Most patients are treated on an outpatient basis. Complications include acute secondary cellulitis and hyperpigmentation of the skin. Several commercial over-the-counter medicines are available that may be applied to the skin prior to possible exposure. These "blocking agents" have a variable degree of protection from future rhus dermatitis.

VI. ERYTHEMA NODOSUM

A. **Discussion**
   1. **Definition.** Erythema nodosum is an inflammatory disease of the skin and subcutaneous tissue characterized by tender red nodules.
   2. **Etiology.** Causes include:
      a. **Bacterial infections** (e.g., *Streptococcus*, *Salmonella*, *Neisseria gonorrhoeae*, *Mycobacterium tuberculosis*, and *Chlamydia*)
      b. **Deep fungal infections** (e.g., histoplasmosis, coccidioidomycosis)
      c. **Viral diseases** (e.g., mononucleosis)
      d. **Drugs** (e.g., sulfonamides, oral contraceptives)
      e. **Idiopathic**

B. **Clinical features**
   1. **Rash.** The pretibial region is most often involved, but the forearms or thighs may be involved as well. Raised, warm, tender red nodules appear that have a bluish discoloration and resemble bruises later on. Healing occurs in 3 to 6 weeks without scarring, atrophy, or ulcers (Figure 11-6).
   2. **Hilar adenopathy** is occasionally noted. Fever, malaise, myalgias, and arthralgia are common.

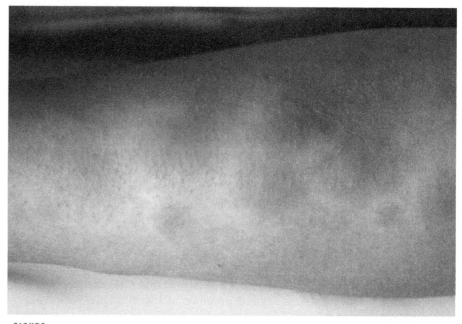

FIGURE
11-6 Erythema nodosum rash.
(Courtesy of Lawrence B. Stack, MD.)

Dermatologic Emergencies

C. **Differential diagnoses** include cellulitis, lymphoma, and superficial thrombophlebitis.

D. **Evaluation.** An elevated erythrocyte sedimentation rate is a common laboratory finding, but the diagnosis is made based on the typical clinical findings. Throat and stool cultures may be indicated. Skin biopsy can be performed but is seldom needed.

E. **Therapy**

1. **General measures** include bed rest and elevation of the extremities. Causative drugs should be discontinued, and underlying disease treated.

2. **Pain relief** can be achieved by administering naproxen (500 to 1,000 mg/day in two divided doses) or enteric aspirin (350 mg, 8 to 12 tablets per day).

3. **Potassium iodide** is administered (400 to 900 mg daily in three divided doses for 3 to 4 weeks).

4. **Corticosteroids** are used in patients with severe, refractory disease.

F. **Disposition.** Most patients are treated as outpatients.

VII. FUNGAL SKIN INFECTIONS

A. **Candidiasis**

1. **Discussion.** *Candida albicans* is part of the normal flora but can become pathogenic in pregnant women, infants, elderly patients, diabetic patients, immunosuppressed patients (e.g., patients with AIDS, patients taking steroids), patients who are using oral contraceptives, and patients who are taking antibiotics.

2. **Clinical features**

a. **Oral candidiasis (thrush)** appears as a white exudate or adherent plaque on the buccal mucosa, tongue, or esophagus. Dysphagia can occur.

b. **Cutaneous candidiasis** favors warm, moist areas like skinfolds, the diaper area, the axilla, and the groin. It appears as a glistening red plaque. Satellite lesions are vesicles or pustules peripheral to the main area.

3. **Evaluation.** KOH slide preparations show hyphae or blastospores (oval yeast forms).

4. **Therapy**

a. **Oral candidiasis.** Treatment options include:

i. **Nystatin oral suspension** (1 mL applied to the inside of each cheek four times daily for 10 days in children, 4 to 6 mL four times daily for 10 days in adults)

ii. **Clotrimazole troches** (dissolved in the mouth five times daily for 14 days)

iii. **Oral itraconazole or terbinafine**

b. **Cutaneous candidiasis** is treated with **miconazole nitrate**, applied twice daily. **Wet aluminum acetate compresses** can be used first to help dry the lesions. **Talcum powder** can be used to keep the area dry throughout treatment.

5. **Disposition.** Patients are followed as outpatients.

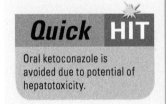

Quick HIT

Oral ketoconazole is avoided due to potential of hepatotoxicity.

B. **Tinea**

1. **Discussion**

a. **Etiology.** The many types of tinea (dermatophytoses) are caused by fungi from the genera *Microsporum*, *Epidermophyton*, and *Trichophyton*.

b. **Pathogenesis.** Dermatophyte infections can be acquired from another person, from fomites, from pets, and, rarely, from soil. The fungi invade the stratum corneum and liberate a toxin. They can also produce an allergic reaction.

2. **Clinical features**

a. **Tinea pedis ("athlete's foot").** Blisters or dry scales are noted on the soles and sides of the feet and between the toes.

b. **Tinea unguium** results in thick, opaque, crumbled nails that can detach laterally.

c. **Tinea cruris ("jock itch")** is characterized by red scaly patches with a sharp raised border on the perineum, thighs, and buttocks. The scrotum is usually spared.

d. **Tinea corporis (ringworm)** is common in children. Ringworm is characterized by round, scaly patches with a raised border and can occur anywhere on the body.

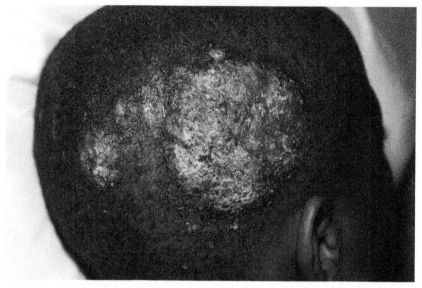

11-7 Kerion.
(Courtesy of Lawrence B. Stack, MD.)

e. **Tinea capitis.** Gray, scaly, round patches occur on the scalp; the hairs in the areas of the lesions are broken off, and the patches may become bald. A **kerion** is an inflammatory reaction with a boggy, indurated mass that exudes pus (Figure 11-7).
3. **Differential diagnoses** include eczema, psoriasis, erythema migrans, and cellulitis.
4. **Evaluation**
   a. **Wood's lamp examination.** *Microsporum* or *Trichophyton* species invade hair shafts. Infected hairs will appear bright green when illuminated with a Wood's lamp.
   b. **KOH preparation.** In patients with tinea corporis, a KOH slide preparation of the scaly, red border will show hyphae.
5. **Therapy**
   a. **Tinea pedis, tinea corporis,** and **tinea cruris**
      i. **Topical treatment**
         a) **Miconazole cream** applied twice daily for 1 month is effective.
            1) **Wet aluminum acetate compresses** should be applied to macerated skin for 30 minutes twice daily before applying antifungal creams.
            2) After the inflammation has resolved, **tolnaftate powder** can be applied to keep the area dry.
            3) **Cotton** should be placed between the toes.
         b) **Clotrimazole cream**
         c) **Topical steroids** (or combination creams containing steroids) can exacerbate dermatophyte infections and should be avoided.
      ii. **Oral treatment** may be necessary for treating resistant infections (except tinea pedis).
         a) **Griseofulvin** (250 mg twice daily in adults, 10 mg/kg/day in children) for 6 to 8 weeks is used. Side effects include headache, urticaria, photosensitivity, and stomach upset.
         b) **Terbinafine 250 mg** daily for 7 to 10 days for acute infestations. Chronic onychomycosis can take up to 3 months to treat and requires periodic laboratory evaluation.
   b. **Tinea unguium**
      i. **Toenails.** Tinea unguium of the toenails is rarely cured. **Debridement** of the affected nails and application of **clotrimazole lotion** four times daily may help if less than half the nail is affected. **Griseofulvin** (500 mg twice daily) is administered for 6 to 9 months.

Dermatologic Emergencies

      ii. **Fingernails.** Tinea unguium of the fingernails is treated for
6 to 9 months with **griseofulvin**. **Terbinafine** (250 mg daily) is an
alternative to griseofulvin.

   c. **Tinea capitis** is treated with **griseofulvin microcrystalline** (10 mg/kg/day
twice daily for 6 to 12 weeks). If no improvement is seen after 1 month, the
dose can be increased to 15 mg/kg/day. **Selenium sulfide 2.5% shampoo**
may also be used. Shaving or cutting the hair is not necessary.

  6. **Disposition.** Patients are treated on an outpatient basis. Patients given griseofulvin and other similar medicines need to have routine hepatic blood tests to
monitor for possible liver inflammation.

VIII. PARASITIC SKIN INFECTIONS

  A. **Scabies**

    1. **Discussion.** The mite *Sarcoptes scabiei* causes a hypersensitivity reaction
("scabies") as it burrows into the skin and lays eggs. Scabies is associated with
poor hygiene and is transmitted by direct contact with an infested person or
infested clothing or bedding. Primary infections have an incubation period of
1 month.

    2. **Clinical features.** Excavations and "S"-shaped burrows (2 to 15 mm) occur
on the waist, buttocks, back, axilla, pubic area, breasts, extremities, and finger
webs (Figure 11-8). Vesicles and papules are often present. Severe itching
occurs at night.

    3. **Differential diagnoses** include herpes simplex, pediculosis pubis, and syphilis.

    4. **Evaluation.** Mites, eggs, and feces are visible when scrapings from the lesion
are mounted on a slide with mineral oil and viewed using a microscope. The
mite is a third of a millimeter long, is oval, and has eight legs.

    5. **Therapy**

     a. **Topical therapy.** Options include:

      i. **Permethrin 5% cream** is applied and washed off after 14 hours. Appli-
cation can be repeated in 7 days if symptoms are not improved.

      ii. **Crotamiton** can be applied once daily for 5 days and washed off
48 hours after the last application.

      iii. **Lindane lotion** can be used but is associated with neurotoxicity.

      iv. **Oral ivermectin** can be used for resistant cases.

     b. **Supportive therapy**

      i. **Diphenhydramine** (25 mg for adults, 5 mg/kg/24 hours in four
divided doses for children) can be administered every 6 hours to
relieve itching, which can persist even after successful eradication of
the parasite.

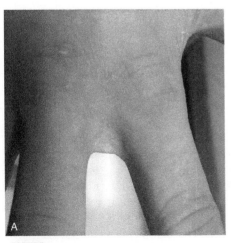
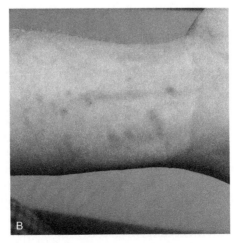

FIGURE 11-8 (A) Scabies burrow in interdigital space. (B) Scabies skin lesion on forearm.
(Courtesy of Jessica Dennison, MD.)

Dermatologic Emergencies

ii. **All beddings, towels, and clothes** should be washed in hot water.

iii. **Antibiotics** may be necessary to treat secondary infections, a common complication.

6. **Disposition.** Most patients are treated on an outpatient basis. Close contacts and sexual partners may be coinfected and should be counseled to seek medical care.

B. **Pediculosis**

1. **Discussion.** Lice, wingless insects with six legs, are spread by close personal contact or by sharing combs, linen, or clothing with an infested person. Lice feed on human blood five times a day.

2. **Clinical features.** Lice should be suspected when a patient complains of itching in a localized area, but no rash is present. Uninfected bites present as red papules and can be seen on the axilla, groin, trunk, or scalp.

   a. **Pediculosis capitis** (infestation of the scalp and eyelashes) is common in children. Lice eggs (nits) are found on hair shafts. Scratching produces infection characterized by pustules, crusting, and cervical adenopathy.

   b. **Pediculosis pubis** (infestation of the pubic area) results in pruritus and adenopathy. Nits are visible in the pubic hair. Gray-blue macules (macula cerulea) can be seen.

   c. **Pediculosis corporis** (infestation of the buttocks, shoulders, and waist) is most often seen in patients unable to change or launder clothing.

3. **Differential diagnoses** include scabies, dermatitis, eczema, tinea, impetigo, and folliculitis.

4. **Evaluation.** Lice and nits can be seen under a microscope. Live nits fluoresce when viewed under a Wood's light.

5. **Therapy**

   a. **General measures.** Clothing, towels, and bedding should be laundered in hot water.

   b. **Pediculosis capitis** and **pediculosis pubis**

      i. A **permethrin cream rinse** is applied, saturating the hair and scalp, and washed out after 10 minutes. **Formic acid 8%** is then applied and left in for 10 minutes before being washed out. The hair is then combed with a **metal nit removal comb.**

      ii. Eyelashes can be treated with **petroleum jelly** or **baby shampoo** rubbed into the lids and brows three times daily for 5 days.

      iii. Resistant head lice in adults can be treated with **co-trimoxazole** (1 tablet twice daily for 3 days).

   c. **Pediculosis corporis.** Body lice are treated with pyrethrin or permethrin, which is applied to the affected areas and washed off after 10 minutes. Treatments should be repeated in 7 days.

6. **Disposition.** Patients are followed as outpatients.

IX. VIRAL EXANTHEMS

A. **Measles (rubeola)**

1. **Discussion.** Measles is spread by respiratory droplets. The incubation period is 10 to 14 days. The patient ceases to be a source of infection 5 days after the rash appears.

2. **Clinical features**

   a. **Cough, coryza, conjunctivitis,** and **fever** occur 3 to 4 days before the rash.

   b. **Koplik spots** (blue-white papules with a red halo) appear on the buccal mucosa 2 days before the rash develops (Figure 11-9).

   c. **Rash.** Elevated red maculopapules appear on the fourth or fifth day behind the ears, spreading to the face, trunk, and extremities. Discrete lesions become confluent on the upper body. The rash fades within 5 to 10 days.

3. **Differential diagnoses** include scarlet fever, German measles, infectious mononucleosis, roseola, and secondary syphilis.

4. **Therapy** is with supportive care only (i.e., fluids, rest, antipyretics).

5. **Disposition.** Patients with complications (e.g., pneumonia, otitis media, encephalitis) may need to be admitted to the hospital.

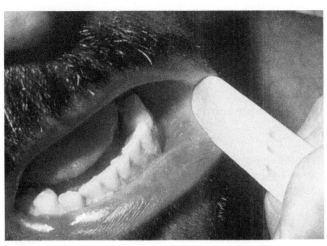

FIGURE
11-9 **Measles-related Koplik spots in mouth.**
(From Goodheart HP. *Goodheart's Photoguide of Common Skin Disorders: Diagnosis and Management.* 2nd ed. Philadelphia: Lippincott Williams & Wilkins; 2003.)

B. **German measles (rubella)**
1. **Discussion**
   a. Rubella is an RNA virus that is spread by respiratory droplets. The incubation period is 14 to 21 days.
   b. Complications include encephalitis and arthritis. In pregnant women, rubella exposure during the first trimester can result in fetal cardiac defects, cataracts, and deafness. Spontaneous abortion, premature delivery, and growth retardation are also common complications of rubella exposure during pregnancy.
2. **Clinical features**
   a. **Malaise**, **headache**, and a **low-grade fever** precede the rash. **Adenopathy** of the posterior auricular, suboccipital, and cervical lymph nodes is present.
   b. **Rash.** The rash consists of small, round, red macules and papules that begin on the neck and face and spread to the trunk and extremities. The rash resolves in 3 days.
3. **Differential diagnoses** include measles, scarlet fever, and drug eruption.
4. **Therapy** is supportive care only.
5. **Disposition.** Most patients are treated on an outpatient basis.
C. **Erythema infectiosum**
1. **Discussion.** Erythema infectiosum is a parvovirus infection that affects children between the ages of 5 and 14 years. The incubation period is 13 to 18 days. Complications include polyarthritis.
2. **Clinical features**
   a. **Malaise**, **sore throat**, and a **low-grade fever** are present.
   b. **Rash.** Red papules appear on the face, sparing the nose and mouth. This "slapped cheek" appearance fades in 4 days.
   c. **Erythema.** A reticulated pattern of erythema appears on the extremities and spreads to the trunk and buttocks. The eruption fades in 6 to 14 days but may reappear in the next 2 to 3 weeks.
3. **Differential diagnoses** include measles, rubella, and scarlet fever.
4. **Therapy** is supportive care only, with fluids, rest, and antipyretics.
5. **Disposition.** Patients are treated on an outpatient basis.
D. **Roseola infantum**
1. **Discussion.** Roseola infantum is caused by herpesvirus 6. Children between the ages of 6 months and 4 years are most often affected. The incubation period averages 12 days.
2. **Clinical features**
   a. The sudden onset of a **high fever** (103°F to 106°F) occurs with few symptoms other than **vomiting**; patients usually appear well despite the high temperature. **Febrile seizures** can occur. **Occipital adenopathy** may be present.

Dermatologic Emergencies

   b. **Rash.** Pale pink, almond-shaped macules appear on the trunk and neck as the fever subsides. The rash clears in 1 to 2 days.
   3. **Differential diagnoses** include measles, scarlet fever, and infectious mononucleosis.
   4. **Therapy** is supportive. Acetaminophen (15 mg/kg every 4 hours) can be administered to reduce the fever.
   5. **Disposition.** Most patients are treated on an outpatient basis.
 E. **Hand-foot-and-mouth syndrome**
   1. **Discussion.** Hand-foot-and-mouth syndrome is caused by a **coxsackievirus.**
   2. **Clinical features.** A **maculopapular confluent rash** is seen on the palms and soles, and **vesicles** are seen in the mouth. **Fever, vomiting, diarrhea,** and a **sore throat** may be present.
   3. **Differential diagnoses** include measles, scarlet fever, infectious mononucleosis, and drug eruption.
   4. **Therapy** is with supportive care only.
   5. **Disposition.** Patients with complications (e.g., myocarditis, meningitis, pneumonia) need to be admitted.

X. BACTERIAL SKIN INFECTIONS

 A. **Scarlet fever**
   1. **Discussion.** Children are most often affected. The rash results from infection with a group A β-hemolytic streptococcus, which produces an erythrogenic toxin. The infection usually originates in the pharynx or the skin and the incubation period is 2 to 4 days.
   2. **Clinical features.** A syndrome characterized by **fever, pharyngitis, vomiting,** and **headache** is followed in 48 hours by the development of a **rash.** **Lymphadenopathy** and **palatal petechiae** are usually present.
     a. The rash consists of fine, pinhead-sized macules that feel like sandpaper. It spares the palms, soles, and circumoral region. **Linear petechiae (Pastia sign)** can be found in skinfolds in the antecubital area.
     b. **Desquamation** begins on the face and trunk and spreads to the palms and soles. The desquamation lasts as long as 8 weeks.
   3. **Differential diagnoses** include measles, drug eruption, rubella, and infectious mononucleosis.
   4. **Evaluation.** A throat culture should be obtained.
   5. **Therapy.** Antibiotic therapy is necessary to reduce the risk of developing rheumatic fever.
     a. **Penicillin G benzathine** (1.2 million U in adults; 600,000 U in children) can be administered intramuscularly as a one-time dose.
     b. **Penicillin VK** (250 mg four times daily in adults; 50 mg/kg/day in four divided doses for children) or **erythromycin** (40 mg/kg/day) can be used for patients who are allergic to penicillin.
   6. **Disposition.** Most patients are treated on an outpatient basis.
 B. **Impetigo**
   1. **Discussion.** Impetigo is commonly seen in children and is caused by group A β-hemolytic streptococci or *Staphylococcus aureus* infection of the skin. Lesions are very contagious. Poor hygiene, malnutrition, and antecedent dermatoses (e.g., scabies, varicella, contact dermatitis) predispose patients to impetigo.
   2. **Clinical features.** Vesicles erode into honey-colored crusts. A bullous form is caused by *S. aureus.* Regional lymphadenopathy is present, and fever is rare (Figure 11-10).
   3. **Differential diagnoses** include tinea, contact dermatitis, varicella, and herpes simplex.
   4. **Evaluation.** Cultures of the pharynx and skin lesions can be tested for group A streptococci.
   5. **Therapy**
     a. **Topical therapy.** Skin should be cleansed daily with **antibacterial soap**, and crusts removed daily. **Mupirocin** is applied three times daily to the lesions.

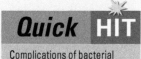

Quick **HIT**

Complications of bacterial skin infections include glomerulonephritis, rheumatic fever, pneumonia, otitis media, and peritonsillar abscess.

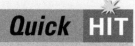

Quick **HIT**

A white coating on the tongue sheds in 2 days to leave a red **"strawberry tongue"** with prominent papillae.

Dermatologic Emergencies

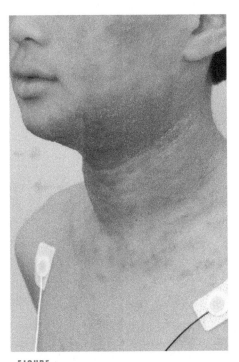

FIGURE
11-10 Impetigo rash.
(Courtesy of Lawrence B. Stack, MD.)

    b. **Oral antibiotics.** Pediatric dosages of cloxacillin (50 to 100 mg/kg/day) or cephalexin (25 to 50 mg/kg/day) for 10 days result in higher cure rates than topical therapy.

  6. **Disposition.** Patients are treated on an outpatient basis.

C. **Cutaneous abscesses**

  1. **Discussion.** *Staphylococcus aureus* and *Streptococcus* are the most common causes of cutaneous abscesses. Methicillin-resistant *Staphylococcus aureus* is increasing in prevalence. Abscesses may form in association with hair follicles or sweat glands, in perineal and perirectal areas, under skin lesions, and following transcutaneous drug use.

  2. **Clinical features**

    a. **Hidradenitis suppurativa** is a disorder of recurrent abscess formation of apocrine sweat glands in the axilla and groin.

    b. **Folliculitis** is inflammation of the hair follicle caused by infection, physical injury, or chemical irritation.

    c. **Furuncle (abscess** or **boil).** A furuncle is a walled-off collection of pus that forms a painful fluctuant mass. Furuncles are characterized by a greater degree of inflammation than folliculitis; the inflammation extends from the follicle into the surrounding dermis.

    d. **Carbuncle.** A carbuncle is a collection of infected hair follicles that have multiple follicular openings on the skin surface. Therefore, a carbuncle is a collection of furuncles. Malaise, chills, and fever may be present.

  3. **Differential diagnoses** include acne, tinea, molluscum contagiosum, and warts.

  4. **Evaluation.** Gram stain and culture of abscess aspirate may be considered.

  5. **Therapy**

    a. **Warm compresses** should be applied three times daily.

    b. **Incision, drainage,** $+/-$ **packing** of the abscess with iodoform gauze is the treatment of choice. The skin over the abscess is anesthetized with lidocaine and incised with a surgical blade. The abscess should be irrigated; it may be necessary to break up loculations.

    c. **Antibiotic therapy** is not indicated unless the infection is recurrent, cellulitis or septicemia is present, or the patient has diabetes or is immunocompromised. If antibiotic therapy is necessary, **dicloxacillin** (500 mg orally four times daily for 10 days) can be used.

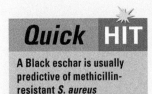

Quick HIT

A Black eschar is usually predictive of methicillin-resistant *S. aureus* involvement.

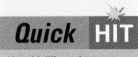

Quick HIT

If methicillin-resistant *S. aureus* is suspected, doxycycline or trimethoprim-sulfamethoxazole should be used.

Dermatologic Emergencies

6. Disposition
   a. **Discharge.** Most patients can be followed up as outpatients at 24 hours.
   b. **Admission**
      i. Patients with diabetes, immunocompromised patients, or patients with abscesses on the hands and face should be admitted to the hospital for intravenous antibiotic therapy.
      ii. Intravenous drug users at risk for septicemia or endocarditis require admission.

XI. LIFE-THREATENING DERMATOSES

A. **Toxic epidermal necrolysis (TEN)**
   1. **Discussion**
      a. **Definition.** TEN is a severe form of erythema multiforme where complement–immunoglobulin complexes are deposited in the cutaneous microvasculature. TEN is more common in adults.
      b. **Etiology.** Common causes include **drugs** (e.g., aspirin, penicillins, sulfonamides, phenytoin, phenobarbital) and **infections** (e.g., *Mycoplasma*, herpesvirus). TEN can also develop **following vaccination** against polio, measles, diphtheria, and tetanus.
      c. **Complications** include secondary bacterial infection, dehydration, pneumonia, blindness, renal failure, and gastrointestinal hemorrhage.
      d. **Mortality.** The mortality rate associated with TEN in elderly patients approaches 25%.
   2. **Clinical features**
      a. Headache, fever, and a sore throat can precede skin lesions by 1 week. Myalgias, arthralgias, vomiting, and diarrhea also occur.
      b. Diffuse, painful, warm erythema develops. The skin separates easily into sheets (**Nikolsky sign**). Pigment is removed from the skin as it desquamates.
      c. Mucous membranes blister and form erosions. Severe conjunctivitis is present.
   3. **Differential diagnoses**
      a. **Early presentations** may be confused with an early drug eruption, toxic shock syndrome, or scarlet fever.
      b. **Late presentations** resemble staphylococcal scalded skin syndrome (SSSS) or erythema multiforme.
   4. **Evaluation.** Skin biopsy shows separation at the dermoepidermal junction.
   5. **Therapy. First-line treatment is to identify and stop offending medication.**
      a. **Fluids and electrolytes** should be replaced as necessary.
      b. **Debridement.** Loose or necrotic skin and blisters are surgically debrided and covered with porcine xenografts.
      c. **Applying dressings soaked in 0.5% silver nitrate** and bathing the affected skin in **potassium permanganate** are useful. Silver sulfadiazine should be avoided because it delays reepithelialization.
      d. **Antibiotic therapy** is indicated to treat the conjunctivitis. An ophthalmologist should be consulted. Erythromycin ointment is usually used.
      e. **Corticosteroids.** The role of systemic corticosteroids (e.g., prednisone, 300 mg/day) is controversial.
      f. Intravenous immunoglobulins
   6. **Disposition.** Admission for intravenous fluid therapy is indicated. Isolation in a burn unit is needed for patients with greater than 10% skin loss to protect them from developing septicemia or gram-negative pneumonia.

B. **Staphylococcal scalded skin syndrome** (see also Chapter 6.VI.A.)
   1. **Discussion.** SSSS is caused by *S. aureus* phage group II exotoxin, which cleaves the epidermis in the stratum granulosum. It is common in children younger than 6 years.
   2. **Clinical features.** Painful erythema and blistering of the skin are seen in association with fever. There is no mucous membrane involvement. The skin

TABLE **11-1**	Comparison of Staphylococcal Scalded Skin Syndrome and Toxic Epidermal Necrolysis		
	Population	**Pathology**	**Cause**
SSSS	Children younger than 6 years	Split in epidermis	*Staphylococcus aureus*
TEN	Adults	Split in dermis	Drug reaction (most common)

SSSS, staphylococcal scalded skin syndrome; TEN, toxic epidermal necrolysis.

wrinkles and peels off in large sheets, leaving a moist, glistening surface. **Nikolsky sign** is present.

3. **Differential diagnoses** include scarlet fever, TEN, and erythema multiforme. SSSS and TEN are compared in Table 11-1.
4. **Evaluation.** Biopsy of the skin shows splitting of the epidermis. Cultures from the lesions, the throat, and the blood should be taken.
5. **Therapy.** Intravenous fluids should be administered to combat dehydration from fluid loss. Nafcillin (50 to 100 mg/kg/day) can be administered intravenously. Unaffected skin should be moisturized with Nutraderm (Galderma, Fort Worth, TX); bathing should be kept to a minimum. Steroids are contraindicated.
6. **Disposition.** Patients with extensive disease should be hospitalized for the admission of intravenous antibiotics.

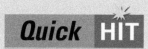

Quick HIT

Every patient with an eye complaint should have a documented visual acuity.

I. EYE

A. Examination of the eye

1. **Evaluation of visual acuity** is analogous to evaluation of a patient's vital signs during a general physical examination.

   a. **Snellen eye chart.** The patient is asked to read the chart from a distance of 20 feet.

   b. **Finger test.** If a patient is unable to see the chart, the examiner should hold his or her hand 3 feet away from the patient and the patient should be asked to count the number of fingers that the examiner is holding up.

   c. **Motion and light perception**

      i. **Motion.** If a patient is unable to count fingers at a distance of 3 feet, then the examiner should wave his or her hand from side to side in front of the patient, asking the patient if he or she can "see hand motion."

      ii. **Light.** The patient should also be asked if he or she can perceive light.

      iii. **Peripheral vision.** The patient's peripheral vision should be checked and documented.

2. **Inspection of the soft tissues**

   a. The **brows, eyelashes,** and **eyelids** are evaluated for swelling, redness, discharge, or abnormal appearance.

   b. The **conjunctivae** are inspected for redness, infection, papillae, follicles, or discharge.

3. **Inspection of the pupils**

   a. **Appearance.** The size and shape of the pupils should be evaluated.

   b. **Reaction to light.** Both direct and consensual constriction should be evaluated.

   c. **Accommodation.** The patient is asked to watch the examiner's finger as the examiner brings his or her finger toward the patient's nose. The patient's eyes should converge, and the pupils should constrict.

4. **Evaluation of extraocular motion.** The **six eye movements** are controlled by three cranial nerves and six muscles (Table 12-1).

5. **Inspection of the cornea.** The cornea should be inspected for clarity and smoothness. If injury to the cornea is suspected, fluorescein stain should be placed in the eye and then the cornea should be examined for abrasions using a slit lamp under cobalt blue light.

6. **Inspection of the iris.** The iris should be examined for any irregularity.

7. **Examination of the fundus** is performed with an ophthalmoscope and is best accomplished after instilling a mydriatic (e.g., tropicamide 0.5%) to dilate the pupil.

   a. The **optic disc** is inspected for cupping, inflammation, and edema.

   b. The **retina** is inspected for abnormalities (e.g., hemorrhages, exudates, cotton wool spots).

   c. The **arteries** and **veins** are inspected for arteriovenous nicking, copper wiring, and engorgement or paucity of blood.

8. **Evaluation of intraocular pressure.** A tonometer should be used to record the pressures in both eyes.

Table **12-1**	Eye Movements	
Movement	**Responsible Muscle**	**Innervation**
Adduction	Medial rectus	Cranial nerve III
	Inferior rectus	Cranial nerve III
Abduction	Lateral rectus	Cranial nerve VI
	Inferior oblique	Cranial nerve III
	Superior rectus	Cranial nerve III
	Superior oblique	Cranial nerve IV
Elevation	Superior rectus	Cranial nerve III
	Inferior oblique	Cranial nerve III
Depression	Inferior rectus	Cranial nerve III
	Superior oblique	Cranial nerve IV
Intorsion	Superior oblique	Cranial nerve IV
	Superior rectus	Cranial nerve III
Extorsion	Inferior oblique	Cranial nerve III
	Inferior rectus	Cranial nerve III

B. **Disorders characterized by severe ocular pain**
  1. **Angle closure glaucoma**
    a. **Discussion**
      i. **Pathogenesis.** Angle closure glaucoma occurs when the outflow of aqueous humor through the trabecular meshwork is obstructed by forward displacement of the iris. The pressure in the eye continues to increase. Unless the condition is treated, damage to the optic nerve can lead to blindness.
      ii. **Predisposing factors.** African Americans, Asians, and women are at increased risk.
    b. **Clinical features.** The presentation may be chronic or acute.
      i. **Symptoms**
        a) **Chronic angle closure glaucoma.** Patients may be asymptomatic, or they may report a dull ache and blurred vision.
        b) **Acute angle closure glaucoma.** Patients report severe ocular pain, blurred vision, seeing halos around lights, lacrimation, nausea, vomiting, and headache.
      ii. **Physical examination findings** vary according to presentation.
        a) **Chronic angle closure glaucoma.** The patient's pupils are normal. The intraocular pressure is normal to elevated, and the cup:disc ratio is increased.
        b) **Acute angle closure glaucoma** is characterized by lid edema, conjunctival hyperemia, and circumcorneal injection.
          1) The cornea appears cloudy as the result of microcystic edema.
          2) The anterior chamber is shallow and cell, and flare (i.e., hazy fluid), secondary to an inflammatory reaction, is noted on slit-lamp examination.
          3) The pupil is midsized, fixed, and often ovoid.
          4) The intraocular pressure is markedly elevated.
    c. **Differential diagnoses** include anterior uveitis, miotic-induced glaucoma, neovascular glaucoma, and traumatic glaucoma.
    d. **Evaluation.** The diagnosis is usually based on the clinical scenario.
    e. **Therapy**
      i. **Chronic angle closure glaucoma** is treated with topical medications, **peripheral iridectomy,** or **laser iridotomy** on an outpatient basis.
      ii. **Acute angle closure glaucoma** is an emergency. The main goal of treatment is to reduce the intraocular pressure (see Clinical Pearl 12-1).

CLINICAL PEARL 12-1

Pharmacologic Management of Acute Angle Closure Glaucoma

1. **Hyperosmotic agents** are used to draw fluid back into the blood by increasing the osmolarity of the blood. These agents must be used with caution in patients with congestive heart failure or renal failure.
   a. **Oral agents** include **50% glycerin** (0.1 to 0.15 g/kg) or **isosorbide**.
   b. **Intravenous agents** include **mannitol 20%** (1 to 2 g/kg over 45 minutes).
2. **Carbonic anhydrase inhibitors** are used to reduce the production of aqueous humor by the ciliary body. **Acetazolamide** (500 mg) is administered intravenously, followed by 500 mg orally, and then 250 mg orally every 6 hours.
3. **β Blockers** increase aqueous outflow. **Timolol 0.5%** (one drop every 12 hours)
4. **Miotics** constrict the pupil and increase the flow of aqueous humor through the trabecular meshwork. **Pilocarpine 2% to 4%** solution (one drop) is the agent of choice, except in the setting of recent eye surgery.
5. **Corticosteroids** are used to reduce inflammation. **Prednisolone acetate 1%** (one drop every 4 to 6 hours) is the agent of choice.
6. **Antiemetics** should be used to control nausea and vomiting, as this can increase intraocular pressure.

  f. **Disposition**
   i. **Chronic angle closure glaucoma.** Patients can be discharged with instructions to consult an ophthalmologist for treatment.
   ii. **Acute angle closure glaucoma.** Ophthalmology should be consulted upon recognition of condition.

 2. **Anterior uveitis**
  a. **Discussion**
   i. **Definitions.** Anterior uveitis is inflammation of the anterior segment of the eye.
    a) **Iritis** is inflammation that involves only the iris.
    b) **Iridocyclitis** is inflammation of both the iris and ciliary body.
   ii. **Etiology.** The causes of uveitis are many:
    a) **Infection** (e.g., tuberculosis, syphilis)
    b) **Systemic disease,** including autoimmune disorders and immune complex–mediated disorders (e.g., sarcoidosis, Lyme disease, ankylosing spondylitis, Reiter syndrome, systemic lupus erythematosus, Sjögren syndrome, interstitial nephritis)
    c) **Idiopathic**
    d) **Trauma**
  b. **Clinical features**
   i. **Symptoms** include the acute onset of deep eye pain and decreased visual acuity. Patients often develop photophobia.
   ii. **Physical examination findings**
    a) **Funduscopic examination. Ciliary flush** (i.e., circumcorneal perilimbal injection of the episcleral and scleral vessels) and **conjunctival injection** are noted. **Flare and cells** may also be present.
    b) **Pupils.** The pupil on the affected side is small. Testing both the direct and consensual light reflex will cause the pain in the affected eye to increase.
  c. **Differential diagnoses** include conjunctivitis, episcleritis, scleritis, keratitis, and acute angle closure glaucoma.
  d. **Evaluation.** Because more than 50% of cases are the result of systemic disease, the underlying disease should be sought.
  e. **Therapy**
   i. **Treatment of the underlying disease process** should be initiated by the emergency physician if the diagnosis is obvious.
   ii. **Symptomatic treatment**
    a) **Cycloplegics.** A cycloplegic agent should be administered to reduce pain and photophobia by dilating the pupil and relaxing the ciliary muscles. The formation of synechia (i.e., adhesions between the iris

and lens) is prevented by dilatation as well. Cycloplegia can be accomplished using one of the following agents:

1) Homatropine hydrobromide 2% (one drop twice daily)
2) Scopolamine hydrobromide 0.25% (one drop twice daily)
3) Cyclopentolate hydrochloride 1% (two drops twice daily)

b) **Steroids.** The administration of steroids to reduce inflammation is best left to the ophthalmologist because the use of steroids can exacerbate infectious causes.

f. **Disposition.** Follow-up should be arranged with an ophthalmologist as soon as possible.

C. **Disorders characterized by vision loss**
1. **Central retinal artery occlusion (CRAO)**
   a. **Discussion.** Occlusion of the central retinal artery (e.g., by a thrombus, thromboemboli, cholesterol plaque, talc, calcium, or vasospasm) interferes with the major supply of blood to the retina, causing vision loss. In 25% of individuals, the cilioretinal arteries supply the macula as well; in these people, some central vision is spared in the event of CRAO.
   b. **Clinical features**
      i. **Symptoms.** CRAO is characterized by a **sudden, painless, monocular loss of vision** (Figure 12-1). Occasionally, it is preceded by **amaurosis fugax** (i.e., episodes of transient vision loss).
      ii. **Physical examination**
         a) **Visual acuity.** The patient is often only able to perceive light.
         b) **Examination of the pupils** shows a relative afferent pupillary defect (i.e., **Marcus Gunn pupil**; Figure 12-2).
         c) **Funduscopic examination**
            1) A **pale retina** with a **red spot** is visible on funduscopic examination. The red spot is the pigment of the choroid showing through the thin macula.
            2) The appearance of **emboli** may help identify the cause of the CRAO: **yellow** = cholesterol plaque; **white** = calcium plaque or talc (the latter is most often seen in intravenous drug abusers); **fluffy** = platelet fibrin; and **red** = sickle cells, thrombus, or thromboembolism.

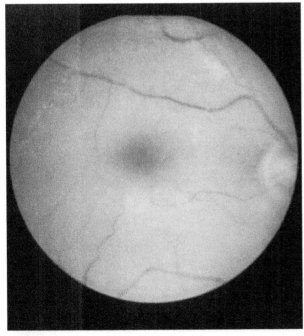

FIGURE 12-1 Central retinal artery occlusion fundus.

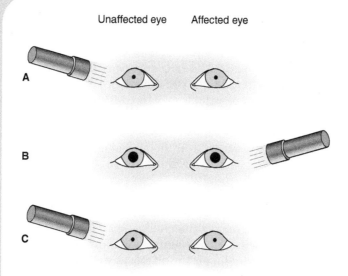

Unaffected eye   Affected eye

FIGURE
12-2 Relative afferent pupillary defect (Marcus Gunn pupil). (A) A penlight directed at the unaffected eye causes constriction of both pupils because both direct and consensual constriction occurs. (B) As the light is directed at the affected eye, which does not detect light, the direct and consensual responses do not occur and both eyes dilate. (C) When the light is swung back toward the unaffected eye, both pupils again constrict.

c. **Differential diagnoses** include other causes of painless visual loss, including central retinal vein occlusion (CRVO), retinal detachment, retrobulbar neuritis, snowblindness, and hysteria.

d. **Evaluation**
    i. If thrombi are seen, the workup should include evaluation of the carotids, heart, and especially the cardiac valves as a source of the thrombi.
    ii. In elderly patients, a sedimentation rate should be ordered. If the sedimentation rate is elevated, giant cell arteritis or temporal arteritis is the likely underlying cause.

e. **Therapy** is usually not particularly effective but should be attempted emergently to try to save the patient's sight. An attempt must be made to **reduce the intraocular pressure**, thereby increasing the pressure gradient in the artery. Increasing the pressure gradient in the artery may force the embolus further along in the artery, leading to the restoration of some vision. Methods to decrease the intraocular pressure include the following:
    i. **Application of digital pressure** to the cornea through the closed eyelid may help force aqueous fluid into the canals of Schlemm, reducing the intraocular pressure. Pressure should be applied for 30 seconds and then released and repeated.
    ii. **Pharmacologic intervention**
        a) **Carbonic anhydrase inhibition** with **acetazolamide** (500 mg orally) reduces aqueous humor production.
        b) **β Blockade** (e.g., with timolol 0.5%, one drop every 12 hours) increases the flow of aqueous humor out of the anterior chamber.
    iii. **Paracentesis** of the anterior chamber may be performed by ophthalmology to decrease the amount of aqueous humor.

f. **Disposition.** Admission to the hospital is necessary, both for treatment and for workup of the underlying cause.

2. **Branch retinal artery occlusion.** A painless partial loss of vision may result if an embolus lodges in a branch retinal artery (either originally, or following treatment for CRAO). The patient complains of loss of peripheral vision and, if the macula is involved, of the loss of central vision as well.

3. CRVO
   a. **Discussion.** The major cause of CRVO is an atheromatous artery that, because of increasing size and rigidity, presses on the vein, leading to collapse of the vein wall and occlusion of the vein.
   b. **Clinical features**
      i. **Symptoms.** The patient notes a **painless, monocular decrease in vision**. Because some vision often remains, the history helps differentiate CRVO from CRAO.
      ii. **Physical examination findings**
         a) **Examination of the pupils.** A relative afferent pupillary defect may be noted. Many times, enough light perception remains to allow both direct and consensual light reflex.
         b) **Funduscopic examination** can reveal anything from a few scattered flame hemorrhages and cotton wool spots to a florid, hemorrhagic blood-streaked retina with prominent dilated veins. The optic disc is often edematous (Figure 12-3).
   c. **Differential diagnoses** include CRAO, branch retinal artery occlusion, retinal detachment, retrobulbar neuritis, and stroke.
   d. **Evaluation** is mainly by history and physical examination.
   e. **Therapy.** Little can be done to reverse the damage that has occurred. Often, there is only branch retinal vein occlusion; in this case, laser photocoagulation by an ophthalmologist can reduce the incidence of later complications (e.g., neovascular glaucoma, vitreous hemorrhage).
   f. **Disposition.** Urgent follow-up with an ophthalmologist is required.
4. **Retinal detachment**
   a. **Discussion.** A tear in the retina allows vitreous fluid to seep behind the retina, detaching it from the underlying choroid.
   b. **Clinical features**
      i. **Symptoms**
         a) **Prodromal symptoms** (e.g., flashing lights in the peripheral visual field, especially at night; floating "spider webs" moving across the visual field)
         b) The patient may report that the **actual detachment** was like "**having a curtain drawn up or down**" the visual field.

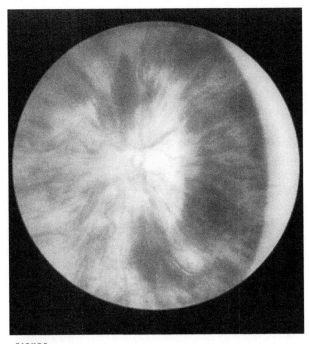

FIGURE 12-3 Central retinal vein occlusion fundus.

   ii. **Physical examination**
    a) **Visual acuity.** The blindness will be in the peripheral fields unless the macula is involved, in which case, central vision will be affected as well.
    b) **Funduscopic examination** will reveal an undulating, pale, detached retina.
  c. **Differential diagnoses** include CRAO, CRVO, retrobulbar neuritis, and strokes in the visual pathway.
  d. **Evaluation** is by physical examination. A good funduscopic examination is essential. Ocular ultrasound may also assist in diagnosis.
  e. **Therapy** is with **photocoagulation** and is carried out by an ophthalmologist.
   i. If the detachment is inferior, the patient should rest with his or her head elevated.
   ii. If the detachment is superior, then the patient's head should not be elevated while resting.
  f. **Disposition.** Prompt evaluation and treatment by an ophthalmologist are essential. If the patient's central vision is intact, there is an excellent chance of preserving the vision.
 5. **Optic neuritis**
  a. **Discussion**
   i. **Definitions**
    a) **Papillitis** is involvement of the optic nerve head.
    b) **Retrobulbar neuritis** is involvement of the optic nerve.
   ii. **Etiology.** Optic neuritis can have multiple causes, the most common being **multiple sclerosis.** Other causes include **sarcoidosis, leukemia, a previous viral illness, syphilis, collagen vascular disease, tuberculosis, and heavy metal intoxication.**
   iii. **Predisposing factors.** Women are more often affected than men.
  b. **Clinical features**
   i. **Symptoms**
    a) The **loss of visual acuity** can occur over hours but generally worsens over the course of 1 week. **Central scotomata** are quite common, and **color vision is more affected.**
    b) Patients often report **pain** in the region of the globe, especially with movement.
   ii. **Physical examination.** There may be no findings in retrobulbar neuritis, hence the expression, "The patient sees nothing, and the doctor sees nothing." However, a relative afferent pupillary defect may be noted, and funduscopic examination may reveal optic disc swelling or papillitis.
  c. **Differential diagnoses** include other causes of painless loss of vision. Because the onset of visual loss is usually gradual, the differential diagnosis list also includes papilledema, ischemic optic neuropathy, orbital tumors or tumors compressing the optic nerve, and severe systemic hypertension.
  d. **Evaluation** is usually focused on identifying systemic underlying causes, such as multiple sclerosis, viral infections, granulomatous inflammations (e.g., syphilis, tuberculosis, sarcoidosis, *Cryptococcus* infection), and toxic causes (e.g., lead poisoning, chloramphenicol toxicity).
  e. **Therapy** is directed toward the underlying cause. Systemic steroids seem to work best in retrobulbar neuritis, shortening the course of recovery. The recovery period can be as short as 1 week or as long as 2 to 3 months but is generally approximately 6 weeks.
  f. **Disposition** is according to the underlying illness.
 D. **Eye infections**
  1. **Blepharitis**
   a. **Discussion.** Blepharitis is chronic inflammation of the lid margins.
    i. **Infectious blepharitis** is caused by *Staphylococcus aureus* or *Staphylococcus epidermidis*.
    ii. **Seborrheic blepharitis** is associated with *Pityrosporum ovale* infection.

b. Clinical features
    i. **Symptoms** are irritation, burning, and itching of the lid margins.
    ii. **Physical examination** reveals red-rimmed eyelids, with scale and debris clinging to the lashes.
       a) In the **staphylococcal type**, the scales are dry, the lashes tend to fall out, and occasionally tiny ulcerations are found along the lid margin.
       b) In the **seborrheic type**, the scales are greasy and the margins are not as inflamed.
c. **Differential diagnoses** include conjunctivitis, hordeolum, dacryocystitis, allergic conjunctivitis, and foreign bodies.
d. **Evaluation** is by history and careful physical examination.
e. **Therapy**
    i. **Cleansing.** The eyebrows and lid margins should be cleaned daily using baby shampoo and a cotton swab to remove the debris on the lid margin.
    ii. **Antibiotics.** Staphylococcal blepharitis is treated with **sulfacetamide ophthalmic drops**.
f. **Disposition.** The patient may be sent home with instructions to follow-up with a primary care physician in 1 to 2 weeks.

2. Hordeola
  a. **Discussion**
    i. **Definition.** A hordeolum is an infection (abscess) of the glands of the eyelid.
       a) An **internal hordeolum** is an infection of the deep **meibomian glands**.
       b) A **superficial hordeolum (stye)** is an infection of the smaller, more external and superficial **Zeis** or **Moll glands**.
    ii. **Etiology.** Most hordeola are caused by *S. aureus*.
  b. **Clinical features**
    i. **Symptoms** include pain, redness, and swelling of the eyelid.
    ii. **Physical examination** reveals redness, swelling, and, often, pointing of the abscess on the lid.
       a) **Internal hordeola** may point to the skin or conjunctival surface.
       b) **Superficial hordeola** always point to the skin.
  c. **Differential diagnoses** include blepharitis and tumors of the eyelid.
  d. **Evaluation** is by physical examination.
  e. **Therapy**
    i. **Conservative measures** include the application of warm compresses to increase blood supply and facilitate spontaneous drainage. In adults, application of an erythromycin-containing ophthalmic ointment every 3 hours may hasten resolution.
    ii **Complicated cases**
       a) If cellulitis develops, systemic antibiotics may be needed.
       b) An abscess that does not resolve in 48 hours may need to be surgically drained.
          1) Incisions made on the conjunctival surface must be vertical to avoid the other meibomian glands.
          2) Incisions made on the skin surface must be horizontal to follow the lines of the face and to reduce scarring.
  f. **Disposition.** The patient should be sent home with instructions to follow-up in 2 days if the abscess has not spontaneously drained. If cellulitis develops, the patient should be advised to return to the emergency department (ED) immediately.

3. Dacryocystitis
  a. **Discussion**
    i. **Definition.** Dacryocystitis is an infection of the lacrimal sac.
    ii. **Etiology**
       a) **Acute infections**
          1) *Haemophilus influenzae* is the most common cause in infants.

2) Acute infections in adults most often occur in postmenopausal women and are usually caused by *S. aureus*. Occasionally, **β-hemolytic streptococci** are the culprits.

    b) **Chronic infections** are usually the result of *Streptococcus pneumoniae* or *Candida albicans*.

  b. **Clinical features**

    i. **Symptoms.** The patient typically experiences tearing and discharge as well as swelling and pain in the medial canthus.

    ii. **Physical examination findings.** The lacrimal sac is tender, and purulent material can often be expressed from the duct.

  c. **Differential diagnoses** include blepharitis, hordeolum, and conjunctivitis.

  d. **Evaluation** is by physical examination. Cultures are needed if therapy fails.

  e. **Therapy**

    i. **Warm compresses** are used to increase blood supply.

    ii. **Antibiotic therapy**

      a) **Children.** Oral antibiotics are used in children:

        1) **Amoxicillin–clavulanate** (40 mg/kg/day, divided, three times daily)

        2) **Second- or third-generation cephalosporin,** such as **cefdinir**

        3) **Trimethoprim–sulfamethoxazole** (8 mg/kg/day, divided, twice daily) for patients who are allergic to penicillin

      b) **Adults.** Acute infections can be treated with oral **penicillin or cephalosporin,** unless methicillin-resistant *S. aureus* coverage is needed.

4. **Cellulitis**

  a. **Periorbital (preseptal) cellulitis** occurs anterior to the orbital septum, a broad layer of fascia that separates the orbit from the eyelids.

    i. **Clinical features**

      a) **Symptoms** include warmth, redness, swelling, and tenderness over one or both of the eyelids. There should never be eye pain.

      b) **Physical examination findings**

        1) Inflammation of the conjunctiva and swelling of the eyelids are noted. Chemosis is often seen.

        2) Fever is common, but its absence does not rule out the diagnosis.

        3) Extraocular motions are full and no pain is elicited on motion. On palpation of the globe, there should be no tenderness.

    ii. **Differential diagnoses.** It is important to differentiate between preseptal cellulitis and orbital cellulitis (see I.D.4.b and Figure 12-4).

    iii. **Evaluation**

      a) **Computed tomography (CT).** A CT scan with intravenous contrast should be performed to look for evidence of orbital involvement.

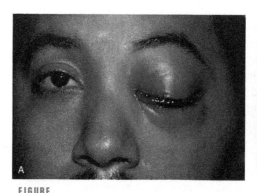
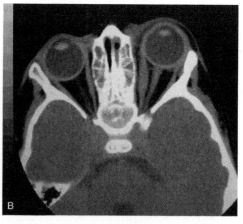

FIGURE
12-4 **Periorbital or orbital cellulitis. (A) Swelling and proptosis on physical examination. (B) CT image.**
(Courtesy of Mark Silverberg, MD; from Greenberg MI, et al. *Greenberg's Text-Atlas of Emergency Medicine.* Philadelphia: Lippincott Williams & Wilkins; 2005.)

b) **Blood cultures** may help identify an organism but are often negative, even with orbital cellulitis.

iv. **Therapy**

a) **Oral antibiotics.** If one is certain that the cellulitis is periorbital, then outpatient therapy can be initiated with one of the following agents:

1) **Clindamycin** (children 30 to 40 mg/kg/day divided every 8 hours, adults 300 mg every 8 hours) or **trimethoprim–sulfamethoxazole** (children 8 mg/kg/day, adults two double-strength tablets every 12 hours) plus one of the following:

2) **Amoxicillin** (children 80 to 100 mg/kg/day divided every 8 hours, adults 875 mg every 12 hours), **amoxicillin-clavulanic acid** (children 45 mg/kg/day divided every 12 hours, adults 875 mg every 12 hours), or **cefdinir** (children 7 mg/kg/day every 12 hours, adults 300 mg every 12 hours).

v. **Disposition.** Next-day follow-up and reexamination are mandatory. The patient should be instructed to return to the ED immediately if he or she experiences pain in the eye, double vision, or other vision problems.

b. **Orbital cellulitis** extends deep to the fascia and into the orbit.

i. **Discussion**

a) **Etiology.** *H. influenzae* is the most common organism, found in over 50% of cases. Other causative organisms include *Staphylococcus aureus*, *Staphylococcus epidermidis*, *Staphylococcus pneumoniae* and other streptococci, *Corynebacterium diphtheriae*, and *Pseudomonas*.

b) **Predisposing factors.** Approximately 75% of patients with orbital cellulitis have recently had sinusitis, an upper respiratory tract infection, or otitis media with effusion.

ii. **Clinical findings.** Physical examination findings may include those found in Clinical Pearl 12-2.

iii. **Differential diagnoses** include the less serious periorbital (preseptal) cellulitis and cavernous sinus thrombosis. Dilatation of the episcleral vessels is the first sign of extension into the cavernous sinus. Late signs are pupillary fixation and venous engorgement of the fundus.

iv. **Evaluation**

a) **CT.** A CT scan of the orbit is important to identify orbital involvement and locate any abscesses that need to be drained.

b) **Blood cultures** are only positive approximately one-third of the time, but they can help identify the organism.

c) **Lumbar puncture** is indicated if the patient has altered mentation or nuchal rigidity (which may suggest spread to the central nervous system).

v. **Therapy.** Orbital cellulitis is a true emergency, and **intravenous antibiotics** should be started as soon as the diagnosis is entertained, even before CT evaluation.

a) The initial antibiotic of choice is **vancomycin** (in children 40 to 60 mg/kg/day every 6 or 8 hours, in adults 30 to 60 mg/kg/day every 8 to 12 hours).

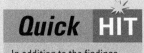

Quick **HIT**

In addition to the findings noted for periorbital cellulitis, ocular pain and limitation of eye movement are the hallmarks of orbital cellulitis.

Eye, Ear, Nose, Throat, and Dental Emergencies

CLINICAL PEARL **12-2**

Physical Exam Findings in Orbital Cellulitis

1. Lid edema, erythema, and even ecchymoses
2. Painful extraocular movements
3. Proptosis and marked tenderness of the globe
4. Decreased visual acuity, possibly even to the point of blindness
5. Pupillary paralysis
6. Increased ocular pressure
7. Loss of sensation along the trigeminal nerve distribution (rare)

b) In addition to vancomycin, coverage should be supplemented by one of the following: **ceftriaxone** (children 50 mg/kg every 12 hours, adults 2 g every 24 hours), **cefotaxime** (children 150 to 200 mg/kg divided every 8 hours, adults 2 g every 4 hours), **ampicillin/sulbactam** (children 300 mg/kg divided every 6 hours, adults 3 g every 6 hours), or **piperacillin-tazobactam** (children 240 mg/kg divided every 8 hours, adults 4.5 g every 6 hours).

5. Conjunctivitis
   a. **Viral conjunctivitis** can be caused by adenoviruses, coxsackieviruses, enterovirus, and herpesviruses.
      i. **Clinical features**
         a) **Symptoms.** The most common symptoms are itching, profuse tearing, and redness of the eyes. In most patients, the infection is bilateral, but unilateral viral conjunctivitis does occur. Many patients have associated systemic symptoms of fever, neuralgia, and pharyngitis.
         b) **Physical examination findings**
            1) The conjunctiva is injected, with minimal exudate.
            2) Preauricular lymphadenopathy is often noted.
      ii. **Differential diagnoses** include bacterial conjunctivitis, foreign bodies, iritis, corneal ulcer, and keratoconjunctivitis. **Fluorescein staining** should be performed to rule out keratitis of herpes infection.
      iii. **Therapy** mainly consists of the application of warm compresses. If the diagnosis is in doubt or one wishes to prevent secondary bacterial infection, an antibacterial agent can be prescribed. Frequent hand washing is advised to prevent spread to others.
   b. **Bacterial conjunctivitis** is most commonly caused by *Staphylococcus aureus*, *H. influenzae*, *Streptococcus pneumoniae*, and *N. gonorrhoeae*.
      i. **Clinical features.** The infection is usually in one eye but may have been spread to the other eye by autoinfection.
         a) **Symptoms** include pruritus, the sensation of a foreign body, tearing, and photosensitivity. A mucopurulent discharge is usually present and may be profuse when *N. gonorrhoeae* is the causative organism.
         b) **Physical examination findings** include conjunctival hyperemia or chemosis and tarsal plate papillae (seen on eversion of the eyelid).
      ii. **Differential diagnoses** include viral conjunctivitis, foreign bodies, iritis, corneal ulcer, and keratoconjunctivitis.
      iii. **Therapy**
         a) Initial empiric therapy with **erythromycin** ophthalmic ointment (0.5 inch every 6 hours) or **polymyxin-trimethoprim** drops (one or two drops every 6 hours)
         b) Fluoroquinolone ophthalmic drops (one or two drops every 6 hours) are the preferred treatment in contact lens wearers.
      iv. **Disposition**
         a) **Admission.** Patients with suspected or confirmed gonorrhea conjunctivitis need to be admitted for intravenous antibiotic therapy and irrigation.
         b) **Discharge.** Patients with other types of bacterial conjunctivitis are treated on an outpatient basis with instructions to follow-up in 24 hours if the infection has not improved.
6. Corneal ulcers
   a. **Discussion**
      i. **Etiology.** Corneal ulcers occur when an infective organism invades the cornea and breaks down the protective epithelial layer (Figure 12-5). Commonly implicated organisms include:
         a) **Bacteria**
            1) Gram-positive organisms (e.g., staphylococci, streptococci, bacilli)

Quick HIT

Fluorescein staining should be undertaken for patients with superficial ocular infection to look for corneal ulcers or keratitis.

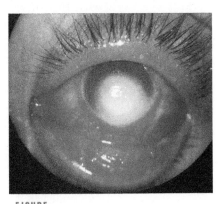

FIGURE
12-5 Corneal ulcer.

     2) Gram-negative organisms (e.g., *Pseudomonas* [common among contact lens wearers], diplococci, bacilli, anaerobes)
     3) Anaerobes (e.g., cocci, bacilli)
   b) **Viruses** (e.g., herpesvirus)
   c) **Fungi**
  ii. **Predisposing factors.** Ulceration is often secondary to infection following burns, abrasions, extended-wear contact lens overuse, or inappropriate use of topical anesthetics.
  b. **Clinical features**
   i. **Symptoms** include a foreign body sensation, blurred vision (especially if the ulcer is in the line of vision), light sensitivity, and mucopurulent discharge.
   ii. **Physical examination findings** include conjunctival injection and irregularity of the cornea. Fluorescein staining reveals uptake of dye in the denuded area of cornea.
  c. **Differential diagnoses** include corneal abrasions, foreign bodies, and conjunctivitis.
  d. **Therapy.** Covering the eye or administering steroids can worsen the infection.
   i. **Topical antimicrobial therapy** should be instituted immediately.
    a) Fluoroquinolone (e.g., moxifloxacin) ophthalmic drops (one or two drops every 6 hours) are the preferred treatment in contact lens wearers.
    b) **Herpesvirus infections** are treated with **antiviral agents** (see I.D.7.e.i.a) and **prophylactic topical antibiotics** to cover gram-negative and gram-positive organisms.
    c) **Fungal infections** are treated with **intravenous amphotericin B**.
   ii. **Cycloplegia** with **homatropine 2.5%** (two drops every 6 to 24 hours) reduces pain and photophobia.
  e. **Disposition.** Prompt consultation with an ophthalmologist is advised.
7. **Herpes infections**
  a. **Discussion.** Any of the herpesviruses can infect the eye.
   i. In neonates, **herpes simplex virus-type 2 (HSV-2)** is most common, but **herpes simplex virus-type 1 (HSV-1)** is becoming more prevalent. HSV-1 and HSV-2 infections cause **conjunctivitis** or **keratoconjunctivitis**.
   ii. In adults, **varicella-zoster virus** is the most common viral cause of eye infections and should be suspected if there is a lesion at the tip of the nose (nasociliary branch of cranial nerve V) or if the eyelid is involved. Herpes zoster infection usually occurs in older patients and may be recurrent.
   iii. **Epstein-Barr virus** may cause **conjunctivitis** or **keratitis in association with mononucleosis**.
   iv. **Cytomegalovirus** can cause a **severe retinitis** in patients with AIDS.
  b. **Clinical features**
   i. **Symptoms** include pain, foreign body sensation, photophobia, decreased visual acuity, and tearing. Constitutional symptoms, especially malaise, may also be present.

Eye, Ear, Nose, Throat, and Dental Emergencies

ii. **Physical examination** reveals marked conjunctival injection and possibly vesicles on the inner aspect of the lid.

c. **Differential diagnoses** include bacterial keratoconjunctivitis, *Chlamydia* (inclusion) conjunctivitis, corneal abrasion, uveitis, and recurrent corneal erosion.

d. Evaluation

   i. **Slit-lamp examination**

   ii. **Scrapings**

     a) **Rose bengal staining** is positive in herpes zoster and HSV-1 or HSV-2 infection.

     b) **Giemsa staining** of scrapings will show multinucleated giant cells.

   iii. **Cultures** can help identify the virus.

e. Therapy

   i. **Antiviral agents**

     a) **HSV-1 or HSV-2 infection.** Acceptable regimens include:

       1) **Vidarabine 3%** (0.5 inch applied five times daily)

       2) **Trifluridine 1%** (two drops every 2 hours while awake)

       3) **Idoxuridine 0.5% ointment** (applied every 4 to 6 hours)

     b) **Varicella-zoster virus infection** is treated with **oral acyclovir,** 800 mg five times daily.

   ii. **Cycloplegia. Cyclopentolate 1% solution** applied three times daily may relieve some of the photophobia.

   iii. **Steroids** have been shown to be beneficial, but prescribing them should be left to the ophthalmologist. They are particularly helpful for reducing inflammation in the anterior chamber.

f. Disposition

   i. **Discharge.** The patient can usually be discharged with instructions to consult an ophthalmologist.

   ii. **Admission.** Patients with severe or systemic infections should be admitted, especially if the patient is immunocompromised.

E. Trauma

  1. **Corneal abrasion**

   a. **Etiology.** Causes include **foreign bodies** under the eyelid, **accidental self-inflicted wounds** (e.g., babies often scratch their own corneas with their fingernails), and **contact lenses,** which may leave multiple abrasions in the central cornea.

   b. **Clinical features**

     i. **Symptoms** include a sharp, stabbing pain or a foreign body sensation aggravated by lid movement, tearing, and photophobia.

     ii. **Physical examination findings**

       a) The conjunctival fornices should be inspected for a foreign body. The eyelid should also be everted to check for a foreign body.

       b) A drop of tetracaine instilled in the eye will cause a burning sensation at first, but then the pain will be temporarily relieved. The relief of pain points to a corneal problem. In addition, the relief of pain facilitates the rest of the examination.

       c) Instillation of fluorescein stain and examination under a cobalt blue light source will reveal an abrasion (Figure 12-6).

   c. **Differential diagnoses** include corneal abrasions, corneal ulcers, corneal laceration, foreign bodies, and keratoconjunctivitis.

   d. **Evaluation.** Physical examination findings should be adequate for diagnosis.

   e. **Therapy**

     i. **Foreign body removal.** If a foreign body is identified, it should be removed by irrigation or by wiping the everted eyelid with a moistened cotton swab. If the foreign body is impeded in the cornea, removal with a corneal spud or a hypodermic needle (guided by the slit lamp) may be necessary.

     ii. **Cycloplegia** with **cyclopentolate 1%** or **homatropine 5%** (two drops) will help relieve photophobia and pain.

     iii. **Antibiotic therapy. Erythromycin** ophthalmic ointment or **polymyxin-trimethoprim** drops should be initiated.

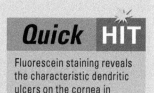

Quick HIT

Fluorescein staining reveals the characteristic dendritic ulcers on the cornea in HSV-1 or HSV-2 infection.

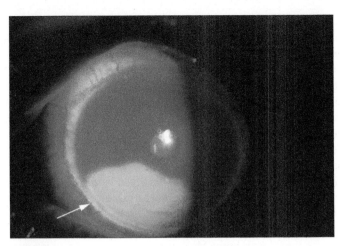

FIGURE
12-6 Corneal abrasion with fluorescein uptake.

    iv. **Analgesia.** The patient can be advised to take an **over-the-counter pain medication** to relieve pain once the anesthetic has worn off. Anesthetic drops are traditionally not prescribed for use on an outpatient basis because repeated use can soften the cornea and lead to corneal ulcer; however, recent studies have indicated a short course of judicial use may be safe.
   f. **Disposition.** The patient can be discharged with instructions to make an appointment with an ophthalmologist for an examination within 24 hours.
2. **Corneal laceration**
   a. **Etiology.** Corneal lacerations can result from impeded foreign bodies, high-energy injuries to the cornea, or intraocular foreign bodies (see I.E.3).
   b. **Clinical features**
     i. **Symptoms** are similar to those of corneal abrasion.
     ii. **Physical examination findings.** Care should be taken to avoid applying pressure to the cornea or the globe because doing so will express aqueous fluid through the laceration.
       a) The pupil may be shaped like a teardrop as a result of prolapse of the iris through the cornea. The prolapsed tissue may look like a foreign body at the edge of the cornea.
       b) On fluorescein staining, streaming of aqueous fluid from a corneal abrasion may be noted (positive Seidel sign), signifying that fluid is flowing through the laceration.
   c. **Differential diagnoses** include foreign bodies, intraocular foreign bodies, and corneal abrasion.
   d. **Evaluation**
     i. **Laboratory studies** are not routinely needed, unless required for evaluation in anticipation of operative management.
     ii. **Imaging studies.** Orbital radiographs or CT scans may be needed to rule out an intraocular foreign body.
   e. **Therapy.** A rigid eye shield should be placed over the orbit to protect the eye, and the patient should be referred emergently to an ophthalmologist for surgical repair. Antibiotics should be initiated after consultation.
3. **Intraocular foreign body**
   a. **Etiology.** Penetration of the globe by a foreign body is usually associated with a history of an object propelled at high velocity (e.g., a pellet from an air gun, a projectile from hammering).
   b. **Clinical features**
     i. **Symptoms.** The initial injury may be painful, but often, there may not be much pain after the object is imbedded.
     ii. **Physical examination findings.** Care should be taken to avoid applying pressure on the globe.

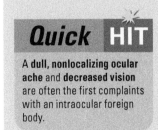

Quick **HIT**

A dull, nonlocalizing ocular ache and decreased vision are often the first complaints with an intraocular foreign body.

Eye, Ear, Throat, and Dental Emergencies

a) **Pupils.** The presence of a "**teardrop pupil**" suggests laceration and protrusion of the iris near the limbus.

b) **Sclera.** Small points of hemorrhage in the sclera may represent a penetration. If bright light is directed in the pupil and a glow is seen at the site of hemorrhage, penetrating injury is likely.

c) **Slit-lamp examination** is performed to search for minute perforations.

d) **Funduscopic examination** should be performed through a dilated pupil. The retina and the area immediately in front of the retina should be examined for foreign bodies.

c. **Differential diagnoses** include corneal abrasion, corneal laceration, subconjunctival hemorrhage, foreign body on the cornea or on the conjunctiva, and a nonpenetrating impeded foreign body.

d. **Evaluation.** Radiographs, tomograms, or a CT scan of the orbit may be necessary to locate the foreign body. Magnetic resonance imaging is contraindicated because if the foreign body is ferrous, attraction of the foreign body by the magnet can be disastrous.

e. **Therapy** is **surgical removal** of the foreign body by an ophthalmologist.

f. **Disposition.** An ophthalmologist should be consulted as soon as possible.

4. **Hyphema**

a. **Etiology and pathogenesis.** Blunt injury to the eye (e.g., by a direct hit from a ball or a fist) can cause small tears in the vessels supplying the iris, leading to the accumulation of blood in the anterior chamber. The blood then forms a layer (i.e., a hyphema) in the lower pole of the chamber.

b. **Clinical features**

   i. **Symptoms** include blurred vision and ocular pain.

   ii. **Physical examination** may reveal a cloudy anterior chamber. Slit-lamp examination will reveal the layer of blood in the lower portion of the anterior chamber.

c. **Differential diagnoses** include conjunctival hemorrhage, traumatic iritis, corneal abrasion, and lens dislocation.

d. **Evaluation** is by the patient history and careful slit-lamp examination. Laboratory tests are not needed.

e. **Therapy**

   i. **Bed rest** is mandatory.

   ii. **Cycloplegia** is usually instituted with homatropine 5% drops.

   iii. **Monitoring.** The affected eye should be reexamined daily for evidence of rebleeding (which occurs in approximately 20% of patients in the first 3 days after the injury). The intraocular pressure should be measured to monitor for the development of glaucoma.

   iv. **Minimization and treatment of complications**

      a) **Rebleeding.** Some ophthalmologists use **aminocaproic acid** (100 mg orally every 4 hours) to reduce the risk of rebleeding by stabilizing the clot.

      b) **Glaucoma** should be treated with β blockers, acetazolamide, and hyperosmotic agents. If pressures remain high, the clot may need to be surgically removed.

f. **Disposition.** Patients should be admitted to the hospital for treatment.

5. **Orbital fractures**

a. **Discussion.** Blunt trauma to the globe transmits forces to the entire orbital cavity. The bones of the floor and medial wall are particularly fragile. When the floor fractures, the orbital fat and inferior rectus muscle can prolapse through the fracture and become entrapped. The infraorbital nerve also traverses the floor and may be involved in injury.

b. **Clinical features**

   i. **Symptoms** include orbital pain, episodes of double vision, and, possibly, tingling along the distribution of the infraorbital nerve (i.e., the cheek and along the side of the nose).

Quick HIT

Complications of blood in the anterior chamber are staining of the corneal epithelium with blood and blockage of the trabecular meshwork, which can lead to the development of glaucoma.

Eye, Ear, Nose, Throat, and Dental Emergencies

ii. **Physical examination findings** may include:
   a) Swelling and ecchymoses about the eye
   b) Enophthalmos
   c) Sensory deficits in the infraorbital nerve distribution
   d) Signs of hyphema

c. **Differential diagnoses** include globe rupture, hyphema, lens dislocation, and zygomatic arch fracture.

d. **Evaluation** by radiograph may be considered but the diagnostic modality of choice is CT of the orbital bones.

e. **Therapy** is usually conservative and most ophthalmologists wait until the swelling and edema have subsided before attempting surgical repair. If clinical signs and symptoms of rectus muscle entrapment are present, **urgent surgical repair is indicated**. It is also important to watch for delayed development of hyphema.

f. **Disposition**
   i. **Discharge.** If no hyphema is present, the patient can usually be discharged with instructions to follow up with an ophthalmologist. Obviously, other consequences of trauma should be addressed before the patient is discharged.
   ii. **Admission.** If the patient develops hyphema, admission is usually required.

6. **Chemical burns**
   a. **Etiology and pathogenesis.** Burns to the eye can occur with both acids and alkalis. The substance does not necessarily have to be a liquid; some powders and solids (e.g., lye, lime, potassium hydroxide, magnesium hydroxide) mix with water to form alkali, and the wet eye is a source of water.
      i. Therefore, these substances can penetrate deeper (i.e., they can penetrate the globe).
      ii. **Acid burns** cause a protein coagulation, which often limits deeper acid penetration.
   b. **Clinical features**
      i. **Symptoms** are ocular pain and blurred vision.
      ii. **Physical examination findings.** The eye can be quickly assessed to rule out frank rupture, but immediate irrigation should be instituted. Assessment of the degree of damage should be carried out after therapy.
         a) **Minor burns** are characterized by:
            1) Erythema and edema of the eyelid
            2) Superficial punctate keratitis of the corneal epithelium
            3) Chemosis, hyperemia, and hemorrhages
         b) **Moderate to severe burns** are characterized by:
            1) Second- or third-degree burns of the eyelids
            2) Corneal edema, opacification, and epithelial defects on fluorescein staining
            3) Chemosis and perilimbal blanching of the conjunctiva
            4) A marked anterior chamber reaction and clouding of the fluid
            5) Possibly, increased intraocular pressures
   c. **Differential diagnoses** include a foreign body, corneal ulcers, and chemical conjunctivitis.
   d. **Evaluation** is mainly by patient history. Therapy should not be delayed for a thorough physical examination if the cause of the patient's complaint is obvious.
   e. **Therapy**
      i. **Irrigation.** It is **impossible to overirrigate**. Irrigation can be done with a Morgan lens, a cup-like device that is placed on the eye and attached to a saline intravenous bag. Alternatively, saline can be directly irrigated into the eye using intravenous tubing.
         a) **pH.** During irrigation, the pH of the inferior cul-de-sac should be repeatedly checked until it registers neutral. After irrigation is completed, it should be rechecked in 5 to 10 minutes to ensure that the pH has remained neutral.
         b) **Visual acuity.** Following irrigation, the visual acuity is checked and the eye is inspected by both direct and slit-lamp examination.

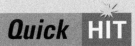

Quick HIT

Restricted extraocular movement, especially upward and laterally, and the presence of diplopia should alert to the possibility of orbital fracture and rectus muscle entrapment.

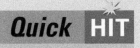

Quick HIT

Alkali burns are generally worse than acid burns. Alkali burns cause saponification of tissues, leading to liquefaction necrosis.

Eye, Ear, Nose, Throat, and Dental Emergencies

Provided the pH remains stable and there is not a penetrating injury, additional therapy can be undertaken.

     ii. **Supportive therapy**

        a) **Cycloplegics** (e.g., cyclopentolate 1%, three times daily) help reduce photophobia.

        b) **Broad-spectrum antibiotic ointment** or **drops** should be prescribed prophylactically.

        c) **Tear substitutes** should be prescribed as well.

        d) **Steroids**, both topical and systemic, are helpful but are probably best prescribed by the ophthalmologist.

   f. **Disposition**

     i. **Discharge.** Patients with mild burns can be discharged with instructions to follow-up the next day with an ophthalmologist.

     ii. **Admission.** Patients with more severe burns may need to be admitted. If the globe has been penetrated, the ophthalmologist needs to see the patient in the ED.

II. EAR

   A. **Infections**

     1. **Otitis externa**

       a. **Discussion**

         i. **Definition**

          a) **Otitis externa** is inflammation of the auditory canal.

          b) **Necrotizing (malignant) otitis externa** is a severe form of otitis externa that involves the surrounding tissues. It is almost always caused by *Pseudomonas* and occurs in patients with diabetes and other debilitating diseases.

         ii. **Etiology.** Otitis externa is usually caused by a bacterial infection (most often *Pseudomonas*, *Staphylococcus*, *Streptococcus*, or a gram-negative rod). Other, less common causes include fungal infection (most commonly *Aspergillus*) and eczema.

         iii. **Predisposing factors** include trauma to the epithelium; swimming; hot, humid weather; cotton ear swabs; and the use of a hearing aid.

       b. **Clinical features**

         i. **Symptoms** include otalgia, pruritus, plugging of the ear, and decreased hearing.

         ii. **Physical examination findings**

          a) The canal is erythematous, often with a purulent discharge.

          b) The preauricular lymph nodes may be swollen.

          c) When the tragus pinna is pulled to open the canal for visualization, there is often pain.

       c. **Differential diagnoses** include eczematous otitis externa, necrotizing otitis externa, otitis media, mastoiditis, and a foreign body.

       d. **Evaluation.** Diagnosis is usually made on the basis of the physical examination. The only time additional testing is warranted is if necrotizing otitis externa is suspected; in this situation, a CT scan to evaluate the deep tissues may be appropriate.

       e. **Therapy**

         i. **Cleansing.** The canal should be cleaned of debris by gentle irrigation with tepid water or 2% acetic acid solution (vinegar).

         ii. **Antimicrobial therapy**

          a) **Uncomplicated otitis externa.** A topical antibiotic with steroids (e.g., **polymyxin B otic suspension**) should be instilled in the ear (four drops three times daily for 10 days).

          b) **Necrotizing external otitis media** is treated intravenously with **ciprofloxacin** (400 mg every 12 hours) and in this instance also used in pediatric patients.

          c) **Fungal infection. Amphotericin B** should be used in consultation with an infectious disease specialist.

f. **Disposition.** Patients with uncomplicated otitis externa can be sent home with instructions to follow up with a primary care physician in 3 to 5 days. The ear should be kept clean and dry, and the patient should be educated about minimizing use of cotton swabs. Patients with necrotizing otitis externa must be admitted for intravenous antibiotic therapy.

2. Otitis media
   a. **Discussion**
      i. **Definition.** Otitis media is a bacterial infection of the middle ear.
      ii. **Etiology.** The organisms that usually cause otitis media are *S. pneumoniae, H. influenzae, Moraxella catarrhalis*, and group A streptococci; however, the incidences of each are changing due to changes in the pediatric immunization schedule.
      iii. **Predisposing factors.** Otitis media is often preceded by a viral upper respiratory infection that produces Eustachian tube dysfunction secondary to swelling of the mucous membranes. The middle ear then fills with fluid, which becomes infected with bacteria.
   b. **Clinical features**
      i. **Symptoms**
         a) In young patients, the only symptoms may be fever and irritability. Infants may bat at or play with the affected ear.
         b) Older children and adults complain of pain and fullness in the ear and trouble hearing.
      ii. **Physical examination findings**
         a) Fever is often present but not necessary for diagnosis.
         b) The tympanic membrane will be bulging and erythematous and is often yellow in color. A poor light reflex on the tympanic membrane is noted. If the eardrum has ruptured, pus may be noted in the canal. Pneumatic insufflation reveals an immobile tympanic membrane.
   c. **Differential diagnoses** include otitis externa, malignant otitis externa, and a foreign body. If there is swelling behind the ear, mastoiditis should be considered.
   d. **Evaluation.** In general, no additional testing is needed. If a pediatric patient appears very ill or dehydrated, then additional workup may be warranted to rule out septicemia and bacteremia.
   e. **Therapy**
      i. **Nonsteroidal anti-inflammatory drugs** are indicated to treat fever and pain.
      ii. **Antibiotics**
         a) **Children.** Most infections are viral. Older than age 4, clinicians may perform a watchful waiting where no antibiotics are started in the first 48 hours. If treating immediately or the patient is still symptomatic after 48 hours, acceptable regimens include:
            1) **Amoxicillin** (90 mg/kg, divided every 12 hours), the drug of choice, except in patients who are allergic to penicillin and those with recently recurrent infections
            2) **Azithromycin** (10 mg/kg on day 1, 5 mg/kg on days 2 to 5)
            3) **Cefdinir** (14 mg/kg/day, divided every 12 hours)
            4) **Ceftriaxone** (50 mg/kg intramuscularly)
         b) **Adults.** Acceptable regimens include:
            1) **Amoxicillin** (500 mg every 12 hours or 875 mg every 12 hours in more complicated infections; treatment of choice in nonallergic patients)
            2) **Cefdinir** (300 mg every 12 hours)
            3) **Azithromycin** (500 mg on day 1, 250 mg on days 2 to 5)
   f. **Disposition**
      i. **Discharge.** Most patients can be discharged with instructions to return to a primary care physician in 2 weeks for a follow-up examination. However, if the patient still has a fever or other symptoms after 3 days

of therapy, a return visit to the ED or follow-up with the patient's own physician is advised.

ii. **Admission.** Very ill or dehydrated children with otitis may require admission to the hospital.

3. **Mastoiditis**

a. **Discussion.** Mastoiditis is an inflammatory process in the mastoid air cells.

i. **Acute mastoiditis** is a suppurative process that is usually preceded by an acute episode of otitis media.

ii. **Chronic mastoiditis** is usually associated with a cholesteatoma or chronic ear disease.

b. **Clinical features**

i. **Symptoms** include otalgia, fever, and pain behind the ear. Hearing may be impaired.

ii. **Physical examination findings**

a) Fever is almost always present.

b) The tympanic membrane is bulging and erythematous, except when perforation has occurred; with perforation, otorrhea is seen.

c) Postauricular erythema, edema, swelling, and tenderness may be seen.

d) Altered mental status or meningeal signs may be present.

c. **Differential diagnoses** include otitis externa, malignant otitis externa, otitis media, and a foreign body.

d. **Evaluation**

i. **Laboratory studies.** A complete blood count (CBC) shows elevation of the white blood cell count with a left shift in the differential.

ii. **Imaging studies.** CT scan may reveal thickening of the mastoid air cell epithelial membrane, air–fluid levels, and a subperiosteal abscess.

iii. **Other studies.** In a patient with altered mental status or signs of meningeal irritation and no evidence of an abscess on the CT scan, a lumbar puncture should be performed to rule out meningitis, which can result from progression of the mastoiditis. Immediate antibiotic therapy directed at an abscess or meningitis (ceftriaxone or cefotaxime in children and adults and high-dose penicillin in elderly patients) should be instituted without awaiting the results of testing.

e. **Therapy**

i. **Antibiotic therapy**

a) **Adults.** Appropriate regimens include intravenous **vancomycin** (15 to 20 mg/kg daily and follow levels) and **ceftriaxone** (2 g every 12 hours).

b) **Children.** Appropriate regimens include intravenous **vancomycin** (60 mg/kg/day divided every 6 hours) plus one of the following if history of recurrent otitis media:

1) **Ceftazidime** (150 mg/kg/day, divided every 8 hours)

2) **Cefepime** (150 mg/kg/day, divided every 8 hours)

3) **Piperacillin-tazobactam** (300 mg/kg/day divided every 8 hours)

ii. **Myringotomy** with **tube placement** is performed by an otolaryngologist.

a) Following the procedure, **daily cleaning** of the ear is necessary to ensure patency.

b) **Topical antibiotics** (e.g., polymyxin B otic suspension) are often instilled after cleaning.

iii. **Mastoidectomy** is reserved for patients who do not respond to treatment and patients with meningeal signs.

f. **Disposition.** Admission to the hospital and consultation with an otolaryngologist in the ED are indicated.

B. **Foreign body**

1. **Discussion.** Foreign bodies in the ear are a common presenting complaint in the ED. Children and mentally handicapped patients often present with objects

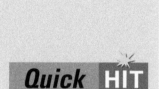

Quick HIT

An auricle that is protruded forward, causing the ear to "stick out" should be considered a warning sign for mastoiditis.

Eye, Ear, Nose, Throat, and Dental Emergencies

such as beads, erasers, and small toys lodged in the ear canal. Insects in the ear, usually cockroaches and often alive, are also seen in a number of cases.

2. **Clinical features**
   a. **Symptoms**
      i. If the foreign body has been present for a relatively long time, the presenting complaint may be discharge from the ear.
      ii. Live insects can cause pain, and patients are often anxious to have something done immediately.
   b. **Physical examination findings**
      i. Signs of otitis externa may be present if the foreign body has been in the ear for some time.
      ii. The object may be impacted in cerumen. A live or dead insect may be seen.
3. **Differential diagnoses** include otitis externa, malignant otitis externa, and otitis media with perforation.
4. **Evaluation** is by physical examination.
5. **Therapy**
   a. **Object removal.** Children need to be restrained or sedated to prevent struggling while attempting removal.
      i. **Irrigation.** Often, objects can be flushed out with warm water and an irrigating bulb or a syringe attached to an 18-gauge angiographic catheter.
      ii. **Alligator forceps** can be used to remove objects. Care should be used not to perforate the tympanic membrane. Beads often have a hole and can be rotated to allow easier grasping with the forceps.
      iii. A **whistle-tip suction catheter** can sometimes be used to remove beads or other round objects. Care should be taken to avoid indiscriminate suctioning, which can lead to perforation of the tympanic membrane.
   b. **Supportive care.** Reexamination after the object is removed may reveal abrasions, otitis externa, or both, in which case proper therapy should be instituted.
6. **Disposition.** In most cases, patients can be discharged with instructions to follow-up with a primary care physician in 3 to 5 days. If attempts in the ED to remove the object are unsuccessful, the object may need to be surgically removed, which requires admission.

C. **Tympanic membrane rupture.** Disarticulation of the ossicles and rupture of the round or oval windows may be seen in addition to tympanic membrane rupture.
1. **Etiology**
   a. **Increased pressure in the external ear canal,** such as can result from a slap to the ear, while scuba diving, or from an explosion, can lead to rupture of the tympanic membrane.
   b. **Penetrating injuries** can result from overambitious cleaning of the external ear canal with a cotton swab and from flying debris (e.g., explosions, welding sparks).
2. **Clinical features**
   a. **Symptoms** include otalgia, hearing loss, and bloody otorrhea.
   b. **Physical examination findings**
      i. The perforation may range from small and linear to stellate.
      ii. Inflammation of the underlying epithelium may occur as a result of infection. Infection is more likely to occur in association with diving and welding accidents.
      iii. Rinne-Weber (tuning fork) hearing tests reveal conductive hearing loss. Bone conduction is better than air conduction.
      iv. Evidence of vertigo or spontaneous nystagmus must be sought. These findings could represent a more serious injury to the inner ear.
3. **Evaluation** is by physical examination. In patients with evidence of vertigo, severe hearing loss, or facial nerve palsy, immediate consultation with an otolaryngologist is indicated.

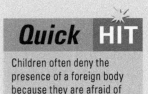

Quick HIT

Children often deny the presence of a foreign body because they are afraid of punishment.

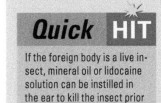

Quick HIT

If the foreign body is a live insect, mineral oil or lidocaine solution can be instilled in the ear to kill the insect prior to attempting removal.

Eye, Ear, Nose, Throat, and Dental Emergencies

4. **Therapy**
   a. **Simple, noncontaminated perforations.** The patient should be advised to keep water out of the affected ear until the perforation heals spontaneously.
   b. **Simple, contaminated perforations** are treated with **ofloxacin.** Patients should be advised to avoid getting water in the affected ear.
   c. **Complicated perforations.** Patients with marked destruction of the tympanic membrane and debris in the middle ear should be seen by an otolaryngologist for debridement.

5. **Disposition.** Most patients can be discharged with instructions to follow up with an otolaryngologist. If marked destruction of the tympanic membrane or vertigo is present, consultation with an otolaryngologist in the ED is appropriate.

III. NOSE

A. **Sinusitis**
   1. **Discussion**
      a. **Definition.** Sinusitis is an inflammation of the paranasal (ethmoid, frontal, maxillary, or sphenoid) sinuses. It is classified as acute or chronic, depending on how long the infection has been present.
      b. **Etiology and pathogenesis.** Sinusitis occurs when pus is trapped in the sinus and is unable to drain completely through the ostia into the nasal cavity.
         i. **Bacterial causes** include *H. influenzae, S. pneumoniae,* streptococci, and *M. catarrhalis.*
         ii. **Fungal causes** are most common in patients with diabetes. Mucormycosis is particularly life-threatening.
      c. **Predisposing factors** include chronic nasal edema, nasal polyps, nasal allergies, preceding upper respiratory tract infection, and upper tooth abscess.
   2. **Clinical features**
      a. **Symptoms**
         i. **Pain.** Nasal congestion increases the **pressure** in the sinus, leading to pain that often worsens when the patient bends over. Patients may complain of a **headache. Facial pain** often corresponds to the affected sinus:
            a) Cheeks and upper teeth—maxillary sinus
            b) Eyebrow area—frontal sinus
            c) Eyes or behind the eyes—ethmoid sinus
         ii. **Generalized malaise** and **periorbital edema** are common complaints.
         iii. **Nasal discharge** is often blood-tinged and purulent. A postnasal drip may cause **coughing** and a **sore throat.**
      b. **Physical examination findings**
         i. **Fever** is often present in acute sinusitis but is rare in chronic sinusitis.
         ii. **Tenderness to percussion** may be present over the affected sinus.
         iii. **Opacity of the affected sinus** may be evident on **transillumination.** A negative transillumination does not rule out sinusitis because the test is only positive when the sinusitis is advanced.
   3. **Differential diagnoses** include viral rhinitis, allergic rhinitis, vasomotor rhinitis, tumors, foreign bodies, and Wegener granulomatosis.
   4. **Evaluation**
      a. **Laboratory studies.** Typically not indicated. In acute sinusitis, a CBC may reveal an elevated white blood cell count.
      b. **Imaging studies**
         i. **Radiographs.** Plain sinus films may reveal air–fluid levels, cloudiness, or thickening of the sinus mucosa.
         ii. **CT scans** may identify an underlying predisposing anatomic condition (e.g., abnormally narrowed outlets, tumorous or cystic obstructions).
   5. **Therapy**
      a. **Supportive measures**
         i. An effort should be made to **avoid air-borne irritants** (e.g., smoke, pollen).

      ii. Although steam inhalation and environmental humidification are useful adjuncts, **aggressive systemic rehydration** is essential to mobilize and prevent reaccumulation of the thickened secretions.

      iii. **Analgesics, decongestants, antihistamines,** and **steroids** may also be helpful.

    b. **Antibiotic therapy.** Not indicated in most cases. If determined necessary, acceptable regimens include:

      i. **Amoxicillin clavulanate** (500 mg three times daily for 2 to 3 weeks)

      ii. **Doxycycline** (100 mg twice daily for 10 days)

    c. **Surgery.** Surgical drainage of the sinus may be indicated if medical treatment fails. Surgery may also be indicated to correct underlying anatomic defects.

6. **Disposition.** All patients diagnosed with sinusitis should be followed up until clinically cured.

    a. **Discharge.** In the absence of complications (e.g., orbital cellulitis, osteomyelitis, septic cavernous thrombosis, contiguous spread to involve the nervous system), patients can be sent home with instructions to follow up in 1 to 2 days.

    b. **Admission** is indicated for extremely ill patients, patients with orbital edema, and patients with nuchal rigidity or altered mental status.

B. **Foreign body**

1. **Discussion.** Nasal foreign bodies are seen most often in children.

2. **Clinical features**

    a. **Patient history.** Sometimes, a parent brings the child to the ED after witnessing the child or the child's sibling place an object (e.g., a bead, bean, sponge, toy) in the child's nose. However, more often the parent brings the child to the ED after noticing a foul-smelling, purulent discharge from the child's nose.

    b. **Symptoms.** The patient may be asymptomatic, or foul, purulent rhinorrhea or epistaxis may be present.

    c. **Physical examination findings.** Often, the foreign body can be identified using a nasal speculum and a headlamp. It may be necessary to suction the nares to clean away purulent secretions in order to visualize the foreign body.

3. **Differential diagnoses** include sinusitis and rhinitis.

4. **Evaluation.** Physical examination is usually adequate for diagnosis. Fiberoptic evaluation may be necessary if the object is in the posterior or turbinate areas.

5. **Therapy**

    a. **Object removal.** Pediatric patients need to be restrained in a papoose or rolled in a sheet to minimize movement during examination and removal. Some children may require sedation.

      i. **Forceful expulsion.** One method that often works is to have the parent seal off the opposite naris and blow into the child's mouth in a manner similar to that used during mouth-to-mouth resuscitation. The result is the expulsion of the object and a fair amount of mucus through the other naris.

      ii. A **suction catheter** with the tip cut off flat can be introduced into the nasal passage until the tip contacts the object, at which point suction is applied.

      iii. **Alligator forceps** can be used to grab the object. With beads, it is best to rotate the bead so that the hole can be grasped with the forceps.

    b. **Supportive care.** After removal of the object, saline drops can be instilled to moisten the nasal passage. If pus is present, a course of antibiotics should be prescribed to treat possible purulent rhinitis or sinusitis.

6. **Disposition.** If attempts at removing the object in the ED are successful, the patient can be sent home. If the object cannot be removed in the ED, an otolaryngologist should be consulted because the patient may need admission to the hospital for surgical removal of the object.

C. **Epistaxis**

1. **Discussion**

    a. **Etiology.** There are many causes of nosebleeds; most can be classified as belonging to one of the following three groups.

    i. **Local causes** include trauma (e.g., nose picking, foreign bodies, nasal fractures), inflammation, upper respiratory tract infection, and environmental irritants.

    ii. **Regional causes** include vascular abnormalities, neoplasms, and ectopic endometriosis.

    iii. **Systemic causes** include intrinsic and drug-induced coagulopathies, thrombocytopenia, leukemia, hepatic disease, and infections. Hypertension is not in itself a cause of epistaxis because the relative frequency in patients with hypertension is the same as in the general population.

  b. **Location.** It is important to differentiate anterior bleeds from posterior bleeds because anterior bleeds are generally easy to treat, whereas posterior bleeds are more difficult.

    i. **Anterior bleeds** usually occur in Kiesselbach plexus on the anterior nasal septum and account for 90% of all nose bleeds. They may also occur on the anterior inferior turbinate.

    ii. **Posterior bleeds** occur from the sphenopalatine artery or in the nasopharynx, often from branches of the carotid arteries.

2. **Clinical findings**

  a. **Anterior bleeds** are almost always unilateral, unless the nasal septum is perforated. Asking the patient to pinch his nose (thereby applying pressure to Kiesselbach plexus) will tamponade most anterior bleeds, whereas posterior bleeds will continue to bleed unabated.

  b. **Posterior bleeds.** Because posterior bleeds occur behind the septum, the blood will often exit both nares and large clots can accumulate in the nasopharynx.

3. **Evaluation.** Most patients with epistaxis do not require any laboratory testing. However, additional studies may be indicated in patients with a history of bleeding problems, oral anticoagulant use, possible hepatic disease, or bleeding that is difficult to control.

  a. A **CBC** to check hemoglobin and look for thrombocytopenia or leukemia

  b. A **prothrombin time** and **partial thromboplastin time** to look for overanticoagulation or hepatic dysfunction

  c. A **blood type and cross-match** in case transfusion is necessary to compensate for ongoing blood loss

4. **Therapy**

  a. **Initial stabilization.** In a patient who presents with hypotension and tachycardia, an intravenous line should be started, blood samples should be drawn, and fluid resuscitation should be initiated immediately. An adequate airway should be ensured in all patients.

  b. **Terminating bleeding**

    i. **Preliminary preparations.** Hospital staff should be gloved, gowned, and wearing protective eyewear. The following equipment should be readied:

      a) A bright light source

      b) Suction (turned on and connected)

      c) A nasal speculum, Bayonet forceps, 4″ × 4″ gauze pads, cotton swabs, cotton balls, a medication cup, silver nitrate sticks, Surgicel (Ethicon, Somerville, NJ) or a nasal tampon, petroleum jelly gauze strips, and two no. 10 Foley catheters

      d) Cocaine 4% solution or viscous solution, lidocaine 1% solution, and phenylephrine 1% solution

    ii. **Clearing the nasal passages.** The patient should be seated in a protective gown with a basin to collect blood. While waiting for treatment, the patient should pinch his or her nose to attempt to slow the bleeding. Once the necessary equipment is assembled, the patient should be asked to gently blow his or her nose and clear his or her throat to get as much blood and clot out of the nasal cavity as possible.

    iii. **Anesthesia.** Cocaine-soaked pledgets or cotton swabs are placed in the nares to anesthetize the mucous membranes and cause

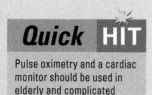

Quick HIT

Pulse oximetry and a cardiac monitor should be used in elderly and complicated epistaxis patients.

vasoconstriction. (These effects usually occur after 5 to 10 minutes.) Alternatively, a mixture of lidocaine and phenylephrine can be used.

    iv. **Inspection.** When adequate anesthesia has been obtained, a headlamp with a bright light source is used to insert the nasal speculum in the nares. The anterior septum should be inspected for the source of the bleeding (a clot may be seen if the bleeding has stopped). Suctioning may be necessary to visualize the source. The absence of an anterior bleed and continued epistaxis point to a more serious posterior bleed.

       a) If the bleeding has stopped, the patient should be observed for 15 to 30 minutes. No additional treatment is necessary.

       b) If the bleeding has not stopped, the evaluation must continue.

    v. **Tamponade and cautery.** When the source of the bleeding is found, an attempt to tamponade the bleeding with an applicator or phenylephrine should be made. If an anterior bleed cannot be stopped by applying pressure, cautery can be attempted with the silver nitrate stick.

    vi. **Anterior packing.** If both tamponade and cautery fail, it will probably be necessary to pack the anterior nose. Often both nares need to be packed to get adequate tamponade with nasal tampons, Vaseline (Unilever, Rotterdam, Netherlands) gauze, or Gelfoam (Pfizer, New York, NY).

    vii. **Posterior packing** is necessary for posterior bleeds.

       a) There are two common methods:

          1) Commercially available posterior packing balloons can be inserted in both nares and inflated as per the insert instructions.

          2) The alternative is posterior gauze packing (Figure 12-7).

       b) Failure to control the posterior bleeding may require operative management or angiography and embolization.

  5. Disposition

    a. Discharge

      i. **Bleeds controlled by pressure tamponade.** Patients should be observed for 15 to 30 minutes to ensure that rebleeding does not occur. The patient can be discharged with "nosebleed instructions" (i.e., no picking or blowing the nose, no sneezing through the nose, no bending forward or lifting). Patients should be advised to use a humidifier and to coat the nares with petroleum jelly the next day.

      ii. **Bleeds controlled by anterior packs.** Patients should be observed for 15 to 30 minutes to ensure tamponade. An antibiotic (e.g., amoxicillin) should be prescribed to prevent sinusitis and the patient should have an appointment with an otolaryngologist 2 to 3 days later to have the packing removed.

    b. Admission

      i. Patients with **multiple recent bleeds, severe anemia, debilitating illnesses, or hepatic dysfunction**, or those who are taking **anticoagulants and are supratherapeutic** probably need to be admitted for observation.

      ii. Patients with **posterior bleeds** require hospital admission, usually in a monitored setting (i.e., the intensive care unit or a step-down unit). These patients are at risk of rebleeding, airway obstruction, and profound hypoxemia. Prophylactic antibiotics should be administered to prevent sinusitis and toxic shock syndrome.

D. Nasal fractures

  1. Discussion. Nasal fractures are the most common fractures of the face and are often misdiagnosed. Nasal fractures are often associated with epistaxis and septal hematomas.

  2. Clinical features include pain in the nasal bridge with swelling, ecchymosis, and deformity. A septal hematoma should be ruled out by directly visualizing the septum.

  3. Differential diagnoses include more severe fractures involving the cribriform plate, ethmoidal bones, or lacrimal bones. More severe fractures may be associated with the leakage of cerebrospinal fluid into the nasal cavity.

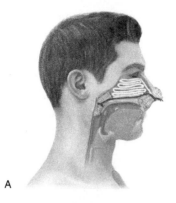

A

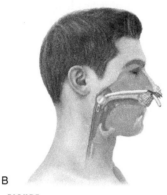

B

FIGURE
12-7 Management of posterior epistaxis. (A) Use of gauze packing in posterior nasopharynx with anterior anchoring to prevent migration of the gauze. Note vaseline gauze layering for tamponade of bleeding. (B) Use of Foley catheter packing in posterior nasopharynx with anterior anchoring to prevent migration of the bulb. An umbilical clip attached to the end of the catheter can alternately be used externally to prevent migration.

4. **Evaluation.** Usually, the clinical findings of pain, crepitance, and deformity are adequate for diagnosis. Radiographs can be used if uncertainty regarding the diagnosis remains.
5. Therapy
   a. Repair
      i. **Minimally displaced fractures** are usually treated pain control alone.
      ii. **More severely displaced fractures** are treated with immediate or delayed reduction.
         a) **Immediate reduction** is recommended if the patient is hemorrhaging or if there is marked deformity.
         b) **Delayed reduction.** Often, delayed reduction is preferable because it is performed after the swelling has subsided, facilitating evaluation of outcome.
   b. **Supportive care.** Epistaxis must be controlled, and septal hematomas require evacuation. A patient requiring packing should be given prophylactic antibodies to prevent sinusitis.
6. Disposition
   a. **Discharge.** Most patients with nasal fractures can be discharged with instructions to follow-up with an otolaryngologist.

   b. **Admission.** Indications for admission include:
      i. Failure to control hemorrhage
      ii. The presence of other injuries requiring hospitalization
      iii. The presence of a cerebrospinal fluid leak associated with deeper
           fractures in the nasal cavity, the cribriform plate, or the ethmoidal bones

IV. THROAT
A. **Pharyngitis** and **tonsillitis** are discussed in Chapter 6.V.A.
B. **Peritonsillar cellulitis** and **peritonsillar abscess**
   1. **Discussion**
      a. **Definitions.** When an acute bacterial tonsillitis is present, there is always
         the possibility of spread to surrounding tissue in the pharynx.
         i. **Peritonsillar cellulitis** is an infection that has spread to the surrounding
            area, causing inflammation and edema in the peritonsillar area.
         ii. **Peritonsillar abscess** is present when the infection progresses to form
             an abscess or collection of pus in the pharyngeal pillar.
      b. **Etiology.** The most common cause is β-hemolytic *Streptococcus*, but often
         the infection is polymicrobic, involving *Streptococcus pneumoniae*, *H. influ-
         enzae*, and *Staphylococcus*, as well as anaerobes such as *Bacteroides fragilis*.
      c. **Complications.** Local extension of the cellulitis or abscess can lead to more
         serious conditions:
         i. Extension of the abscess into contiguous neck spaces, including the
            retropharynx, subglossal spaces, and mediastinum
         ii. Erosion into the carotid artery, leading to life-threatening hemorrhage,
             or into the internal jugular vein, leading to septic thrombosis
   2. **Clinical features**
      a. **Symptoms**
         i. The **classic features of tonsillitis—fever, sore throat, and
            odynophagia**—are present for 2 to 3 days. The throat pain localizes to
            one side. The patient may drool because of an inability to swallow.
         ii. The patient may also complain of **dysphagia, dysphonia,** and **referred
             pain to the ear.**
      b. **Physical examination findings**
         i. **Trismus** (spasm of the muscles of mastication) may be present and the
            patient may have difficulty opening the mouth.
         ii. **Marked swelling of the pharyngeal pillar** displaces it downward. The
             uvula is pushed to the opposite side.
             a) In **peritonsillar cellulitis**, the pillar will be soft and not as enlarged
                as it is in patients with a peritonsillar abscess.
             b) In **peritonsillar abscess**, the pillar is larger and firm or fluctuant
                (Figure 12-8).
   3. **Differential diagnoses**
      a. Epiglottitis does occur in adults, and an absence of pharyngeal findings or
         the presence of stridor should warrant consideration of this diagnosis.
      b. If a noninfectious asymmetrical swelling is present, squamous cell carcinoma,
         lymphoma, a vascular lesion, or other neoplasms should be considered.

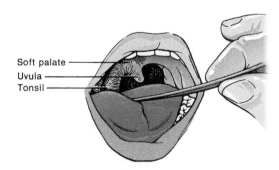

Soft palate
Uvula
Tonsil

FIGURE
12-8 Illustration of peritonsillar abscess.

    c. Mononucleosis and other viral infections, as well as diphtheria, must be ruled out.

4. **Evaluation**
    a. **Needle aspiration of the tonsillar pillar** allows differentiation between cellulitis and an abscess. Failure to aspirate pus in a soft pillar will indicate cellulitis, whereas the diagnosis is peritonsillar abscess if pus can be aspirated.
    b. **Laboratory studies** are of little value in the diagnosis. However:
       i. In a septic, dehydrated, or diabetic patient, additional workup, including a CBC, serum electrolyte panel, and a glucose level, may be appropriate.
       ii. If mononucleosis is suspected, a monospot test may be of value.
    c. **Imaging studies.** CT scan can delineate the size and location of cellulitis/abscess and the risk of impending airway compromise.

5. **Therapy**
    a. **Abscess drainage.** If an abscess is present, it needs to be drained.
       i. **Needle aspiration** without opening the abscess is advocated by some.
       ii. **Incision** and **drainage** by opening the abscess with a scalpel and gently opening the space with a forceps is the second option.
    b. **Antibiotic therapy**
       i. Patients who are able to swallow and are not dehydrated or toxic can be administered **oral antibiotics**. Acceptable regimens include:
         a) **Amoxicillin-clavulanate** (875 mg every 12 hours)
         b) **Clindamycin** (450 mg every 6 hours)
       ii. Dehydrated patients who are unable to swallow should receive **intravenous fluids** and **antibiotics**.
         a) **Ampicillin-sulbactam** (3 g every 6 hours)
         b) **Clindamycin** (600 mg every 6 hours)
    c. **Supportive therapy**
       i. **Saltwater gargles** often help soothe the throat and rinse the incised pillar. Mouthwashes should be avoided because they are irritating.
       ii. An **analgesic/antipyretic agent** should be prescribed.

6. **Disposition**
    a. **Discharge.** Patients who are discharged after initiating intramuscular or oral antibiotic therapy should be seen in 24 hours for reevaluation. These patients should be instructed to return to the ED if they experience trouble swallowing or breathing.
    b. **Admission** is required for any patient who is unable to swallow, dehydrated, toxic, or immunocompromised.
    c. **Referral.** Consultation with an ear, nose, and throat specialist should be arranged if the patient was not seen by a specialist in the ED.

C. **Ludwig angina**
1. **Discussion**
    a. **Definition.** The fascial planes within the head and neck are potential spaces for abscess formation. Ludwig angina is cellulitis with or without fluctuance of the submaxillary, sublingual, and submental spaces accompanied by elevation of the tongue.
    b. **Etiology.** The lower second and third molars are the usual source of infection. The usual causes are β-hemolytic streptococci, staphylococci, and mixed anaerobic and aerobic infection.
    c. **Pathogenesis.** Ludwig angina is a serious infection that can lead to airway compromise. There is also the potential for the infection to spread inferiorly and invade the mediastinum.

2. **Clinical features**
    a. **Symptoms.** The patient presents with swelling in the jaw, stiffness of tongue movements, and trismus, accompanied by fever, chills, and difficulty swallowing.
    b. **Physical examination findings**
       i. There is swelling beneath the chin, which is often tense and brawny without fluctuance.

      ii. The tongue is displaced up and posteriorly. Often, trismus makes opening the mouth for examination difficult.

     iii. If the presentation is late, airway obstruction and edema of the larynx may be present.

  3. Differential diagnoses

    a. Other causes of swelling in the area of the tongue include tumors of the tongue and salivary glands, and salivary duct obstructions.

    b. Other causes of neck swelling include mumps, salivary duct obstructions, tuberculous cervical lymphadenitis (scrofula), and Sjögren syndrome of the salivary glands.

  4. Evaluation should be carried out after airway patency is ensured. **CT scan** of the neck with intravenous contrast may be necessary to determine the extent of abscess formation and extension in to the next and mediastinum.

  5. Therapy

    a. **Initial stabilization.** Ensuring airway competence should be the first concern. Often oral intubation is not possible; therefore, cricothyrotomy or tracheostomy may be required.

    b. **Abscess drainage** is by incision and drainage. An otolaryngologist or oral maxillofacial surgeon should be consulted as soon as the diagnosis is made.

    c. **Intravenous antibiotic therapy** should be instituted as soon as possible.

      i. **Ampicillin-sulbactam** (3 g every 6 hours)

      ii. **Penicillin G** (2 million U every 4 hours) is one acceptable regimen; **metronidazole** (500 mg every 6 hours) may be added to provide anaerobic coverage against *B. fragilis.*

     iii. **Clindamycin** (600 to 900 mg every 8 hours) provides better anaerobic coverage than penicillin alone.

  6. Disposition. Patients are generally sent to the operating room for incision and drainage. If an abscess is not yet present, admission to a monitored setting is appropriate. The airway should be closely watched and intubation performed before trouble develops.

D. Parapharyngeal abscess

  1. Discussion

    a. **Definition.** Pharyngeal abscess is abscessation of the lateral pharyngeal space, which lies lateral to the pharynx and medial to the masticator space. It extends from the base of the skull to the hyoid bone. The space is lateral to the superior pharyngeal constrictor muscle and medial to the mandible and internal pterygoid muscle.

    b. **Pathogenesis.** Airway compromise can occur as well as spread to the mediastinum.

  2. Clinical features include the rapid onset of a high fever, chills, and swelling. The swelling in the neck can proceed rapidly, and swallowing may be difficult. Trismus is usually present, and there is marked pain as the space distends.

  3. Differential diagnoses include posterior pharyngeal abscess, masticator space abscess, Ludwig angina, and angioedema.

  4. Evaluation. Because the abscess can spread to the mediastinum, CT scans of the neck and chest are often needed prior to incision and drainage.

  5. Therapy

    a. **Initial stabilization.** Airway patency is the first concern, and oral intubation or cricothyrotomy may be necessary.

    b. **Incision and drainage** are usually performed in the operating room after making an external incision.

    c. **Antibiotic therapy** is the same as for Ludwig angina.

  6. Disposition. Patients are generally sent to surgery for incision and drainage.

E. Retropharyngeal abscess

  1. Discussion

    a. **Definition.** The retropharyngeal space is the fascial plane between the posterior pharyngeal muscles and the paraspinous muscles.

    b. **Etiology and pathogenesis**

  i. **Children.** Retropharyngeal abscess is mostly a pediatric problem because there are lymph nodes in the retropharyngeal space that can become suppurative.

  ii. **Adults.** The lymph nodes in the retropharyngeal space involute in adolescence. Infections in adults are usually secondary to trauma (e.g., foreign body perforations from chicken or fish bones, iatrogenic injuries from intubation or endoscopy).

2. **Clinical features.** The patient usually appears ill and presents with a fever, sore throat, and neck pain. The neck is often stiff, and motion at the neck is painful. The voice may be muffled and airway compromise is possible. If the abscess extends into the mediastinum, chest pain is a likely symptom.

3. **Differential diagnoses.** The lack of trismus helps differentiate retropharyngeal abscess from Ludwig angina and parapharyngeal abscess.

4. **Evaluation.** Imaging studies may be indicated after ensuring a patent airway.
   a. **Lateral soft tissue radiographs** of the neck will show swelling posterior to the airway.
   b. **CT scans** of the neck and chest are needed to identify the extent of the abscess.

5. **Therapy**
   a. **Initial stabilization.** An open airway must be ensured.
   b. **Incision and drainage** are carried out in the operating room.
   c. **Antibiotic therapy** is administered intravenously. Regimens include:
      i. Adults
         a) **Ampicillin-sulbactam** (3 g every 6 hours)
         b) **Ceftriaxone** (1 g every day) plus **metronidazole** (500 mg every 8 hours)
         c) **Vancomycin** (15 to 20 mg/kg, follow levels for dosing)
      ii. Children
         a) **Ampicillin-sulbactam** (50 mg/kg per dose every 6 hours)
         b) **Clindamycin** (13 mg/kg per dose every 8 hours)

6. **Disposition** is to the operating room for incision and drainage.

V. TEETH, MAXILLA, AND MANDIBLE

A. **Dental anatomy.** The tooth consists of a crown and root. The crown consists of the enamel, dentin, and pulp above the gingiva. The root has no enamel, and the dentin is fixed to the periodontal ligament by the cementum. The neurovascular bundle leaves the root at the apex. **Identification** of the teeth for charting purposes is illustrated in Figure 12-9.

B. **Dental caries (cavities)** result from bacterial erosion through the enamel into the dentin and pulp.
   1. **Clinical features**
      a. **Symptoms.** The chief complaint is usually a "toothache" or jaw pain. The pain is exacerbated by hot and cold liquids or food. The tooth is often sensitive to touch as well. Pain can be referred to the jaw or ear.
      b. **Physical examination** reveals pitting of the tooth surface. Percussion of the tooth or probing of the caries may elicit pain.
   2. **Differential diagnoses** include apical abscess, periodontal abscess, and fracture of the tooth. Myocardial infarction can present as tooth or jaw pain and should be considered in a patient who is short of breath or ill-appearing and in whom no caries can be readily identified.
   3. **Evaluation.** Physical examination is the sole means of evaluation.
   4. **Therapy.** In the ED, supportive care can be provided (e.g., analgesics, local anesthesia with a lidocaine or mepivacaine injection at the root of the tooth, and placement of dental wax in the cavity to reduce sensitivity).
   5. **Disposition.** Patients are discharged with instructions to see a dentist as soon as possible.

C. **Dental abscesses**
   1. **Discussion.** A tooth that has caries is susceptible to infection.
      a. **Apical abscesses** occur when the pulp is infected and the infection progresses along the root to form an abscess at the apex of the tooth.
      b. **Periodontal abscesses** result from infection of the gum or periodontium.

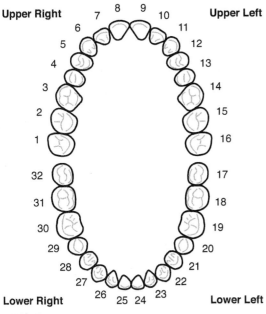

Upper Right   7   8   9   10   Upper Left

Lower Right   26   25   24   23   Lower Left

FIGURE 12-9   **Number designation of adult teeth.**
(Courtesy of Brenton Kathman.)

2. **Clinical features**
   a. **Symptoms.** The chief complaint is usually a "toothache" or pain in the gums.
   b. **Physical examination findings.** A fluctuant, tender gingival area at the base of the infected tooth is palpable.
3. **Differential diagnoses** include caries, gingivitis, and gingival foreign bodies.
4. **Evaluation** is by physical examination.
5. **Therapy**
   a. **Drainage of the abscess** is best performed by incision with a no. 15 scalpel blade.
   b. **Antibiotic therapy.** An antibiotic effective against anaerobes, such as penicillin VK (250 mg four times daily) or clindamycin (300 mg four times daily), should be administered.
6. **Disposition.** Patients can be discharged with instructions to follow-up with a dentist.

D. **Trauma**
   1. **Dental trauma**
      a. **Tooth fractures.** Dental trauma can lead to a tooth being chipped or broken. The Ellis classification scheme is used to classify dental fractures (Figure 12-10 and Clinical Pearl 12-3).
         i. **Evaluation** entails careful inspection. The tooth should be blotted (to improve visibility), but never probed, because probing can introduce bacteria to exposed pulp.
         ii. **Therapy**
            a) **Ellis class I fractures** are a minor problem and often do not require any treatment. If there is a bothersome sharp edge, it can be rounded with an emery board.
            b) **Ellis class II fractures** in older children and adults should be covered with calcium hydroxide and a dressing. In children, some class II fractures require emergent treatment by a dentist to reduce the risk of infection.
            c) **Ellis class III fractures** should be treated emergently by a dentist to reduce the risk of infection. Often, a root canal must be performed.

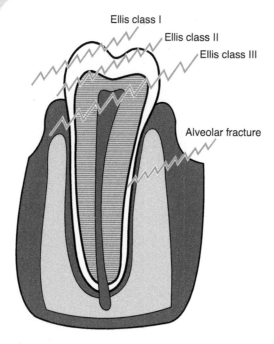

Ellis class I
Ellis class II
Ellis class III
Alveolar fracture

FIGURE
12-10 Ellis classification scheme for dental fractures. In Ellis class I fractures, the enamel is fractured. In Ellis class II fractures, the enamel and dentin are fractured. In Ellis class III fractures, the enamel, dentin, and pulp are fractured.
(Courtesy of Brenton Kathman.)

iii. **Disposition.** Generally, patients with Ellis class I or II fractures are referred to a dentist for follow-up the next day. Patients with class III fractures, children with class II fractures, and patients with suspected root fractures should be referred emergently to the dentist.

b. **Tooth subluxation or intrusion**
   i. **Discussion**
      a) **Subluxation** occurs when an injured tooth is loose or displaced in the socket.
      b) **Intrusion** occurs when a tooth is impacted in the socket.
   ii. **Clinical features.** The tooth may be loose, painful, and maloccluded. On physical examination, the tooth will be loose and it may be impacted into the gum. Often, there is blood in the gingival crevice.
   iii. **Differential diagnoses.** Subluxation must be differentiated from root fracture and avulsion.

CLINICAL PEARL **12-3**

1. **Ellis class I fractures.** Patients complain of a chip or a sharp edge, but no pain. Physical examination will reveal the chip.
2. **Ellis class II fractures.** Patients often complain of sensitivity to changes in temperature or to air. On physical examination, a yellow spot (i.e., the dentin) in the center of the fracture is visible.
3. **Ellis class III fractures** can be painful because the nerve is exposed. On physical examination, the fracture has a pink center (representing bleeding from the disturbed blood vessels and nerves in the pulp). Class III fractures that occur at the root are often missed because the tooth may seem to be intact. Therefore, any tooth that is loose or painful after trauma should be evaluated by a dentist.

    iv. **Evaluation** often requires dental radiographs, which are not available in most EDs.

    v. **Therapy**

       a) **Reduction** is often painful, and anesthesia (provided by a lidocaine injection at the root) may facilitate the process. Once reduced, the tooth can be immobilized with dental wax.

       b) **Analgesia** should be provided.

    vi. **Disposition.** Patients should be referred to a dentist for definitive treatment as soon as possible.

  c. **Tooth avulsion** occurs when a tooth is knocked out of its socket.

    i. **Differential diagnoses.** Avulsion must be differentiated from an alveolar fracture.

    ii. **Therapy.** An avulsed tooth is a true emergency and must be reimplanted as soon as possible. Each minute that the tooth remains out of its socket reduces the likelihood of the tooth surviving by approximately 1%. It is important to determine whether the tooth is a primary (baby) tooth or a secondary tooth. Primary teeth are not reimplanted because they often ankylose or fuse to the bone, causing permanent deformity.

2. **Maxillary fractures**

  a. **Discussion**

    i. **Etiology.** Most maxillary fractures are the result of motor vehicle collisions.

    ii. **Types** include:

       a) **Simple alveolar fractures**, which run through the alveolar portion of the maxilla, where the teeth are implanted

       b) **Antrum fractures**, which are fractures of the maxilla at the base of the nose

       c) **Le Fort fractures** (Figure 12-11)

  b. **Clinical features.** Le Fort fractures are usually a combination of the three types (e.g., one type may be seen on one side of the face and another type may be seen on the other; see Clinical Pearl 12-4).

  c. **Differential diagnoses** include orbital blow-out fractures, orbital tripod fractures, fracture of the antrum of the maxillary sinus, and Le Fort type I and type II fractures.

  d. **Evaluation.** A CT scan is the standard of care and yields the most information because the three-dimensional image allows clear visualization of the fracture.

  e. **Therapy**

    i. **Airway control** is the most important priority and should be accomplished early, before airway obstruction is present. It is much easier to intubate a patient when the airway is moderately swollen; when the airway is obstructed, cricothyrotomy often becomes necessary.

    ii. **Control of epistaxis** is often difficult. If packing is unsuccessful, emergent reduction of the fracture may be needed to control the bleeding.

    iii. **Fracture reduction** and **internal fixation** are accomplished by a facial specialist.

    iv. **Antibiotic therapy** is needed to minimize the risk of central nervous system infection.

  f. **Disposition**

    i. **Alveolar fractures** should be stabilized using dental wax or arch wires. Urgent follow-up with an oral surgeon is necessary.

    ii. **Antrum fractures** can be repaired on an outpatient basis if no other injuries are present.

    iii. **Le Fort fractures.** Patients require admission for open reduction and internal fixation. Often, these patients have other injuries and require a complete trauma evaluation anyway.

3. **Mandibular fractures**

  a. **Discussion.** Mandibular fractures (Figure 12-12) are relatively common and are usually the result of a direct blow.

Eye, Ear, Nose, Throat, and Dental Emergencies

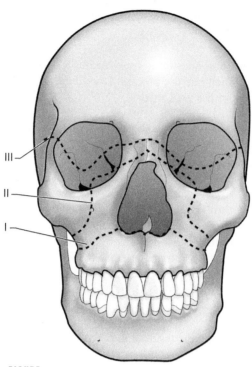

FIGURE
12-11 Le Fort fractures of the midface. In Le Fort fracture type I, the maxilla is separated from the upper face by a horizontal fracture though each nostril above the hard palate. In Le Fort fracture type II, the fracture is oblique and runs from the nasomaxillary area through the orbit, separating the zygoma and orbits from the nose. In Le Fort fracture type III (craniofacial dysjunction), the facial bones are separated from the cranium. The fracture runs through the maxillary sinus, orbits, and zygoma.

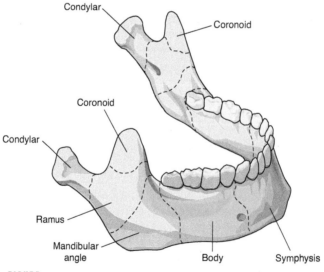

FIGURE
12-12 The most common locations of mandibular fractures are the body, the angle, the condyle, and the symphysis. In more than 50% of patients, the mandible is broken in two places.

CLINICAL PEARL 12-4

Types of Le Fort Fractures

1. Le Forts type I fractures

　a. **Symptoms** include malocclusion (manifested as an inability to bite) and facial tingling (as a result of infraorbital nerve involvement).

　b. **Physical examination findings** include a bilateral epistaxis, a long-appearing face, a mobile hard palate, and crepitance. Airway obstruction may occur secondary to swelling in the area of the soft palate.

2. Le Fort type II fractures

　a. **Symptoms** include malocclusion, facial tingling, and often diplopia.

　b. **Physical examination findings**

　　i. Bilateral epistaxis, periorbital ecchymosis, and a long-appearing face are noted.

　　ii. The central region of the face will be mobile between the bridge of the nose and teeth, and crepitance is present.

　　iii. A step-off defect at the inferior orbital rim, a medial canthal deformity, enophthalmos, and restricted extraocular motion (resulting from entrapment of the inferior oblique muscle) may be noted.

　　iv. Airway obstruction can occur as a result of swelling in the nasopharynx.

3. Le Fort type III fractures

　a. **Symptoms** include malocclusion, tingling in the face, diplopia, and facial pain.

　b. **Physical examination findings**

　　i. Bilateral epistaxis and cerebrospinal fluid rhinorrhea are noted.

　　ii. The face is unstable, moving laterally through the orbits with stress.

　　iii. Marked facial swelling, ecchymosis, a medial canthal deformity, a lateral orbital rim defect, and enophthalmos may be noted.

　　iv. Significant retropharyngeal swelling can lead to airway obstruction.

　　b. Clinical features

　　　i. **Symptoms** include pain, the inability to open the mouth, malocclusion, and tingling of the lip if the inferior alveolar nerve is affected.

　　　ii. **Physical examination findings**

　　　　a) Trismus, deviation of the jaw, an inability to bite down, and malalignment of the teeth are usually noted. Lip and chin sensation may be impaired.

　　　　b) In patients with a condylar fracture, blood may be noted in the external auditory canal.

　　　　c) The teeth should be inspected. Bleeding at the base of a tooth signifies an open fracture through the socket.

　　c. **Differential diagnoses** include an alveolar fracture, dislocation of the jaw, and trismus from a zygoma fracture.

　　d. **Evaluation. CT scan** is again the standard method and provides more anatomic information in terms of displacement and angulation.

　　e. **Therapy**

　　　i. **Fractures that displace the mandible forward** are more amenable to treatment because the muscles help to stabilize the fracture. These fractures can be stabilized with arch wire supports to the teeth. The patient should be placed on a diet of soft foods.

　　　ii. **Fractures that displace the mandible backward** are more difficult to treat because the masseter, medial pterygoid, and temporalis muscles displace the fracture. These fractures often require open reduction and internal fixation.

　　　iii. **Open fractures.** Prophylactic antibiotics must be prescribed to prevent infection of the bone.

　　f. **Disposition**

　　　i. **Discharge.** Patients with closed fractures amenable to treatment can be discharged with instructions to follow-up with an ear, nose, and throat specialist.

　　　ii. **Admission.** Patients with open fractures that are amenable to treatment require admission for prophylactic antibiotics and open irrigation of the wound. Patients with complicated fractures also require admission for open reduction and internal fixation.

Eye, Ear, Nose, Throat, and Dental Emergencies

13 PSYCHIATRIC EMERGENCIES

Joseph Bales • Jessica Dennison

I. ORGANIC BRAIN DISORDERS AND PSYCHOSIS

A. **Discussion and clinical features**

1. **Organic brain disorders.** Characterized by impaired orientation and cognitive brain function

   a. **Dementia.** Typically older patients with progressive memory loss plus a decline in executive function, aphasia (speech), agnosia (use of objects), or apraxia (organization). May be agitated due to inability to understand their surroundings and often have an overlying component of psychosis or delirium

   b. **Delirium.** Characterized by the rapid onset (hours to days) of impaired orientation and cognition. These patients may have a readily treatable and reversible condition (e.g., hypoglycemia).

2. **Psychosis.** Typically characterized by abnormal thought patterns, often with intact cognition. These patients often have the ability to perform calculations, memorize items, or converse, but they have bizarre ideas and thoughts. For a diagnosis of psychosis, one should have hallucinations, delusions, catatonia, thought disorder, or social impairments. Psychosis is usually secondary to one of the mental disorders listed below but may be a result of drug intoxication or abuse (e.g., methamphetamine abuse, alcohol abuse or withdrawal, prescription drugs). Psychosis typically presents for the first time in a patient's teens to mid-30s; patients presenting with psychosis at older ages should be highly suspicious for organic causes.

   a. **Schizophrenia.** Characterized by delusions and hallucinations and is the most common cause of psychosis. These patients may present to the emergency department (ED) in a flattened mood and withdrawn state (catatonia), or they may be violent, paranoid, and suspicious of health care workers. Antipsychotic medications are the mainstay of treatment, both emergently and on a chronic basis.

   b. **Mania.** Associated with bipolar disorder, wherein patients have cyclical mood swings that vary from depression to mania. Mania is characterized by elevated mood and energy. Acutely manic patients will exhibit pressured speech, agitation, grandiose delusions, and insomnia. Sedating neuroleptics are often needed in the emergent setting to control the patient.

   c. **Depression.** Patients may present with psychotic features, although this is rare. Delusions are the most common psychotic feature seen in depressed patients; these patients are not usually violent or agitated.

B. **Evaluation.** EDs should have a defined plan for dealing with violent or abusive patients. If the patient is threatening, evaluation and treatment should always take place with several people in the room.

1. **History and physical examination.** An attempt should be made to obtain as much information about the patient's condition as possible from relatives, friends, paramedics, and other health care workers. If possible, perform the history or physical examination before restraining or sedating the patient.

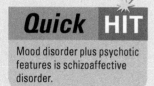

Quick HIT

You must rule out delirium before making a diagnosis of dementia.

Quick HIT

Most common causes of delirium: *d*ementia; *e*lectrolyte imbalances; *l*ung/liver/heart/kidney/brain; *i*nfection; *R*x drugs; *i*njury/stress/pain; *u*nfamiliar surroundings; *m*etabolic.

Quick HIT

Mood disorder plus psychotic features is schizoaffective disorder.

Psychiatric Emergencies

306

2. **Laboratory studies** and other studies (e.g., radiography) should be guided by the history and physical examination findings. Patients with known psychiatric disorders or dementia may require minimal workup. Standard tests for these patients often include an ethanol level, drug screen, and basic blood work.

C. **Therapy**

1. **Restraint and sedation.** The first priority in dealing with patients with organic brain disorders or psychosis is ensuring the safety of both health care workers and the patient. This can be accomplished in several ways.

   a. **Environmental seclusion.** Placement of the patient in a quiet, darkened room will often prevent escalation of agitation in patients who are mildly agitated.

   b. **Physical restraint.** Violent and severely agitated patients may require physical restraints. At least five or six ED personnel must be present to restrain each of the patient's limbs and his or her trunk in unison. Physical restraints are only justified if the patient is an imminent threat to himself or herself or others.

   c. **Chemical restraint.** Sedation may be required if the patient remains agitated. Quick and safe sedatives to use include droperidol, ziprasidone, haloperidol, or lorazepam.

      i. Patients on phencyclidine or methamphetamines may require substantial doses (e.g., 10 mg droperidol, 6 to 10 mg haloperidol, 10 to 15 mg lorazepam) before control is achieved.

      ii. Because some antipsychotics may lower the seizure threshold, the use of benzodiazepines may be more appropriate in certain circumstances (e.g., cocaine intoxication).

      iii. Patients with acute uncontrolled psychosis often require the rapid administration of antipsychotics to gain control.

2. **Glucose, oxygen, thiamine, naloxone, and flumazenil** should be considered for the altered patient. These agents may rapidly correct causes of coma, delirium, or psychosis. Note: Flumazenil should only be considered for the benzodiazepine-naive patient who has overdosed.

D. **Disposition**

1. Acutely psychotic patients usually need inpatient psychiatric care. An involuntary psychiatric hold may need to be invoked.

2. Patients with delirium should be admitted to the hospital unless a readily reversible or minor cause is found in the ED.

3. Many patients with drug or alcohol intoxication can be observed in the ED until they are appropriate for discharge.

4. Suicidal or homicidal thoughts should be ruled out prior to discharge.

II. ANOREXIA NERVOSA AND BULIMIA NERVOSA

A. **Discussion.** Approximately 80% to 85% of patients are women younger than 25 years of age. Others are men or older women.

1. **Anorexia nervosa.** Syndrome of self-starvation

2. **Bulimia nervosa.** Characterized by frequent episodes of binge eating. The patient usually consumes large amounts of food during a defined period of time (e.g., less than 2 hours) and then uses compensatory measures (e.g., laxatives, diuretics, induced vomiting) to prevent weight gain.

B. **Clinical features**

1. **Anorexia nervosa.** The patient usually weighs less than 85% of the expected weight (e.g., body mass index <19).

   a. The patient may present with life-threatening malnutrition, hypotension, or bradycardia.

   b. Endocrine abnormalities are present, usually amenorrhea.

2. **Bulimia nervosa.** These patients are often of normal weight or are overweight.

   a. Serious complications of repeated vomiting (e.g., esophageal rupture, Mallory-Weiss tears, dental decay) may be the presenting complaint.

   b. Electrolyte imbalances (e.g., hypokalemia) are fairly common secondary to repeated vomiting or laxative or diuretic abuse.

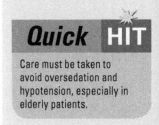

Quick HIT

Care must be taken to avoid oversedation and hypotension, especially in elderly patients.

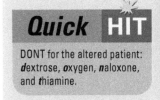

Quick HIT

DONT for the altered patient: *d*extrose, *o*xygen, *n*aloxone, and *t*hiamine.

C. **Differential diagnoses**
1. Medical causes of excessive weight loss (e.g., diabetes, Crohn disease, cancer, thyroid disorders, lupus) must be excluded.
2. Anxiety, schizophrenia, body dysmorphic disorder, and depression can all lead to significant weight changes. Criteria for depressive disorder are found in nearly 50% patients.
D. **Evaluation**
1. **History and physical examination** form the basis for the diagnosis of these disorders
    a. There is often a family history of eating disorders or job pressures to be thin (e.g., professional dancers, gymnasts).
    b. The patient is often evasive about purging or the use of laxatives or diuretics. Friends or family members are more likely to mention these behaviors.
2. **Laboratory studies.** Appropriate studies include a serum electrolyte panel and glucose level as well as renal and thyroid function tests.
3. **Electrocardiography.** An electrocardiogram is warranted especially in a symptomatic patient.
E. **Therapy.** Intensive psychiatric therapy and frequent monitoring of weight are the cornerstones of treatment for patients with these disorders. Antidepressants have been shown to be effective in certain patient populations.
F. **Disposition**
1. **Discharge.** Most patients will require outpatient treatment.
2. **Admission** to the hospital is indicated for any patient with substantial electrolyte imbalances or signs of cardiac abnormalities.

III. ANXIETY DISORDERS AND PANIC ATTACKS

A. **Discussion.** Anxiety disorder is characterized as feelings of uneasiness, danger, tension, stress, irritability, or fatigue. Panic disorder is a form of anxiety that is characterized by recurrent panic attacks (i.e., sudden episodes of intense fear or impending doom associated with a variety of somatic symptoms).
1. Panic attacks are often unpredictable, although they may occur commonly in certain situations.
2. First-time panic attacks are rarely seen in patients older than 35 years; organic disorders should be considered in these cases.
B. **Clinical features.** Symptoms associated with both generalized anxiety and panic attacks may mimic life-threatening conditions (see Table 13-1) but include palpitations or pounding heart, diaphoresis, sensation of shortness of breath or

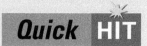

Quick HIT

Electrolyte abnormalities, prolonged QTc, and bradycardia are some potentially life-threatening complications of eating disorders.

Quick HIT

Almost half of patients with anxiety eventually find some organic reason for their anxiety.

TABLE 13-1 Differential Diagnoses for Panic Disorder
Acute myocardial infarction
Cardiac arrhythmias
Pulmonary emboli
Hyperthyroidism and thyroid storm
Pheochromocytoma
Mitral valve prolapse
Alcohol withdrawal
Use of central nervous system stimulants
Hypoglycemia
Asthma exacerbation
Stroke or serious intracranial abnormalities

choking, chest pain or discomfort, nausea, dizziness, light-headedness, numbness, tingling, or chills.

C. **Differential diagnoses.** Many serious medical conditions can mimic the symptoms of panic disorder and need to be considered (Table 13-1), especially in patients older than 45 years.

D. **Evaluation**

1. **Patient history.** A careful history of recurrent, short-lived episodes of panic will usually lead to the correct diagnosis of panic attacks. Anxiety may be harder to determine but is often a diagnosis of exclusion in the ED.

2. **Laboratory studies** should be guided by the patient history and physical exam as well as age and presentation and may include a serum electrolyte panel and glucose level, and a drug screen. Older patients or those with atypical symptoms should have a thorough workup to detect conditions with a medical basis.

3. **Electrocardiography and radiology.** An electrocardiogram or chest radiograph may be warranted.

E. **Therapy.** Generally, both medications and behavioral therapy are used for patients with anxiety and panic disorders. Usually, medical therapy for panic attacks should be started by the patient's primary care physician or a psychiatrist, not in the ED. However, commonly used medications include the following:

1. **Selective serotonin reuptake inhibitors** are first-line therapy for long-term control of anxiety and panic attacks.

2. **Benzodiazepines** are both useful for panic attacks and usually produce a response within several hours to days of beginning the medication but should be used sparingly due to abuse and withdrawal potential.

F. **Disposition.** Most will be discharged, although patients with risk factors for significant disease should be admitted to the hospital to rule out a life-threatening condition.

IV. CONVERSION REACTIONS

A. **Discussion.** A conversion reaction is the transformation of a stressor into a physical symptom. To diagnose a conversion reaction, the following five elements must be present (see Clinical Pearl 13-1):

1. Physical dysfunction or symptom that suggests a neurologic or medical condition
2. The onset of the symptom is preceded by a stressful situation or conflict.
3. The patient does not knowingly produce the symptom.
4. The symptom cannot be explained by a known medical condition
5. The symptom is not limited to sexual dysfunction or pain and is not explained by another psychiatric disorder.

B. **Clinical features.** The symptom associated with a conversion reaction is usually a neurologic complaint, but other systems may be affected. Typical symptoms include blindness, paralysis, sensory loss, seizures, vomiting, or diarrhea.

C. **Differential diagnoses.** In some studies, up to 25% of patients diagnosed with conversion reactions eventually are found to have a medical cause of their

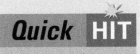

Quick HIT

Atypical presentation or older patients without a history of panic attacks warrant a workup to rule out life-threatening medical conditions.

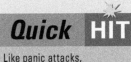

Quick HIT

Like panic attacks, conversion reactions may present with potentially life-threatening symptoms; a thorough history and physical is necessary.

Psychiatric Emergencies

CLINICAL PEARL 13-1

Compare All Four

1. **Conversion disorder** typically causes true physical dysfunction or symptoms. Patients desire medical care, but in contrast to Munchausen syndrome, symptoms are not under voluntary control.

2. Patients with **factitious disorder (Munchausen syndrome)** strongly seek medical care or hospital admission with self-induced or no medically warranted reason in order to assume the sick role.

3. **Munchausen syndrome by proxy** is a medical condition induced often in children or disabled by someone else (often a parent or caregiver) with the goal to vicariously assume the sick role; this has a mortality rate of 9% to 31%.

4. **Malingering** patients seek medical care for secondary gain (e.g., to get out of work).

TABLE 13-2	Differential Diagnoses for Conversion Reaction
Multiple sclerosis	
Myasthenia gravis	
Guillain-Barré syndrome	
Brain tumor	
Dystonia	
AIDS	
Stroke or serious intracranial abnormality	
Myopathy	
Seizure disorder	

symptoms. Therefore, it is important to consider organic causes for the patient's symptoms (Table 13-2).

D. **Evaluation.** The evaluation of a possible conversion reaction necessitates a complete neurologic or symptom-related examination.
1. A patient with conversion reaction will often have an inconsistent examination over brief periods of time.
2. A patient with conversion reaction will often fail tests designed to evaluate the symptom. For example, a patient who complains of blindness may avoid a visual threat.

E. **Therapy.** After thorough workup and life-threatening conditions have been excluded, ED therapy entails reassurance that there is no disease process present and the assurance that the symptom will resolve with time. The patient should not be confronted with the suspicion that his or her symptoms are completely psychogenic. Long-term counseling may be required.

F. **Disposition.** With a supportive, nonconfrontational approach, 90% to 95% of patients will experience relief of their symptoms in a short period of time. Patients should be discharged to a supportive environment and psychiatric referral.

V. DEPRESSION AND SUICIDE

A. **Discussion.** Depression and suicide attempts or ideation are often seen together.
1. **Depression** is the most common psychiatric disorder, occurring in approximately 2% to 3% of the population at a given time.
2. **Suicide** is the second leading cause of death among adolescents and young adults.

B. **Clinical features**
1. **Psychiatric symptoms of depression.** Depressed patients usually express feelings of guilt, worthlessness, and hopelessness and report that they have thoughts of death or suicide.
2. **Physiologic symptoms that may accompany depression** include:
   a. A change in appetite or weight
   b. Insomnia or excessive sleep
   c. Fatigue
   d. Difficulty concentrating

C. **Differential diagnoses**
1. Medical causes of depression include pain, cancer, medical disorders such as hypothyroidism, drug and alcohol abuse, and certain medications.
2. **Situational/loss depression.** Depression may also be situational (e.g., death of a spouse or parent, loss of a job).

D. **Evaluation**
1. **Patient history.** The patient's past medical and psychiatric problems and medication history should be carefully reviewed.

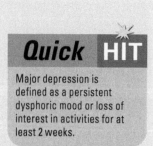

Quick HIT

Major depression is defined as a persistent dysphoric mood or loss of interest in activities for at least 2 weeks.

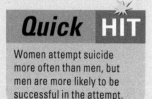

Quick HIT

Women attempt suicide more often than men, but men are more likely to be successful in the attempt.

The SAD PERSONS suicide risk scale has high sensitivity and specificity. **S**ex, **a**ge, **d**epression (2); **p**revious attempts or hospitalizations, **e**xcessive alcohol or drug use, **r**ational thinking loss (2); **s**ingle (separated, divorced or widowed), **o**rganized or serious attempted (2); **n**o social support, **s**tated future intent (2)

2. **Risk assessment.** In patients who are brought to the ED because of an attempted suicide, the physician should assess the patient's risk of successfully carrying out a suicide attempt in the future (see Clinical Pearl 13-2).
   a. **High risk.** Patients who have made an organized or serious suicide attempt (e.g., hanging, gunshot) are classified as high risk. Patients at high risk for successfully carrying out plans of suicide generally make the attempt in an isolated area and do not seek help.
   b. **Low risk.** Patients who have attempted to overdose with over-the-counter medications or present with superficial cuts are classified as low risk. These patients often want to be rescued; they tend to make immediate calls to friends or relatives, and their attempt is usually in a highly visible location.

E. **Treatment.** Therapy with antidepressant medications is best initiated by the patient's primary care physician or psychiatrist, not by the ED physician.

F **Disposition**
   1. **Admission.** Patients who have attempted suicide and meet any of the following criteria should be admitted to an inpatient psychiatric facility:
      a. High SAD PERSONS score
      b. Moderate risk with poor social support system
      c. Actively suicidal
   2. **Discharge.** Patients who present to the ED as the result of a low-risk suicide attempt and who have good social support can usually be treated as outpatients with early follow-up. To be treated as an outpatient, the patient should no longer exhibit any active suicidal ideation.

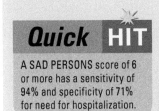

Quick HIT

A SAD PERSONS score of 6 or more has a sensitivity of 94% and specificity of 71% for need for hospitalization.

Psychiatric Emergencies

Obstetric and Gynecologic Emergencies

I. PELVIC PAIN

A. **Discussion.** There are many reasons for the female patient to have pelvic pain. In general, there are two types of pelvic pain.

1. **Visceral pain** results from stimulation of the nerves innervating the splanchnic organs. Pain is vague, dull, and poorly localized.

2. **Somatic pain** results from stimulation of the peripheral somatic nerves. The pain is dermatomal or localized. Pain is sharp and usually involves the skin, muscle, or parietal peritoneum.

B. **Clinical features.** There are four patterns of pelvic pain that can be helpful to know when trying to isolate the cause of the pain.

1. **Mild visceral pain** results from visceral inflammation due to infection or distention. Causes include the following:

   a. **Pelvic inflammatory disease (PID)** is characterized by vague lower abdominal pain and diffuse cervical, uterine, and adnexal tenderness.

   b. **Early appendicitis** is characterized by diffuse abdominal pain, primarily epigastric or periumbilical, with right lower quadrant tenderness on direct palpation. Symptoms include fever, nausea, and anorexia, usually evolving over 24 to 48 hours.

   c. **Vaginitis** or **cervicitis** can cause diffuse, lower abdominal pain focused around the suprapubic region. Tenderness is appreciated on vaginal and cervical examination with no adnexal findings. Other symptoms include vaginal discharge, dyspareunia, and dysuria.

   d. **Urinary tract infection** is characterized by suprapubic fullness and crampy pain, possibly referred to the flank. Patients may describe dysuria or hematuria associated with painful, burning urethral irritation.

   e. **Ovarian cyst** symptoms usually occur around midcycle or during the postovulatory phase. Fluid engorgement and distention cause dull, constant, achy pain in the lower abdominal adnexal region. Adnexal tenderness may be noted around the affected ovary.

   f. **Early ectopic pregnancy.** The growing trophoblast causes distention at the implantation site, vague lower abdominal pain, and/or adnexal tenderness. Other findings include vaginal bleeding and a positive pregnancy test.

   g. **Menstrual cramps** are vague, cramping, sometimes sharp pains, lasting several days before to several days after cycle begins. This is a diagnosis of exclusion.

   h. **Uterine fibroids** are associated with pubic pressure, pain, and dysmenorrhea or menorrhagia. Uterine tenderness may be noted, and fibroids may be palpable.

   i. **Endometriosis.** Growth of ectopic endometrial tissue may cause a dull, constant ache that worsens late in the menstrual cycle due to hormone shifts and tissue breakdown. Pain may intensify during menstruation as the lesions "slough," causing local inflammation. Exam may note adnexal or cul-de-sac tenderness without cervical motion tenderness. Endometriosis is a diagnosis of exclusion in the emergency department (ED), typically only diagnosed after laparoscopic surgery.

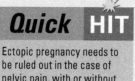

Quick HIT

Ectopic pregnancy needs to be ruled out in the case of pelvic pain, with or without vaginal bleeding, in the setting of a positive pregnancy test.

j. **Dysmenorrhea** is cyclic, painful menstruation thought to be mediated by prostaglandins. The patient may describe a dull, progressive pelvic ache that radiates to her back or thighs.

2. **Severe visceral pain** is an intense, restless pain often associated with nausea and vomiting. Underlying causes include severe infection, inflammation, obstruction, and visceral ischemia.

a. **Ovarian torsion** is characterized by sudden, severe pain that is out of proportion to the concomitant adnexal tenderness. Symptoms usually occur around midcycle and can also occur in pregnant patients. The patient may have a history of ovarian cysts.

b. **Nephrolithiasis** is characterized by colicky, intermittent, restless pain that usually begins in the flank but may progress or radiate to the lower quadrant, suprapubic, and groin regions. Associated nausea, vomiting, and hematuria are possible. Examination may reveal flank and/or lower quadrant tenderness without peritoneal signs.

c. **Bowel obstruction** is associated with diffuse, crampy pain, bloating, nausea, and vomiting. Examination may reveal a distended abdomen, decreased or high-pitched bowel sounds, and diffuse tenderness without peritoneal signs. Inability to pass stool or flatus should alert the physician to this diagnosis. Previous abdominal surgery, hernia, or cancer are risk factors.

3. **Visceral pain progressing to somatic pain.** Organ inflammation causes the adjacent peritoneum to become progressively irritated. The inflamed parietal peritoneum may produce localized, somatic pain sensation.

a. **Appendicitis.** Progression of appendiceal inflammation or rupture may induce parietal peritoneal inflammation. The patient describes diffuse, crampy pain that becomes progressively more localized to the right lower quadrant. Tenderness in that region becomes more sharp, intense, and focal. The incidence of appendicitis is unchanged during pregnancy, but the location of pain and tenderness may vary due to uterine displacement.

b. **Complicated PID.** Extension of salpingeal infection to involve the parietal peritoneum can produce local peritonitis. Gonococcal or chlamydial seeding of Glisson capsule (in the liver) may produce severe, right upper quadrant pain and tenderness, and right pleuritic chest pain due to diaphragmatic irritation (Fitz-Hugh–Curtis syndrome).

c. **Advanced ectopic pregnancy.** As trophoblastic tissue erodes the implantation site, hemorrhage can occur, causing local peritoneal pain, progressive adnexal and cul-de-sac tenderness, abdominal distention, diffuse peritonitis, and even shock.

4. **Sudden somatic pain.** Parietal peritoneal inflammation from blood, cystic fluid, pus, urine, or feces can induce severe local abdominal pain that can progress to diffuse peritonitis.

a. **Ruptured ectopic pregnancy.** Small amounts of hemorrhage may produce sudden, severe, localized abdominal pain and tenderness. As bleeding continues, the peritoneum becomes diffusely involved, causing significant peritoneal findings on examination.

b. **Ruptured ovarian cyst.** Cyst rupture spills fluid or blood onto the adjacent parietal peritoneum, producing sudden, significant unilateral adnexal pain and tenderness that may become diffuse.

    i. **Follicular cysts** rupture midcycle; rupture is associated with ovulatory pain (**mittelschmerz**).

    ii. **Luteal cysts** rupture late in the menstrual cycle and may be associated with significant hemorrhage and shock.

C. **Evaluation**

1. **Stabilization.** Airway, respiratory, and cardiovascular status should be assessed, and shock should be treated immediately before making a diagnosis.

2. **Patient history.** It is imperative to obtain a menstrual history in all women of childbearing age.

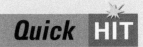

Quick HIT

Primary dysmenorrhea is idiopathic, whereas secondary dysmenorrhea may be related to endometriosis, uterine fibroids, pelvic adhesions, or ovarian cysts.

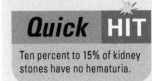

Quick HIT

Ten percent to 15% of kidney stones have no hematuria.

Obstetric and Gynecologic Emergencies

3. **Physical examination.** Consider the type of pain and tenderness the patient is experiencing. Is there an associated fever, abdominal distention, or vaginal discharge? Peritonitis is best demonstrated by percussion, gentle motion of the bed, or asking the patient to cough.
4. **Laboratory studies**
   a. **Pregnancy test.** All women of childbearing age should undergo a pregnancy test. This can help but cannot completely rule out ectopic pregnancy or miscarriage.
   b. **Blood work.** A blood type and screen and a complete blood count (CBC) should be obtained.
   c. **Urinalysis** should be performed on a sample obtained by catheterization.
   d. **Culture.** Cervical and vaginal swabs are sent for culture, potassium hydroxide, and wet prep as indicated. Blood and urine cultures can be considered in patients with fever.
5. **Other diagnostic tools**
   a. **Abdominal and pelvic ultrasonography** may be indicated to search for free fluid in the cul-de-sac, uterine fibroids, ectopic pregnancy, ovarian cyst, ovarian torsion, tubo-ovarian abscess, or an inflamed appendix.
   b. **Computed tomography** scanning can be considered in the nonpregnant patient where ultrasound is unable to definitively identify the cause.
   c. **Laparoscopy** and **biopsy** may be necessary to definitively diagnose endometriosis, dysfunctional uterine bleeding, uterine or ovarian cancer, and complicated PID.

D. **Therapy** is directed at the underlying cause. Therapies for gynecologic causes of pelvic pain are summarized here; therapies for other causes of pelvic pain are discussed in Chapter 4 (Gastrointestinal Emergencies) and Chapter 5 (Urogenital Emergencies).
   1. **Vaginitis, cervicitis, and PID.** Treatment is discussed in section VII.A.5, VII.B.5, and VII.C.5, respectively.
   2. **Ectopic pregnancy.** Therapy is discussed in section II.E.
   3. **Ovarian cyst.** A patient with confirmed cyst may go home with pain control or if sonographic evidence of free fluid in the cul-de-sac may be observed without intervention. Patients with suggestion of active hemorrhage or hemodynamic instability should undergo surgical intervention.
   4. **Ovarian torsion.** Patients with suggestive history, examination, and sonographic findings should undergo laparoscopy or laparotomy for exploration and attempted salvage.
   5. **Endometriosis.** Oral contraceptive regimens, methyltestosterone, or progesterone may be used to suppress ectopic endometrial growth. Surgical excision is performed in refractory cases.
   6. **Dysmenorrhea.** Oral contraceptive therapy may be attempted to suppress endometrial growth. Pain control is attempted using nonsteroidal anti-inflammatory drugs such as ibuprofen or naproxen. Narcotics are typically avoided.

E. **Disposition**
   1. Hemodynamically unstable patients are treated with aggressive fluid resuscitation (with blood products) and taken to the operating room.
   2. Hemodynamically stable patients are admitted for observation and treatment when an evolving surgical disease is suspected or the patient is at risk for systemic toxicity.
   3. All patients who are discharged must have follow-up arranged and verified prior to leaving the ED.

II. ECTOPIC PREGNANCY

A. **Discussion.** Ectopic pregnancy is the development of a fertilized ovum outside of the uterine cavity (e.g., in the fallopian tube, ovary, cervix, or abdominal cavity). The ectopic site can rarely sustain the pregnancy beyond several weeks, at which time the implantation site ruptures.
   1. **Pathogenesis.** The fertilized ovum implants at the ectopic site, stimulating a persistent corpus luteum. The resultant elevated estrogen levels stimulate

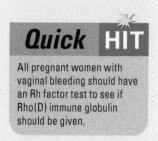

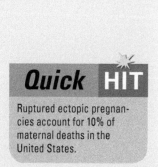

Obstetric and Gynecologic Emergencies

endometrial growth, and progesterone maintains this lining for a uterine implantation that never arrives. The ectopic pregnancy continues to proliferate until it outgrows its blood supply and involutes or ruptures.

2. **Risk factors** are generally related to tubal dysfunction or injury and include:
   a. **Tubal anomalies** (e.g., hypoplasia, diverticula)
   b. **Salpingitis** (characterized by inflammation, scarring, and lumen narrowing)
   c. **Tubal adhesions** (e.g., from infection or endometriosis)
   d. **Previous tubal surgery** (e.g., salpingostomy, tubal ligation)
   e. **Intrauterine device use**
   f. **Previous ectopic pregnancy**

B. **Clinical features.** The "classic triad" of a missed period, abdominal pain, and a palpable mass on examination is present in fewer than 30% of patients. Important historical and clinical findings include the following:

1. **Menstrual history.** A history of amenorrhea or a late period is common in patients with ectopic pregnancy. Only 10% of patients describe a normal last menstrual period.

2. **Abdominal pain or tenderness.** Ninety percent of patients complain of abdominal or pelvic pain.
   a. Pain usually begins as colicky and diffuse (as a result of ectopic distention and inflammation) and later becomes localized (as a result of inflammation of the adjacent abdominal wall and local bleeding).
   b. Peritoneal symptoms may be noticed if the bleeding causes diffuse peritoneal irritation. With severe bleeding and peritonitis, the abdomen will be rigid, distended, and tender.

3. **Cervical motion tenderness** or **adnexal tenderness** is highly suggestive of a pathologic process. Adnexal tenderness is a likely finding in ectopic.

4. **Vaginal bleeding.** Fifty percent to 90% of patients will note abnormal bleeding, ranging from spotting to heavy flow with large clots.

5. **Uterine enlargement.** In pregnancy, the uterus softens and grows in response to hormonal stimulation regardless of the site of conceptus implantation. One cannot assume the pregnancy is intrauterine on the basis of uterine size.

6. **Palpable mass.** Experienced examiners may note a unilateral or cul-de-sac mass, although the absence of such a mass does not rule out an ectopic pregnancy.

7. **Volume depletion.** Tachycardia, orthostatic hypotension, near-syncope, abdominal pain, and a positive pregnancy test in an otherwise healthy woman are indicative of a ruptured ectopic pregnancy until proven otherwise.

C. **Differential diagnoses** include miscarriage, ovarian cyst, vaginitis, cervicitis, salpingitis, PID, combined pregnancy (i.e., intrauterine and ectopic, may be seen in patients taking infertility medications), normal intrauterine pregnancy, appendicitis, urinary tract infection, acute nephrolithiasis, enteritis, and diverticulitis.

D. **Evaluation.** The incidence of detected ectopic pregnancies has increased fivefold over the last 20 years due to increasingly sensitive screening aids.

1. **Stabilization.** It is important to establish the airway, respiratory, and cardiovascular status immediately before making a diagnosis. Two large-bore peripheral lines are secured for fluid and blood resuscitation.

2. **Laboratory studies**
   a. **Urine pregnancy test.** A urine sample can provide a quick qualitative β–human chorionic gonadotropin (β-hCG) screen and most screens with increasing sensitivity, now at approximately 4 weeks' gestational age.
   b. **Blood work.** Blood typing and screening, Rh sensitivity, quantitative β-hCG level, and a CBC are sent immediately. β-hCG levels normally double every 36 to 48 hours. Levels in abnormal pregnancies do not increase as rapidly and may plateau or decline. Thus, if they are available, serial levels are useful in establishing a growth pattern.

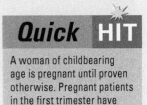

Quick HIT

A woman of childbearing age is pregnant until proven otherwise. Pregnant patients in the first trimester have ectopic pregnancies until proven otherwise.

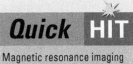

Quick HIT

Magnetic resonance imaging is safe for the growing fetus and may be necessary if ultrasound is unable to detect the etiology.

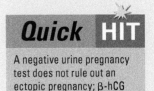

Quick HIT

A negative urine pregnancy test does not rule out an ectopic pregnancy; β-hCG levels can be zero.

Obstetric and Gynecologic Emergencies

Obstetric and Gynecologic Emergencies

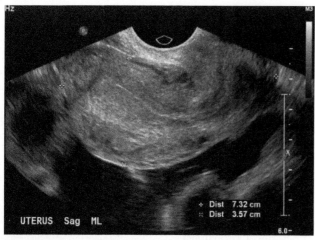

A

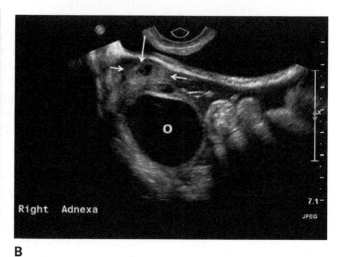

B

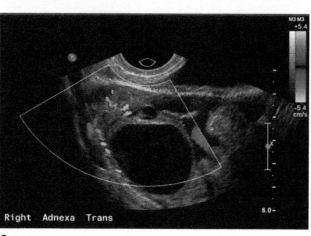

C

FIGURE
14-1 Ultrasound of ectopic pregnancy versus an intrauterine pregnancy.

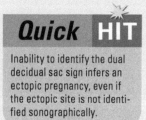

Inability to identify the dual decidual sac sign infers an ectopic pregnancy, even if the ectopic site is not identified sonographically.

3. **Ultrasonography.** A distinct fetal body and fetal cardiac activity can be detected ultrasonographically by 6 weeks' gestation (transvaginal) or 7 weeks' gestation (transabdominal), making the search for the ectopic site a bit easier at this stage (Figure 14-1). There must be two distinct echogenic layers (i.e., the decidua vera and the decidua capsularis) surrounding the gestational sac before the diagnosis of intrauterine pregnancy can be made.

E. **Therapy**

1. **General therapy.** All Rh-negative mothers are given Rho(D) immune globulin in a single intramuscular dose to prevent potential maternal Rh antibody formation. Can be within 72 hours of initial bleeding episode

2. **Specific therapy**

   a. **Unruptured ectopic pregnancy.** These patients are hemodynamically stable. Treatment options include:

      i. Laparoscopic salpingostomy and ectopic excision

      ii. Nonsurgical treatment with methotrexate, leucovorin, or mifepristone

      iii. Salpingocentesis (i.e., transvaginal needle aspiration of the gestational sac, potentially with direct injection of methotrexate)

   b. **Ectopic pregnancy without cardiac activity.** Patients with serial decline of β-hCG levels and no evidence of erosion or rupture on repeat sonography may be managed nonoperatively by the obstetrician. Medications may be used to induce expulsion. Laparoscopic intervention is performed if there is any sign of erosion or rupture.

c. **Ruptured ectopic pregnancy.** These patients may be hemodynamically unstable and therefore require aggressive fluid and blood resuscitation and control of bleeding. Laparoscopic ectopic excision via salpingectomy is indicated.

F. **Disposition**
1. A hemodynamically stable patient with a history of abdominal pain, vaginal bleeding, or both; a benign examination; and ultrasound revealing no clear evidence of ectopic or intrauterine pregnancy may be discharged with strong ectopic precaution warnings. These patients should see an obstetrician in 48 hours for a repeat examination and quantitative β-hCG levels. Ultrasound is repeated in 2 to 7 days to search for pregnancy.
2. A hemodynamically stable patient with a history of abdominal pain, vaginal bleeding, or both with abdominal or adnexal tenderness on physical examination, and evidence of cul-de-sac fluid accumulation on ultrasound but no clear evidence of intrauterine pregnancy should be admitted for observation, serial abdominal examinations, repeat quantitative β-hCG levels (in 36 to 48 hours), and repeat sonography.
3. A hemodynamically stable patient with or without abdominal or adnexal tenderness and sonographic evidence of ectopic pregnancy is admitted.
4. A hemodynamically unstable patient with a pregnancy by qualitative β-hCG requires aggressive resuscitation en route to the operating room.

III. VAGINAL BLEEDING DURING PREGNANCY

A. **First-trimester bleeding**
1. Ectopic pregnancy is discussed in section II.
2. **Abortion/miscarriage**
   a. **Discussion.** Approximately 20% of all pregnancies spontaneously terminate, and 80% to 90% of these end as miscarriage during the first trimester (weeks 1 to 14). Risk factors include previous miscarriage, increased maternal parity, and increased maternal age.
   b. **Clinical features.** Fetal demise usually occurs 2 to 3 weeks prior to the onset of clinical symptoms. Different types of abortions are described in Clinical Pearl 14-1.

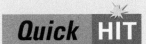

Quick HIT

A FAST scan (focused assessment with sonography for trauma) done by the ED physician can quickly make the diagnosis of free fluid in the abdomen.

Obstetric and Gynecologic Emergencies

CLINICAL PEARL   14-1

1. **Threatened abortion** is most common in the ED. The patient complains of vaginal bleeding, which may be accompanied by abdominal pain. Examination reveals blood in the vaginal vault, a closed internal cervical os, and an enlarged, tender uterus. Quantitative β-hCG levels may not correlate with the gestational age according to the last menstrual period.
2. **Inevitable abortion** presents in the same manner as threatened abortion, except the internal cervical os is open on examination.
3. **Incomplete abortion** may yield findings similar to inevitable abortion, except blood or gestational products are noted in the cervical canal and vaginal vault on examination. The internal cervical os is open.
4. **Completed abortion** is rarely diagnosed in the ED and not without obstetric consultation. The patient may report a history that would suggest vaginal passage of large amounts of blood and gestational products. Upon examination, the internal cervical os is closed and the uterus is nontender. Diagnosis cannot be made unless the patient actually miscarries in the ED, allowing identification of an intact gestational sac and products.
5. **Missed abortion** occurs when fetal products are retained in utero despite their demise. The patient may complain of frequent episodic abdominal cramping and vaginal spotting. Examination reveals a closed internal cervical os. Quantitative β-hCG levels are low for the gestational age, and ultrasound reveals no fetal cardiac activity. Fetal products may remain for prolonged periods and may need to be surgically removed.
6. **Septic abortion** usually begins as an inevitable abortion complicated by intrauterine infection due to prolonged os opening, repeated examinations, or instrumentation. The patient is febrile and has an elevated white blood cell count, with cervical motion and uterine tenderness noted on examination.

c. **Differential diagnoses.** Although 15% of first-trimester pregnancies terminate as miscarriage, ectopic pregnancy must top the differential list until it can be ruled out by examination, ultrasonography, or surgical findings. Other differential diagnoses include normal intrauterine pregnancy, molar pregnancy, vulvovaginitis, cervicitis, urinary tract infection, PID, and vaginal foreign body.

　i. **Molar pregnancy (hydatidiform mole)** is defined as placental proliferation without fetal tissues.

　　a) **Pathogenesis.** Hydatidiform mole is associated with chromosomal anomalies producing trophoblastic hyperplasia and vascular, grape-like chorionic villi. Hydatidiform mole carries the risk of subsequent choriocarcinoma.

　　b) **Risk factors** include maternal age greater than 40 years or less than 20 years.

　　c) **Features** include painless vaginal bleeding, most commonly before 20 weeks' gestation. Uterine size is large for gestational age. Rarely, patients may exhibit symptoms of preeclampsia before they reach the 20-week gestation mark.

d. **Evaluation**

　i. **Patient history.** The date of the last menstrual period must be identified. The patient should be questioned about the amount, character, and time course of the bleeding. A history of trauma, fevers, and associated pain should be sought.

　ii. **Laboratory studies.** The workup should proceed as for ectopic pregnancy (see II.D).

　iii. **Microscopic examination.** All expulsed products of conception must be examined microscopically for the presence of a gestational sac, chorionic villi, or fetal material before miscarriage can be diagnosed.

　iv. **Molar pregnancy.** Ultrasound is usually diagnostic, revealing a "snowstorm" intrauterine pattern and absence of fetal heart activity (Figure 14-2).

e. **Therapy**

　i. A hemodynamically stable patient with no clinical evidence suggesting inevitable or incomplete abortion and no clinical or sonographic evidence supporting ectopic or intrauterine pregnancy has an ectopic pregnancy until proven otherwise. These patients must undergo repeated quantitative β-hCG levels every 48 hours and sonograms every week until the pregnancy is located and β-hCG levels dictate viability or demise.

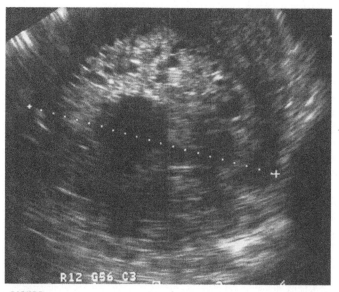

FIGURE
14-2 Ultrasound image of molar pregnancy.

ii. Intrauterine abortion may occur spontaneously and requires little intervention.

   a) Patients with clinical evidence of inevitable, incomplete, or missed abortion may typically undergo expectant management. Medical management is an option but may require dilatation and curettage to reduce the risk of retained products, continued bleeding, and infection. Misoprostol or oxytocin may be used after dilatation and curettage to induce uterine contraction and reduce bleeding.

   b) Patients who are hemodynamically unstable despite an aggressive resuscitative effort require surgical intervention (e.g., dilatation and curettage, hysterectomy).

iii. **Molar pregnancy.** After sonographic documentation, dilatation and curettage is necessary to ensure complete removal, which reduces the risk of subsequent choriocarcinoma. Follow-up serial β-hCG levels should be obtained.

  f. Disposition

    i. Hemodynamically stable patients with no evidence of ongoing hemorrhage, pelvic bleeding, or intraperitoneal bleeding and no findings suggesting inevitable or incomplete miscarriage may be discharged after obstetric follow-up has been arranged. These patients should see an obstetrician within 24 to 48 hours for repeat quantitative β-hCG and sonography.

    ii. Hemodynamically unstable patients are admitted for definitive operative therapy and observation.

3. **Normal intrauterine pregnancy** may be associated with vaginal bleeding, especially during the first trimester. Patients may experience abdominal cramping with vaginal spotting, but on examination, the cervical os is closed and the uterus is nontender. This bleeding is not from the cervical os and is typically from local inflammation, infection, or trauma.

  a. Serial quantitative β-hCG levels should still be trended and increase normally (i.e., they double every 36 to 48 hours, peaking at 100,000 mIU by 8 to 11 weeks).

  b. After 6 weeks' gestation, ultrasound reveals an intrauterine pregnancy with fetal heart activity.

B. Second- and third-trimester bleeding

  1. **Discussion**

    a. Placenta previa

     i. **Pathogenesis.** Placenta previa occurs when a portion of the placenta implants on the lower uterine segment. As the uterus grows or as the cervix dilates, more or less of the os may be covered by placenta.

     ii. **Risk factors** include increasing maternal age, increasing maternal parity, and prior uterine scarring from surgery.

    b. Placental abruption (abruptio placentae) and subchorionic hemorrhage occurs when the placenta separates from the decidua basalis of the uterus prior to stage III of labor. Separation can be partial (subchorionic hemorrhage) or complete. Vaginal bleeding may occur, or the hemorrhage may be concealed under the placenta away from the cervical os.

     i. **Pathogenesis.** Associated with defective placental vasculature

     ii. **Risk factors** include multiparity, increased maternal age, previous abruption, pregnancy-induced hypertension, a short umbilical cord, trauma, smoking, and cocaine abuse.

    c. Uterine dehiscence and rupture is failure of the myometrial wall to adequately contain the contents of the uterus.

     i. **Pathogenesis.** Typically occurs during labor but also can occur during late pregnancy. Weakness in myometrium may allow blood and uterine wall (dehiscence) or all uterine contents (rupture) into the abdominal cavity.

     ii. **Risk factors** include any type of uterine surgery, use of medications to induce labor, and multiparity.

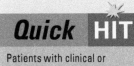

Quick HIT

Patients with clinical or sonographic data suggesting pelvic intraperitoneal hemorrhage must undergo surgical exploration.

Obstetric and Gynecologic Emergencies

2. Clinical features
   a. **Placenta previa.** Patients present with spontaneous, painless, bright red vaginal bleeding, either slight or profuse. Initial bleeding may cease suddenly, only to recur.
   b. **Placental abruption or subchorionic hemorrhage**
      i. Fetal distress or vaginal bleeding are cardinal signs. Sudden abdominal or pelvic pain is seen in 90% of patients with abruption. Shock is variably present, and fetal well-being should be monitored.
      ii. The uterus may be tender, hypertonic, or enlarged for gestational age (due to bleeding). Premature labor may be present. Fetal compromise is variably present.
   c. **Uterine dehiscence or rupture.** Symptoms can initially be mild abdominal pain but quickly lead to fetal compromise, shock, and death.
3. **Differential diagnoses** include trauma, blood dyscrasias and cirrhosis, and estrogen excess state.
4. **Evaluation**
   a. **Stabilization.** Maternal resuscitation is the highest priority. Once the patient's airway, breathing, and circulatory status have been stabilized, historical information should be obtained. Blood typing and screening (including ABO and Rh sensitivity), quantitative β-hCG studies, a CBC, and coagulation profile are sent immediately. Fetal monitoring is established as appropriate for gestational age.
   b. **Physical examination** of patients with second- or third-trimester bleeding should be performed in consultation with an obstetrician in the operating room to minimize the potential for hemorrhagic catastrophe, particularly when uterine rupture or placental abruption is suspected.
   c. **Laboratory studies**
      i. **Quantitative β-hCG levels** are abnormally high (500,000 to 1,000,000 mIU; the normal peak is 100,000 mIU) in molar pregnancy.
      ii. **Coagulation studies** may reveal low fibrinogen, diminished factors V and VIII, and a low platelet count in patients with placental abruption.
   d. **Ultrasonography.** Uterine ultrasound can make the distinction between placenta previa and placental abruption. Its use is paramount, especially in patients with second- or third-trimester bleeding, because complete pelvic examination is contraindicated in these patients until placenta previa and placental abruption are ruled out.
      i. **Placenta previa.** Ultrasound is the diagnostic test of choice to document the location and extent of previa. The placental margin covers part or all of the os.
      ii. **Placental abruption.** Ultrasonography is not sensitive and should be used in conjunction with tocometry to measure fetal distress. It may reveal retroplacental clots.
5. **Therapy**
   a. **Rho(D) immune globulin** is given to all Rh-negative mothers experiencing hemorrhage in pregnancy to prevent maternal Rh antibody formation and risk of hydrops fetalis with any future pregnancy.
   b. **Hemodynamically stable patients with no evidence of fetal distress.** Strict bed rest and observation with frequent fetal checks until the fetus reaches maturity are indicated for stable patients with no evidence of fetal distress but who have ultrasonographic evidence of placenta previa or abruption. Fetal maturity is documented by dates, sonography, and amniotic phospholipid ratios (see VI.B.1.c.ii).
   c. **Hemodynamically stable patients with fetal distress.** If the fetus is less than 23 weeks, the maternal environment should be optimized with expectant management. A fetus younger than 23 weeks cannot survive outside of the uterus and is considered a second-trimester miscarriage. If the fetus is greater than 23 weeks and cannot be stabilized, emergent cesarean section is warranted.
   d. **Hemodynamically unstable patients with or without evidence of fetal distress.** Aggressive fluid and blood resuscitation, positioning of the mother in

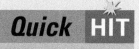

Quick HIT

Babies need their mother to survive in utero, so maternal stabilization is the first priority.

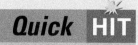

Quick HIT

In a viable fetus, a quick history and physical can necessitate emergent cesarean section in cases of uterine rupture (peritonitis) and placental abruption (tender, hard uterus).

the left lateral decubitus position, and emergent delivery by cesarean section if the fetus is older than 23 weeks are indicated. Oxytocin is administered after placental delivery to reduce further bleeding.

e. **Placenta previa** typically is managed by cesarean section when time for delivery comes, although in cases of mild previa, vaginal delivery is still possible.

f. **Uterine rupture or complete placental abruption** with or without maternal instability with cause fetal compromise and necessitates immediate delivery.

6. **Disposition.** Patients with placenta previa and mild bleeding do not always get admitted but should have obstetrical consultation. All other patients with second- or third-trimester bleeding should be admitted for further sonographic evaluation, fetal maturity studies, maternal–fetal monitoring, bed rest, observation, delivery, and/or surgery.

IV. HYPERTENSION IN PREGNANCY

A. **Discussion.** Untreated hypertensive disorders are associated with fetal compromise resulting in growth retardation, progressive placental insufficiency, placental abruption, and fetal demise.

B. **Clinical features.** The American College of Obstetrics and Gynecology has classified hypertensive disorders in pregnancy on the basis of the onset of clinical findings, associated symptoms, and previous (prepregnancy) hypertension.

1. **Gestational hypertension** occurs after the 20-week gestation mark. Patients develop a mean arterial pressure greater than 100 to 106 mm Hg but have no associated edema or proteinuria. The blood pressure returns to baseline postpartum.

2. **Chronic hypertension** is defined by a blood pressure that exceeds 140/90 mm Hg or a mean arterial pressure greater than 100 to 106 mm Hg that was present prepregnancy or before the 20-week gestation mark. Chronic hypertension is not associated with edema or proteinuria.

3. **Preeclampsia** is similar to worsened gestational hypertension. It is noted after the 20-week gestation mark and is associated with peripheral edema, proteinuria, and any of the following findings: hepatic dysfunction, hypoalbuminemia, coagulation abnormalities, hemoconcentration, or hyperuricemia. The disorder usually improves within 48 hours of delivery but may persist for days to weeks.

a. **Risk factors** include nulliparity, diabetes mellitus, multiple gestations, extremes of age, a family history of preeclampsia, hydrops fetalis, and hydatidiform mole.

b. **Classification.** Preeclampsia is classified as follows:
   i. **Mild to moderate preeclampsia** is characterized by recurrent blood pressures greater than 140/90 mm Hg in a previously normotensive patient. The elevated blood pressures are often accompanied by proteinuria, lower extremity edema, and possibly mildly abnormal laboratory tests.
   ii. **Severe preeclampsia** is characterized by markedly elevated blood pressures (greater than 160/110 mm Hg), generalized edema, and symptoms of headache, blurred vision, epigastric pain or tenderness, pulmonary edema, impaired liver function, significant proteinuria (greater than 1 g/24 hours), and/or oliguria.
   iii. **HELLP syndrome** (*h*emolytic anemia, *e*levated *l*iver enzymes, and *l*ow *p*latelet count). As the plasma volume is reduced, vasoconstriction (and, therefore, blood pressure) is enhanced.

4. **Preeclampsia superimposed on chronic hypertension.** Hypertension develops before the 20-week gestation mark and is accompanied by proteinuria and edema later in the pregnancy. This disorder is found in 10% of patients with hypertension despite continued treatment during pregnancy.

5. **Eclampsia** is severe preeclampsia complicated by generalized seizures. Eclampsia carries the risk of aspiration and maternal–fetal hypoxia.

C. **Differential diagnoses**
1. **Chronic hypertension** caused by renal artery stenosis, chronic renal insufficiency, systemic lupus erythematosus, pheochromocytoma, primary aldosteronism, essential hypertension, and anxiety should be considered.

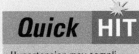

Hypertension may complicate 10% of all pregnancies (20% of nulliparous pregnancies and 40% of twin gestations).

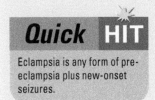

Eclampsia is any form of preeclampsia plus new-onset seizures.

Obstetric and Gynecologic Emergencies

2. **Seizures.** In addition to being caused by eclampsia, generalized seizures can be caused by drugs, substance intoxication or withdrawal, epilepsy, cerebrovascular accident, or trauma.

D. **Evaluation**

1. **Patient history.** Important questions to address include:
   a. What was the patient's prepregnancy or first-trimester blood pressure?
   b. Is the patient on an antihypertensive regimen?
   c. Has a cause for the patient's hypertension been identified?
   d. Has the patient noted progressive swelling of the feet or hands?
   e. Has the patient experienced headache, visual changes, or abdominal pain?

2. **Physical examination**
   a. **Vital signs.** A blood pressure greater than 140/90 mm Hg in a previously normotensive patient should raise concern or a systolic pressure greater than 30 mm Hg and a diastolic greater than 15 mm Hg above the patient's baseline.
   b. **General examination.** Generalized pitting edema may be noted, especially of the extremities and face. A petechial rash or ecchymosis suggests hepatic dysfunction with platelet destruction.
   c. **Ocular examination.** Findings may range from the "retinal sheen" of pregnancy to arteriovenous nicking, "copper wire" arteries, or spot hemorrhages and exudates.
   d. **Abdominal examination** may reveal epigastric, right upper quadrant tenderness, and ascites.
   e. **Neurologic examination.** The patient may have hyperreflexia.

3. **Laboratory studies**
   a. **Blood work**
      i. A CBC may reveal an elevated hematocrit, suggesting hypovolemia and worsening of preeclampsia. A low platelet count (less than 100,000/μL) is suggestive of HELLP.
      ii. Smears may show evidence of hemolysis.
      iii. Elevated liver transaminases and lactic dehydrogenase and a prolonged prothrombin time or partial thromboplastin time are indicative of hepatic dysfunction in patients with severe preeclampsia.
   b. **Urinalysis** reveals significant proteinuria, large proteinuria on urinalysis, or more than 1 g/L in a 24-hour collection.

E. **Therapy**

1. **Chronic hypertension.** A careful balance must be maintained between controlling the blood pressure and minimizing the side effects and teratogenic risk of antihypertensive agents or compromising uterine blood flow. Clinical Pearls 14-2 outlines antihypertensive management in chronic hypertension and preeclampsia.

CLINICAL PEARL **14-2**

a. **Methyldopa**, a central α-adrenergic agonist, reduces the effects of norepinephrine, thereby lowering arterial resistance without seriously affecting uterine blood flow. **Side effects** include postural hypotension, depression, liver dysfunction, and hemolytic anemia.

b. **β Blockers**, especially mixed α-/β-adrenergic antagonists, are often used because they reduce both cardiac contractility and cause smooth muscle relaxation; examples include labetalol and propranolol. **Side effects** include a potential reduction in uterine blood flow, bronchospasm in patients with asthma, and hepatotoxicity.

c. **Hydralazine** acts by direct smooth muscle vasodilatation. **Side effects** include reflex tachycardia, headache, nausea, and diarrhea.

d. **Diuretics** are often used for symptomatic treatment of fluid overload but do not prevent preeclampsia or its complications.

e. **Calcium channel blockers** (e.g., **nifedipine**) reduce both cardiac contractility and cause smooth muscle relaxation. **Side effects** include dizziness, light-headedness, and tachycardia.

f. **Angiotensin-converting enzyme inhibitors and angiotensin receptor blockers** have known teratogenic effects and have been shown to reduce uterine blood flow; they are contraindicated.

2. **Preeclampsia.** Definitive treatment is by fetal delivery, but treatment of maternal blood pressure and end-organ pathology prior to fetal maturity is paramount. Prevention of eclampsia is vital to health of mother and fetus. The following regimens may be considered:

a. **Magnesium sulfate** has a direct vasodilator effect as well as anticonvulsant properties and is usually reserved for patients with severe preeclampsia or those patients who are unresponsive to other regimens.

   i. **Dose.** The loading dose is 4 to 6 g intravenously over 20 minutes, followed by 1 to 3 g/hour.

   ii. **Side effects** include those of hypermagnesemia (i.e., serum magnesium levels greater than 9 μg/dL): muscle relaxation and hyporeflexia. Hypermagnesemia can lead to depressed deep tendon reflexes and apnea. (Treatment of magnesium toxicity is calcium gluconate, 1 g administered intravenously [IV].)

b. **Labetalol** (initial dose 10 mg IV) and **hydralazine** (initial dose 5 mg IV) may be used by the ED physician in severe preeclampsia.

c. **Diuretics** are used only in patients with congestive heart failure or pulmonary edema.

3. **Coagulopathies and laboratory abnormalities** that must be managed attentively along with other symptoms of severe preeclampsia

a. **Volume expansion** is provided slowly to maintain urine output at 0.5 to 1 mL/kg/hour while avoiding volume overload and pulmonary edema.

b. **Albumin** administration to maintain plasma volume may be considered.

c. **Transfusion.** In patients with severe thrombocytopenia (less than 20,000/dL), a platelet transfusion can be considered. Patients with coagulopathy may require fresh frozen plasma or plasmapheresis.

4. **Eclampsia** is managed acutely by maintaining adequate oxygenation and monitoring cardiovascular status. Fluid input and output are monitored carefully to avoid overload.

a. **Seizures** are treated initially with a benzodiazepines (e.g., diazepam, 5 to 10 mg; midazolam, 2 to 5 mg IV; or lorazepam, 1 to 2 mg IV) due to fast onset of action.

b. **Magnesium sulfate** infusion is initiated as described in IV.E.2.a (therapeutic levels are 4 to 7 mEq/L). Patients with seizures refractory to therapeutic levels of magnesium may need barbiturates (e.g., phenobarbital), phenytoin, or increasing doses of magnesium. In these cases, airway management and intensive monitoring is likely necessary.

F. **Disposition**

1. **Chronic hypertension.** Patients with a history of chronic hypertension are screened for superimposed preeclampsia and admitted for blood pressure control on an as needed basis.

2. **Preeclampsia.** All patients displaying criteria for preeclampsia are admitted to obstetrics and screened for fetal growth retardation, oligohydramnios, and maternal end-organ damage.

3. **Eclampsia.** Patients require emergent treatment and admission to obstetrics for continued monitoring and treatment.

V. COMPLICATIONS OF PARTURITION

A. **Approach to the pregnant patient with complications of labor.** Upon presentation of a mother after 24 weeks' gestation, one is dealing with two patients. Both maternal and fetal monitoring are indicated, searching for potential hemodynamic compromise.

1. **Maternal resuscitation** is paramount to maintaining fetal stability—the greatest cause of fetal demise is failure to treat the mother first. Administration of supplemental oxygen, positioning in the left lateral decubitus position (to relieve inferior vena cava compression, ensure venous return, and maximize placental perfusion), and establishment of peripheral intravenous access should be carried out immediately.

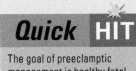

Quick HIT

The goal of preeclamptic management is healthy fetal delivery at an optimal time while preventing progression to eclampsia.

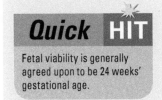

Quick HIT

Fetal viability is generally agreed upon to be 24 weeks' gestational age.

Obstetric and Gynecologic Emergencies

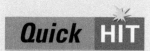

Quick HIT

Variable deceleration is a sign of head or cord compression, and late decelerations or persistent fetal bradycardia is a sign of fetal hypoxia.

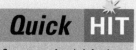

Quick HIT

Symptoms of early infection may include malodorous, cloudy discharge, maternal fever, tachycardia, uterine tenderness, frequent contractions, and fetal distress.

2. A blood type and screen, Rh sensitivity screen, and CBC should be sent as quickly as possible.
3. The fetal heart rate is recorded continuously. The normal basal rate is approximately 140 to 160 beats/min, with beat-to-beat variability. During uterine contractions, a quick return to the baseline rate should be observed after each contraction deceleration.
4. Vaginal and cervical examinations are performed using sterile technique to reduce the risk of infection. The cervix is examined for effacement and dilatation, and the fetal presenting part is checked for position relative to the cervix (station).
5. Fetal ultrasonography is useful in evaluating fetal activity, amniotic fluid volume, uterine anatomy, and placental abnormalities.

B. **Complications of labor**

1. **Premature rupture of membranes**
   a. **Discussion.** Premature membrane rupture complicates less than 5% of pregnancies but causes 30% to 40% of premature births. At term, 90% of mothers go into labor within 24 hours of membrane rupture. However, preterm rupture may not induce labor immediately and carries a high risk of maternal and fetal infection prior to delivery. Chorioamnionitis is a common complication that is directly related to both delay of labor onset and the number of digital cervical examinations the patient has undergone.
   b. **Clinical findings.** The patient usually reports a sudden leak or gush of vaginal fluid. The fluid may be clear, cloudy (indicating the presence of infection), or green (indicating the presence of meconium).
   c. **Evaluation**
      i. Sterile pelvic exam may reveal the following:
         a) Amniotic fluid, which will cause an alkaline reaction on Nitrazine paper (i.e., the color changes from yellow to blue) and ferning (i.e., the development of fern-like crystals) when the fluid sample is smeared on a microscope slide.
         b) Vaginal swabs are also necessary to check for signs of vaginitis, cervicitis, or chorioamnionitis.
         c) In known placenta previa, pelvic examination should be reserved for the obstetrician.
      ii. An abdominal examination may reveal a tender, firm uterus in the setting of infection. Frequent contractions are possible even in very early pregnancy.
   d. **Therapy**
      i. **Antibiotic therapy.** Fever, tachycardia, malodorous vaginal discharge, and cervical or uterine tenderness all suggest chorioamnionitis, and antibiotic therapy may be appropriate. Prophylactic antibiotics are controversial but may be advocated to lengthen the latent interval prior to labor (in an attempt to give the fetus more time to mature).
      ii. **Rho(D) immune globulin.** All Rh-negative mothers are given a single intramuscular injection of Rho(D) immune globulin to prevent maternal Rh antibody formation.
2. **Premature labor**
   a. **Discussion.** Premature labor (i.e., preterm uterine contractions leading to progressive cervical effacement and dilatation) complicates 8% to 10% of pregnancies and is associated with high neonatal morbidity and mortality rates. If the gestational age is less than 37 weeks, a cause must be identified and tocolysis considered if initial treatment fails to cease cervical dilatation. Causes include:
      i. **Premature rupture of membranes**
      ii. **Genitourinary tract infections**
      iii. **Placenta previa, placental abruption, or subchorionic hemorrhage**
      iv. **Maternal hypertension or preeclampsia**
      v. **Diabetes mellitus** (longstanding or gestational)
      vi. **Uterine or fetal anomalies**

b. **Clinical features.** Patients may complain of progressive frequency, intensity, and duration of contractions. Complaints of fluid loss, vaginal bleeding, vaginal discharge, or dysuria are possible.

c. **Evaluation.** Preterm labor requires close maternal–fetal monitoring.

   i. A maternal CBC, urinalysis, and cervical culture are obtained to screen for infection.

   ii. In patients with ruptured membranes and prematurity (less than 37 weeks), fetal maturity must be taken into account for appropriate therapy.

d. **Therapy**

   i. **Supportive therapy** entails control of the underlying cause (e.g., hypertension, hyperglycemia, infection).

   ii. **Corticosteroid therapy** may be required to enhance fetal lung maturity, typically given if fetus is less than 34 weeks.

   iii. **Tocolysis** is not attempted without consultation with an obstetrician. Therapy consists of β agonists (e.g., terbutaline) or nifedipine.

3. **Prolapsed umbilical cord**

   a. **Discussion.** Prolapse of the umbilical cord may occur with uterine contractions and low amniotic intrauterine volumes following membrane rupture. The cord may pass through the cervix before the fetal presenting part, causing cord compression and compromising fetal circulation.

   b. **Clinical findings.** The mother usually presents in labor after membrane rupture with increasingly frequent uterine contractions. The cord is noted on vaginal or cervical inspection. Deep variable decelerations or persistent bradycardia on fetal monitoring are concerning signs.

   c. **Therapy.** Prolapsed umbilical cord is an obstetric emergency. Cord prolapse warrants prompt elevation of the presenting part and maternal positioning to the left lateral decubitus or knee–chest position. The examiner's hand must remain in position until the fetus is delivered by cesarean section.

4. **Abnormal presentation**

   a. **Discussion**

   i. **Shoulder dystocia** is an increasingly common presentation in which the fetal shoulder breadth exceeds the anteroposterior pelvic diameter. The fetal shoulder is caught behind the pelvic outlet, while the head is engaged or presenting, leading to fetal hypoxia. Retraction of the head after its delivery (the turtle sign) is highly suggestive.

   ii. **Breech** (i.e., presenting with the buttocks), **frank breech** (i.e., presenting with hip flexion and knee extension), **shoulder presentation**, and **transverse lie** are other abnormal presentations.

   b. **Therapy.** Shoulder dystocia is an obstetric emergency requiring emergent consultation; however, fetal compromise is likely and delivery should not be delayed.

   i. **McRoberts maneuver** (i.e., hyperflexion of the mother's hips) and the application of suprapubic pressure are performed to dislodge the shoulder from under the pubic symphysis.

   ii. **Other procedures,** including **episioproctotomy, posterior shoulder delivery, Wood maneuver** (i.e., axis rotation of the shoulders), **Zavanelli maneuver** (i.e., pushing head back in with eventual cesarean section), or the often used episiotomy procedure

5. **Postpartum hemorrhage**

   a. **Discussion.** Postpartum hemorrhage can be profuse and, in 90% of patients, is caused by uterine atony. Postpartum hemorrhage can also be caused by vaginal lacerations or retained placental structures.

   b. **Clinical features.** Complete inspection of the vault will reveal reparable lacerations. A soft, boggy uterus despite direct massage suggests atony.

   c. **Therapy**

   i. Prompt fluid and blood resuscitation may be indicated.

   ii. Direct stern palpation and massage of the uterus may stimulate its contraction and reduce bleeding.

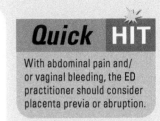

Quick HIT

With abdominal pain and/or vaginal bleeding, the ED practitioner should consider placenta previa or abruption.

Obstetric and Gynecologic Emergencies

    iii. The patient should be examined for signs of vaginal trauma, and any damage should be surgically repaired.

    iv. Missing portions of the placenta suggest retained contents, which must be removed.

    v. Oxytocin (10 to 20 U) is infused over 30 minutes to stimulate uterine contraction.

C. **Disposition.** All mothers are admitted for continued maternal and fetal monitoring. Newborns are evaluated by the pediatrician or neonatologist for admission to the nursery or neonatal intensive care unit.

VI. VAGINITIS, CERVICITIS, AND PELVIC INFLAMMATORY DISEASE

A. **Vaginitis**

1. **Discussion.** Vaginitis is inflammation of the vulva and vaginal vault.

a. **Predisposing factors** include multiple unprotected sexual exposures, high estrogen states (e.g., use of oral contraceptives, pregnancy), antibiotic use, diabetes, and immunosuppression.

b. **Etiology**

    i. **Infection** is the leading cause of vaginitis.

        a) *Candida albicans*, a fungus, is not usually sexually transmitted.

        b) *Trichomonas vaginalis* is a sexually transmitted, protozoal infection involving the cervical and vaginal epithelium.

        c) *Gardnerella (Haemophilus) vaginalis*, a bacterium, is not generally sexually transmitted, although this infection is common in sexually active women. Symptoms occur when there is overgrowth of normal flora in the vaginal vault (e.g., in immunocompromised or diabetic patients).

    ii. **Foreign bodies** (e.g., tampons, sanitary napkins) may produce vaginal irritation and a malodorous discharge.

    iii. **Chemical irritation** (e.g., from medications, douches, perfume) can cause local irritation and acute tenderness during intercourse (dyspareunia). Physical examination may reveal an erythematous, inflamed vaginal vault without discharge or cervical motion tenderness.

    iv. **Reduced estrogen levels** in postmenopausal women result in a more friable vaginal mucosa, leading to atrophic vaginitis (characterized by pruritus, erythema, and tenderness).

2. **Clinical features.** Inflammation of the vulva and vaginal vault leads to itchy, tender, erythematous tissues and increased vaginal discharge. Patients may also complain of dyspareunia or dysuria.

a. *C. albicans* **vaginitis** is characterized by a "cottage-cheese" discharge in the cervix and in the vaginal vault. The patient may have mild cervical motion tenderness but no uterine or adnexal tenderness.

b. **Trichomoniasis.** Patients complain of a thin, "frothy," malodorous discharge, vaginal pruritus, dysuria, and dyspareunia. Examination reveals an erythematous, tender vagina and cervix ("strawberry cervix").

c. **Bacterial vaginitis.** Patients complain of a thin, foul "fishy-smelling" discharge, vaginal pruritus, and dyspareunia. Cervical motion tenderness may be present.

3. **Differential diagnoses** include pinworm infection, acute cystitis, cervicitis, and sexually transmitted infections, such as gonorrhea and chlamydia.

4. **Evaluation**

a. **Patient history.** It is important to obtain a complete gynecologic and menstrual history.

b. **Laboratory studies**

    i. **Culture.** Vaginal and cervical discharge should be cultured and evaluated microscopically.

        a) *C. albicans* **vaginitis.** A potassium hydroxide preparation, sodium chloride preparation, or Gram staining may reveal yeast buds.

        b) **Trichomoniasis.** A sodium chloride microscope slide preparation reveals round, flagellated, motile protozoa.

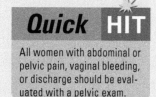

Quick HIT

All women with abdominal or pelvic pain, vaginal bleeding, or discharge should be evaluated with a pelvic exam.

      c) **Bacterial vaginitis.** A sodium chloride preparation may reveal "clue" cells (i.e., epithelial cells studded with bacteria).

    ii. **Syphilis serologies** should be sent when a sexually transmitted agent is suspect.

    iii. **Urinalysis** (on a sample obtained by catheterization) and culture should be performed to rule out concurrent urinary tract involvement.

5. **Therapy**
   a. **Infectious vaginitis**
      i. **Fungal vaginitis**
         a) *C. albicans* **vaginitis** is treated with miconazole suppositories (200 mg each evening for 3 to 7 days), oral fluconazole (150 mg orally once), or terconazole suppositories (80 mg each evening for 3 days).
         b) **Other fungal agents of vaginitis** (e.g., *Torulopsis glabrata*) may be resistant to conventional antifungal treatment and may need longer therapy, repeated dosing, or systemic antifungal treatment.
      ii. **Trichomoniasis** is treated with oral metronidazole (2 g administered in a single dose). In pregnant patients, a 7-day course of metronidazole (500 mg twice daily) or clotrimazole suppositories (inserted each evening for 7 days) can be used.
      iii. **Bacterial vaginitis** is treated in similar fashion to trichomoniasis. Metronidazole (500 mg twice daily for 7 days). Treatment with clotrimazole suppositories can be considered for pregnant patients with severe infections.
   b. **Foreign object vaginitis.** Object removal and proper hygiene education.
   c. **Contact vaginitis** is treated by terminating exposure to the offending agent.
   d. **Atrophic vaginitis** is improved by applying topical estrogen cream daily for 5 to 10 days.
6. **Disposition.** Patients require short-term follow-up with a gynecologist after evaluation in the ED.

B. **Cervicitis**
1. **Discussion.** Cervicitis involves inflammation of the cervix, producing dyspareunia and cervical motion tenderness on examination. The following microorganisms can cause cervicitis:
   a. *Neisseria gonorrhoeae* is a gram-negative diplococcus that infects up to 90% of patients after a single sexual encounter with an infected partner.
   b. *Chlamydia trachomatis*, the most common sexually transmitted organism in the United States, is an obligate, intracellular bacterium.
   c. **Herpes simplex virus** is a DNA virus of two serotypes. Type 2 is predominantly associated with genital lesions, although type 1, more commonly causing stomatitis, may be found in 20% of patients. Transmission is via direct mucous membrane contact.
2. **Clinical features**
   a. **Gonococcal cervicitis.** The incubation period is 2 to 5 days, although up to 75% of patients with gonococcal cervicitis may be asymptomatic for months. Patients with symptoms note abnormal vaginal discharge, lower abdominal pain, and dyspareunia. Examination reveals a yellowish, mucopurulent discharge from the cervix and tenderness on digital manipulation. No adnexal tenderness is noted.
   b. **Nongonococcal cervicitis.** The incubation period for *Chlamydia* is 6 to 21 days, and 60% to 70% of patients may have an asymptomatic "latent" period. Patients with acute cervicitis may complain of an abnormal vaginal discharge. Examination reveals an erythematous, friable cervix with motion tenderness.
   c. **Viral cervicitis.** Most patients have lesions involving the vulvovaginal and cervical region. The development of hyperesthetic tissues and red, papular eruptions, which evolve into ulcerating vesicles that eventually crust and heal, occurs after an incubation period of 3 to 7 days. Constitutional symptoms include malaise, fever, myalgias, and headache. Herpetic lesions are exquisitely tender to touch, making pelvic examination difficult. Symptoms may persist for 7 to 20 days with gradual resolution and also reactivation later.

3. **Differential diagnoses** include bacterial or protozoal vaginosis, PID, and cervical cancer.
4. **Evaluation**
   a. **Gonococcal cervicitis.** Gram stain of the discharge may show gram-negative intracellular and extracellular diplococci.
   b. **Nongonococcal cervicitis.** Gram stain of the discharge is rarely revealing. Diagnosis is usually confirmed with a cervical culture.
   c. **Viral cervicitis.** Tzanck smear of an ulcer crater may reveal multinucleated giant cells. Viral polymerase chain reaction for herpes simplex virus DNA is becoming test of choice in many laboratories.
5. **Therapy.** Due to high rates of coinfection, treatment for bacterial infection is directed at gonococcal and chlamydial infection.
   a. **Gonococcal.** Ceftriaxone (250 mg in one intramuscular dose) plus doxycycline (100 mg orally every 12 hours for 7 days). Doxycycline and tetracyclines should be avoided in pregnant women.
   b. **Chlamydial.** Azithromycin (1 g administered in a single oral dose) or a 7-day course of doxycycline.
   c. **Viral.** Herpes virus becomes latent inside neuronal cells and is impossible to eradicate from the body. Acyclovir (200 mg orally five times daily or 400 mg three times daily for 10 days) or valacyclovir (1 g orally twice daily for 10 days) are used to limit initial and reactivation symptoms.

C. **PID**
1. **Discussion.** PID is an ascending infection (from the lower genital tract) that involves acute infection of the uterus and fallopian tube. PID rarely occurs during pregnancy because the cervical mucus plug prevents infection from traveling beyond the cervix.
   a. **Incidence.** The incidence is 1 in 100 women of childbearing age (i.e., between the ages of 15 and 40).
   b. **Risk factors** include unprotected intercourse, multiple partners, prior infection, pelvic procedures (e.g., dilatation and curettage), and intrauterine device use.
   c. **Etiology.** Over 75% of infections are sexually transmitted. Causative organisms include *C. trachomatis*, *N. gonorrhoeae*, and *Mycoplasma hominis*. Normal vaginal flora may also ascend through the cervix, causing symptoms.
   d. **Complications** include infertility (20% risk after first infection), ectopic pregnancy, recurrent infection, and chronic pelvic pain. PID may also be complicated by gonococcal perihepatitis (Fitz-Hugh–Curtis syndrome) or the development of tubo-ovarian abscess.
2. **Clinical features.** PID is characterized by vague, lower abdominal pain with diffuse cervical, uterine, and adnexal tenderness. A vaginal or cervical discharge and a fever may also be noted.
3. **Differential diagnoses** include pyelonephritis, appendicitis, tubo-ovarian abscess, ovarian cyst, ovarian torsion, endometritis, enteritis, inflammatory bowel disease, cholecystitis, and diverticulitis.
4. **Evaluation.** Symptoms range from severe to subclinical (no overt symptoms): lower abdominal tenderness, dyspareunia, fever, irregular bleeding, abnormal discharge, cervical motion tenderness, and unilateral or bilateral adnexal tenderness.
5. **Therapy**
   a. **Outpatient therapy.** Ceftriaxone (250 mg administered in a single, intramuscular injection) plus doxycycline and metronidazole for 14 days
   b. **Inpatient therapy.** Appropriate regimens include:
      i. A cephalosporin (e.g., ceftriaxone, 1 g every 24 hours; cefotetan, 2 g every 12 hours; or cefoxitin, 2 g every 6 hours) plus doxycycline (by mouth or IV)
      ii. Clindamycin (900 mg every 8 hours) plus gentamicin (an initial loading dose of 2 mg/kg followed by a maintenance infusion of 1.5 mg/kg every 8 hours intravenously)
      iii. Ampicillin/sulbactam (3 g IV four times daily) plus doxycycline
6. **Disposition.** Admission criteria include severe, systemic toxicity; an inability to tolerate oral antibiotic or pain medications; suspected or confirmed

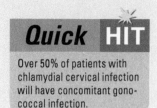

Quick HIT

Over 50% of patients with chlamydial cervical infection will have concomitant gonococcal infection.

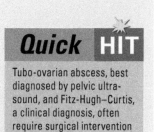

Quick HIT

Tubo-ovarian abscess, best diagnosed by pelvic ultrasound, and Fitz-Hugh–Curtis, a clinical diagnosis, often require surgical intervention and admission.

Obstetric and Gynecologic Emergencies

tubo-ovarian abscess or Fitz-Hugh–Curtis Syndrome; failed outpatient treatment; and concomitant pregnancy. Inpatient therapy should also be considered for patients who have no history of PID and for infected nulliparous patients who desire pregnancy at a later date.

VII. ABNORMAL VAGINAL BLEEDING IN NONPREGNANT PATIENTS

A. **Discussion.** Bleeding that differs in cyclic interval, duration, or flow from the patient's normal menstrual pattern must be evaluated. Infection, trauma, or hormonal imbalances may explain bleeding in premenarchal girls. Causes of abnormal vaginal bleeding in nonpregnant patients include:

1. **Bleeding disorders**
2. **Trauma** to genital structures may occur from straddle injuries, coitus, vaginal delivery, self-manipulation, or sexual assault.
3. **Neoplasia**, either benign or malignant, can cause significant bleeding. Malignancy should be suspected in all postmenopausal woman who have vaginal bleeding of pelvic discomfort. Clinical Pearl 14-3 has a list of common malignant and benign neoplasia.
4. **Ovarian cysts** can result from anovulatory cycles (follicular cysts) or occur following ovulation (luteal cysts).
   a. **Follicular cysts** enlarge due to continued hormonal stimulation as a result of failed ovulation. They are usually multiple, bilateral, and associated with endometrial hyperplasia (leading to breakthrough bleeding).
   b. **Luteal cysts** may persist long after implantation. Continued hormonal secretion from the cyst maintains an amenorrheic state. Cyst enlargement and hemorrhage can occur, producing a tender, adnexal mass or peritonitis from cyst rupture. Symptoms may mimic those of ectopic pregnancy; however, a β-hCG screen will be negative.
5. **Intrauterine devices** may cause irregular and/or excessive bleeding due to local inflammation or erosion of an endometrial vessel and exogenous hormones.
6. **Endogenous or exogenous anovulation** may cause dysfunctional uterine bleeding.
   a. **Endogenous anovulation** is caused by unopposed estrogen inducing endometrial hyperplasia. These patients may be amenorrheic for several months followed by episodes of moderate to heavy breakthrough bleeding. Estrogen excess may be due to central hypothalamic or pituitary dysfunction, tumor secretion, or androgen aromatization (seen in some patients with liver disease).
   b. **Exogenous anovulation** can be caused by failure to comply with an oral contraceptive regimen. Variable hormone levels are attained with different

> **Quick HIT**
>
> Perineal or periurethral ecchymosis or vaginal vault or perianal lacerations, abrasions, and excoriations should raise suspicion for sexual assault.

Obstetric and Gynecologic Emergencies

CLINICAL PEARL 14-3

1. **Malignant neoplasia.** Malignancy is most common in older patients.
   a. **Cervical cancer** carries a high mortality rate if left untreated. It is difficult to distinguish the lesions of cervical cancer from those caused by infection. Risk factors include unprotected intercourse and multiple partners.
   b. **Endometrial carcinoma.** Although more common in perimenopausal women, endometrial carcinoma has a 25% incidence in the reproductive age group. Diabetes mellitus, hypertension, obesity, and history of anovulation are risk factors.
   c. **Ovarian carcinoma** is most common in postmenopausal women. Common symptoms include abnormal vaginal bleeding, increased abdominal girth, and weight loss. Endometrial hyperplasia may be present due to hormone excess from the tumor. A palpable mass is highly suggestive.
2. **Benign neoplasia**
   a. **Cervical polyps** may produce metrorrhagia (i.e., noncyclic bleeding), especially after intercourse. The polyps are red, ulcerated lesions that protrude from the cervical os. They rarely become malignant.
   b. **Uterine leiomyomas (fibroids)** are benign lesions affecting 20% of women older than 35 years. Submucosal or interstitial lesions commonly cause menorrhagia (i.e., painfully prolonged or heavy menses). Fibroids may be palpated during pelvic examination.
   c. **Adenomyosis**, more common in older women, results in hyperplastic, benign, globular infiltration of the myometrium, producing heavy menses, dysmenorrhea, local uterine enlargement, and tenderness.

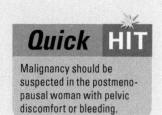

oral contraceptive preparations. Hormone excess or deficiency may induce endometrial hyperplasia or withdrawal bleeding.

B. **Clinical features.** Use of an increased number of pads/tampons or the passage of blood clots suggests an abnormality. Changes in the nature of menstrual cramping also increase suspicion of a pathologic process.

C. **Differential diagnoses** include pregnancy, endometriosis, molar pregnancy, cystitis, bladder tumor, hemorrhoids, diverticulosis, hemorrhagic enteritis, inflammatory bowel disease, gastrointestinal tumors, bleeding disorders, liver diseases, and hypertension.

D. **Evaluation**
1. **Stabilization.** Attention should be directed to the patient's airway, respiratory, and cardiovascular status, and shock should be treated before making a diagnosis.
2. **Patient history.** After initial resuscitation, a detailed gynecologic history should be obtained:
   a. When was the patient's last "normal" menses and the menses prior to that?
   b. What is different regarding this episode?
   c. When was the patient's most recent sexual contact?
   d. Which, if any, contraceptive method does the patient use?
3. **Physical examination.** The presence of clotting blood (abrupt, acute hemorrhage) and vaginal or cervical lesions should be noted during the pelvic examination. An open internal cervical os suggests a uterine process. Uterine or adnexal tenderness or enlargement may be noted.
4. **Laboratory studies**
   a. **Blood work.** A blood type and screen, CBC, coagulation profile, and β-hCG should be sent immediately.
   b. **Urinalysis.** A urine specimen should be obtained via catheterization (to avoid contamination with vaginal flora).
   c. **Vaginal** and **cervical cultures** are sent from the ED.
5. **Other diagnostic tools**
   a. **Ultrasound** may be helpful in locating a pelvic mass or fluid in cul-de-sac. A FAST scan (*f*ocused *a*ssessment with *s*onography for *t*rauma) may be performed looking for free fluid in the abdomen.
   b. **Computed tomography** is useful for detecting abnormalities not seen on ultrasound in the nonpregnant patient.

E. **Therapy**
1. **Acute therapy.** Hypotensive patients are resuscitated using a crystalloid boluses. Blood products are used if the hypotension is refractory to crystalloid infusion.
2. **Definitive therapy**
   a. **Ruptured ovarian cysts,** specifically hemorrhagic cysts, require operative repair to terminate severe bleeding. Even extremely large ovarian cysts without rupture in asymptomatic patients can be set up for outpatient surgery.
   b. **Intra-abdominal hemorrhage.** All patients with significant hemodynamic compromise and examination findings consistent with intra-abdominal hemorrhage are taken to the operating room without delay.
   c. **Uterine leiomyomas.** Dilatation and curettage with biopsy may be diagnostic or leiomyomectomy for definitive treatment. All material removed is evaluated for dysplasia or malignant changes.
   d. **Dysfunctional uterine bleeding** may require curettage followed by prophylactic hormone therapy. Such a regimen should be chosen with gynecologic consultation.
   e. **Exogenous anovulation.** Hemodynamically stable patients with minimal bleeding may be placed on continual progesterone therapy after consultation and follow-up arranged with gynecologist.

F. **Disposition**
1. Hemodynamically unstable patients are admitted for observation, workup, or surgery.
2. Hemodynamically stable patients with no evidence of surgical emergency or continued bleeding may be discharged. Short-term follow-up with a gynecologist should be arranged.

15

PEDIATRIC EMERGENCIES

Sandra Herr

I. APPROACH TO THE ILL PEDIATRIC PATIENT

A. **Discussion.** Approximately 30% to 35% of patients seen in the emergency department (ED) are within the pediatric age range. Most of these children require urgent care or office care for self-limited illnesses but are unable to gain access to the primary provider's office. Thus, they present for care in the ED. Between 3% and 6% of ED visits are true emergencies in which children could suffer death or serious disability if not cared for in a timely fashion.

B. **Clinical features.** Children in rapid need of assessment are often referred to as "septic" or "sick" by experienced pediatric emergency physicians, who rapidly make the assessment based on a constellation of symptoms and signs that are difficult to teach without first-hand experience (see Clinical Pearl 15-1).

C. **Differential diagnoses.** Children who suffer true, life-threatening emergencies fall into several distinct categories of illness. Children with any of the following life-threatening emergencies usually have initial respiratory compromise resulting from increased metabolic demands and cardiac compromise as a secondary event:
   1. Acute respiratory distress
   2. Cardiovascular disorders
   3. Shock syndromes
   4. Traumatic disorders
   5. Environmental injuries
   6. Injuries and emergencies with altered states of consciousness

D. **Evaluation**
   1. A **primary survey** should be performed immediately.
      a. **Airway.** The airway should be assessed for patency.
         i. The airway should be opened with external maneuvers to relieve tongue obstruction.
         ii. Obstruction from foreign bodies should be recognized and relieved.
         iii. Gas exchange should be assessed and optimized.
         iv. Aspiration of gastric or oral contents should be prevented.
         v. An artificial airway should be provided if no protective reflexes exist.
      b. **Breathing.** The adequacy of ventilation should be assessed, including the equality of chest rise and breath sounds.
         i. A determination of whether air entry is impaired from a central or pulmonary cause should be made.
         ii. Ventilation should be enhanced if necessary with mouth-to-mouth breathing, bag-mask ventilation, or endotracheal intubation with or without bag assistance.
         iii. A surgical airway should be provided if an oral or endotracheal airway cannot be established.
      c. **Circulation** should be assessed, including the quality and intensity of pulses in the upper and lower extremity and blood pressure.
         i. Hemorrhage should be controlled with direct pressure until surgical intervention can be accomplished.

331

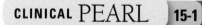

CLINICAL PEARL 15-1

Signs and Symptoms of a Sick Child

1. Lethargy with little or no apprehension to examination or painful procedures; failure to interact appropriately with their environment
2. Irritability, particularly when held by parents, with inability to be comforted
3. Poor feeding associated with weak suck and poor interest in feeding
4. Weak cry or no cry when painful procedures or examination maneuvers are performed
5. Elevated temperature or hypothermia
6. Poor capillary refill with mottled skin appearance or poor turgor
7. Persistent vomiting with or without feedings
8. Complaint of headache and photophobia (in older children); stiff neck is not a reliable sign in children younger than 18 months, and these children are unlikely to be able to report subjective complaints.
9. Seizures, which may be prolonged or focal in nature and are often associated with fever
10. Altered mental status, particularly with combativeness or inappropriate thoughts
11. Respiratory distress, particularly with nasal flaring, grunting respirations, tachypnea, intercostal and subcostal retractions, or diaphragmatic breathing
12. Drooling or stridor with severe air hunger
13. Cyanosis of lips and extremities with poor perfusion and absent pulses in the lower extremities
14. Extreme hypotension
15. Any presentation of trauma that may be associated with a blunt injury to the head or thorax or with a penetration injury to the chest
16. Petechiae or purpura associated with fever

    ii. Intravenous vascular access and a resuscitative fluid bolus should be provided; if intravenous access cannot be rapidly achieved, intraosseous access should be performed.

    iii. External cardiac massage should be provided if no pulse exists.

    iv. Pharmacologic management of circulation should be provided if fluid status is adequate and cardiac output is impaired because of either vascular or pump instability.

    v. Conversion of dangerous cardiac rhythm disturbances should be provided if hypotension and unresponsiveness ensue.

  d. Neurologic examination. A preliminary assessment should be made according to the following simple scale:

    i. Alert and responsive to verbal stimuli

    ii. Responsive to verbal stimuli but no spontaneous alertness

    iii. Responsive only to painful stimuli

    iv. Unresponsive to any stimuli

  e. Overall examination. Infants should be unclothed and examined rapidly for injuries. Passive heat loss should be prevented by removing wet clothing and by providing external warmth. The patient's core temperature should be obtained to monitor for hypo- or hyperthermia.

2. A **secondary survey**, entailing a detailed physical examination and history, is then performed.

  a. Head

    i. Evidence of trauma is determined by palpating bony prominences and the maxillae and by inspecting the nose and ears for drainage of cerebrospinal fluid (CSF).

    ii. The existence of dehydration is determined by inspecting the mucosae for evidence of decreased tearing or moisture or sunken eyes.

    iii. The eyes should be inspected for pupillary size and extraocular movements. A funduscopic examination should be performed if possible to assess for central nervous system (CNS) or toxic involvement.

    iv. The oral cavity should be inspected for odor or discoloration that may imply a toxicologic basis for the condition.

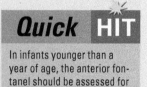

Quick HIT

In infants younger than a year of age, the anterior fontanel should be assessed for bulging (intracranial hypertension, bleeding) or depression (dehydration).

Pediatric Emergencies

b. **Neck**
   i. The neck should be palpated for midline tenderness or deformity.
   ii. Flexion, extension, and rotation should be performed only after injury has been excluded either clinically or by radiographic means.
c. **Chest**
   i. The chest wall should be inspected for symmetric expansion or disarticulation.
   ii. Palpation for change in respiratory fremitus or inequality should be performed.
   iii. Auscultation of the chest for breath sounds and for evidence of adventitial sounds such as rales, rhonchi, or wheezes should be performed.
   iv. Penetrating or blunt chest trauma is treated immediately.
d. **Abdomen**
   i. The abdominal wall should be inspected for bruising, penetration, or hematoma.
   ii. Palpation for trauma, masses, or guarding and rigidity, which may indicate peritonitis, should be performed.
   iii. Palpation of the flanks to search for hematoma or an expanding mass should be performed.
e. **Pelvis**
   i. The pelvis should be palpated laterally and in an anteroposterior position for tenderness or instability.
   ii. The perineum should be inspected for lacerations, active bleeding, or hematoma. The urethra and rectum should be inspected for trauma or blood.
   iii. In age-appropriate females, a pelvic and rectal examination should be performed, and pregnancy should be excluded.
f. **Extremities**
   i. The extremities should be inspected for signs of abrasion, hematoma, laceration, or deformity.
   ii. Palpation of the bones for instability, tenderness, or deformity should be performed.
g. **Neurologic assessment**
   i. Attention should be focused on cranial nerve function, motor function, and sensory function, along with the patient's level of consciousness.
   ii. The presence or absence of reflexes should be noted.
   iii. Serial examinations for changes in level of consciousness or loss of neurologic function should be performed.

3. **Additional studies** are often nonspecific but may provide clues to the diagnosis.
   a. **Laboratory studies**
      i. Complete blood count (CBC) and differential
      ii. Electrolytes and bicarbonate
      iii. Blood urea nitrogen and creatinine
      iv. Immediate fingerstick glucose and serum glucose
      v. Aerobic and anaerobic cultures of blood
      vi. Arterial blood gas (ABG) determination
      vii. Urinalysis and urine culture
      viii. Stool culture
   b. **Radiologic studies**
      i. Chest radiography
      ii. Abdominal radiography
      iii. Abdominal ultrasonography
      iv. Computed tomography (CT) of head and/or abdomen
   c. **Ancillary studies**
      i. Echocardiography
      ii. Electrocardiography
      iii. Urine for toxicologic analysis
      iv. Lumbar puncture

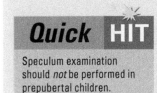

Quick HIT

Speculum examination should *not* be performed in prepubertal children.

Pediatric Emergencies

E. **Therapy**
1. **Stabilization** is the first priority. Prior to admission or transport, all life-threatening conditions (in particular, tenuous airway or circulatory dysfunction) must be addressed fully.
   a. Any possibility of airway compromise must be addressed and stabilized prior to admission or transport, and endotracheal intubation must be secured, if in question.
   b. Circulatory status must be addressed fully; resuscitative fluid boluses or blood transfusions may be indicated.
   c. Vasoactive drugs (e.g., dopamine, dobutamine) should be administered only in the presence of a physician or of a nursing staff qualified in critical care. The environment should be monitored and should have intravenous pump capabilities.
2. **Supportive care** is essential.
   a. **Fluid resuscitation.** A fluid bolus of 20 mL/kg should be provided to establish blood volume and increase efficiency of the heart. Care must be taken to avoid cerebral edema of fluid overload when vascular volume is restored.
   b. **Anticonvulsant therapy** is indicated to control seizures.
   c. **Assisted ventilation** may be necessary to control respiratory failure or cerebral edema.
   d. **Surgical consultation** should be obtained promptly in all cases of suspected trauma or when the diagnosis is in doubt in a critically ill infant with non-specific physical signs.
3. **Antibiotic therapy** should be initiated for children with presumed sepsis, meningitis, or pneumonia.
   a. **Agent selection.** The patient should be treated with an antibiotic that is effective against the pathogens that most often cause disease in the patient's age group.
      i. **Neonates and infants younger than 2 months** are usually given ampicillin sodium and either an aminoglycoside or cefotaxime.
      ii. **Infants and older children** may be treated with ceftriaxone in single or daily divided doses or cefotaxime. Vancomycin should be added in unstable patients to cover for resistant *Streptococcus pneumoniae* and methicillin-resistant *Staphylococcus aureus*.
   b. **Duration of therapy** is based on the patient's age and the causative organism.
      i. Infants with sepsis but without meningitis are usually treated with intravenous antibiotics for 7 to 10 days.
      ii. Infants with meningitis receive 10 to 14 days of parenteral therapy depending on the causative organism. Meningitis caused by *Neisseria meningitidis* may be treated for fewer than 7 days under certain circumstances.
4. **Corticosteroid therapy** is indicated for patients with meningitis to reduce the incidence of hearing loss. These drugs also may augment survival in children with sepsis or meningitis, but the effective dosage is unknown.

F. **Disposition**
1. **Critically ill infants** must be evaluated and treated in a timely manner and admitted to the hospital for further treatment.
   a. Such children should be cared for by the highest level of provider available, preferably a pediatrician able to care for critically ill infants.
   b. When higher level care is unavailable, transport should be arranged to a referral center with the capability to care for critically ill children.
2. **Seriously ill infants** who may have the possibility of a bacterial process should not have antibiotics withheld pending hospital admission or transfer. All seriously ill infants should be accompanied by the admitting physician to the admitting ward or be attended by another physician during transfer and transport.

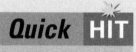

Quick HIT

Reassessment should be performed after each 20-mL/kg fluid bolus to assess need for ongoing fluid resuscitation and any signs or symptoms of fluid overload.

II. PAIN

A. Discussion

1. **Definition.** Pain is a **subjective experience** of superficial or visceral sensation that is sensory as well as emotional and relates to the degree of the injury, anticipation of a procedure, and previous experiences with painful procedures.

2. **Misconceptions about pain and its management in children** include:

a. Children will not remember painful events.

b. Pain sensation is decreased because of neurologic immaturity.

c. Children are more sensitive to analgesics, particularly when parenterally administered.

3. **Quantification of pain in children** is difficult because of neurologic immaturity and expressive immaturity, but it can be partially characterized by facial expression, excess motor activity, and autonomic responses (e.g., diaphoresis, tachycardia, hypertension, intensity of cry). Pain can be measured roughly, depending on the age of the patient.

a. In children **younger than 3 years**, no good visual guideline is available.

b. In children **older than 3 years**, a visual analog scale consisting of drawn facial expressions may be useful.

c. In **older children and adolescents**, a numerical scale may be used relative to pain that the child has perceived prior to this episode.

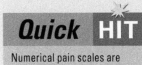

Numerical pain scales are not useful for small children and may have limited validity for adolescents because of their emotional and psychologic lability.

B. **Clinical features.** Pain may be made evident by withdrawal of the injured parts, fleeing the immediate treatment situation, extreme facial expressions, crying, or excess verbal or motor aggressive behavior.

C. **Differential diagnoses**

1. Preoperative pain from a painful injury

2. Postoperative pain following a difficult procedure

3. Chronic pain syndromes associated with malignancy or chronic conditions

D. **Evaluation**

1. **Prompt intervention** to prevent loss of life or limb should take place, including:

a. Airway support and control

b. Assessment of quality of breathing

c. Support of circulation and control of hemorrhage with replacement of fluid loss

2. A **thorough secondary survey** is performed following the initial assessment and stabilization of the patient.

a. An appropriate **physical examination** is necessary to assess the degree of injury or the site of pain as it may relate to visceral pathology (e.g., appendicitis).

b. An **analog scale** appropriate to the patient's age should be used to assess the severity of pain.

E. **Therapy.** Treatment of pain should be instituted based on the injury and emotional distress. Throughout treatment, monitoring is necessary to assess the quality of intervention and the potential side effects of medications.

1. **Local anesthesia** is a safe and effective method of pain relief during painful procedures or injuries, particularly those involving lacerations or fractures. Toxicity is determined by the total amount of drug absorbed into the circulation and the rapidity of administration. Local anesthetic may be applied topically to provide minimal anesthesia for simple procedures.

a. **Eutectic mixture of local anesthetics (EMLA)**, such as lidocaine 2.5% and prilocaine 2.5%

i. EMLA must be applied 60 to 90 minutes before procedures.

ii. EMLA requires an overlay of occlusive dressing.

iii. Safety in open wounds is not established.

b. **Lidocaine, epinephrine, and tetracaine solution or gel**

i. Mixture concentrations are variable from institution to institution.

ii. Lidocaine, epinephrine, and tetracaine solution or gel may be applied to open wounds.

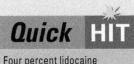

Four percent lidocaine (LMX-4 [Ferndale Laboratories, Inc., MI]) is an alternative to EMLA which is effective 20 to 30 minutes after application.

iii. Contact with the eyes should be avoided.
iv. Effectiveness of anesthesia is visible by the appearance of skin blanching.

c. **Subcutaneous infiltration** may be used to effect regional anesthesia at the site of the injury. Buffering of the injected agent with **sodium bicarbonate** may lessen the sensation of pain caused by the acidic nature of the anesthetic. Smaller gauge needles (30 or 27) and slower infiltration also decreases pain with injection. **Epinephrine hydrochloride** may be added to increase the duration of a block but should not be used in areas supplied by end arteries (e.g., the distal digits, nose, pinna, penis).
  i. **Lidocaine** (1% or 2%) can be infiltrated locally.
  ii. **Bupivacaine** (0.25% or 0.5%) may be used for prolonged anesthesia, particularly for nerve blocks.

d. **Peripheral nerve block** is achieved by local infiltration of a nerve supplying a wounded or painful area. Usually, 1% or 2% lidocaine is used without adrenaline. A peripheral nerve block should be used only by skilled personnel with prior training.

e. **Regional nerve block** is achieved by local infiltration of a nerve supplying an extremity. Usually, longer acting local anesthetics such as 0.5% bupivacaine or ropivacaine is used without epinephrine. This method is attempted by specially trained individuals to control painful procedures.

2. Sedation
   a. **Nitrous oxide** calms the emotional reaction to pain perception. It requires patient cooperation in the form of holding the mask to the face and is usually not indicated for children younger than 3 years of age. Nitrous oxide should be used only with continuous (transcutaneous) monitoring of the oxygen tension and cardiorespiratory function monitoring.

   b. **Ketamine** is a dissociative anesthetic that interrupts electrophysiologic perceptions between higher thalamocortical centers and limbic and medullary centers. Ketamine is most often used in combination with either local or regional anesthesia to induce amnesia during painful procedures. It is also useful for children with anxiety-induced bronchospasm.

   c. **Midazolam** may be used intranasally, orally, parenterally, or rectally. It is useful as an anxiolytic and has no analgesic effect. It may be used in combination with other medications (e.g., fentanyl, meperidine) to achieve a combination effect.
     i. Continuous monitoring is necessary for patients receiving combination therapy because of the degree of anesthesia. After the painful procedure is completed, care must be taken not to forget about the patient because a lack of pain drive afterward can result in profound respiratory depression.
     ii. At the bedside, midazolam plus fentanyl should be used only with the narcotic antagonist naloxone and the benzodiazepine antagonist flumazenil.

   d. **Propofol** is useful for rapid and deep induction of anesthesia within 40 seconds of injection but requires maintenance infusion for continued sedation. The incidence of apnea in 5% to 7% of patients necessitates cardiorespiratory monitoring and airway equipment at the bedside. There is a rapid emergence of alertness (within 3 to 5 minutes) after cessation of anesthesia. Propofol must be used only by physicians skilled in its usage; dosage guidelines are usually individualized to patient need.

   e. **Chloral hydrate** cannot be recommended because of its safety profile. The dosage is far too speculative for safety and usually provides for excessive recovery times in children. Chloral hydrate has been associated with aspiration syndromes.

(sidebar, left margin)

Pediatric Emergencies

Quick HIT

Ketamine may be associated with emergence phenomena that can manifest as psychosis.

Quick HIT

Midazolam plus **fentanyl** is extremely useful for very painful procedures (e.g., reduction of a fracture or dislocation).

Quick HIT

Chloral hydrate has in almost all cases been replaced by safer sedative agents.

E. **Disposition**
1. **Discharge.** Patients who have received anesthetics or sedatives may be discharged, provided that all immediate life threats have been addressed and the following have taken place:
   a. **Stable airway and cardiorespiratory function** are documented after careful monitoring.
   b. The patient has **full function** of the injured area and neurologic assessment of the area reveals **no deficits**.
   c. The patient is **neurologically intact** and has demonstrated **protective airway reflexes**.
   d. The patient is **able to function** commensurate with age and **able to walk** without staggering or falling (if age appropriate).
   e. The patient has **full truncal control** consistent with growth and development, is able to **sit unaided** (if age appropriate), and is able to **take liquids**.
2. **Additional monitoring or admission.** Any patient who does not return to functional baseline responsiveness should be monitored for additional time or admitted for further evaluation.

III. SUDDEN INFANT DEATH SYNDROME

A. **Discussion**
1. **Definition.** Sudden infant death syndrome (SIDS) is the sudden death of any infant or child younger than 1 year of age that is unexpected by history and not explained by findings on postmortem examination, examination of the past medical history, or a review of the death scene.
2. **Statistics**
   a. SIDS accounts for 40% to 60% of infant deaths between the ages of 1 month and 12 months and is the **most common cause** of postneonatal infant death in developed countries.
      i. Approximately 6,000 deaths occur each year with a peak age of incidence of 2 to 4 months.
      ii. Between 95% and 98% of all cases occur before or by 6 months of age, with almost no cases seen prior to 1 month of age.
   b. The rate in the general population in the United States is 1.3 to 2.5/1,000 live births.

B. **Clinical features**
1. **History**
   a. Children are usually discovered by parents or caregivers in the early morning hours lifeless and cyanotic with no cardiorespiratory effort. Most infants show signs of struggle and are often wrapped in bed clothing, suggesting entanglement. Vomitus is often found in the mouths of infants with SIDS, which suggests aspiration and apnea induced by secretions in the oral cavity.
   b. SIDS has been associated with nonspecific illnesses in the last 2 weeks of life and increased incidence of gastrointestinal illness preceding death. Fatigue during feedings in the week prior to death and profuse sweating during sleep are often present.

C. **Differential diagnoses**
1. **Infectious disorders** include primary or secondary meningitis or sepsis.
2. **Cardiovascular disorders** include undiagnosed critical coarctation of the aorta, severe tetralogy of Fallot, prolonged QT syndrome, or unrecognized arrhythmia.
3. **Environmental disorders** include hypothermia and hyperthermia or hyperthermia associated with undiagnosed cystic fibrosis.
4. **Inborn errors of metabolism** not previously diagnosed include branched-chain aminoacidopathy and many forms of fatty-acid metabolic defects, including medium-chain acetylcoenzyme A dehydrogenase deficiency.
5. **CNS disorders** include prolonged idiopathic seizures, unrecognized CNS hemorrhage due to arteriovenous malformation, or aneurysm rupture.

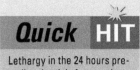

Quick HIT

Lethargy in the 24 hours preceding death is frequently seen and is associated with an intercurrent upper respiratory tract infection.

6. **Traumatic disorders** include particularly nonaccidental trauma that results in CNS events such as intraventricular and intracerebral hemorrhages and subarachnoid and subdural collections of blood.

7. **Asphyxiating injuries** can occur in infants who sleep with large, overweight parents who inadvertently roll onto the infant during sleep and in those who sleep in adult beds or in cribs with inappropriate bedding or other suffocation risks.

8. **Fluid and electrolyte disorders**, particularly following gastrointestinal illnesses, include hyponatremia, hypernatremia, hyperkalemia secondary to adrenal insufficiency, or profound dehydration with renal vein thrombosis.

9. **Toxicologic disorders** include inadvertent or purposeful administration of prescription drugs, such as diphenoxylate hydrochloride and atropine for diarrhea, or accidental ingestion of or poisoning with illicit drugs (e.g., cocaine, heroin).

10. **Idiopathic disorders** include Ondine curse and other hypoventilation syndromes.

D. **Evaluation**

1. **Antemortem evaluation.** Survivors of an apparent life-threatening event (ALTE) should be evaluated as follows:

    a. **Physical examination.** A careful physical examination should be performed to search for signs of nonaccidental trauma, such as unexplained bruising, retinal hemorrhages, strangulation marks, or handprints on the neck.

    b. **Laboratory studies** should include a CBC; serum electrolyte panel; creatinine phosphokinase determination; prolactin serum concentration; ABG determination; urinalysis for microscopic and amino acid analysis; and culture of blood, CSF, and urine. Urine should also be obtained for toxicologic analysis.

    c. **Radiologic studies** should include a full skeletal survey including two views of all body areas. A single "babygram" is *not* acceptable and will frequently miss rib and metaphyseal fractures. Repeat imaging in 10 to 14 days may be indicated in cases of suspected abuse because acute fractures, particularly of the ribs, may not be visible on initial X-rays.

2. **Postmortem examination.** A thorough postmortem examination must be performed on all infants who are suspected to have died of SIDS (see Clinical Pearl 15-2). The emergency physician should not allow attending physicians of the deceased infant to take responsibility for the death, even in children with chronic and protracted neonatal illnesses such as bronchopulmonary dysplasia.

E. **Therapy**

1. **Resuscitation.** Most infants found cold and with dependent lividity are essentially dead at the scene, and all resuscitation attempts are futile.

    a. Infants who respond to maternal or first-responder **cardiopulmonary resuscitation** are salvageable in 80% to 90% of cases when provided with adequate pediatric emergency care.

    b. No medications are effective in preventing SIDS. **Caffeine** is administered to infants with apnea of prematurity as a respiratory stimulant and is effective for improving the arousal responsiveness in some, but not all, infants.

CLINICAL PEARL 15-2

Autopsy Findings in Patients with SIDS

a. Mild pulmonary edema

b. Intrathoracic petechia

c. Evidence of chronic asphyxia

d. Brain stem dendritic spines with reactive astrocytosis

e. Elevated substance P, which is a neurotransmitter

f. Hypoplasia of the arcuate nucleus in the medulla

g. Prenatal and postnatal growth retardation

2. **Monitoring.** Survivors of an ALTE should be offered home monitoring after risks and benefits are fully explained to parents. Children should be monitored under the direction of a specialist with expertise in SIDS. Monitoring should be discontinued only under the direction of the primary physician and never by an emergency physician.

F. **Disposition.** In all cases, the appropriate authorities should be notified, including police and child protective agencies. A thorough investigation of the death scene should be performed by individuals skilled in such investigations. Photographs should be taken for later correlation with findings on postmortem examination.

1. **Survivors** of an ALTE should be admitted to the hospital for a thorough and complete medical and cardiorespiratory evaluation and monitoring.

   a. Prior to hospital discharge, **parents of infants who have survived** an initial ALTE should fully understand home monitoring and should be taught cardiopulmonary resuscitation according to American Heart Association standards.

   b. Infants who were under the care of a private physician should be referred back to them. **Private-practice physicians** should be intimately involved in all decisions with regard to monitoring and other apparent concerns of the parents of such children.

   c. Survivors of ALTE should be fully evaluated in established centers for SIDS with appropriate sleep and awake pneumograms and other studies as clinically indicated.

2. **Infants who do not survive.** Considerations for the remaining family members include the following:

   a. A careful evaluation of other siblings should be performed following the death of the index infant.

   b. Appropriate social services counseling should be offered to the parents and immediate family members following such events and in the weeks after the event.

   c. A follow-up visit for the physician caring for the infant at death as well as the parents and immediate family members should be arranged after the results of all toxicologic and postmortem studies are completed. This meeting is crucial because many unwarranted fears and concerns may be dispelled by such a meeting.

IV. FOREIGN BODIES

A. **Discussion**

1. **Definition.** A foreign body is any substance that is not natural to the body passage in which it is found. Foreign bodies are common in infants and young children because of their common exploration and experimentation by putting things in the mouth, ears, or nasal passages, and occasionally inadequate supervision by adults. The majority of foreign bodies placed in the mouth are swallowed. A smaller percentage of objects are aspirated into the respiratory tree; approximately 50% of aspiration episodes are unwitnessed by caregivers.

2. **Severity.** Although most foreign objects are expelled immediately by the cough reflex and never require medical attention, foreign body injury is the most common cause of injury-related death in children younger than 1 year of age. Factors that influence the severity of the situation include:

   a. **Size of the foreign body.** Large foreign objects that nearly or completely occlude the upper airway pose an immediate life threat and must be emergently removed.

   b. **Location of the foreign body.** The location is directly related to the size of the pediatric airway. The younger the child is, the greater the chance that the site of obstruction will be more proximal. Large esophageal foreign bodies can produce respiratory compromise due to compression of the adjacent airway structures (see Clinical Pearl 15-3).

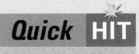

Quick HIT

Similar-aged infant siblings have a 20-fold greater risk of sudden infant death than the general population and should be offered interventional monitoring or further study for risk factors.

Pediatric Emergencies

CLINICAL PEARL **15-3**

1. Esophageal foreign objects are most likely to become lodged at one of three sites of natural narrowing in the esophagus: the thoracic inlet, the level of the aortic arch, and the gastroesophageal junction.
2. The **larynx** and **cricopharyngeus muscle** are the most common sites of airway involvement in children younger than 1 year.
3. The **trachea** and **bronchi** are the most common sites involved in children between the ages of 15 and 48 months. Despite the acute angle of the left main stem bronchus, the propensity for the object lodging in either side is approximately 50%.

    c. **Composition of the foreign object.** Plant and other organic matter usually is much more tenacious and irritating than inorganic materials. Long, sharp objects (such as sewing needles) pose a risk of perforation if ingested. Caustic materials, such as disc batteries, can cause erosion leading to scarring and stenosis or perforation if they remain in the nose or gastrointestinal tract for a prolonged period of time.

B. **Clinical findings.** A high index of suspicion for foreign body aspiration must be held for any child who presents with unexplained respiratory symptoms.
  1. Many patients with aspiration events may have a **symptom-free interval** during which the body attempts to wall off the object. Walling off leads to definitive symptoms.
  2. The **symptoms**, **physical findings**, and **complication rate** depend on the nature of the aspirated foreign object, the location of the obstruction, and the degree of obstruction.
    a. **Laryngeal foreign bodies** cause an **obstructive cough** that becomes hoarse and brassy, resembling the sound of croup.
      i. This cough must be recognized quickly and managed correctly.
      ii. Hot dogs and bread are the two most commonly aspirated substances that lodge in the larynx. Bread and peanut butter are particularly irritating and tenacious, making removal difficult.
    b. **Tracheal foreign bodies** cause **cough** and **wheezing, intermittent cyanosis**, and a peculiar **precordial thud**, caused by the object impacting against the subglottic area.
    c. **Bronchial foreign bodies** often present with **blood-streaked sputum, cough**, and **dyspnea** with or without wheezing or absent air sounds.
      i. Initially, the child may be symptom-free, but later, unilateral wheezing or prolongation of the expiratory phase may be noted.
      ii. Edema and lodging of the foreign body in a smaller subsegmental airway may result in obstruction to outflow of air and air trapping or atelectasis and mediastinal shift toward (with air trapping) or away from (with atelectasis) the side of the obstructing foreign body.

C. **Differential diagnoses**
  1. **Pneumonia syndrome** (see V.E). The sudden onset of symptoms will usually not confuse the astute clinician but may well be confused with more protracted symptoms seen in smaller foreign body aspirations. Physical examination findings are helpful only if air trapping or unilateral wheezing is noted.
  2. **Croup syndrome** (see V.A). The sudden onset of symptoms is often confused with this entity acutely, but the lack of fever mitigates against the diagnosis.
  3. **Acute epiglottitis** (see V.D) usually occurs in older children and is usually heralded by high fever (i.e., greater than 103°F), toxicity, and air hunger. Epiglottitis is rarely seen because of the widespread use of vaccine preparations specific for *Haemophilus influenzae*.

D. **Evaluation**
  1. **History and physical examination.** A suggestive history and confirmatory physical examination are the most important diagnostic tools initially.

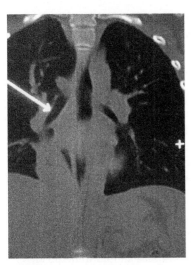

FIGURE 15-1 CT chest showing foreign body (whistle) in right mainstem bronchus.

2. Imaging studies
   a. **Roentgenographic examination** is truly useful only for radiopaque foreign bodies but may be beneficial for asymmetric lung expansion or collapse.
   b. **Radiographic examination**
      i. **General considerations**
         a) The **plane** in which the foreign object lies aids in differential location of the object (Figure 15-1).
            1) If the object is in the **sagittal** plane, it is probably in the larynx.
            2) If in the **coronal** plane, it is probably in the esophagus.
         b) The **administration of contrast agents** may also guide the location of the foreign object if it is in the esophagus.
      ii. **Plain films** are often helpful for diagnosing bronchial foreign bodies, especially in patients with overinflation syndromes and collapse. If an object causes complete obstruction in the expiratory phase but allows air to pass in the inspiratory phase, air becomes trapped and hyperinflation is seen. This appears as a hyperlucency of the involved side.
   c. **Bronchoscopy** is usually the only way to definitively diagnose and treat tracheal foreign bodies
3. **Laboratory studies** are seldom helpful in the management of acute or subacute obstructions with foreign bodies but may be useful with chronic obstructions that were missed. **Blood cultures** are usually not warranted, except for chronic foreign body ingestion of vegetable matter, particularly peanuts, which produces a cough, a septic type of fever, dyspnea, and chronic suppuration.
E. **Therapy**
1. **Object removal.** Patients with acute, life-threatening foreign body aspirations should be treated emergently at the scene by either chest blows and thrusts or abdominal thrusts, depending on the age of the patient, while attempting to maintain oxygenation. Most ingested foreign bodies can be addressed nonemergently; proximal esophageal foreign bodies causing respiratory compromise require emergent endoscopy. Any foreign body remaining in the esophagus requires urgent removal. Button batteries and long (>5 cm), sharp objects (such as sewing needles) pose special risks and require urgent surgical or gastroenterology consultation; if they are beyond the stomach, serial X-rays should be obtained every 2 to 3 days to document progression and ultimate clearance of the foreign body.
   a. In a child who can cough, breathe, or speak, **nonintervention** is essential. A natural cough is more effective than airway or chest-compressive maneuvers. Blind sweeps of the pharynx and hypopharynx in an awake and

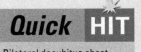

Quick **HIT**

Bilateral decubitus chest films can demonstrate unilateral air trapping in a patient who cannot cooperate to perform inspiratory/expiratory films.

Pediatric Emergencies

alert child may induce vomiting and may further lodge the object deeper into the airway, producing complete obstruction.

b. For a child younger than 1 year of age who is unresponsive, **back blows** and chest thrusts are recommended in concert with attempts at ventilation.

c. For an unresponsive child older than 1 year, **abdominal thrusts** may be performed in accordance with published standards in addition to attempts at ventilation. Abdominal thrusts are not used for children younger than 1 year of age because of the risk of perforating the abdominal viscus.

d. Children in whom abdominal thrusts or chest thrusts fail to dislodge the object may require **advanced airway adjuncts** to bypass the site of the obstruction until the object can be removed. Airway adjuncts include:

   i. Needle cricothyrotomy
   ii. Surgical cricothyrotomy
   iii. Rigid bronchoscopy
   iv. Open bronchotomy

e. **Endoscopy.** Children with more distal foreign bodies should undergo endoscopy as soon as practical. A delay doubles the morbidity and mortality.

f. **Surgery** may be necessary to remove the object.

2. **Bronchodilator therapy** is not recommended because of the risk of dislodging a distal foreign body and having it lodge in a larger airway.

3. **Antibiotic therapy** may be indicated if a secondary infection has developed, or in patients with subacute or chronic obstructions. Initiation of antibiotic therapy should not delay the removal of foreign objects.

F. Disposition

1. **Discharge.** Children in whom the foreign body has been expelled, or in whom a swallowed foreign body has entered the stomach, may be discharged to home without further intervention or therapy except for accident counseling.

2. **Admission.** Children in whom surgical manipulation is necessary to clear obstructions warrant admission to the hospital for 24 hours or less.

3. **Referral.** Children with chronic unrecognized aspiration syndromes should have consultation with not only an otolaryngologist but also a surgeon with regard for the need for lobectomy.

V. RESPIRATORY TRACT INFECTIONS

A. Laryngotracheobronchitis (croup syndrome) is the most common form of non–life-threatening acute upper airway obstruction in childhood.

1. Discussion

   a. **Cause.** Nearly all cases of croup are caused by viral pathogens in only three distinct viral groups: influenzae, adenovirus, and parainfluenza viruses.

   b. **Incidence.** Boys are affected more often than girls. Croup is more common during the colder months of the year, paralleling the prevalence of the most common viral causes of this entity.

   c. **Predisposing factors.** Approximately 20% of affected children have a strong family history of similar illness, and 5% to 10% of children have recurrences of similar symptoms. Recurrences are infrequent after age 7 years, as the size of the airway increases.

2. Clinical features

   a. **Course.** Most patients have an **upper respiratory syndrome** for several days preceding the onset of the characteristic symptom complex. The disease is usually prolonged over 7 days. Characteristically, croup syndrome is worse over the first 3 days, and then gradual improvement occurs over the next 4 days.

   b. **Symptoms** and **signs** are characteristically worse at night, with a propensity for 10:00 p.m., and children are most often brought to the ED following the initial event.

      i. A **"seal-like" barking** or **brassy cough with agitation** is characteristic of croup and is usually diagnosed by parents prior to arrival at treatment facilities. The characteristic cough results from edema in the immediate subglottic region of the trachea.

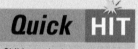

Quick HIT

Children who have severe croup or continued recurrences after 7 or 8 years of age should undergo otolaryngology evaluation to exclude airway anomalies, mass, or foreign body.

ii. As obstruction increases, **stridor** develops that is initially inspiratory only. With progression of disease, stridor becomes both inspiratory and expiratory in nature.

iii. With worsening disease, the bronchi and bronchioles are affected. The **respiratory effort becomes more labored**, and fatigue ensues. Such worsening is usually seen in younger infants. Most infants are usually comfortable at rest in the caregiver's arms and usually do not display air hunger or drooling.

iv. **Temperature elevations** are common with croup.

3. **Differential diagnosis**

   a. **Acute epiglottitis** (see V.D) is characterized by a rapid and fulminant course of high fever with temperatures in excess of 103°F, sore throat, skin mottling, progressive air hunger, and drooling.

   b. **Acute infectious laryngitis** is usually preceded by a viral upper respiratory syndrome (e.g., laryngotracheobronchitis) but with little or no fever. Hoarseness or vocal loss is usually seen without the stridor or brassy cough. Physical examination usually does not demonstrate any accentuation of hoarseness with activity or signs of cardiovascular compromise.

   c. **Acute spasmodic laryngitis** is clinically indistinguishable from acute infectious laryngotracheobronchitis except for absence of fever. Acute spasmodic laryngitis tends to occur rapidly and is often associated with hoarseness in addition to stridor. Patients usually appear well. Illness usually lasts only 24 to 36 hours and abates without treatment. Recurrences are common and aid in the diagnosis in most cases.

   d. **Bacterial tracheitis** is associated with high fever and profound toxicity shortly after clinical symptoms occur. Initially, bacterial tracheitis usually is indistinguishable from acute laryngotracheobronchitis, but progressive worsening over 48 hours and prostration usually point to the correct diagnosis. Copious, thick purulent secretions are the rule.

   e. **Foreign body aspiration** usually occurs suddenly with choking and coughing and without antecedent upper respiratory infection or fever. Foreign body aspiration may be associated with unilateral or bilateral wheezing or may progress to complete airway obstruction.

   f. **Peritonsillar abscess.** Usually, visible upper airway extrinsic compression is evident. This condition is rare in children younger than 10 years. Drooling is seen that is associated with hoarseness but little or no stridor.

   g. **Retropharyngeal abscess.** This condition is seen in toddlers and young children and rarely occurs after 10 to 12 years of age. Infection involving the deep neck tissues and prevertebral lymph nodes causes airway compression, limited extension and rotation of the neck, high fever, and drooling. Neck swelling is often noted on examination.

4. **Evaluation**

   a. **Laboratory studies** are rarely needed and are seldom helpful in management. A **CBC** may reveal lymphocytosis and occasionally neutropenia. **Bacterial** and **viral cultures**, although beneficial for epidemiologic inference, are costly and do not affect care.

   b. **Pulse oximetry** is more beneficial for the child who is stridulous at rest and may provide a better guide to respiratory fatigue in the comfortable and nonthreatening environment of a caregiver's arms. **Hypoxemia**, as measured by pulse oximetry, is **usually not a feature** of this disease. If present in an older child, it suggests another diagnosis.

   c. **Radiographic studies** including chest and soft tissue radiography are confirmatory but often do not definitively differentiate any diagnosis except for epiglottitis.

5. **Therapy**

   a. **Vaporization.** Most children with mild to moderate laryngotracheobronchitis can be managed safely at home if their only manifestation is a brassy cough and stridor with agitation only.

      i. **Cool mist vaporization** at home is the preferred treatment because of its intrinsic safety and because of its efficacy for providing some

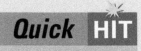

Quick HIT

Profound hypoxemia, air hunger, drooling, and hypotension suggest another diagnosis and mandate immediate referral for specialty care.

humidification to the upper airway. Ultrasonic home nebulizers are best when available but are cost prohibitive for many families.

    ii. In addition to vaporization, a **bathroom filled with the steam from a hot shower** is often therapeutic and can avert a trip to the hospital. Safety is a concern for the unattended child. Cool or warm mist devices may also be helpful.

    iii. Perhaps the cheapest and easiest home remedy is to **take the child outside into the moist, cool air for a period of 30 to 60 minutes**. Often the simple act of driving in the family car with the windows down is enough to allay an attack of coughing for several hours.

  b. **Nebulization.** Children with stridor at rest must be seen and evaluated in a hospital by practitioners experienced in the care of such children. Research has failed to demonstrate any measureable improvement with mist or nebulized saline treatments.

    i. **Racemic epinephrine.** Children with **moderate to severe stridor at rest** and those with labored breathing should be treated with nebulized racemic epinephrine (2.25% solution diluted 1:5 or 1:8 with water and given 4 mL nebulized over 15 minutes).

      a) Children treated in this manner should be observed in the ED for at least 2 hours prior to discharge.

      b) Past literature suggested that such children may need hospital admission because of the rebound of stridor and potential worsening.

        1) Most children rebound in 2 hours.

        2) Children with extenuating circumstances should be considered for admission, particularly children in poor social situations, for whom shower facilities are unavailable or long commuting distances to the hospital exist.

  c. **Administration of dexamethasone.** Dexamethasone is preferred over prednisone or prednisolone because of its half-life of 36 to 55 hours, which frequently is all that is necessary for treatment for most cases of stridor.

    i. Children who received 0.6 to 1.0 mg/kg of dexamethasone were much improved over children who received cool mist nebulization alone and for longer periods. Studies have demonstrated that oral dexamethasone is as effective as intramuscular or intravenous dosing, without the additional pain and anxiety associated with injection or intravenous placement. Dosing of 0.15, 0.3, and 0.6 mg/kg resulted in similar outcomes.

    ii. Side effects are very rare and do not warrant additional monitoring with single-dose therapy. Anecdotal reports of corticosteroid use worsening the presentation of common childhood illnesses (e.g., varicella) exist but have not been substantiated in more rigorous prospective studies.

  d. **Intubation** may be necessary for children who present in marked respiratory distress.

    i. The endotracheal tube should be one size smaller than the ideal size required for the age of the child.

    ii. The use of paralytic agents for such intubated children is beyond the scope of this text but may be required because of agitation.

    iii. The addition of repeated doses of dexamethasone should be considered in children who require prolonged intubation.

6. **Disposition**

  a. **Discharge**

    i. Most patients can be managed at home with humidification procedures as outlined above, particularly children who have only **stridor with agitation** or **cough** and are otherwise well. Dexamethasone (0.6 mg/kg) may markedly improve outcome and prevent worsening.

    ii. Children with **stridor at rest** and/or labored breathing may be treated with nebulized racemic epinephrine and a single dose of dexamethasone 0.15 to 0.6 mg/kg. Such children are observed in the department for a minimum of 2 hours and, if free of symptoms, are discharged to close follow-up evaluation within 24 to 48 hours.

   b. **Admission**

      i. Children who require multiple racemic epinephrine doses or are **worse** or **unchanged** 2 hours after treatment should be considered for hospital admission and further treatment with additional doses of dexamethasone or an inhaled corticosteroid.

      ii. Children rarely present in **marked respiratory distress** but may require endotracheal intubation and hospitalization in an intensive care setting.

B. Bronchiolitis is a common disease of the lower respiratory tract of infants. It is the most common cause of acute respiratory distress and wheezing in small infants and the most common cause of hospitalization for infants between the ages of 6 and 20 months.

  1. **Discussion**

    a. **Cause.** Bronchiolitis is predominantly a viral illness.

      i. **Respiratory syncytial virus** accounts for more than 50% of cases.

      ii. **Parainfluenza virus 3** and **adenovirus** account for 30% to 40% of cases.

      iii. *Mycoplasma* and *H. influenzae* cause fewer than 5% of all cases.

    b. **Incidence.** Bronchiolitis occurs during the first 48 months of life, with a peak incidence in patients between the ages of 6 and 8 months. Incidence is highest in winter and early spring months, but it occurs throughout the year in more temperate climates with less epidemic periodicity.

    c. **Predisposing factors.** Bronchiolitis is most common in boys who have not been breastfed and who live in crowded family quarters with heavy cigarette smokers.

    d. **Pathogenesis.** Bronchiolitis is characterized by bronchiolar obstruction caused by edema and accumulation of mucus and debris, leading to a dramatic increase in airway resistance.

      i. There is no evidence for bacterial infection as a primary event.

      ii. Usually, the course of bronchiolitis is benign but may be severe.

        a) **Bronchiolitis obliterans**, a sclerosing bronchiolitis, is most often caused by adenovirus.

        b) **Unilateral hyperlucent lung syndrome** (Swyer-James syndrome), a unilateral variant of bronchiolitis obliterans, results in a radiographic picture that suggests lobar emphysema.

      iii. Respiratory rates in excess of 60 breaths/min are directly correlated with hypoxemia and hypercapnia.

  2. **Clinical features**

    a. **Symptoms**

      i. Bronchiolitis begins with a **serous nasal discharge**, **sneezing**, and a **mild fever** (101°F to 102°F). Gradually, respiratory distress develops that is characterized by **wheezing**, **cough**, **intercostal retraction**, and **irritability**.

      ii. **Decreased appetite** follows increasing respiratory rates in infants 6 months of age or younger because of obligate nasal breathing patterns and because of the coordinated efforts required to suck and breathe simultaneously.

      iii. **Posttussive emesis** may occur and may mimic the postcough whoop or stridor of pertussis; paroxysmal cough similar to pertussis is also common with bronchiolitis.

    b. **Physical examination findings** include tachypnea, flaring of the nasal alae, and retractions; pallor and cyanosis are associated with more severe disease. Rales and expiratory wheeze are common. Artifactual hepatosplenomegaly may be detected because of air trapping with a decrease in the diaphragmatic movement and increased downward excursion of the diaphragm.

  3. **Differential diagnoses**

    a. **Reactive airway disease** is the most commonly confused entity. This condition is usually associated with a positive family history of reactive airway

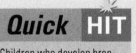

Quick HIT

Children who develop bronchiolitis usually had an exposure to older children with minor respiratory symptoms 1 to 2 weeks prior to illness.

Pediatric Emergencies

CLINICAL PEARL 15-4

Congestive Heart Failure Signs and Symptoms

1. **Slowed feeding** for weeks prior to the onset of respiratory symptoms is common in children with CHF.
2. **True organomegaly** is seen and is characterized by not only an increase in the ability to palpate the organ but also by an actual enlargement of the organs caused by stasis that can be demonstrated by percussion of the span on the body surface.
3. The history is usually positive for **sweating** during feedings or **cyanosis** with feedings or increased activity.
4. **Precordial deformity** with or without thrill or murmur is often seen with a shift in the point of maximum impulse laterally.
5. **Isolated tachypnea** without other respiratory symptoms or fever is often the earliest clinical finding.
6. **Hypoxia that fails to improve with oxygen therapy is indicative of a cardiac mixing lesion with right to left shunting of blood flow.**

disease in immediate family members or parents. Repeated bouts of wheezing in the same infant within the same respiratory season are highly suggestive for reactive airway disease. The onset is sudden without antecedent viral syndrome. One or two treatments of nebulized albuterol sulfate usually produce an immediate response.

b. **Congestive heart failure (CHF)** is often confused with bronchiolitis initially, but associated other symptoms often guide the clinician (see Clinical Pearl 15-4).

c. **Foreign body aspiration** is usually not difficult to differentiate initially. There is a sudden onset of dyspnea and unilateral or bilateral wheezing without antecedent upper respiratory symptoms and little or no response to nebulized bronchodilator therapy. The history is usually positive for choking immediately preceding the onset of wheezing and dyspnea.

d. **Pertussis syndrome.** A catarrhal stage of pertussis initially appears similar to early bronchiolitis, but copious secretions that are thick and tenacious are uncommon in bronchiolitis. The characteristic staccato cough and expiratory whoop or stridor usually are not confused with bronchiolitis. Prolonged illness for 4 to 5 weeks is usual in children with pertussis, with periods of profound apnea seen in infants.

e. **Cystic fibrosis** is not usually confused with bronchiolitis except in severely affected smaller infants. Family history of a previously affected child may be helpful in differentiation. Recurrent episodes of wheezing and pneumonia associated with failure to thrive suggest the diagnosis, as does a positive sweat chloride test. Cystic fibrosis is most common in Caucasian infants.

f. **Bronchopneumonia with bronchospasm** is commonly confused with bronchiolitis in small wheezing infants. Chest radiography is helpful in half of cases with perihilar, segmental, or subsegmental infiltrates. Other signs of consolidation are often seen, such as dullness to percussion, decreased air entry, and diminished breath sounds.

4. **Evaluation.** Patients with **known cardiac problems** or **bronchopulmonary dysplasia** should be promptly evaluated regardless of the severity of symptoms. Most patients with mild bronchiolitis require no testing.

a. **Radiographic examination** reveals hyperinflation and scattered areas of consolidation in 30% to 40% of patients.

b. **Laboratory studies** are seldom helpful acutely.

  i. **CBC.** A CBC usually reveals a normal white blood cell (WBC) count and differential.

  ii. **ABG determinations** are seldom indicated; the severe pain associated with the procedure often predisposes to exaggerated hypoxemia due to segmental collapse. **Transcutaneous oximetry** provides a more reliable method of assessing trends in oxygen saturation.

  iii. **Nasopharyngeal washings** allow retrieval of cells from which a diagnosis of the specific etiologic agent can be made. Outside of the neonatal period, viral testing is unlikely to change the patient's management or disposition; neonates with respiratory syncytial virus are at an increased risk for apnea and should be hospitalized for monitoring.

    iv. **Viral culture** is of no cost-effective proven benefit.

    v. **Serology.** Increases in specific **antibody titers**, although of epidemiologic importance, may not be of distinct clinical importance.

5. **Therapy.** The most **critical phase** of illness is the first 48 to 72 hours after the beginning of cough and dyspnea. In infants who are not affected by feeding difficulties at 48 to 72 hours into the illness, the illness will most likely resolve without consequence.

  a. **Supportive care** is usually all that is indicated; nasal suctioning, smaller and more frequent feeds, and close follow-up with their primary care provider are adequate for most infants. Intravenous fluids, deep suctioning, and oxygen therapy may be necessary in those with more severe illness

  b. **Antibiotics** have no value except when the possibility of a secondary bacterial pneumonia is likely.

  c. **Corticosteroids** have no place in therapy; multiple clinical trials of these agents have failed to demonstrate benefit in patients with bronchiolitis.

  d. **Bronchodilators** administered by nebulized routes are often used empirically with no proven effect. Albuterol may be effective for those infants (approximately 20%) with reactive airways; racemic epinephrine can improve work of breathing in those infants with severe **respiratory distress**. Hypertonic saline nebulizations has shown benefit in some studies.

6. **Disposition**

  a. **Discharge.** Infants with **mild wheezing** and **dyspnea** may be evaluated and managed at home with close follow-up evaluation, provided parents are able to understand the illness and the need for appropriate intervention if the condition worsens.

  b. **Admission.** Infants with **severe dyspnea**, **hypoxia** (<92%), **extreme tachypnea** (>70), or **dehydration** secondary to feeding difficulties should be considered for hospitalization.

C. **Pharyngitis**

1. **Discussion.** Pharyngitis describes any infection of the pharynx, including tonsillitis, pharyngotonsillitis, and uvulitis. Most commonly, pharyngitis occurs as part of an upper respiratory tract infection with secondary involvement.

  a. **Incidence.** Pharyngitis is uncommon in children younger than 2 years. There is a peak incidence in children 4 to 7 years of age.

  b. **Etiology**

    i. Pharyngitis is caused by **viruses** in approximately 85% to 90% of cases.

    ii. **Group A β-hemolytic streptococci** are the only common and significant bacterial pathogens, accounting for approximately 10% to 15% of cases.

2. **Clinical features** differ depending on whether bacteria or viruses are the cause.

  a. **Viral pharyngitis** is a disease of gradual onset usually with malaise, upper respiratory symptoms, and myalgias.

    i. A **sore throat** usually begins 1 to 3 days after the onset of symptoms. **Hoarseness**, **cough**, and **rhinitis** are common and are the reason for primary medical attention.

    ii. **Inflammation** may be relatively minor.

    iii. **Small ulcerations** may be visible on the palate and posterior pharyngeal wall.

      a) Ulcerations that start posteriorly and extend **anteriorly** are usually caused by coxsackievirus.

      b) Ulceration that begins at the gingival margins is usually caused by herpes simplex.

    iv. Exudates are rarely present, and no uvula edema or palatal petechiae occur.

  b. **Bacterial (streptococcal) pharyngitis** is usually seen in children 2 years of age or older. Associated symptoms include the following:

    i. **Fever** in excess of 104°F

    ii. **Tonsillar enlargement** and exudates; **fetid odor** of breath

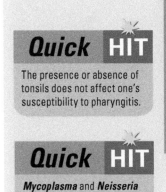

Quick HIT

The presence or absence of tonsils does not affect one's susceptibility to pharyngitis.

Quick HIT

Mycoplasma and *Neisseria* species also cause pharyngitis but usually in adolescents.

Pediatric Emergencies

       iii. **Cervical adenopathy**, usually moderate and painful but not fluctuant

       iv. **Palatal petechiae** and **uvula edema** (40% to 60% of cases); diagnostic when present

       v. **Cough**, **rhinitis**, or **hoarseness** (rare)

3. **Differential diagnoses**

   a. **Viral syndrome** is associated with hoarseness and cough. The course is usually mild, and often there are no exudates.

   b. **Infectious mononucleosis** is a nonspecific illness in children younger than 10 years. In adolescents, it is often confused with a streptococcal infection. Associated splenomegaly and generalized adenopathy are helpful in making the diagnosis. The monospot or heterophile antibody tests are not helpful for children younger than 6 years. However, a positive test in young children remains diagnostic.

   c. **Diphtheria.** In patients with diphtheria, a very adherent membranous exudate is present on the tonsils, posterior pharynx, or palate. This disease may be associated with cardiac symptoms and signs of tachycardia out of proportion to fever.

   d. **Herpangina.** A tonsillar exudate is not usually seen. However, multiple shallow ulcerations are seen on the pillars, palate, and fauces (throat).

4. **Evaluation.** Laboratory studies are seldom useful. However:

   a. **Rapid antigen detection methods** for streptococcal infection are accurate in 85% to 90% of cases.

       i. Children with **negative rapid antigen detection** should have a definitive **culture** performed.

       ii. Children with **positive rapid antigen detection** should be considered to have a proven streptococcal infection and should be treated appropriately.

   b. **Serologic testing** for streptococcal antibody response is not warranted.

5. **Therapy**

   a. **Antibiotic therapy.** If antigen detection methods are available, treatment should be guided by results of such testing. Treatment usually results in rapid improvement if it begins before the fifth day of the illness. Reculture is usually not necessary unless symptoms do not abate after 7 to 10 days of effective therapy.

       i. **Penicillin V potassium** (125 to 250 mg/dose, administered four times daily) for 10 days is usually the cheapest alternative.

       ii. **Amoxicillin (40 to 45mg/kg/day, given once or twice daily) for those patients who cannot swallow pills due to the poor tolerance of liquid penicillin**

       iii. **Erythromycin** (50 mg/kg/day, divided into three doses) or azithromycin (10 mg/kg/day for 5 days) is effective for penicillin-allergic patients.

       iv. **Intramuscular long-acting benzathine penicillin** as a single one-time treatment is indicated when compliance is an issue or the patient is vomiting or refusing oral medications.

   b. **Supportive therapy**

       i. **Saline gargles** and **cool liquids** are beneficial for relief of symptoms.

       ii. **Topical anesthesia** with viscous anesthetic agents is usually not warranted, particularly when the possibility for systemic absorption is possible in younger children.

6. **Disposition.** Most patients with pharyngitis can be managed with conservative antibiotic therapy.

D. **Epiglottitis**

1. **Discussion**

   a. Epiglottitis is a dramatic, potentially life-threatening condition that occurs in children between the ages of 2 and 7 years. Previously, the peak age of incidence was 36 to 42 months, but the widespread use of the conjugated *H. influenzae* vaccine has shifted the age of incidence toward adolescent and adult age groups.

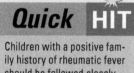

Quick **HIT**

Children with a positive family history of rheumatic fever should be followed closely and considered for prophylactic therapy.

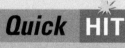

Quick **HIT**

The widespread use of the conjugated *H. influenzae* vaccine has significantly decreased the incidence of this disease.

b. Approximately 70% of children who develop epiglottitis have bacteremia caused by *H. influenzae* type b. Children who develop epiglottitis have a qualitatively and quantitatively different antibody response to the causative organism. Since the advent of the *H. influenzae* vaccine, staphylococcal and streptococcal species cause the majority of cases of epiglottitis.

2. **Clinical features.** Epiglottitis has a fulminant course characterized by a high fever, sore throat, dysphagia, progressive dyspnea, and stridor.

a. **Symptoms**

    i. **Respiratory symptoms.** The characteristic presentation is abrupt onset of high fever, drooling, relative aphonia, and inspiratory stridor. Older children may have only sore throat and dysphagia as the presenting symptoms; as a result, epiglottitis may mimic peritonsillar abscess in that age group. Within 1 to 2 hours of presentation, airway obstruction becomes more severe and may progress to complete obstruction if not managed properly.

    ii. **Posture.** Children appear apprehensive, with their posture usually upright and forward in the tripod position (the chin and neck extended forward and mouth open, often with the tongue extruded forward).

    iii. **Skin tone.** Children may have a mottled or ashen skin coloration, which implies serious illness and, in most instances, bacteremia.

b. **Physical examination findings** include moderate to severe respiratory distress with inspiratory and (rarely) expiratory stridor. Retraction of the suprasternal, intercostal, and supraclavicular areas is a sign of impending respiratory failure.

3. **Differential diagnoses**

a. **Bacterial tracheitis.** Children with bacterial tracheitis are usually profoundly ill with temperature elevation in the range of 106°F to 107°F. Their cough is productive of thick, purulent secretions that are seen on establishment of an endotracheal airway.

b. **Diphtheric croup** is usually characterized by a gray adherent membrane. There may be evidence of cardiotoxicity.

c. **Measles croup** is seen always in conjunction with cough, coryza, conjunctivitis, and the classical morbilliform eruption.

d. **Acute spasmodic laryngotracheobronchitis** occurs in children between the ages of 1 and 5 years. Often, there is a previous history of similar attacks. The child is usually afebrile and not drooling.

e. **Acute infectious laryngotracheobronchitis.** Hoarseness and a barking, seal-like cough are seen with mild fever in a well-appearing infant.

f. **Foreign body aspiration.** There is a sudden onset of symptoms, usually in the daylight hours, after the child has been awake for some time. The age of highest incidence is 6 to 24 months. Usually, there is no fever or other evident signs of infection.

g. **Retropharyngeal abscess** is usually a disease of toddlers with a subacute onset of symptoms. Radiographic examination of the lateral cervical airway is often helpful. This condition is usually associated with a muffled voice but not stridor.

h. **Peritonsillar abscess** may mimic epiglottitis only in dysphagia, but there usually is no stridor. A muffled voice is characteristic but usually is seen only in the adolescent and older age group.

4. **Evaluation.** Epiglottitis is a **true medical emergency**; evaluation and treatment must occur in tandem.

a. Children with **severe symptoms** should not be subjected to routine diagnostic procedures but should be **evaluated in an operating room** by a team of physicians skilled in airway management, such as:

    i. Pediatric intensive care physician or skilled pediatrician

    ii. Otolaryngologist with skills in placement of tracheostomy if necessary

    iii. Anesthesiologist capable of intubation of the complicated airway

b. **Laryngoscopy.** Definitive diagnosis is by direct visualization of the large edematous epiglottis using **direct laryngoscopy** or **fiberoptic laryngoscopy**

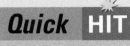

***Quick* HIT**

Restlessness, agitation, and air hunger follow shortly after retractions and are the earliest, but most severe, signs of impending obstruction.

***Quick* HIT**

Bacterial tracheitis usually is misdiagnosed initially and presents late in a shock-like state.

***Quick* HIT**

The child may have a fulminant course complicated by measles pneumonia.

***Quick* HIT**

The hoarseness and loss of voice are out of proportion to the degree of illness in infectious laryngotracheobronchitis.

Pediatric Emergencies

in the controlled environment of the operating room. Occasionally, a co-operative child will allow the visualization of a red epiglottis on tongue protrusion, but no attempt should be made to use a tongue blade for visualization. Manipulation of the airway with tongue blades or other instruments should not be attempted without supervision and with airway-adjunctive equipment at the bedside.

c. **Radiography.** Children who appear acutely ill with suspected epiglottitis should *not* undergo radiographic evaluation. In children with **mild stridor** who are not acutely ill, a single lateral neck radiograph helps with the diagnosis of epiglottitis. Physical evidence includes:
   i. Ballooning of the hypopharynx
   ii. Swollen anterior-to-posterior diameter of the epiglottis with the appearance of a thumb (thumb sign)

d. **Laboratory studies**
   i. **Culture of the epiglottis** and **blood** should be obtained but only after the airway is secure. Culture and cell analysis of other sites, such as the CSF, are not warranted because no association with meningitis has ever been reported.
   ii. **Antigen-detection methods** are not useful acutely.
   iii. A **CBC** and **electrolyte determinations** are not beneficial.

5. **Therapy**
   a. **Airway stabilization.** Following visual confirmation of epiglottitis, the child should be intubated and provided with humidified air via a T tube or by ventilator until edema of the upper airway subsides in 2 to 3 days. Intrinsic lung disease is usually not present, and mechanical ventilation is not usually necessary unless paralysis and sedation are needed.
      i. **Nasotracheal intubation** is preferable to orotracheal intubation because it provides anatomic support for the tube and allows the child to feed while it is in place.
      ii. **Sedation** is necessary while the child is intubated to provide for comfort with the endotracheal tube and to prevent extubation.
   b. **Intravenous antibiotic therapy** should be instituted in the operating room only after the airway is secure.
      i. **Cefuroxime sodium** can be used safely because of the infrequency of secondary infection at sites such as the meninges.
      ii. **Ceftriaxone** is also highly efficacious and can be used once daily intravenously or intramuscularly.
   c. **Corticosteroids** are not useful.
   d. **Bronchodilators,** administered by nebulization, are not warranted unless wheezing is present. **Racemic epinephrine** has no place in therapy, even as a temporizing measure, because any short-term benefit obtained may result in severe rebound after cessation of such therapy.

6. **Disposition.** Children with **no evidence of epiglottitis** on direct visualization of the upper airway may be discharged if other causes are not found.

E. **Pneumonia syndrome**
1. **Discussion**
   a. **Definition.** Pneumonia is an inflammation of the lung parenchyma including the bronchioles, alveolar ducts and sacs, and the alveoli. The anatomic area of involvement classifies pneumonia as **lobar**, **lobular**, or **interstitial**.
   b. **Etiology.** There are numerous causes of pneumonia, although most childhood cases are caused by viral pathogens.
      i. **Common respiratory viruses** are the most common cause of pneumonia during the first several years of life.
      ii. **Bacterial pathogens** cause more severe infection and more clinical findings.
      iii. **Fungi, parasites,** *Mycoplasma,* and **rickettsia** may cause pneumonia but are rare and unusual causes in most children.

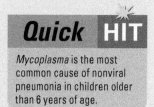

Quick HIT

Mycoplasma is the most common cause of nonviral pneumonia in children older than 6 years of age.

Pediatric Emergencies

2. **Clinical features** depend on the causative organism.

    a. **Bacterial pneumonia** presents with mild upper respiratory symptoms followed by abrupt onset of fever, chills, tachypnea, and chest discomfort. A physical examination reveals decreased breath sounds and rales on the affected side. Cough, intercostal retractions, grunting respirations, and nasal flaring may be seen in younger individuals. Abdominal pain and vomiting are common with basilar infiltrates due to diaphragmatic irritation.

    b. **Viral pneumonia** causes several days of rhinitis and cough followed by fever and coryza but usually no decreased breath sounds and no rales or rhonchi. In younger infants, tachypnea may be the only sign.

    c. **Other causes of pneumonia**

        i. *Mycoplasma pneumoniae.* Symptoms including fever and headache have a gradual onset. A nonproductive protracted cough and dyspnea are hallmarks of the disease.

        ii. *Pneumocystis carinii*

            a) Progressive desaturation with dyspnea may occur in an immunocompromised host.

            b) Pneumonia caused by *P. carinii* can produce an asymptomatic infection that mirrors viral pneumonia in normal children.

3. **Differential diagnoses**

    a. Cystic fibrosis (see V.B.3.e)

    b. Congenital bronchiectasis

    c. Ciliary dyskinesia syndrome

    d. Tracheoesophageal fistula

    e. Foreign body aspiration (see IV)

    f. Atelectasis

    g. Pulmonary abscess

    h. Acute asthma exacerbation

    i. Allergic bronchitis

4. **Evaluation**

    a. **Physical examination.** Diagnosis often is based on the clinical presentation and physical examination findings on chest examination.

    b. **Laboratory studies**

        i. A **CBC** reveals leukocytosis but a predominance of neutrophils in bacterial pneumonia.

        ii. **Cold agglutinin titer.** *M. pneumoniae* may be diagnosed by cold agglutinin titer elevation during the first week of the illness but may be falsely negative in children younger than 5 years.

        iii. **Culture or rapid diagnostic testing.** Specific diagnosis can be made by culture of or rapid diagnostic testing of serum, urine, bronchial wash specimens, or pleural fluid.

        iv. **Immunofluorescence or culture.** Viral pneumonitis can be specifically diagnosed by immunofluorescence or culture of nasopharyngeal wash.

        v. **Silver staining.** The specific diagnosis of *Pneumocystis* pneumonia can be made only by silver staining of specimens from tracheal or bronchial washings, lung aspirate, or lung biopsy.

        vi. **Blood cultures** are positive in 40% to 60% of bacterial pneumonias, but the cost of testing is difficult to justify because it rarely changes therapy acutely.

    c. **Chest radiography.** Dense focal infiltration is noted on chest radiography in bacterial pneumonia. Bilateral, streaking perihilar infiltrates are characteristic of viral pneumonia.

5. **Therapy**

    a. **Bacterial pneumonia.** There is no universally accepted antibiotic regimen for presumed pneumonia.

        i. **Neonates** should be hospitalized and treated intravenously with ampicillin and either an aminoglycoside or cefotaxime.

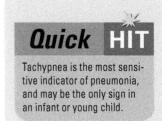

Quick **HIT**

Tachypnea is the most sensitive indicator of pneumonia, and may be the only sign in an infant or young child.

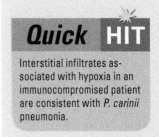

Quick **HIT**

Interstitial infiltrates associated with hypoxia in an immunocompromised patient are consistent with *P. carinii* pneumonia.

Pediatric Emergencies

      ii. **Children older than 3 months** with **mild to moderate illness** and no evidence of desaturation may be treated with oral amoxicillin for presumed bacterial pneumonia.

      iii. **Children with more severe illness**, particularly with respiratory rates in excess of 60 breaths/min and desaturation, should be hospitalized and given intravenous antibiotics. Ampicillin is first-line therapy for community-acquired pneumonia in a normal host.

      iv. **Children older than 6 years** with **mild to moderate illness** and **dyspnea** but no desaturation may be presumed to have *Mycoplasma* illness and should be treated with azithromycin.

      v. **Immunocompromised children.** Children who are immunocompromised and at high risk for *P. carinii* pneumonia should be treated only after appropriate diagnostic studies.

        a) **Trimethoprim–sulfamethoxazole** is the drug of choice at a dosage of 20 mg/kg/day of the trimethoprim component.

        b) Those who do not tolerate trimethoprim–sulfamethoxazole may be treated with **pentamidine isethionate** parenterally or by inhalation after appropriate consultation.

    b. **Viral pneumonia** is usually treated with supportive care alone.
      Acyclovir is useful for varicella zoster or herpes simplex pneumonia.

  6. **Disposition**

    a. **Discharge.** Children with **mild to moderate illness** and **no desaturation** may be managed conservatively at home with oral antibiotics appropriate for the likely pathogen according to age.

    b. **Admission**

      i. Children with **moderate to severe illness**, with failure to feed or take oral therapy, or with desaturation should be admitted for further study and treatment.

      ii. Any **immunocompromised child with pneumonia** should be hospitalized for further evaluation, consultation, and definitive treatment.

      iii. **Neonates up to 2 months of age with pneumonia** should be considered for admission and parenteral antibiotics due to the risk of associated sepsis or multifocal infection.

VI. OTITIS MEDIA

  A. **Discussion.** Otitis media is a common diagnosis in the ED.

    1. **Incidence.** One in three children will have otitis media before his or her sixth birthday. The peak age of incidence is between 6 and 13 months of age. Children with recurrent otitis media frequently have a positive family history for the same type of problems in the parents or siblings.

    2. **Clinical forms.** Otitis media is a clinical syndrome consisting of several forms that overlap in pathophysiology and treatment.

      a. **Acute suppurative otitis media.** Acute otitis media can present with purulent drainage from the external canal making differentiation from otitis externa difficult.

      b. **Otitis media with effusion**

      c. **Recurrent acute suppurative otitis media**

    3. **Etiology.** Major causative organisms include *Streptococcus pneumoniae, H. influenzae, Moraxella catarrhalis,* and *Staphylococcus aureus.*

  B. **Clinical features**

    1. **Symptoms**

      a. **Local symptoms.** Children with otitis media complain of ear pain, decreased hearing, and ear discharge. Infants may exhibit ear pulling, head banging or rubbing, or apparent ataxic gait.

      b. **Systemic symptoms** such as fever, abdominal pain, vomiting, fussiness, and decreased feeding may be seen.

2. **Physical examination findings.** Marked redness, lack of normal landmarks, splaying, or absent light reflex and lack of (or abnormal) mobility on pneumatic otoscopy are noted.

    a. Children with recurrent otitis media often have only dullness of the tympanic membrane without obvious redness.

    b. Children with surgically placed tympanostomy tubes often present a confusing picture of ear drainage without pain, which can lead to a misdiagnosis of otitis externa.

    c. In a child with a fair complexion who is crying, there is no good diagnostic test except for the lack of mobility of the tympanic membrane.

C. **Differential diagnoses**

  1. **Primary ear disease**

    a. **External otitis,** an inflammatory process of the external canal that produces ear pain and a decrease in hearing, is associated with pain on movement of the pinna of the involved ear.

    b. **External infections** of the auricle, pinna, or helix result in a superficial cellulitis.

  2. **Referred pain** along nerves supplying common areas, including:

    a. Pain fibers from the distribution of cranial nerves V, VII, IX, and X, which innervate the posterior pharynx

    b. Pain resulting from postherpetic neuralgia as a result of cutaneous herpes zoster infection

D. **Evaluation**

  1. **Laboratory studies** are rarely needed and seldom helpful in the diagnosis.

  2. **Tympanometry** provides a useful adjunct to diagnosis as well as a visual confirmation of diagnosis that can be placed in medical records for future reference regarding response to treatment.

  3. **Cultures of the nasopharynx or purulent drainage** from the perforation of an acute suppurative otitis media or from tympanostomy tubes is unrewarding and should be discouraged.

E. **Therapy**

  1. **Antibiotic therapy**

    a. **Selection of agents.** Many antibiotics are useful for the treatment of otitis media, varying only in interval of dosing and palatability—there is little difference regarding the microbiologic spectrum. The advantage of one antibiotic over another is entirely speculative. Children who have tympanostomy tubes and who develop acute suppurative otitis media can be treated with topical therapy alone; clinical trials have shown similar rates of resolution with decreased side effects compared to systemic therapy.

      i. **First-line agents.** Generally, a first-line drug is chosen, with amoxicillin being the drug of first choice. Other first-line drugs may be useful, depending on the presence of sulfa allergy or prior episodes of otitis media within the past 3 months that have been treated with antibiotics.

        a) **Amoxicillin** (80 to 90 mg/kg/day, administered every 12 hours) is the most frequently prescribed and cost-effective initial therapy; it has an acceptable and safe side effect profile.

        b) **Erythromycin–sulfisoxazole** (30 to 50 mg/kg/day, administered every 6 hours) is a safe alternative drug with a broad microbial spectrum.

        c) **Trimethoprim–sulfamethoxazole** is effective, and it is safe when penicillin allergy exists.

      ii. **Second-line agents.** Other more expensive agents should be considered when failure with a first-line agent or allergy precludes the use of another agent.

        a) **Cefdinir** (14 mg/kg/day, given once or twice daily). An extended spectrum cephalosporin, Omnicef (Abbott Laboratories, Chicago, IL) provides excellent microbiologic coverage and offers the advantage of once daily dosing.

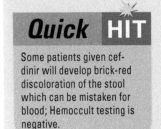

Quick HIT

Some patients given cefdinir will develop brick-red discoloration of the stool which can be mistaken for blood; Hemoccult testing is negative.

b) **Amoxicillin with clavulanate** (90 mg/kg/day, administered every 12 hours); Augmentin-ES has high-dose amoxicillin combined with standard-dose clavulanate to avoid an increased rate of diarrhea.

c) **Azithromycin** (10 mg/kg for 5 days) can be used for penicillin- and cephalosporin-allergic patients, although failure rates are higher than with the medications listed earlier.

d) **Trimethoprim–sulfamethoxazole** (10 mg/kg/day divided twice daily) can be used as a second-line agent, particularly if methicillin-resistant *Staphylococcus aureus* is suspected.

e) **Ceftriaxone** (50 mg/kg, administered intramuscularly in one to three daily doses) is attractive to parents and clinicians because of the parenteral dosing and a higher than 90% cure rate. Data on recurrences or resolution of serious effusions are not yet available.

f) **Ciprofloxacin or ofloxacin drops**, with or without corticosteroids, can be used for otitis media with tympanostomy tubes in place.

b. **Duration of therapy.** Children should be treated for **10 days** for acute suppurative otitis media. Longer treatment courses offer no advantage.

i. Most patients have no relief of fever before 72 hours of effective antibiotic therapy.

ii. On average, redness decreases substantially by 72 hours of therapy, but effusion persists with limited mobility. All children should be reevaluated at 28 to 42 days after therapy to ensure resolution of effusion. Normally, 50% of children have persistent effusion at 14 to 21 days after therapy.

2. **Decongestants** have no place in the management of either acute otitis media or persistent effusion. Literature suggests that such treatment may actually prolong effusion.

3. **Tympanostomy tube placement.** Despite the frequency of operations for placement of tympanostomy tubes, such devices do not prevent infection. They serve only to improve hearing by allowing better middle ear ventilation. Most children appear to outgrow their episodes of otitis media because of complex growth of the eustachian tube diameter, the orientation of the tube within the bony skull, and enhanced secretory and cell-mediated immunity.

F. **Disposition.** Most patients can be treated on an outpatient basis.

VII. CONGENITAL HEART DISEASE

A. **Discussion.** Many types of congenital heart disease are appreciated and are beyond the scope of this text. Only those entities that are likely to present to an ED are covered here.

1. **Incidence.** Congenital heart disease occurs in approximately 8 in 1,000 live births; 2 to 4 of those 1,000 newborn infants are symptomatic with heart disease in the first year of life.

a. The diagnosis is established by 1 week of age in 40% to 50% of patients with congenital heart disease.

b. The diagnosis is made by 1 month of age in 60% to 70% of infants with serious congenital heart disease.

2. **Types.** Congenital heart disease can be divided into cyanotic and acyanotic types.

a. **Acyanotic.** The majority of cases of congenital heart disease involve acyanotic lesions that are usually discovered on examination for other reasons. They usually are not the reason for an ED visit.

b. **Cyanotic.** The cyanotic congenital heart disease variants are true life-threatening emergencies and often result in such children presenting to the ED in extremis. Cyanosis results when obstruction to right ventricular outflow causes shunting at the cardiac level from right to left or when left ventricular outflow is impeded. Because of decreased ventilatory reserve, profound acidosis is common. Circulatory collapse is imminent after the development of acidosis.

B. **Clinical features**
  1. **Cyanotic lesions associated with decreased pulmonary blood flow**
      a. **Tetralogy of Fallot** is the most common cyanotic congenital heart defect, accounting for 10% of congenital defects.
          i. **Pathogenesis.** The primary lesion involves hypoplasia of the infundibulum, resulting in outflow tract obstruction. Variable **right ventricular outflow obstruction** results in functional **pulmonary stenosis**. Dextroposition of the aorta results in overriding of the ventricular septum. Ventricular septal defect and right ventricular hypertrophy may also be evident.
          ii. **Manifestations** reflect the degree of severity of the right ventricular outflow obstruction.
              a) Cyanosis is variable and may be absent.
              b) Hypoxemic or "tet spells" characterized by irritability, hyperpnea, cyanosis, and syncope occur and may be fatal if not managed properly.
              c) A harsh systolic ejection murmur is often heard along the sternal border.
              d) Because of the functional pulmonary banding that occurs with the anatomy of this syndrome, CHF does not usually develop.
      b. **Pulmonary atresia with or without ventricular septal defect** is an extremely severe form of tetralogy of Fallot.
          i. **Pathogenesis.** The main pulmonary artery is atretic, and pulmonary blood flow depends entirely on a patent ductus arteriosus or bronchial collateral vessels.
          ii. **Manifestations.** Patients present with findings of severe cyanosis and are usually profoundly ill. Often no murmur is heard, and a single first heart sound (S_1) is all that is appreciated in the syndrome when associated with a ventricular septal defect.
      c. **Transposition of the great vessels with ventricular septal defect and pulmonary stenosis** may mimic tetralogy of Fallot in clinical presentation.
          i. **Pathogenesis.** This condition is caused by transposition of the vessels; therefore, the obstruction is in the left ventricle instead of the right ventricle. The heart is usually enlarged, and there may be pulmonary congestion, depending on the degree of pulmonary stenosis.
          ii. **Manifestations.** The most common presentation is poor feeding and lethargy, with mild cyanosis present on physical examination.
      d. **Ebstein anomaly of the tricuspid valve**
          i. **Pathogenesis.** Ebstein anomaly is caused by downward displacement of the right atrium and tricuspid valve into the right ventricle, which results in an enormous right atrium and a regurgitant tricuspid valve.
          ii. **Manifestations.** The severity of symptoms depends on the degree of displacement of the tricuspid valve.
              a) In most patients, the only complaint is fatigue and cardiac dysrhythmias, of which paroxysmal atrial tachycardia is the most common.
              b) Some severely affected children may have cyanosis due to the admixture of blood through an open foramen ovale.
              c) The characteristic murmur is a loud systolic murmur maximal at the right heart border.
  2. **Cyanotic lesions associated with increased pulmonary blood flow**
      a. **Total anomalous pulmonary venous return** is characterized by partial or complete anomalous drainage of the pulmonary veins with no direct connection with the left atrium. All blood returns to the right atrium or a tributary that drains into it.
          i. **Types of anomalous drainage**
              a) **Infracardiac with obstruction of pulmonary venous return** is usually seen in neonates who present with severe cyanosis and tachycardia and marked pulmonary hypertension.
              b) **Infracardiac or intracardiac pulmonary venous return with only mild to moderate obstruction** results in intermittent bouts of CHF that appear to improve with oxygenation and then recur.

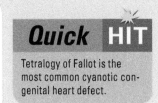

Quick **HIT**

Tetralogy of Fallot is the most common cyanotic congenital heart defect.

Pediatric Emergencies

c) **Infracardiac or intracardiac anomalous venous return with no obstruction** results in admixture but only mild or no cyanosis and no pulmonary hypertension.

ii. A **murmur** may be present and depends on the degree of pulmonary obstruction and the degree of pulmonary hypertension.

b. **Truncus arteriosus** is characterized by a single outflow vessel arising from the heart to supply systemic, pulmonary, and coronary circulations. It is always associated with ventricular septal defect.

i. In **early infancy**, only a murmur and minimal cyanosis are present as pulmonary vascular resistance is high.

ii. In **later infancy**, when pulmonary resistance falls, signs of CHF predominate but only mild cyanosis is noted. A loud murmur is usually heard at the left sternal border and is usually associated with only a single second heart sound (S_2).

c. **Hypoplastic left heart syndrome** is characterized by atresia of the aortic or mitral valve and hypoplasia of the ascending aorta associated with hypoplasia or atresia of the left ventricle. All blood flow to the systemic circulation is via a patent ductus arteriosus. Closure of the patent ductus arteriosus results in immediate and profound shock and hypoperfusion associated with pronounced acidosis.

i. A peculiar gray coloration of the lips and skin is seen before frank cyanosis develops.

ii. Peripheral pulses are either weak or absent.

iii. A nondescript systolic murmur is often heard but is nondiagnostic.

iv. If a ventricular septal defect is also present, hypotension is not seen but increasing cyanosis and pulmonary hypertension develop.

C. **Differential diagnoses.** Few things present so dramatically as an infant with cyanosis and lethargy. It is imperative to consider all possible differential diagnostic points in critically ill infants and not become fixated on one diagnosis to the exclusion of others. Infants who are profoundly ill should be treated with age-appropriate antibiotics, pending more definitive cardiac evaluation.

1. **Sepsis.** Presentation of infants with sepsis or congenital heart disease often is identical and particularly confusing because of poor perfusion and absent pulses. Pulse pressure that is widened may be very helpful. Frequently, profoundly ill children with congenital heart disease are placed on antibiotics before a primary diagnosis is made.

2. **Inborn errors of metabolism.** Profound acidosis is present in children with inborn errors of metabolism, and ketonuria and aminoaciduria are often present. A family history of similarly affected infants can help differentiate an inborn error of metabolism from a congenital heart defect.

3. **CNS disease**

a. **Intracranial hemorrhage** accounts for most presentations that are life-threatening.

b. **Iatrogenic drug administration** or **overdosage** is another possibility but not in the neonatal period.

4. **Hemoglobinopathies.** Methemoglobinemia resulting in arterial desaturation is a rare cause. The arterial oxygen tension (PaO_2) is usually normal or elevated.

D. **Evaluation**

1. **Examination.** Careful physical examination and prolonged observation of breathing patterns should be performed.

a. **Murmurs.** Location and timing should be carefully noted.

b. **Upper** and **lower extremity blood pressure** determinations should be made, as well as a **recording of pulses** in the upper and lower extremities, with particular attention to the amplitude and duration of impulse.

c. **Skin coloration** and **capillary refill** should be noted.

d. **Associated congenital anomalies** should be sought.

2. **Pulse oximetry** should be performed with the patient breathing room air and 100% oxygen.

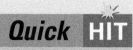

Quick HIT

Lower extremity blood pressures should be higher than upper extremity pressures; a decreased lower extremity blood pressure indicates coarctation of the aorta or other lesion resulting in left outflow tract obstruction.

3. **Chest radiography** should be performed, focusing on cardiac size and shape as well as pulmonary blood flow.
4. **Electrocardiography** and **two-dimensional echocardiography** are indicated.
5. **Cardiac catheterization** may be required for severely ill infants.

E. **Therapy** depends on the diagnosis.
1. **Supportive measures** include:
   a. Supplemental oxygenation
   b. Rapid correction of lactic acidosis
   c. Maintenance of normal temperature
   d. Arrangement for transfer to a center that is equipped to handle such infants
   e. The administration of prostaglandin E_1 (0.05 to 0.2 μg/kg/min) for suspected ductal-dependent lesions to maintain patency
   f. Dobutamine for patients in CHF who do not have ductal-dependent lesions
   g. Medical stabilization prior to definitive cardiac catheterization or palliative surgery
2. **Tetralogy of Fallot.** Patients require a special form of treatment when hypercyanotic attacks occur, including the following:
   a. Placing the infant on the abdomen in the knee–chest position
   b. Administration of supplemental oxygen
   c. Administration of morphine sulfate subcutaneously in a dose not to exceed 0.2 mg/kg
   d. Rapid correction of metabolic acidosis with administration of sodium bicarbonate
   e. Adrenergic blockade by intravenous administration of propranolol (0.1 to 0.2 mg/kg) for infants with tachycardia and cyanosis

F. **Disposition**
1. Infants with a **murmur** but **no evidence of CHF** or **cyanosis** may be referred for pediatric cardiology evaluation in a more controlled fashion after initial telephone consultation.
2. Infants with a **murmur** and **signs of CHF** but **no evidence of cyanosis** must be stabilized after initial diagnostic evaluation. The patient should be referred to a tertiary center for cardiology evaluation.
3. Infants with **cyanosis on room air** who **fail to improve following the administration of 100% oxygen** (as determined by pulse oximetry) most likely have a cyanotic congenital heart lesion and are at high risk for deterioration. Transport to the nearest tertiary center should be emergently arranged, with a physician in attendance during the transport.

VIII. KAWASAKI DISEASE

A. **Discussion.** Kawasaki disease is a febrile condition associated with vasculitis of the large coronary vessels and marked inflammation of the mucous membranes, especially of the eye and mouth. It is the leading cause of acquired heart disease in children and primarily affects children 5 years of age or younger.

B. **Clinical features**
1. **Fever** is abrupt in onset, lasts for at least 5 days, and may be as high as 105°F (the mean temperature is 104°F).
2. **Bilateral nonpurulent conjunctival injection** is present and not associated with discharge or crusting.
3. **Dry, erythematous, fissured lips; injected oral mucosae**; and peculiar "**strawberry tongue**" are noted, which may cause an inappropriate diagnosis as streptococcal infection.
4. **Lymphadenopathy** is present in the cervical and axillary areas. It is usually nonsuppurative and not generalized.
5. **Skin eruptions** are usually present and may be the morbilliform, maculopapular, urticarial, or erythema multiforme type. At times, the skin eruptions may resemble diaper dermatitis.
6. **Swollen feet.** After the third day of the illness, the feet become edematous and painful, with most children refusing to bear weight or walk.

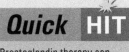

Quick HIT

Prostaglandin therapy can be associated with apnea; preparation for respiratory support should be made during the initiation of this medication.

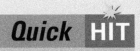

Quick HIT

The cause of Kawasaki disease is unknown—no putative infectious or autoimmunologic cause has been found. There is no evidence for person-to-person transmission.

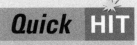

Quick HIT

Sparing of the limbic area immediately surrounding the iris is classic for Kawasaki disease.

Pediatric Emergencies

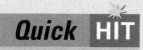

7. **Desquamation.** After several weeks of illness, desquamation of the hands and feet occurs. The first appearance is in the subungual area. Desquamation then spreads to the palms and soles before becoming generalized.

8. **Transient arthritis** is apparent in older children and is characterized by symmetric swelling of the small and large joints of the lower extremities.

9. **Cardiac involvement** is seen in 10% to 50% of untreated children and is usually silent. However, cardiac involvement may present as CHF, complete heart block, or an evolving myocardial infarction.

C. **Differential diagnoses**

1. **Scarlet fever.** The "strawberry tongue" of scarlet fever is similar to that of Kawasaki disease, but the characteristic sandpaper-like papular rash of scarlet fever usually allows differentiation of the two entities. Also, children with scarlet fever have no edema of the hands or feet.

2. **Toxic shock syndrome** is often difficult to differentiate from Kawasaki disease in severely ill children.

3. **Leptospirosis.** Exposure to a vector is a helpful clue. Profuse conjunctivitis with no other symptoms, along with elevated liver enzymes, often aids in the diagnosis. Hepatitis may mimic infectious mononucleosis.

4. **Epstein-Barr virus infection.** A positive heterophil antibody response in older children or elevation of specific Epstein-Barr complement fixation titers in younger children is common. Splenomegaly is common in adolescents but rare in smaller children.

5. **Juvenile rheumatoid arthritis.** The pauciarticular variety common in small children is difficult to differentiate from Kawasaki disease. Rheumatoid factor is not helpful. The presence of iridocyclitis is helpful diagnostically.

6. **Rocky Mountain spotted fever.** The rash usually begins on the wrists and is petechial and vasculitic in type. It occurs only during the months that the tick vector is active.

7. **Measles** (see Chapter 11.IX.A)

8. **Stevens-Johnson syndrome** (see Chapter 11.III.B)

D. **Evaluation**

1. **Laboratory studies.** There are no definitive diagnostic laboratory studies available to diagnose Kawasaki disease. Testing for autoimmune disease is unnecessary.
    a. **CBC.** Leukocytosis is marked in the second to third week of the illness with immature forms.
    b. **Sedimentation rate** and **C-reactive protein level** are usually elevated.
    c. **Hepatic panel.** Enzyme levels may be mildly elevated, but liver tests are nondiagnostic.
    d. **Urinalysis.** Sterile pyuria without bacteriuria is common.

2. **Imaging studies.** A chest radiograph is usually not helpful, but **two-dimensional echocardiography** is essential for the diagnosis. It obviates the need for coronary arteriography in most children and allows rapid assessment of coronary artery size.

3. **Electrocardiography** is usually not helpful.

E. **Therapy**

1. **Intravenous immunoglobulin.** Patients with Kawasaki disease respond dramatically and predictably to the administration of immunoglobulin during the febrile phase. A single dose of 2 g/kg is given over a 12-hour period. Severe side effects of intravenous immunoglobulin are rare.
    a. Fever abates 24 hours after therapy.
    b. This therapy prevents the formation of coronary artery aneurysms and coronary vasculitis if given within 48 hours of diagnosis. If given after 10 days of illness, the intravenous immunoglobulin ameliorates most symptoms in severely ill infants but will not change coronary vasculitis.
    c. If given within 10 days of onset, aneurysm formation may not be prevented, but further enlargement is prevented.

2. **Salicylate therapy** is indicated during the initial febrile phase of the illness and for 6 to 8 weeks after active disease subsides.
    a. **Febrile phase.** High doses (80 to 100 mg/kg/day) may be required to achieve serum concentrations of 30 to 40 mg/dL.

b. **Following acute disease.** Salicylate therapy (5 to 8 mg/kg/day) is continued for its antithrombotic effect. In children with coronary lesions discovered at initial echocardiography, aspirin therapy must be continued until they completely resolve.

3. **Coumadin therapy** is advocated for large, persistent, or multiple nonobstructive aneurysms.

4. **Corticosteroid therapy** has no proven value in therapy.

5. **Thrombolytic therapy** has had limited usage in children with acute coronary thrombosis.

F. **Disposition**

1. Children should not be discharged until the acute phase of illness has subsided following salicylate and immunoglobulin therapy.

2. Any child with known coronary artery aneurysms who presents in failure or with chest pain should be considered to have cardiac ischemia until proven otherwise. Acutely ill children should be admitted for monitoring to an intensive care setting until a full evaluation can be performed.

IX. BACTEREMIA, MENINGITIS, AND SEPSIS

A. **Discussion**

1. **Bacteremia** is defined as the presence of bacteria in the blood; most often, bacteremia is asymptomatic.

a. **Occult bacteremia** is usually transient and self-limited. It is most common in children between the ages of 6 and 30 months and is associated with temperature elevation above 103°F and a leukocyte count of 15,000 to 20,000/mm^3 or more. In 15% to 20% of children with occult bacteremia, the leukocyte count is greater than 20,000/mm^3, the fever is higher than 103°F, and there is a primary site of infection (e.g., otitis media, pneumonia).

   i. **Etiology.** *S. pneumoniae* is the most common causative organism. *H. influenzae* is uncommon because of the widespread usage of conjugated *H. influenzae* vaccine.

   ii. **Pathogenesis.** Secondary spread to the meninges occurs in 5% to 15% of patients.

b. **Secondary bacteremia** is caused by spread from a primary site of infection, such as pneumonia or an indwelling medical appliance.

2. **Sepsis** is a life-threatening bacterial invasion of the intravascular compartment that is associated with symptoms of lethargy, irritability, or hypotension, and may or may not be associated with a focus of infection. Sepsis is most common in children younger than 3 months of age. It is usually caused by a group B streptococcal infection in children younger than 1 month of age and by *S. pneumoniae*, *H. influenzae*, or *N. meningitidis* in older children.

3. **Meningitis** refers to any inflammation of the meninges and the subarachnoid space. It can be caused by bacterial, viral, or fungal agents. Meningitis is seen most frequently in children older than 6 months of age. It is associated with an increased CSF WBC concentration, variable elevation of CSF protein, and a low level of CSF glucose.

a. **Bacterial meningitis**

   i. In **neonates**, the most common cause is group B streptococcus and *Escherichia coli*.

   ii. In **older children**, the most common causative organisms are *H. influenzae*, *S. pneumoniae*, and *N. meningitidis*.

b. **Aseptic meningitis** usually is caused by viral agents, predominantly coxsackievirus, echovirus, and the mumps virus. In neonates, herpes simplex should be considered in any child with skin lesions characteristic of the infection, irritability, or focal seizures.

B. **Clinical features**

1. **Sepsis.** In patients with sepsis, signs and symptoms are usually isolated to a temperature elevation of 103°F or higher and irritability with no obvious focus of infection. Sepsis should be considered in any infant younger than 3 months of age with fever, no obvious source of infection, and ill appearance.

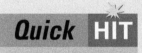

Quick HIT

Occult bacteremia occurred in up to 5% of febrile young children with a high fever and no focal infection prior to routine use of the pneumococcal and *H. influenzae* vaccines; more recent data found rates of occult bacteremia to be <1%.

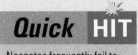

Quick HIT

Neonates frequently fail to mount a febrile response to infection including sepsis; euthermia or hypothermia are common in this age group.

Pediatric Emergencies

2. **Meningitis** often presents with symptoms of vomiting, poor suck and feeding, lethargy, and irritability.
   a. In **older children**, headache, photophobia, and neck stiffness may be seen.
   b. In **young infants**, a bulging fontanelle may be all that is apparent along with lethargy or irritability.

C. **Differential diagnoses** include:
   1. CHF
   2. Arrhythmia
   3. Pericarditis or myocarditis
   4. Ductus-dependent cardiac lesions
   5. Congenital adrenal insufficiency
   6. Electrolyte imbalance (hyponatremia)
   7. Inborn errors of metabolism
   8. Volvulus
   9. Intussusception
   10. Leukemia
   11. Intoxication
   12. Infantile botulism
   13. Nonaccidental trauma with CNS sequelae
   14. Hemolytic–uremic syndrome

D. **Evaluation**
   1. **Laboratory studies**
      a. **No child should be excluded from appropriate evaluation or therapy based on the results of a single laboratory test.**
         i. **Sepsis** is a clinical diagnosis primarily substantiated by laboratory diagnosis and not excluded by a test other than a negative blood culture.
         ii. **Meningitis** is based on analysis of all parameters of the properly performed lumbar puncture, and treatment should not be withheld based on a single test.
      b. **CBC.** The peripheral **WBC concentration** may be remarkable for a leukocytosis in excess of 15,000 cells/mm^3 with left shift. Children with sepsis usually have high-grade bacteremia, leukocytosis, or neutropenia, and a shift of the WBC differential concentration to more immature forms. A low WBC concentration of less than 5,000 cells/mm^3 is also associated with serious infections.
      c. **Quantitative blood cultures** usually reveal low-level bacteremia in children with occult bacteremia.
      d. **Urinalysis** of an unspun urine sample (obtained by catheterization) is useful for children younger than 2 or 3 years of age.
      e. **CSF analysis.** Any child with altered mental status must have an evaluation of the CSF by lumbar puncture to exclude meningitis, which is characterized by the following findings:
         i. Increased CSF WBC concentration (100 to 10,000 cells/μL)
         ii. Increased CSF pressure
         iii. Increased protein concentration (greater than 80 mg/dL)
         iv. Decreased CSF glucose concentration (less than 40 mg/dL)
         v. Positive Gram stain and positive culture of CSF
         vi. Possibly positive antigen detection tests
   2. **Chest radiography** is useful only in children with respiratory symptoms of cough or tachypnea.

E. **Therapy**
   1. **Antibiotic therapy**
      a. **Occult bacteremia**
         i. Children who may have occult bacteremia (i.e., those with a WBC count greater than 20,000/mm^3 and a temperature higher than 103°F) benefit from a single dose of **ceftriaxone** given intramuscularly after a complete diagnostic evaluation. These patients should be seen again in 12 hours to ensure that a secondary infection is not present.

ii. Children with occult bacteremia that resolves in 24 to 48 hours with no clinical findings and no further temperature elevation require no additional therapy.

b. **Sepsis or meningitis.** Children with presumed sepsis or meningitis should be treated with an antibiotic that is effective against the common pathogens (as suggested by the patient's age) after a full diagnostic evaluation is completed.

  i. **Neonates and infants younger than 2 months** of age are usually given ampicillin sodium and either an aminoglycoside or cefotaxime.

  ii. **Infants and older children** may be treated with a single or daily divided dose of ceftriaxone or with cefotaxime. Vancomycin should be given initially for patients with suspected bacterial meningitis or sepsis until cultures and sensitivity are available.

c. **Duration of therapy** is based on patient age and the organism treated.

  i. Children with **occult bacteremia** are usually treated with 3 days of intravenous antibiotics followed by oral therapy for 7 to 10 days.

  ii. Infants with **sepsis but without meningitis** are usually treated with intravenous antibiotics for 7 to 10 days.

  iii. Infants with **meningitis** are treated with parenteral antibiotics for 10 to 14 days, depending on the organism. *N. meningitidis* meningitis may be treated for fewer than 7 days, under certain circumstances (e.g., improving clinical course, afebrile after 3 days of therapy).

2. **Supportive care** is essential and includes:

  a. **Fluid resuscitation** to treat shock and hypoperfusion, with care to avoid cerebral edema when vascular volume is restored

  b. **Anticonvulsant therapy** to control seizures

  c. **Assisted ventilation** to control respiratory failure or cerebral edema

3. **Corticosteroids** are indicated for meningitis to reduce the incidence of hearing loss.

F. **Disposition.** Children with **sepsis** or **meningitis** must be admitted for further therapy.

1. Children with stable vital signs may be admitted to a regular-floor bed with close observation and monitoring.

2. Children who are unstable must be admitted to an intensive care unit.

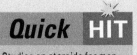

Quick HIT

Studies on steroids for meningitis showed benefit when the steroids were administered before or concomitant with the initial dose of antibiotic.

X. GASTROINTESTINAL DISORDERS

A. Gastroenteritis

1. **Discussion**

  a. **Incidence.** Diarrhea accounts for 3 to 5 million deaths worldwide yearly and for 25 to 35 million episodes per year in the United States.

  b. The major **mechanism of transmission** of the organisms that cause gastroenteritis is the fecal–oral route. Water-borne and food-borne outbreaks also occur, but they are seasonal. Diarrheal pathogens vary by geographic location and season.

  c. **Etiology**

    i. In **underdeveloped countries**, where nutrition is poor, causes are usually diverse and may be bacterial, viral, or parasitic.

    ii. In **industrialized countries**, acute or chronic diarrhea is usually caused by bacterial or viral agents that reflect seasonality, local epidemiology, and age.

      a) **Bacterial agents** can cause inflammatory or noninflammatory disease; inflammatory disease is most important in industrialized countries.

        1) *Salmonella* species
        2) *Shigella* species
        3) *Campylobacter jejuni*
        4) *Yersinia enterocolitica*
        5) *E. coli*

b) **Viral agents.** Most children with diarrhea have a viral etiology for their illness.
1) In **young infants**, **rotavirus** and **enteric adenovirus** can cause severe diarrhea, dehydration, and acidosis, which often necessitates hospitalization.
2) In **older infants and adults**, **Norwalk agent**, **calicivirus**, and **astrovirus** are associated with a short-lived 3- to 4-day illness that usually does not involve dehydration or acidosis.
c) **Parasitic agents** are common in underdeveloped countries. In the United States, *Giardia lamblia* is the most common cause of parasitic diarrhea.

2. **Clinical features.** Enteric infections have local (gastrointestinal), extraintestinal, and systemic manifestations.
   a. **Local symptoms** include diarrhea, abdominal cramping, and emesis.
   b. **Extraintestinal manifestations** may include signs of vulvovaginitis, conjunctivitis, endocarditis, osteomyelitis, or meningitis.
   c. **Systemic manifestations** may include fever and malaise, rash, arthritis, or seizures.

3. **Differential diagnoses**
   a. **Feeding difficulty** with reflux or dumping due to overfeeding
   b. **Anatomic gastrointestinal defects**
      i. Malrotation
      ii. Hirschsprung disease
      iii. Volvulus
      iv. Intussusception
   c. **Malabsorptive states**
      i. Monosaccharidase and disaccharidase deficiency
      ii. Immunoglobulin A deficiency
      iii. Celiac disease
      iv. Cystic fibrosis with pancreatic insufficiency
   d. **Toxigenic food poisoning**
      i. Scombroid poisoning
      ii. Ciguatera poisoning
      iii. *Amanita* mushroom poisoning
   e. **Endocrine deficiency states**
      i. Congenital adrenal insufficiency
      ii. Adrenogenital syndrome
   f. **Inflammatory bowel disease**
      i. Crohn disease
      ii. Ulcerative colitis
      iii. Acrodermatitis enteropathica

4. **Evaluation**
   a. **Laboratory studies**
      i. A **serum electrolyte panel** is necessary for children with significant dehydration.
      ii. A **CBC** is usually not helpful.
      iii. **Fecal analysis.** Stool specimens should be analyzed for blood, mucus, and leukocytes. Blood and leukocytes detected in a stool sample merit culture of the stool for bacterial agents.
      iv. **Serology.** Antigen-detection methods for rotavirus may be helpful for infants with vomiting and diarrhea during the winter months. Nonspecific serologic markers of infection (e.g., febrile precipitins, acute-phase reactants) are not helpful and do not aid in the specific diagnosis.
      v. **Blood cultures** are beneficial in children with fever and studies that may suggest *Salmonella* gastroenteritis.
      vi. **Aspiration of vasculitic lesions** may yield evidence of the organism on Gram stain or culture.

vii. **Urinalysis** is not helpful unless extraintestinal spread is suggested.
b. **Radiographic studies** usually are not warranted unless a bowel obstruction, secondary pneumonia, or osteomyelitis is suspected.

5. **Therapy**
a. **Management of dehydration** is the cornerstone of therapy for diarrhea, regardless of the cause. If symptoms do not resolve in 5 to 7 days with conservative replacement of fluid and electrolytes, cultures or antigen detection may be necessary to determine the cause of the diarrhea.
  i. **Oral rehydration** is the treatment of choice for all but the most severely affected infants.
    a) **Commercially available rehydration solutions** usually have a carbohydrate source that is easily digestible and aids in electrolyte absorption. Ongoing losses should be replaced with oral electrolyte solution.
      1) The **sodium concentration** is usually at least 90 to 140 mmol/L.
      2) The **carbohydrate:sodium concentration** should be approximately 1:8 to 1:2.
      3) The **osmolality** is 300 to 350 mOsm/L.
    b) **Home remedies** (e.g., fruit juices, gelatin, tea, decarbonated soda, sports drinks) should not be used because of their unsuitable low-sodium concentrations and excessive carbohydrates.
  ii. **Intravenous rehydration.** Severely dehydrated children should receive 20 mL/kg of lactated Ringer solution or normal saline to improve perfusion. After the initial resuscitative bolus is administered, further fluid therapy should be guided by serum electrolyte determinations and the clinical response to the infusion. Additional boluses (20 mL/kg) of the previously used fluid administered over 1 hour may be necessary to establish urine flow.
b. **Serum electrolyte disturbances** (e.g., hyponatremia, hypernatremia) should be corrected in the hospital within 16 to 24 hours.
c. **Feeding.** Once rehydration is complete, **introduction of bland foods** such as bananas, apples, rice cereal, or a high-protein source (e.g., chicken) is helpful.
  i. **In patients with symptoms worsened with dairy products, dairy products should be withheld** for 3 to 5 days because of the induced disaccharidase deficiency.
  ii. **Breastfed infants** should resume their feedings as soon as possible.
d. **Antidiarrheal compounds** generally are not warranted for most cases of childhood diarrhea.
e. **Antibiotic therapy** is indicated when certain bacterial pathogens have been implicated, primarily to shorten the clinical course or to decrease excretion of the organism to prevent secondary spread.
f. **Antiviral therapy** (including fractionated albumin, high-titer breastmilk, or egg white) is not useful in otherwise healthy children.
g. **Vaccination** is not warranted in most cases of gastroenteritis in the United States but may be helpful for *Salmonella typhi* or *Vibrio cholerae* infection in other countries.

6. **Disposition**
a. Most children may be easily managed by oral rehydration at home with a commercially available electrolyte solution followed by a bland but protein-rich diet. Early reinstitution of nutrition is critical to avoid prolonged diarrhea due to starvation.
b. Children who are isotonically dehydrated may be discharged to home after appropriate oral or intravenous rehydration and after a trial of oral hydration is effective.
c. Children with hypernatremic or hyponatremic dehydration usually require admission to the hospital for rehydration and correction of deficits over an 18- to 24-hour period.

Quick HIT

Twenty percent to 30% of patients with gastroenteritis may develop a temporary lactase deficiency; the majority of patients with gastroenteritis will tolerate dairy products well.

Quick HIT

In developed countries, antibiotic therapy should not be initiated prior to definitive culture of a bacterial pathogen. Patients infected with *E. coli* 0157-H7 may have an increased rate of developing hemolytic uremic syndrome if treated with antibiotics.

Pediatric Emergencies

B. **Intestinal obstruction**
   1. **Discussion**
      a. **Incidence.** Intestinal obstruction is not common in pediatrics but occurs with a frequency of approximately 1:2,000 live births.
      b. **Etiology.** In adults, intestinal obstruction is usually a complication of fibrotic bands that have formed after surgery. In children, intestinal obstruction usually is the result of maldevelopment of the embryonic intestine or mechanical factors that have allowed the intestine to slide or move.
      c. **Types.** Intestinal obstruction can be partial or complete but the distinction is often difficult.
   2. **Clinical features** vary with the cause of the obstruction, the level and completeness of the obstruction, and the time between the obstruction and the presentation for care.
      a. **Symptoms**
         i. **Nausea and vomiting.** Obstruction is associated with accumulation of intestinal secretions, ingested food, and gas from fermentation of contents of the intestine. This results in dilatation proximal to the obstruction. Because of the osmolality of the obstructed contents, intraluminal fluid shifts occur that result in fluid and electrolyte depletion.
            a) Nausea, vomiting, and abdominal distention are classic signs, with **bilious emesis** found only when the site of obstruction is high in the intestinal tract but distal to the first portion of the duodenum.
            b) Lower intestinal obstruction in adults often results in **feculent vomiting** but is seldom seen in children with similar obstruction.
         ii. **Pain** and **cramping** are intermittent and often positional. Vomiting often provides relief.
         iii. **Obstipation** (intractable constipation) is common but not diagnostic by itself or exclusive of obstruction in children.
      b. **Physical examination findings**
         i. **Fever** usually is not seen unless the blood supply to the obstructed bowel becomes compromised, resulting in bacterial proliferation and the development of sepsis.
         ii. **Peritoneal signs** (i.e., an increasingly tender, distended abdomen with rebound tenderness; involuntary guarding; and rigidity) develop as the obstruction progresses and peritonitis ensues.
         iii. **Profound dehydration** (evidenced by **poor capillary refill**, **hypotension**, and **shock**) may be seen in children who present late in the course of their illness as a result of increasing loss of fluid into the bowel lumen.
   3. **Differential diagnoses**
      a. Hypertrophic pyloric stenosis
      b. Congenital gastric outlet obstruction
      c. Gastric duplication syndromes
      d. Duodenal atresia, which is associated with the "double bubble" sign of intestinal obstruction and often with other congenital anomalies
      e. Duodenal bands and webs
      f. Annular pancreas
      g. Jejunal and ileal atresia
      h. Malrotation, which is usually associated with bilious vomiting and, later, small bowel volvulus
      i. Intestinal duplication syndromes
      j. Meckel diverticulum
      k. Appendicitis
      l. Intussusception
      m. Sepsis
      n. Incarcerated hernia
   4. **Evaluation.** Often, the obstructive process is complete when the patient presents, and little diagnostic skill or laboratory evaluation is required to make the initial diagnosis. Obstructive processes that are incomplete offer a diagnostic

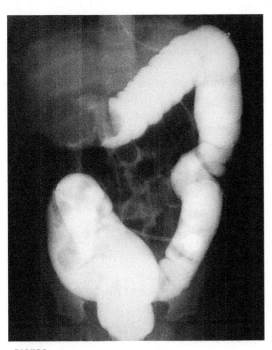

FIGURE 15-2 Barium enema showing intussusception.
(Courtesy of Mark Silverberg, MD; from Greenberg MI, et al. *Greenberg's Text-Atlas of Emergency Medicine.* Philadelphia: Lippincott Williams & Wilkins; 2005.)

challenge of episodic pain and vomiting that have often resolved by the time care is sought.

a. **Physical examination and history findings** are usually suggestive of obstruction.

b. **Laboratory studies** are supportive of the diagnosis but not diagnostic. They often reveal hypochloremic alkalosis with hemoconcentration. A CBC often reveals only leukocytosis; a shift to more immature forms is suggestive of impending peritonitis.

c. **Diagnostic imaging studies**

  i. **Ultrasonography** may be useful for the diagnosis of pyloric stenosis, intussusception, and malrotation. Ultrasound can also reveal evidence of ischemia, abscess formation, and free fluid suggestive of peritonitis associated with other disorders (Figure 15-2).

  ii. **Radiographic studies**

   a) **Plain radiographs.** Flat and upright radiographs of the abdomen reveal distention of the bowel at and above the obstruction and the presence of multiple air–fluid levels in various locations in the abdomen.

   b) **Contrast studies** are indicated only when an obstructive pattern exists on plain radiographs but no obvious source of obstruction is apparent on ultrasonography.

    1) **Water-soluble oral contrast** is useful for recognizing atresia, volvulus, and congenital web or band syndromes as well as some presentations of malrotation. These contrast agents should be used carefully, particularly in ill patients in whom the risk of perforation is high.

    2) **Water-soluble enemas** are useful for the diagnosis of malrotation, intussusception, or colonic duplications.

  iii. **CT examination** of the abdomen is seldom useful in localizing the site of the obstruction, even with contrast.

5. **Therapy**

  a. **Stabilization.** Initial treatment involves **fluid** and **electrolyte resuscitation** to compensate for intraluminal losses.

  b. **Nasogastric decompression** is beneficial for the relief of pain and vomiting.

Quick HIT

If perforation is present, free air is noticeable in the subdiaphragmatic region, but small amounts are not visible unless lateral decubitus radiographs are performed with air layering over the liver edge.

Pediatric Emergencies

c. **Prompt surgical consultation** must be obtained, and additional diagnostic maneuvers should be directed by the surgeon in charge of the case. **Immediate surgical consultation and operation** are imperative for any child who has signs of **peritonitis**.

d. **Hydrostatic reduction of suspected intussusception** is usually not performed by the emergency physician because perforation may result. Air-contrast enema reduction can be performed by interventionalists in radiology; surgery consultation is generally recommended due to the potential for perforation or failure of reduction requiring surgical intervention.

e. **Antibiotic therapy** may be instituted after appropriate cultures are obtained for an ill child with signs of peritonitis. The antibiotic regimen should provide broad coverage against anaerobic as well as fecal aerobic organisms.

6. **Disposition.** Most patients are hospitalized for stabilization and gastrointestinal decompression via nasogastric suction.

a. Most patients with intestinal obstruction but no evidence of peritonitis can be managed conservatively. If there is no response while the patient is hospitalized, the condition requires surgical intervention.

b. **No child with suspected intestinal obstruction is ever discharged home without surgical consultation.**

C. Volvulus

1. **Discussion.** The most common type of volvulus in infants and children involves the small bowel; gastric and colonic volvulus may also occur. A volvulus occurs when a portion of the intestinal tract twists, resulting in luminal obstruction, compression of vascular structures, and possible progression to ischemia and necrosis of the involved segments.

2. **Clinical features**

a. **History.** Volvulus may be intermittent, so a history of poor weight gain or weight loss, episodic pain and vomiting, and/or blood in the stool may indicate recurrent episodes of obstruction.

b. **Symptoms.** Volvulus is characterized by the **acute onset of severe abdominal pain** and **intractable vomiting; depending on the level, degree, and duration of the obstruction, the emesis may be bilious or nonbilious.**

c. **Physical examination findings.** The level and length of the obstructed segment determines the symptoms seen; distension may or may not be present. Bowel sounds are often diminished, and tenderness may be localized or diffuse depending on the duration of the volvulus and degree of ischemia. As ischemia progresses, peritonitis, severe dehydration, and septic appearance occur.

3. **Differential diagnoses are similar to obstruction.**

4. **Evaluation**

a. **Careful physical examination** often reveals signs of acute obstruction but no peritoneal findings unless it is late in the course.

b. **Laboratory studies.** Electrolyte levels and renal function should be assessed; hyponatremia and hypochloremia may be present in proximal obstructions. CBC may reveal hemoconcentration or evidence of infection or diffuse intravascular coagulation in advanced cases.

c. **Radiographic studies**

i. **Plain abdominal radiographs.** Focal dilated loops with air–fluid levels and decreased or absent distal air may be seen.

ii. **Contrast radiographic studies may be performed in stable patients to establish the underlying cause such as malrotation.**

5. **Therapy**

a. **Stabilization**

i. **Intravenous electrolyte** solution should be administered to stabilize the patient's blood pressure and reestablish urine flow.

ii. **Emergent referral for surgery** is necessary to prevent progression of volvulus to perforation and frank peritonitis. All patients with suspected volvulus must have a surgical consultation.

Pediatric Emergencies

      b. **Antibiotic therapy** usually is not warranted. However, in critically ill infants with perforation and peritonitis, coverage for aerobic gram-negative organisms as well as anaerobic infection is justified.

  6. **Disposition.** Patients at **high risk for volvulus** must be emergently taken to surgery or transferred to a center where such care is available.

D. **Incarcerated hernia**

  1. **Discussion.** An incarcerated hernia occurs when the contents of a hernia sac cannot be reduced back into the abdominal cavity. The incarcerated organ is usually intestine but may be any abdominal organ—most commonly the mesentery or the ovary. The vast majority of incarcerated hernias involve the inguinal region; incarceration is rarely seen with umbilical hernias.

  2. **Clinical features.** Painful swelling localized to the area of the herniation is the most common initial symptom. There may be signs and symptoms of intestinal obstruction, such as bilious vomiting, abdominal distention, hematochezia, or constipation in cases with significant bowel entrapment.

    a. **Symptoms.** Children are irritable and often refuse most or all feedings. They may have vomiting that may or may not be bilious in character.

    b. **Physical examination findings**

      i. A tender, edematous, slightly discolored to pale mass is noted in the inguinal area.

      ii. A swollen erythematous mass that becomes erythematous to violaceous and is exquisitely tender is usually a sign of a strangulated hernia.

      iii. Fever and toxicity suggest frank necrosis of the incarcerated organ and impending or completed perforation.

  3. **Differential diagnoses** are the same as for volvulus (see X.C.3). Testicular torsion must be considered as well.

  4. **Evaluation.** Incarcerated hernia must be considered in all children with intestinal obstruction who have no other obvious reason for obstruction, such as antecedent surgery.

    a. **Careful physical examination** is the most useful diagnostic test that can be performed.

    b. **Laboratory studies**

      i. **CBC** may confirm the presence of impending strangulation.

      ii. A **serum biochemistry profile** guides therapy for replacement of fluid and electrolytes but is not helpful diagnostically.

    c. **Radiographic studies.** Air–fluid levels may be visible on plain radiographs; however, radiographs do not localize the source any better than a careful physical examination. Contrast studies are usually not indicated and add nothing to the diagnosis.

  5. **Therapy (see Clinical Pearl 15-5)**

    a. **Stabilization.** Electrolyte solution is administered intravenously to stabilize blood pressure and reestablish urine flow.

    b. **Emergent referral for surgery** to prevent progression of incarceration to perforation and frank peritonitis is mandatory for those patients with hernias that cannot be reduced and for those patients with strangulation. Absolutely **no delay** should occur from the time of diagnosis of an unreduced incarcerated hernia to surgical consultation because the need for surgery increases the morbidity 25-fold.

CLINICAL PEARL 15-5

Reduction of a nonstrangulated hernia can be accomplished in approximately 95% to 98% of cases.

1. The patient is usually best aided by sedation and placement in mild Trendelenburg position.

2. Gentle traction on the hernia and the contents of the sac are usually sufficient to allow for loss of volume and rapid retraction of the contents of the sac into the abdominal cavity.

3. After reduction of the hernia, elective repair may be accomplished 24 to 48 hours after edema subsides.

c. **Antibiotic therapy** usually is not warranted. However, in critically ill infants with perforation and peritonitis, coverage for aerobic gram-negative organisms as well as anaerobic infection is justified.

6. **Disposition**

a. **Discharge.** Children with an incarcerated hernia that is promptly reduced in the ED may be sent home if they are not dehydrated, provided that close surgical care is arranged.

b. **Admission**

   i. Patients at **high risk for strangulation** must be emergently taken to surgery or transferred to a center where such care is available.

   ii. **Dehydrated children** should be hospitalized and scheduled for surgery in the next 48 to 72 hours to allow time to correct fluid and electrolyte imbalances.

E. **Pyloric stenosis**

1. **Discussion.** Pyloric stenosis is the most commonly considered diagnosis in a small infant who is vomiting.

a. **Incidence.** Pyloric stenosis occurs at a rate of 3 to 5/1,000 live births in the United States. Boys, particularly firstborns, are affected four to six times more frequently than girls. Pyloric stenosis is also more common in Caucasian infants.

b. **Etiology.** The cause of pyloric stenosis is unknown, and no direct evidence is available to suggest a preventive strategy. There is an association of other congenital anomalies, particularly tracheoesophageal fistula and trisomy 18. Exposure to macrolide antibiotics in utero or in the neonatal period has been associated with an increased incidence of pyloric stenosis.

c. **Pathogenesis.** Vomiting causes **contraction of the intravascular space** and the development of a marked **hypochloremic alkalosis** with **hypokalemia** and **dehydration**.

2. **Clinical features**

a. **Symptoms** usually begin after the second or third week of life but have occurred as early as the first week. The peak age of onset is 3 to 4 weeks.

   i. The initial manifestation is most often **nonbilious vomiting** that is **nonprojectile** and often confused with feeding intolerance or gastroenteritis. Vomiting is often intermittent and not associated with an ill appearance. Affected infants appear well after an episode of vomiting and are usually hungry and ready to feed again.

   ii. As the disease progresses and the **infant loses weight**, a **visible peristaltic wave is often seen across the abdomen** that parents may notice.

b. **Physical examination findings**

   i. A **pyloric mass** (pyloric olive) that is often firm, movable, and nontender may be palpated immediately under the edge of the liver. Palpating the mass is diagnostic in 60% to 90% of affected infants. With more liberal use of ultrasound and earlier diagnosis, a palpable mass is rarely present at the time of diagnosis.

   ii. **Dehydration.** In the past, infants presented late in their disease course and were often misdiagnosed, which made them more likely to finally present with signs of significant dehydration. Increased awareness of the entity has decreased the incidence of severe dehydration dramatically.

3. **Differential diagnoses** include gastroesophageal reflux, poor maternal–infant bonding or poor feeding technique, congenital gastric outlet obstruction, gastric duplication syndromes, duodenal atresia, malrotation, intussusception, intracranial processes including hemorrhage, and sepsis.

4. **Evaluation**

a. **Laboratory studies.** A CBC is usually not indicated. An electrolyte and renal function panel should be performed to identify electrolyte disturbances common with the disorder. Blood cultures are usually not warranted.

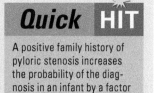

Quick HIT

A positive family history of pyloric stenosis increases the probability of the diagnosis in an infant by a factor of 40.

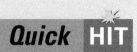

Quick HIT

The development of **projectile vomiting** appears to be related to the degree of obstruction at the pylorus.

Pediatric Emergencies

b. **Diagnostic imaging studies**
   i. **Radiography**
      a) **Plain radiographs** may be obtained to exclude other causes in the differential diagnosis but are not diagnostic of pyloric stenosis.
      b) **Contrast radiographs** are seldom used to make the diagnosis given the ready availability and lack of ionizing radiation associated with ultrasound. Upper gastrointestinal contrast studies were historically used and can reveal a narrowed and elongated pyloric channel; this approach has the advantage of assessing other differential considerations including reflux, malrotation, and gastric or duodenal webs or duplications.
   ii. **Ultrasonography** is safe and has a sensitivity that exceeds 95% when performed by an experienced radiologist. An ultrasonogram can establish the diagnosis on the basis of pyloric thickness and length; normal pyloric dimensions are <3 mm muscle thickness and <15 mm channel length.

5. **Therapy.** The infant must not be given anything by mouth. Vomiting usually subsides with the last bout of emesis after the stomach is empty.
   a. **Stabilization.** Initially, treatment is directed at **correcting fluid and electrolyte disturbances** and **replenishing intravascular volume**. Fluid therapy should be instituted concurrent with obtaining surgical consultation and should be continued until the patient is clinically rehydrated and the serum bicarbonate concentration is near normal. Isotonic saline should be used initially, with early addition of potassium once hyperkalemia and renal dysfunction are excluded.
   b. **Nasogastric suction** is rarely needed.
   c. **Prompt surgical consultation is mandatory**, and most children require hospitalization to correct any electrolyte abnormalities.

6. **Disposition.** Most children who undergo **ultrasound examination** of the pylorus and have **no evidence of stenosis** may be discharged home with appropriate follow-up care.

F. **Intussusception**
   1. **Discussion.** Intussusception is the most common cause of intestinal obstruction in infants and children between the ages of 3 months and 6 years. This condition occurs when a portion of the intestine telescopes into itself at one or more locations. Intussusceptions are most commonly located in the ileocolic junction.
      a. **Incidence.** As is the case with pyloric stenosis, intussusception is more common in boys than in girls by 4:1 or 5:1.
      b. **Etiology.** The cause is unknown, but a viral etiology is suspected because of a seasonal predisposition for spring and autumn months. Only 8% to 10% of children who require surgery for reduction have a recognized lead point, usually Meckel diverticulum, a polyp, duplication, or lymphosarcoma in older children.
      c. **Pathogenesis.** As with volvulus, intussusception causes initial bowel obstruction and progressive vascular compression with early venous and later arterial occlusion. With time, bowel ischemia and necrosis occur, and perforation or peritonitis may occur; the time course for bowel ischemia is highly variable, with some cases occurring within hours and other cases persisting for days without bowel ischemia.
   2. **Clinical features**
      a. **Symptoms**
         i. In typical cases, there is a sudden onset of **severe abdominal pain** that is colicky in nature and often so profound that the child drops to the floor in agony with crying and pain. Children who are so affected appear to be normal between paroxysms of pain.
         ii. As the intussusception progresses, the child becomes progressively more **irritable and lethargic** until **shock** develops.

iii. **Vomiting** initially occurs with the early phase of the illness and is bilious in 30% of cases.

iv. Stools are initially normal early in the course of the disease but become bloody and mucoid within the first 12 hours (**currant jelly stool**).

b. **Physical examination findings.** Palpation of the abdomen usually reveals a **tender, sausage-shaped mass** that is variable in size and firmness with spasms of pain.

3. **Differential diagnoses** include hypertrophic pyloric stenosis, congenital gastric outlet obstruction, gastric duplication syndromes, duodenal atresia, malrotation, appendicitis, sepsis, testicular torsion, incarcerated or strangulated hernia, gastroenteritis with enterocolitis, Henoch-Schönlein purpura, and diabetic ketoacidosis.

4. **Evaluation.** Typically, the **clinical history** and **physical findings** are sufficient for diagnosis.

   a. **Laboratory studies**

   i. A **CBC** and **serum biochemistry profile** are not indicated and are nondiagnostic in the first 12 hours of the illness but may be warranted in children with hypotension and symptoms of greater than 16 hours' duration.

   ii. **Urinalysis** is not helpful, although it may give some idea of fluid status.

   b. **Diagnostic imaging studies**

   i. **Radiography**

      a) **Plain abdominal radiographs** may show areas of increased soft tissue density or scattered air–fluid levels that suggest an ileus or partial obstruction. A soft tissue mass obscuring the liver edge, paucity of gas in the cecum and right colon, target-like mass or meniscus within the ascending, or transverse colon are highly suggestive of intussusception. Fifty percent of plain films are normal or nonspecific but are performed to exclude perforation prior to contrast enema.

      b) **Contrast radiographs.** An air or contrast enema is therapeutic as well as diagnostic, revealing a **filling defect**. A "**coil spring**," caused by the tracking of barium around the lumen of the edematous intestine, is a classic sign.

   ii. **Ultrasonography** has become standard of care for diagnosing intussusception, and has the advantage of avoiding ionizing radiation, being relatively inexpensive and noninvasive, and allowing exclusion of other diagnostic considerations such as malrotation. Sensitivity exceeds 90% when performed by experienced ultrasonographers.

5. **Therapy**

   a. **Stabilization** is the same as for pyloric stenosis (see X.E.5.a). The child should not be given anything by mouth.

   b. **Nasogastric suction** should be instituted to attempt to decompress the obstruction from above.

   c. **Barium or air reduction** is appropriate after surgical consultation if there are no signs of peritonitis. Children who have signs of peritonitis should not be considered candidates for barium or air reduction. These children should be stabilized and taken expeditiously to the operating room because untreated intussusception is almost always fatal.

6. **Disposition**

   a. **Discharge.** Most children who undergo ultrasound examination of the abdomen and have no evidence of intussusception and are well-hydrated without peritoneal signs may be discharged home with close follow-up with their primary care provider.

   b. **Admission. Prompt surgical consultation** is mandatory, and most children require hospitalization to correct any electrolyte abnormalities prior to surgery.

G. **Meckel diverticulum**

1. **Discussion**

   a. **Cause.** Meckel diverticulum is a remnant of the embryonic yolk sac that failed to involute. This results in the presence in the mesenteric or

Pediatric Emergencies

antimesenteric border of a blind pouch that is usually 50 to 75 cm from the ileocolic junction.

b. **Pathogenesis**

i. Diverticula become symptomatic when ectopic mucosae secrete acid, causing intermittent painless rectal bleeding following ulceration of the adjacent mucosa.

ii. Occasionally, Meckel diverticulum may be associated with partial or complete bowel obstruction when the diverticulum becomes edematous and acts as a lead point for an intussusception. Such diverticula may become inflamed and mimic appendicitis or result in perforation and peritonitis.

2. **Clinical features**

a. **Symptoms.** Many diverticula remain clinically silent and are found in approximately 3% to 5% of autopsy cases as an incidental finding.

i. Chronic or **acute abdominal pain** may precede frank bleeding and may be difficult to distinguish from appendicitis or another intestinal obstructive event.

ii. **Melanotic stools** are intermittent and may correlate with clinical symptoms. Symptoms characteristic of intussusception may occur; currant jelly stools can lead to misdiagnosis.

iii. **Nausea, vomiting,** and **abdominal distention** may mirror appendicitis.

b. **Physical examination findings**

i. **Signs of intestinal obstruction** are often present and are associated with bands that may result from inflammation of the diverticula.

ii. **Signs of shock** or **dehydration** are rarely seen and are not usual unless perforation and peritonitis are present from ulceration.

3. **Differential diagnoses** include peptic ulcer disease, caustic ingestions, gastric duplication syndromes, annular pancreas, malrotation, appendicitis, colonic diverticulitis, testicular torsion, incarcerated or strangulated hernia, gastroenteritis with enterocolitis, Henoch-Schönlein purpura, diabetic ketoacidosis, and intussusception.

4. **Evaluation**

a. **Laboratory studies**

i. A CBC usually reveals anemia from chronic blood loss and may show a leukocytosis if inflammation of the diverticulum is present or if there is impending peritonitis.

ii. A **serum biochemical profile** is not useful unless protracted vomiting or signs of peritonitis are evident.

iii. Blood and **urine cultures** are warranted in ill-appearing children with signs of peritonitis.

b. **Diagnostic imaging studies**

i. **Radiography**

a) **Plain radiographs of the abdomen** may be normal but may show evidence of ileus or free air with perforation.

b) **Contrast radiographic studies** rarely demonstrate the diverticula and almost never fill the sac.

ii. A **Meckel radionuclide scan** reveals acid-secreting mucosa and can be enhanced with glucagon, gastrin, or cimetidine; this study is sensitive in 85% to 90% of cases.

iii. **Ultrasonography** is of no value and is not warranted unless the purpose is to exclude other causes.

5. **Therapy** entails **stabilization, nasogastric suction,** and **surgical excision.** The child should not be given anything by mouth. **Broad-spectrum antibiotic therapy** is indicated for children with peritonitis or diverticulitis.

6. **Disposition.** Children at risk for Meckel diverticulum must be hospitalized following surgical consultation for antibiotic therapy and exploration. **Prompt surgical consultation is mandatory,** and most children require hospitalization to correct any electrolyte abnormalities prior to surgery and to treat peritonitis.

> **Quick HIT**
>
> Meckel diverticulum usually becomes clinically apparent during the first 2 years of life but is equally common in the first 10 to 15 years of life.

Pediatric Emergencies

H. **Appendicitis**
  1. **Discussion.** Appendicitis is the most common condition requiring emergency abdominal surgery in childhood.
    a. **Etiology.** Appendicitis is inversely related to the amount of fiber in the diet and is uncommon in third-world countries. The cause of appendicitis is unknown but may be due to luminal obstruction with fecal material, inflammation, enteric bacteria, viruses, or tumor mass.
    b. **Pathogenesis.** Perforation rates are two to five times higher in children when compared with adults because of nonspecific symptoms and delays in presentation. Approximately 50% to 60% of children with perforation were seen by a physician in the preceding 24 hours. Perforation risk is inversely related to age, with the highest risk of perforation being 70% to 80% in the 1- to 4-year-old group and lowest in adolescents (30% to 40%).
  2. **Clinical features**
    a. **Classic symptoms** consist of anorexia, fever, vomiting, and pain that initially begins as vague periumbilical discomfort. Progression of symptoms is usually subacute and occurs over 36 to 48 hours, with perforation rates that exceed 75% at 48 hours.
      i. **Fever** is usually not reported or is low grade but may be elevated with perforation.
      ii. **Pain** usually precedes the development of vomiting and fever and is an important point in differentiating from infectious gastroenteritis. As inflammation progresses, pain becomes more localized to the site of inflammation in the right lower quadrant. A large retrocecal appendicitis may frequently produce pain in the right upper quadrant that resembles cholecystitis in adults and is usually misdiagnosed in children as nonspecific abdominal pain.
      iii. **Diarrhea** is seen in 15% of pediatric patients with appendicitis and is often small, pasty, and mucoid and resembles the stool pattern of *Shigella* but without blood.
    b. **Physical examination findings** are inconsistent.
      i. **Abdominal tenderness may be localized or diffuse; focal tenderness in the right lower quadrant and radiation of pain to that area with palpation of distant locations (Rovsing sign) are suggestive of appendicitis.**
      ii. **Rebound tenderness,** particularly percussion tenderness, is suggestive of impending peritonitis.
      iii. An **inflammatory mass** palpated on rectal examination suggests the diagnosis, particularly if the mass is painful.
  3. **Differential diagnoses** include peptic ulcer disease, caustic ingestions, gastric duplication syndromes, annular pancreas, malrotation, foreign body obstruction, colonic diverticulitis, testicular torsion, incarcerated or strangulated hernia, pyelonephritis, gastroenteritis with enterocolitis, Henoch-Schönlein purpura, diabetic ketoacidosis, intussusception, lower lobe pneumonia, tubal ectopic pregnancy (in adolescents), pelvic inflammatory disease, and inflammatory bowel disease.
  4. **Evaluation**
    a. **Laboratory studies**
      i. A **CBC** may reveal a leukocytosis with left shift; multiple studies have shown that CBC findings are not sensitive or specific for appendicitis.
      ii. **C-reactive protein may be a more reliable predictor of inflammation consistent with appendicitis.**
      iii. **A serum electrolyte determination** is not useful unless protracted vomiting or signs of peritonitis are evident.
      iv. **Blood** and **urine cultures** are warranted in ill-appearing children with signs of peritonitis.
      v. **Urinalysis.** Sterile pyuria and microscopic hematuria are occasionally noted because of irritation of the inflamed appendix on the right ureter or bladder.

Quick HIT

Clinical trials have demonstrated that the use of narcotic pain medication for patients with significant pain and tenderness allows better localization of tenderness and does *not* mask important examination findings.

b. **Diagnostic imaging studies**
  i. **Radiography**
    a) **Plain radiographs of the abdomen** may be normal or may show evidence of ileus or free air with perforation and, in 15% to 20% of cases, may reveal a calcified appendicolith.
    b) **Contrast radiographic studies** rarely demonstrate the appendicitis—they may show indentation of the cecum with the inflammatory mass but almost never fill the sac.
  ii. **Ultrasonography.** A useful study is an **appendiceal compression ultrasound**, which has a false-negative rate of 8% to 10%. Ultrasound can also be used to guide percutaneous drainage of periappendiceal abscesses to allow for delayed appendectomy after a course of antibiotics.
  iii. **CT** is usually helpful and diagnostic. Intravenous contrast should be utilized; use of oral and rectal contrast is controversial and varies from center to center.
5. **Therapy** entails **stabilization**, **nasogastric suction**, and a **barium enema** (if intussusception or Meckel diverticulitis cannot be excluded), as described in X.E.5. Children who have had symptoms longer than 36 to 48 hours or who have signs of peritonitis should not be considered candidates for immediate **surgical exploration**. Children with peritonitis should receive **broad-spectrum antibiotic therapy** and should be hospitalized following surgical consultation.
6. **Disposition**
  a. All children **at risk for appendicitis** must have intravenous access established and be promptly fluid resuscitated if signs of peritonitis or perforation are present. Analgesia should be provided to improve patient comfort and allow localization of maximal pain and tenderness. After surgical consultation, they should be hospitalized for antibiotic therapy and exploration.
  b. Children in whom the **diagnosis is unclear** merit a period of hospital admission and observation or reexamination 6 to 12 hours later, preferably by the same physician.

XI. SEIZURES

A. **Discussion.** Seizures represent abnormal neural discharges in the cerebral cortex or brain stem that are paroxysmal in nature and may be either physically silent or expressed in the form of repetitive movements and actions.
  1. **Etiology.** Seizures are most often caused by birth trauma, congenital infection, or congenital anatomic defects in young infants.
  2. **Classification.** Seizures may be classified according to many schemes, depending on anatomic site of seizure, duration and type of movement disorder (if any), or recurrence patterns.
    a. **Acute nonrecurring seizures**
      i. **Febrile seizures** are seizures that accompany febrile disorders but are not directly caused by CNS infections (see Clinical Pearl 15-6). Febrile convulsions usually occur between the ages of 6 months and 6 years. There is frequently a positive family history of febrile seizures. These events most commonly occur at the onset of the fever and are thought to be related to the rate of rise of the temperature rather than the absolute temperature. Febrile seizures are divided into simple and complex.
      ii. **Seizures secondary to toxic ingestions** (e.g., isoniazid or clonidine toxicity)

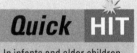

Quick HIT

In infants and older children, there may be no apparent cause (idiopathic), or seizures may be the sequela of an acute infectious process.

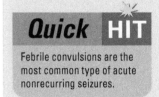

Quick HIT

Febrile convulsions are the most common type of acute nonrecurring seizures.

CLINICAL PEARL 15-6

Simple febrile seizures last <20 minutes, are generalized, consist of a single event within a 24-hour period, and occur in a neurologically normal child who returns to baseline after the event.

iii. **Metabolic disturbances** (e.g., hypoglycemia, hypocalcemia, hyponatremia)

iv. **Intracranial disorders** (e.g., cerebral tumor, meningitis, tumor)

b. **Chronic recurring seizures**

i. **Partial simple seizures** start focally and do not cause loss of consciousness. They usually are motor and nongeneralized and often result in deviation of the eyes and head.

ii. **Partial complex seizures** were previously known as psychomotor or temporal lobe seizures. These seizures usually start focally and classically are associated with a loss of awareness or consciousness but not with loss of motor control.

    a) Minor changes in behavior or affect may be the only visible manifestation.

    b) However, these changes may be dramatic, with repetitive purposeless activity. Some patients may perform acts of which they are unaware for minutes or hours. Often, these activities involve walking or running distances, which may put them in great jeopardy.

iii. **Generalized seizures**

    a) **Generalized tonic–clonic seizures** are the prototype, alternating between the brief tonic phase of generalized muscle contraction and a longer period of rhythmic spasms.

        1) Classically, children old enough to describe their symptoms report a **prodrome** or **aura** that may be characterized by muscular discomfort, gastrointestinal upset, scotomata, or noxious gustatory stimuli.

        2) **Postseizure somnolence** followed by confusion and ataxia (postictal period) is common and may last for several hours.

    b) **Myoclonic seizures** are a variant that consists of sudden movements of the trunk and extremities, causing the patient to fall. Myoclonic seizures are a common presentation of metabolic or neurodegenerative diseases in infancy (infantile spasms).

iv. **Absence seizures** consist of staring and eye-blinking episodes that usually last 10 to 20 seconds. These seizures represent brief interruptions of consciousness without overt loss of motor control. Episodes happen many times per day and are usually precipitated by exertion or emotional upset, with resulting subsequent hyperventilation, or by photic stimulation described by blinking lights.

v. **Akinetic seizures** are central seizures that cause a sudden loss of muscle tone. Previously called "**drop attacks**," these seizures put children in danger of falling at inappropriate times.

vi. **Status epilepticus or serial status**

    a) **Status epilepticus** is a continuous seizure (i.e., the patient does not regain consciousness or function without intervention) lasting more than 20 minutes.

    b) **Serial status** usually represents bursts of status epilepticus that last for variable periods of time only to recur after an interstatus interval.

vii. **Neonatal seizures** are a special form of seizures because of the lack of stereotypic repetitive behavior. They require a high index of suspicion for subtle symptoms of pedaling movements of legs, stiffening, or lip smacking.

B. **Clinical features** depend on the type of seizure. Most seizures are composed of a brief tonic phase of generalized contraction of all or partial muscle groups followed by a more prolonged clonic phase of rhythmic repetitive spasms of the same muscle groups or recruitment of others.

1. **Partial complex seizures** are usually focal and do not generalize but usually are associated with a loss of awareness of surroundings.

2. **Absence seizures** are associated with staring or blinking episodes that last for seconds and with brief interruptions in consciousness but no loss of motor

tone. These seizures usually are precipitated by an emotional event or photic stimulation.

3. **Myoclonic seizures** or infantile spasms are associated with sudden flexion of the trunk at the waist with extension or flexion of the arms or legs, resulting in the child falling to the ground.

4. **Akinetic seizures** are similar to myoclonic seizures in that the child falls to the ground, but these seizures are caused by loss of muscle tone, not flexion or muscle spasms.

5. **Neonatal seizures** may be the most difficult to characterize because of the variable presentation of symptoms. A high index of suspicion must be maintained, particularly with infants who present with stiffening episodes or repetitive movements of the eyes, mouth, or tongue. A hospitalized careful observation period is warranted with video recording to characterize such movements.

C. **Differential diagnoses**

1. **Anatomic and structural defects**
   a. Hydranencephaly
   b. Absent corpus callosum
   c. Dandy-Walker cyst

2. **Metabolic and storage diseases**

3. **Phycomycoses**
   a. Tuberous sclerosis
   b. Neurofibromatosis

4. **CNS tumor**

5. **Infection**
   a. Meningitis
   b. Encephalitis
   c. Brain abscess
   d. Cerebral cysticercosis

6. **Trauma**
   a. Subdural effusion
   b. Intracerebral hemorrhage
   c. Cortical infarct

D. **Evaluation**

1. A careful **physical examination** should be performed, including growth and development parameters, and analysis of perinatal factors and family history.

2. **Laboratory studies.** Appropriate studies vary by seizure type and duration, patient age and underlying risk factors, and exam findings. Simple febrile seizures in a child with a normal examination require no testing other than what would be indicated for the fever in that child (i.e., urinalysis and culture in a patient younger than 2 years). Brief, afebrile seizures in an otherwise healthy child with a normal examination also require no ED testing.
   a. Serum biochemistry profile
   b. Liver tests
   c. ABG analysis
   d. Urinalysis and urine amino acid analysis
   e. Serologic screens (e.g., for cytomegalovirus, toxoplasmosis, HIV, varicella zoster virus)
   f. CSF analysis
   g. Determination of serum anticonvulsant concentrations is important in children with established seizure disorder.

3. **Diagnostic imaging studies**
   a. **Electroencephalography** should be performed alone, with hyperventilation, and with photic stimulation. **Continuous electroencephalogram (EEG) recordings** may provide helpful information. EEG can be performed on an outpatient basis in patients who do not require admission for status epilepticus, multiple seizures, or persistent neurological abnormalities.
   b. **Axial CT scanning** or **magnetic resonance imaging** may be necessary. Emergent CT is only indicated in patients with focal seizures, preceding

signs/symptoms suggestive of increased intracranial pressure, or a persistent abnormal neurologic examination. Magnetic resonance imaging is the preferred imaging modality and can be performed on a nonurgent basis in most cases.

E. Therapy
1. **Simple febrile convulsions** require no further evaluation if patients have no focal neurologic deficits, convulsions lasting fewer than 15 to 20 minutes, a short postictal period, and no neurologic disorders following the seizure.
2. **Recurrent febrile seizures.** Up to 30% of children will have at least one recurrence of a febrile seizure. Antiepileptic medications are rarely utilized and are generally reserved for those patients with multiple events or recurrent febrile status epilepticus.
3. **Seizures** as a result of **toxic ingestions** or **metabolic disorders** require no specific treatment except correction of the underlying cause. Neonatal seizures may be pyridoxine-responsive.
4. **Chronic seizures** are treated in consultation with a neurologist based on the EEG findings and the seizure type.
5. **Status epilepticus** requires emergent treatment with either lorazepam or diazepam intravenously. If intravenous access is not available, intranasal midazolam or rectal valium can be used as abortive therapy.
   a. **Careful monitoring** of pulse oximetry and vital signs is imperative.
   b. If benzodiazepines are ineffective, parenteral loading and maintenance with a second-line agent are indicated. Second-line therapy may include fosphenytoin or levetiracetam (Keppra, UCB, Anderlecht, Belgium), followed by phenobarbital or pentobarbital. Children requiring further therapy should be transferred to a regional pediatric center and to the care of a pediatric neurologist.

F. Disposition
1. **Discharge. Children with simple febrile seizures** who are normal on examination and to parents do not merit further evaluation and may be discharged home.
2. **Admission** is indicated for:
   a. Children who have **prolonged febrile seizures**, **focal deficits**, a **prolonged postictal time**, or **neurologic deficits** after a seizure
   b. Children younger than 2 years with **new-onset seizure** that is not associated with fever should be hospitalized for further evaluation. Older children who have brief, nonfocal seizures and are back to baseline can be managed as an outpatient with EEG and follow-up with their primary care provider.
   c. **Children with status epilepticus** or **serial status**

XII. CHILD ABUSE

A. **Discussion.** Child abuse is one of the leading causes of death in children between the ages of 1 and 12 months. With first episodes of child abuse, the mortality rate is approximately 5% to 8%, but repeated cases of child abuse are associated with a mortality rate higher than 50%.
1. **Types of abuse**
   a. **Physical abuse** is the intentional injury of a child (e.g., beating, shaking).
   b. **Sexual abuse** is any sexual activity between an adult and a child.
   c. **Physical neglect** is the failure of caregivers to provide the necessities of life such as nourishment, shelter, clothing, supervision, medical care, cleanliness, education, or monetary support.
   d. **Emotional neglect** is failure of caregivers to provide the necessities of emotional support for self-esteem and normal development.
   e. **By-proxy neglect (Munchausen syndrome)** is a condition in which the parents induce or fabricate illness, causing the child to undergo unnecessary diagnostic and therapeutic interventions.
2. **Incidence.** Approximately 30% of instances of child abuse occur in children younger than 12 months of age, 33% in children 1 to 6 years of age, and 37%

in children older than 6 years. When the child or family has a life of poverty, crises, or limited access to social resources, the incidence of child abuse is increased.

3. **Characteristics of the abuser.** In 90% to 95% of cases, the abuser is a related adult (average age, 25 years). The most common perpetrators are the father (21%), mother (21%), mother's boyfriend (9%), babysitter (8%), and stepfather (5%).

B. **Clinical features.** Physical abuse should be suspected when an injury is **unexplained** by caregivers, is inconsistent with the stated mechanism, or is **implausible**, or when a **significant delay in seeking medical care** is noted. Bilateral, **symmetric**, or **geometric injuries** increase clinical suspicion for child abuse. **Unexplained falls** from heights, **electrocutions**, or **drowning** is always suspicious for child abuse or neglect.

1. **Bruises** are the most common manifestation of child abuse and may be found on any body surface area. Concerning bruises are those occurring in nonambulatory infants and children, not involving bony prominences, and in areas that cannot be reached or would be unusual in a fall. Bruising may take the shape of the inflicting instrument in the case of a belt buckle, belt, looped electrical cord, flyswatter, coat hanger, or hand.

2. **Fractures** are usually caused by wrenching or pulling injuries that damage the bone metaphysis. The most common abusive fractures are parietal skull and transverse long bone fractures; spiral fractures in children who are not ambulatory are highly concerning. Rib fractures and metaphyseal fractures are unusual accidental injuries and warrant a full evaluation for child abuse.

3. **Damaged hair.** At first, tinea capitis may be suspected, but this diagnosis can be eliminated on the basis of lack of skin involvement, broken hairs of varying lengths, and no evidence of fungal elements on the surface of the hair.

4. **Burns** account for 10% to 15% of all cases of abuse and usually take on characteristics of the burning object.

5. **Head trauma** is the most common cause of death and usually presents as coma, convulsions, apnea, signs of intracranial hypertension, or protracted vomiting.

   a. **Subdural hematomas** are the most frequently seen injury.

   b. **Skull and rib fractures** are common together and indicate slamming of the body and head against a wall or mattress.

   c. **Head and neck petechiae** associated with subconjunctival hemorrhage are commonly caused by choking.

   d. **Retinal hemorrhages** occur with shaking; are often found in association with subdural hematomas; and rarely result from cardiopulmonary resuscitation, accidental falls, or from infectious processes.

6. **Intra-abdominal injuries** are the second most common cause of death and usually result in shock if the liver or spleen ruptures.

C. **Differential diagnoses** include accidental orthopedic trauma (e.g., nursemaid's elbow, shoulder dislocation, humerus fractures, forearm fractures, wrist fractures, cervical spinal injuries), soft tissue trauma, osteochondrosis of the capitellum (Panner disease), epicondylitis of the lateral humeral condyle, septic arthritis of the elbow, hemarthroses secondary to hereditary coagulopathy, accidental burns or immersions, metabolic abnormalities (e.g., osteogenesis imperfecta), accidental trauma to sexual organs, and underlying medical conditions leading to failure to thrive.

D. **Evaluation**

1. A properly performed **physical examination with careful attention to the historical facts of the injury** is perhaps the most important part of the evaluation process.

   a. In girls, when sexual abuse is suspected, **standard rape testing protocols** should be followed (see Chapter 14.X.C.3). In addition, a **colposcopic examination** should be performed. Photographic evidence may be necessary for later forensic examination.

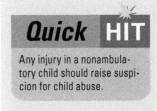

Quick **HIT**

Any injury in a nonambulatory child should raise suspicion for child abuse.

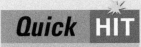

Quick **HIT**

Cigarette burns result in circular punched-out burns, immersion burns result in a line of demarcation on the distal extremities, and steam-iron burns result in V-shaped burns, particularly if they cross joint spaces.

Pediatric Emergencies

b. Suspicious traumatic lesions should be **photographed**; appropriate color correction is necessary.

2. Laboratory studies
   a. **Screening tests** for a bleeding diathesis should be obtained in all cases of bruising, **including a CBC and prothrombin and partial thromboplastin times.**
   b. **Hepatic and pancreatic enzymes and a noncatheterized urinalysis should be performed on cases with abdominal findings and on those with multiple or severe injuries.**
   c. **Urine and stool samples** should be screened for blood in cases of abdominal trauma.
   d. **Cultures of rectal, vaginal, urethral, and pharyngeal smears** may be indicated in suspected cases of sexual abuse.

3. Diagnostic imaging studies
   a. A **radiographic bone survey**, including two views of all body regions should be performed in all cases of suspected abuse <2 years of age.
   b. A **CT scan** of the head and abdomen may be indicated in severely traumatized children. Abdominal CT is indicated on cases with abdominal bruising or tenderness or in those with abnormal liver or pancreatic enzyme levels.

E. **Therapy.** Life-threatening conditions such as seizures, apnea, or respiratory arrest should be treated promptly. All surgically remediable injuries should be quickly evaluated in consultation with a surgeon.

F. **Disposition**
1. **Admission** is indicated when the medical condition requires inpatient management, when the diagnosis is unclear, when no alternative for the safety or well-being of the child can be assured, or when custody is unavailable.
2. In all cases of physical or sexual abuse, the proper **authorities should be notified**, and the case should be reported as mandated in all states. The child should not be released until his or her safety can be assured. The suspected perpetrator should have no unsupervised access to the child or should be in custody pending evaluation.
3. Children suspected of being abused or neglected should receive adequate **psychological support** and **evaluation**.

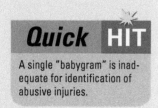

Quick HIT

A single "babygram" is inadequate for identification of abusive injuries.

HEMATOLOGIC AND ONCOLOGIC EMERGENCIES

16

Joseph Bales • Daniel O'Brien

I. APPROACH TO THE BLEEDING PATIENT

A. **Discussion**

1. Patients with spontaneous bleeding or multisite hemorrhage should be suspected of having bleeding diathesis.
2. Delay of bleeding for several hours after trauma, persistent hemorrhage, or bleeding into deep tissues or joints may be signs of hematologic abnormality.

B. **Clinical features**

1. Patients may present with normal-appearing bleeding, which is abnormal only when delayed or persistent.
2. Bleeding may range from visually worrisome, such as appearance of hemarthrosis or petechiae, to hemodynamically threatening, especially if bleeding into potential spaces (e.g., retroperitoneum), which may be life-threatening.

C. **Differential diagnosis** of patients with bleeding disorders primarily involves determination of which one of the multitudes of congenital and hematologic abnormalities is responsible for the patient's presentation.

D. **Evaluation**

1. **Patient history.** Details regarding the patient's current problem, past disease, and family medical history are particularly important in patients who present to the emergency department (ED) with abnormal bleeding.
   a. Most patients with hematologic disease are aware of their diagnosis and are knowledgeable about previous therapy.
   b. Past medical history, including such items as postdental extraction bleeding, may also provide useful information about a patient's hemostatic disease. Chronic liver disease affects hemostasis in many cases.
   c. A medication history is useful because certain drugs (e.g., nonsteroidal anti-inflammatory drugs, ethanol, warfarin) may affect clotting.
2. **Physical examination** includes searches for sites of bleeding and other findings to provide clues to the nature of hemostatic disruption.
   a. Mucocutaneous bleeding (petechiae, ecchymoses, respiratory or gastrointestinal tract hemorrhage) is characteristic of platelet disorders.
   b. Delayed bleeding after trauma and deep tissue or joint hemorrhage are characteristic of disorders of the coagulation cascade.
   c. Postural hypotension and other signs of volume loss may be present on examination of patients with significant blood loss.
3. **Laboratory evaluation** begins with a complete blood count (CBC), platelet count, prothrombin time (PT), partial thromboplastin time (PTT), and international normalized ratio. Other specialized hematologic tests (e.g., coagulation factors, fibrin degeneration products, inhibitor screens) are ordered as indicated by the differential diagnosis, although results may not be obtained while the patient is still in the ED.

Quick HIT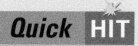

Type AB+ patients may receive any blood type; type O− people are universal donors and any blood type may receive O−. Type A and B patients may also receive blood types A and B, respectively.

Quick HIT

Type O− blood (Rh negative in patients of childbearing age) may be used when there is insufficient time to obtain type- and Rh-specific blood.

Quick HIT

Type-matching and Rh-matching require only 10 to 15 minutes in the laboratory (compared with up to 60 minutes for fully cross-matched blood).

Quick HIT

The most important variable, besides the actual hematocrit or hemoglobin level, is whether blood loss is acute or chronic.

Quick HIT

Symptomatic patients and patients with very low hemoglobin levels (e.g., below 7) should be considered candidates for PRBC transfusion.

E. **Therapy.** Treatment priorities and initial therapy (e.g., normal saline administration to correct hypotension) are the same as those for any other patient in the ED.
  1. **Stabilization**
    a. Airway compromise may be threatened by blood in the upper airway. When indicated, intubation should be performed with an endotracheal tube large enough (preferably 8.0) to allow subsequent bronchoscopy.
    b. Hemodynamic instability should be first treated with crystalloid replacement, with progression to blood component therapy as indicated by the situation.
  2. **Pharmacologic adjuncts** (e.g., steroids for idiopathic thrombocytopenic purpura) may be indicated.
  3. **Blood component therapy** is indicated for some patients with abnormal bleeding in the ED. Blood component therapy is commonly administered in many EDs, necessitating familiarity with infusion indications, methods, and complications.
    a. **Blood type.** Type AB+ patients may receive any blood type; all patients may receive type O− (males receive O+). Type A and B patients may also receive blood types A and B, respectively.
      i. ED patients who may not require immediate transfusion may still require type and cross-match in preparation for impending blood product therapy. Patients with the following disease processes should be typed and crossed: shock, gastrointestinal bleeding, anemia (hemoglobin less than 10 g/dL), significant or continuing blood loss, or impending surgical procedures that pose a risk of hemorrhage.
      ii. Incompletely matched blood may be transfused in some emergency situations. These emergency transfusions may be life-saving, but they also carry significantly increased risks of transfusion reactions.
    b. **Blood components.** Whole blood is essentially unavailable in civilian hospitals because units of donated blood are separated into components to allow optimal storage and directed therapy.
      i. Packed red blood cells (PRBCs) represent the most commonly transfused blood component.
        a) Administration of PRBCs results in increased oxygen-carrying capacity in patients with significant blood loss.
        b) There is no specific threshold for PRBC transfusion.
          1) **Acute blood loss** can be replaced with crystalloid until the lost volume approaches 25% to 30% of circulating volume.
          2) **Chronic blood loss.** Patients with chronic blood loss may tolerate decrements in hemoglobin to 8 g/dL or lower without requiring a transfusion.
      ii. Other formulations of RBCs are transfused in special circumstances.
        a) Leukocyte-poor RBCs are administered to patients who have undergone transplants or who have had febrile nonhemolytic transfusion reactions.
        b) Frozen RBCs represent an expensive method of providing reduced antigen exposure or keeping rare blood types stored for longer periods of time than the usual 42-day shelf life of PRBCs.
        c) Washed RBCs have had plasma proteins and some leukocytes and platelets removed, preventing the precipitation of hemolysis.
      iii. Platelets are another blood component commonly administered in the ED. Usually given in "single donor packs," platelets may also be prepared specially (with human leukocyte antigen matching or radiation) to minimize reactions. Indications for platelet transfusion depend on both the platelet count and the cause of thrombocytopenia.
        a) Thrombocytopenia caused by antiplatelet antibodies is generally refractory to platelet transfusion.
        b) Platelet counts of 10,000 to 50,000/mm³ may be associated with spontaneous bleeding in patients with concurrent hepatorenal disease. *Bleeding* patients with platelet counts at this level should be treated with platelet transfusion.

    c) Prophylactic platelet transfusion (to prevent spontaneous hemorrhage) is indicated in patients with platelet counts below 10,000/mm^3.

  iv. Fresh frozen plasma (FFP) units are used for replacement of coagulation factors and fibrinogen. Indications for FFP transfusion include factor deficiency or other coagulopathy in patients who are bleeding or who will undergo procedures that may induce hemorrhage.

    a) Patients taking warfarin and those with coagulopathy from liver disease or disseminated intravascular coagulation (DIC) may require treatment with FFP.

    b) Patients with acquired or congenital factor deficiency, or antithrombin III deficiency, may be treated with FFP when specific therapy is unavailable.

    c) FFP may be administered to patients with coagulopathy related to massive transfusion therapy.

  v. Cryoprecipitate is derived from FFP and is used for replacement of fibrinogen and von Willebrand factor (vWF).

    a) Cryoprecipitate may be infused when factor VIII therapy is unavailable to treat patients with von Willebrand disease whose bleeding is uncontrolled with desmopressin.

    b) Patients with fibrinogen levels below 100 mg/dL, as may occur with DIC, may be treated with cryoprecipitate.

  vi. Specific factor replacement therapy is the optimal choice for replacement of coagulation factors (see II.B). Specific factor replacement therapy minimizes the risks associated with pooled blood component therapy.

c. Administration protocols

  i. General considerations

    a) The first step is to identify the patient's needs and choose the correct product.

    b) Blood products are infused through large-bore catheters to minimize the risks of hemolysis and to allow rapid infusion of blood products when necessary.

  ii. PRBCs. Transfusion of 1 U of PRBCs is expected to raise the hemoglobin level by 1 g/dL and the hematocrit by 3%.

    a) Normal saline, the only crystalloid compatible with blood, is usually given along with PRBCs for dilution and infusion facilitation.

    b) Transfusion rate. When the clinical situation allows, blood product infusion should proceed slowly for the first half hour, when transfusion reactions are most likely. Patients without a history of congestive heart failure may be administered 1 U of PRBCs over 1 to 2 hours. The rate is halved for patients with congestive heart failure.

  iii. Platelets. Infusion of one pack of single donor platelets is expected to result in a platelet count increment of 60,000/mm^3 as assessed 1 hour after infusion. Platelets, as well as FFP, may be given per protocol during massive transfusion of PRBCs.

    a) ABO blood type compatibility is recommended for platelet transfusions to minimize the risks of transfusion reaction.

    b) Rh-negative females of childbearing age should receive platelets from Rh-negative donors.

  iv. FFP units should also be transfused from ABO-compatible donors. The initial dose is 8 to 10 mL/kg (two bags). Prothrombin complex concentrates in three- or four-factor form will correct the international normalized ratio much more quickly than FFP.

  v. Cryoprecipitate is infused in initial doses of two to four bags per 10 kg body weight.

  vi. Specific factor therapy is guided by the patient's factor levels and desired magnitudes of increment.

  vii. Tranexamic acid is an amino acid analogue of lysine that has significant antifibrinolytic properties, used as early as possible during major trauma or intraoperative at the surgeon's discretion.

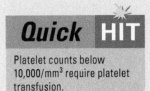

Quick HIT

Platelet counts below 10,000/mm^3 require platelet transfusion.

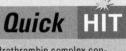

Quick HIT

Prothrombin complex concentrates are preferable to FFP in many cases of bleeding associated with anticoagulation therapy.

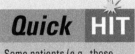

Quick HIT

Some patients (e.g., those with fever, DIC, excessive hemorrhage, hypersplenism, antiplatelet antibodies) may be refractory to platelet transfusion.

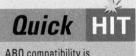

Quick HIT

ABO compatibility is required only if large amounts of cryoprecipitate are administered.

Hematologic and Oncologic Emergencies

    d. Transfusion complications

       i. Acute intravascular hemolysis, usually resulting from ABO blood group incompatibility, represents the most dangerous acute transfusion reaction. Advanced hemolytic reactions may progress to cardiovascular, pulmonary, and renal failure.

         a) Clinical presentation of a hemolytic transfusion reaction includes fever, chills, back pain, dyspnea, or localized burning at the infusion site. Laboratory tests in patients with acute hemolytic reactions reveal elevated free plasma hemoglobin, haptoglobin, and bilirubin; hemoglobinuria is also found. Coombs testing should be performed on pre- and posttransfusion blood samples.

         b) Therapy of hemolytic reactions should begin before confirmative testing and includes cessation of transfusion and institution of aggressive hydration.

      ii. Rh incompatibility hemolysis. A less acute hemolysis, caused by Rh incompatibility, may occur in the extravascular space of the spleen. These patients often are asymptomatic and do not require therapy.

     iii. Febrile nonhemolytic transfusion reactions occur relatively commonly, especially in patients undergoing multiple transfusions. These nonthreatening reactions are caused by antigen–antibody reactions involving donor plasma, platelets, or leukocytes.

         a) Clinically, nonhemolytic reactions begin within the first few hours after transfusion and manifest as temperature elevation and chills.

         b) Because these reactions cannot be differentiated clinically from early acute hemolytic reactions, transfusions must be discontinued when reactions are first suspected, and repeat cross-matching and Coombs testing of blood are indicated.

         c) Patients with previous nonhemolytic reactions may be pretreated with acetaminophen and opioids or may be administered leukocyte-depleted components.

      iv. Allergic reactions to transfused blood components occur in 1 of 100 transfusions. True anaphylaxis is rare. Symptoms are classic for allergic reactions.

         a) Patients with history of allergic transfusion reactions should be premedicated with diphenhydramine before blood product administration.

         b) In patients who develop allergic symptoms, the transfusion should be interrupted and diphenhydramine should be administered. If symptoms improve with diphenhydramine, transfusion may be restarted.

      v. Hypervolemia may result from PRBC or FFP transfusion. Headaches or dyspnea should alert the clinician to the possibility of too rapid intravascular volume enlargement. Diuresis with furosemide (40 mg intravenously) and reduction in infusion rate are therapeutic.

      vi. Hypothermia resulting from transfusion of multiple PRBC units can be ameliorated by using warmed fluids.

     vii. Infection. The risk of contracting HIV is estimated at 1 in 3,000,000 U. Hepatitis B and hepatitis C transmission risks are 1 in 3,000,000 U and 1 in 2,000,000 U, respectively.

    viii. Graft-versus-host disease, which is usually fatal, occurs when non-irradiated (i.e., immunocompetent) leukocytes are administered to, and attack host tissue in, patients without functioning immune systems.

      ix. Electrolyte abnormalities secondary to transfusion are unusual. Hypokalemia or hyperkalemia may occur, necessitating monitoring of potassium in all transfusions. Hypocalcemia is common in massive transfusion and supplement may be necessary.

    x. Noncardiogenic pulmonary edema develops within 4 hours of transfusion and presents as respiratory distress in the setting of fever, chills, and tachycardia. Usually, hospitalization and supportive care are sufficient, although the entity may be life-threatening in patients with significant comorbidity.

    xi. Asymptomatic anemia, caused by a delayed hemolytic transfusion reaction, may occur more than 1 week after transfusion. A previously negative Coombs test is positive.

    xii. Complications of massive transfusion (i.e., transfusion of a volume of blood equal to the patient's normal circulating blood volume over a 24-hour period)

        a) Bleeding, related to platelet and coagulation factor deficiencies, is the most frequent complication of massive transfusion. Routine replacement of platelets and coagulation factors should be guided by clinical situations. Prophylactic transfusion of platelets and FFP may be necessary to prevent these complications.

            1) DIC may occur in the setting of massive transfusion.

            2) Platelet dysfunction. Platelet levels often are not below $100,000/mm^3$, but dysfunction occurs because of coexistent hepatorenal disease or DIC.

            3) Coagulopathy may be exacerbated by the fact that stored blood loses much of its factor activity, especially factors V and VIII.

        b) Citrate toxicity (a product added to help store blood) may occur with transfusion of large amounts of whole blood.

        c) Hypothermia may be a significant component of disease states (e.g., major trauma, burns) that require massive transfusion, and particular attention must be paid to preventing the exacerbation of hypothermia when large-volume transfusions are performed.

F. Disposition. Most patients with significant bleeding require admission; however, some may receive treatment and be discharged. All patients should be monitored for at least 4 to 6 hours after a transfusion.

II. HEMATOLOGIC EMERGENCIES

A. Von Willebrand disease

    1. Discussion. Von Willebrand disease is the most common hereditary bleeding disorder. Genetic transmission is heterogenous because of multiple disease subtypes. Von Willebrand disease is caused by quantitative and/or functional deficiency of vWF, which is necessary for normal bleeding times.

      a. Type I von Willebrand disease. The amount of vWF is low.

      b. Type II von Willebrand disease. The structure of vWF is abnormal.

      c. Type III von Willebrand disease. Patients have little or no functioning vWF.

    2. Clinical features

      a. Bleeding involves primarily the skin and mucosal surfaces.

        i. More than half of patients with von Willebrand disease have a history of epistaxis; 40% report easy bruising and hematoma formation.

        ii. One-third of patients with von Willebrand disease have chronic gingival bleeding; an equal proportion of females with von Willebrand have menorrhagia.

        iii. Gastrointestinal bleeding is less common (10% of patients).

      b. Hemarthrosis occurs primarily in patients with severe disease.

      c. A severe bleeding diathesis, similar to that seen in patients with severe hemophilia, is seen in patients with type III disease.

    3. Differential diagnosis. Mild von Willebrand disease can be difficult to differentiate from mild hemophilia. Severe bleeding in patients with types II and III von Willebrand disease may present similarly to that in patients with hemophilia, but laboratory tests will help differentiate.

4. **Evaluation.** Laboratory evaluation of von Willebrand disease can be difficult because variable results may cause the clinician to confuse vWF deficiency with hemophilia, especially in mild cases.
   a. The PT is normal, and the activated PTT is normal except in cases of severe deficiency.
   b. The bleeding time is prolonged, and the vWF activity is low.
   c. The vWF antigen and factor VIII activity are low or normal.
5. **Therapy**
   a. **Desmopressin.** Primary therapy for patients with bleeding due to von Willebrand disease is desmopressin (0.3 µg/kg every 12 hours) subcutaneously or intravenously.
   b. **Aminocaproic acid** may be used for patients with oral bleeding.
   c. **Blood component transfusion.** For patients with type II or III von Willebrand disease, vWF replacement with cryoprecipitate (two bags per 10 kg) or factor VIII concentrate (10 IU/kg) is usually indicated.
6. **Disposition.** Most patients with von Willebrand disease, and all patients with significant bleeding, require hospital admission (Figure 16-1).

B. **Hemophilias A and B**
   1. **Discussion.** Hemophilias A and B are X-linked recessive disorders that may occur in patients without family history of bleeding disorders. Females are generally asymptomatic carriers of hemophilia with 50% of normal factor activity.
      a. **Types**
         i. Hemophilia A is caused by factor VIII deficiency; 85% of patients with hemophilia have hemophilia A.
         ii. Hemophilia B is caused by factor IX deficiency.

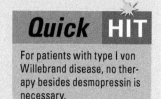

Quick HIT

For patients with type I von Willebrand disease, no therapy besides desmopressin is necessary.

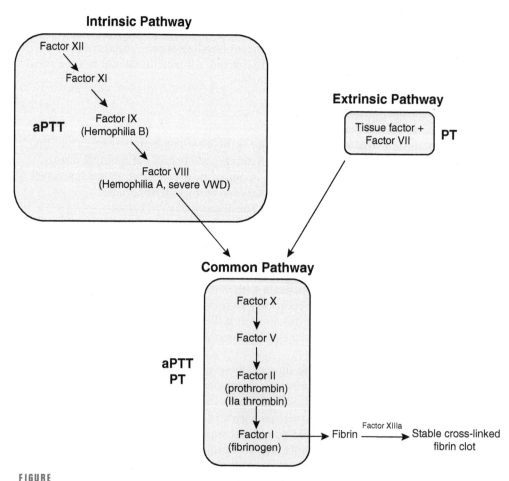

FIGURE
16-1 Schematic photo of coagulation cascade.

  b. Severity depends on the level of factor deficiency.
   i. Patients with mild or moderate disease have 6% to 60% and 1% to 5% of normal factor activity, respectively.
   ii. Severe disease is manifested as less than 1% factor activity.
  c. Pathogenesis. Minor lacerations rarely cause bleeding problems; however, deep hematomas or hemarthroses may occur with minimal or no trauma and may be delayed for hours.
   i. Hemarthroses may lead to chronic arthropathy.
   ii. Soft tissue or muscular hematomas may cause problems such as obstruction, mass effect (e.g., airway composite compartment syndrome), or volume depletion.
   iii. Intracranial bleeding is a major cause of death in people with hemophilia.
2. **Clinical features.** Mucocutaneous bleeding may occur in the respiratory or gastrointestinal tracts. Hematuria is common but rarely severe. Symptoms of compartment syndrome (i.e., pain, paresthesias, neurovascular findings) may accompany intramuscular bleeding in the extremities.
3. **Differential diagnoses.** Hemophilias cause prolongation of the intrinsic pathway, so the initial differential consists primarily of other diseases that result in prolonged activated PTT.
4. **Evaluation**
  a. History should focus on bleeding disorders in the patient or family, including previous requirements for factor replacement.
  b. Physical examination should begin with assessment for volume depletion and should include a thorough search for bleeding sites.
  c. Laboratory tests
   i. Blood work should begin with a CBC (with special attention paid to the hematocrit) and coagulation screening, which reveals prolongation of the activated PTT and a normal PT. In patients with more than 30% factor activity, the activated PTT may be normal, and definitive diagnosis may be difficult.
   ii. Other tests important in the hemophilia workup (factor assays, inhibitor testing) may be ordered after the initial evaluation in the ED.
  d. Diagnostic imaging studies. A cranial computed tomography (CT) scan should be performed in hemophiliacs with headache or neurologic signs. Patients with abdominal, back, groin, or thigh pain may have retroperitoneal bleeding and should undergo an urgent abdominal CT scan.
5. **Therapy** for hemophilia depends on the type of hemophilia, the severity of disease, the presence of factor inhibitors, and the location and severity of the acute bleeding episode.
  a. General measures
   i. Stabilization
    a) Primary (e.g., volume loss) and secondary (e.g., airway compromise) effects of bleeding must be assessed. Early endotracheal intubation is indicated for patients with impending airway compromise. Oral intubation is preferable to nasal intubation to minimize the risk of epistaxis.
    b) The placement of central venous lines, intramuscular injections, and arterial puncture should be avoided in patients with hemophilia.
   ii. FFP contains all clotting factors and is therefore useful for initial therapy for patients with hemophilia A or B when specific factor therapy is delayed or unavailable.
   iii. Factor concentrates, created from large numbers of pooled donors, represent effective hemophilia therapy.
    a) Types
     1) Factor VIII (1 IU/kg) raises the factor activity approximately 2%. The amount of factor VIII required for therapy is determined by the following equation: patient's weight (kg) × 0.5 × percentage increase in factor activity required.

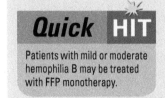

Quick HIT

Patients with mild or moderate hemophilia B may be treated with FFP monotherapy.

Hematologic and Oncologic Emergencies

2) Factor IX (1 IU/kg) raises the factor level approximately 1%. The amount of factor IX required for therapy is determined by the following equation: patient's weight (kg) × percentage increase in factor activity required.

b) Assessment of compartment pressures and fasciotomy (if necessary) should occur after factor replacement to minimize the risk of further bleeding.

iv. Prothrombin complex concentrates may be indicated for factor therapy in some patients with factor VIII inhibition.

v. DDAVP (1-deamino-8-d-arginine vasopressin; desmopressin) is useful for patients with hemophilia A but not hemophilia B. The dose is 0.3 μg/kg intravenously every 12 hours. Response should be seen within 1 hour.

vi. ε-Aminocaproic acid and tranexamic acid are plasminogen inhibitors, which prevent clot lysis. These agents are used primarily for mucosal bleeding (e.g., after dental procedures) because prevention of clot resorption in other areas (e.g., joints) may lead to chronic complications.

vii. Cryoprecipitate. With the advent of factor VIII concentrates, the administration of cryoprecipitate is rarely indicated for patients with hemophilia A.

b. **Therapy for specific conditions in hemophilia**

i. **Lacerations.** Patients with lacerations requiring suturing usually require factor replacement at the time of suturing and also at the time of suture removal.

ii. **Intra-articular and intramuscular bleeds.** Most bleeding in hemophiliacs occurs into the joints and muscles.

a) Intra-articular bleeds. Ice, splinting, and elastic bandages often provide symptomatic relief to patients with intra-articular bleeds. Factor replacement should strive to achieve a level of at least 30% to 40% initially.

b) **Intramuscular bleeds.** Immobilization is also indicated in patients with intramuscular hematomas, and factor replacement often is required in these patients as well.

iii. **Fractures.** Factor replacement to a level of 50% is necessary.

iv. **Dental procedures.** Oozing can usually be controlled with ε-aminocaproic acid.

v. **Hematuria.** Patients with persistent hematuria that does not respond to intravenous fluids usually require factor replacement to 50%.

vi. **Intracranial bleeding** is a major cause of mortality in patients with hemophilia. It may occur without prior history of trauma. In the case of patients with severe disease who suffer any potentially significant cranial trauma, factor replacement to 100% should proceed even before diagnostic imaging is obtained.

vii. Epistaxis can usually be controlled by direct pressure or packing with microfibrillar collagen. Cautery and traditional petroleum packing can lead to rebleeding. In patients who do require factor replacement, levels should be increased to 50%.

viii. Gastrointestinal or retropharyngeal bleeding. Patients should receive factor replacement to a level of 50% to 100%.

ix. Retroperitoneal bleeding is an additional life risk for hemophiliacs. Therapy with factor replacement to 75% to 100% (factor VIII) or at least 50% (factor IX).

6. **Disposition.** Patients with significant bleeding (e.g., retroperitoneal) or those at risk for potentially serious sequelae (e.g., compartment syndrome, airway obstruction) should be admitted for observation and specialist consultation when appropriate.

C. **Anemia**

1. **Discussion.** Causes of anemia include:

a. **Blood loss**, which can be occult, is the most common cause of anemia.

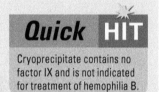

Quick HIT

Cryoprecipitate contains no factor IX and is not indicated for treatment of hemophilia B.

b. **Autoimmune hemolysis** may present as disease occurring in the absence of obvious precipitating factors (warm antibodies) or in the setting of hypothermia (cold antibodies) or drug ingestion (drug-induced hemolysis).

   i. **Warm autoimmune hemolysis** is often idiopathic, but there may be underlying leukemia, lymphoma, or lupus.

   ii. **Cold autoimmune hemolysis** occurs when RBCs interact with abnormal antibodies in the cooler peripheral circulation, resulting in hemolysis on entering the central circulation.

c. **Glucose-6-phosphate dehydrogenase (G6PD) deficiency** is seen in up to 10% of the world population. Resultant weakness in the RBC membrane predisposes these patients to hemolysis in the presence of oxidant stress (e.g., fava bean ingestion, antimalarial medication, acidosis).

d. **Hereditary spherocytosis** with splenic RBC destruction is the most common hemolytic disease found in individuals of Northern European descent.

e. **Aplastic anemia**, manifested as pancytopenia, results from bone marrow failure, usually after exposure to a drug or toxin.

f. **Red cell aplasia** is caused by immunologic disease (e.g., thymoma) and is characterized by decreased numbers of RBCs and other cells derived from erythroid precursors.

g. **Hypochromic disease** is present when RBCs are being produced but are poorly hemoglobinated (see Clinical Pearl 16-1).

h. **Megaloblastic anemia**, resulting from disruption in DNA synthesis, is primarily caused by folate or vitamin B_{12} deficiency.

   i. Because all stem cell lines in the marrow divide rapidly, patients with significant folate or vitamin B_{12} deficiency can present with profound pancytopenia.

   ii. Other rapidly dividing cell lines are affected, and the patient with folate or B_{12} deficiency may present with disease in the skin, gastrointestinal tract, or mucosae.

i. **Alcoholism.** The direct bone marrow suppressive effects of ethanol and the presence of concomitant hepatic dysfunction, combined with chronic nutritional deficiencies, make anemia an entity commonly seen in alcoholics.

j. **Mechanical disruption of RBCs** may result in anemia.

   i. **Following valvuloplasty or vascular surgery.** Patients with implants and increasing anemia should be evaluated for implant dysfunction.

   ii. **Microangiopathic hemolytic anemias** involve fragmentation of morphologically normal RBCs by microvascular fibrin strands; examples of this may be seen in DIC, thrombotic thrombocytopenic purpura (TTP), hemolytic–uremic syndrome, hypertension, renal graft rejection, and mitomycin C toxicity.

2. **Clinical features**

a. **Chronic blood loss anemia.** Patients may be asymptomatic from the gradually developing anemia but may present with fatigue, exercise intolerance, anginal exacerbation, or syncope when hemoglobin levels drop to critical values.

b. **Autoimmune hemolysis**

   i. **Cold agglutinin disease** is usually acute and transient, with rare development of severe anemia or chronic disease. In paroxysmal cold

---

CLINICAL PEARL 16-1

Hypochromic Diseases

1. **Iron deficiency** is the most common cause of hypochromic disease, and it is usually caused by a precipitating disease process.
2. **Anemia of chronic disease** may be seen in almost any chronic disease state. These patients suffer from poor iron utilization.
3. Defective heme or porphyrin synthesis, as is seen with **porphyrias**, is a common cause of hypochromic anemia.
4. Impaired globin synthesis, as is seen in **thalassemias**, may also present as hypochromic anemia.

hemoglobinuria, patients present with urinary discoloration, chills, fever, and abdominal or back pain. The disease is usually transient but may result in severe anemia.

    ii. **Drug-induced hemolytic anemia** may be significant but is usually of moderate severity. Hemolysis may develop weeks after institution of drug therapy, and positive Coombs tests may persist for up to 1 year after drug discontinuation.

c. **Anemia attributed to G6PD deficiency** may present as hemolytic crisis in patients who have ingested oxidant drugs (e.g., sulfa drugs) or who have intercurrent infection or acidosis. Hemolysis may occur up to 3 days after the precipitating insult. Laboratory testing reveals a hemolytic state with hemoglobinuria.

d. **Hereditary spherocytosis** may also present as an acute hemolytic state, although the anemia is usually relatively mild. Hematologic findings expected in hereditary spherocytosis include a normal mean corpuscular volume (MCV) and an elevated mean corpuscular hemoglobin.

e. **Aplastic anemia** presents with a marked pancytopenia, which is easily recognized upon ED laboratory testing.

f. **Pure red cell aplasia** presents with severe anemia and absence of reticulocytosis in patients with normal white blood cell and platelet counts.

g. **Hypochromic anemia.** The presentation is similar to that of other patients with decreased RBC counts; low MCV is the hallmark. Fatigue and generalized malaise are the most common presenting complaints.

h. **Megaloblastic anemia.** Patients may be folate- or vitamin B_{12}–deficient from underlying disease processes.

    i. The most noteworthy findings associated with vitamin B_{12} deficiency are peripheral neurologic abnormalities, which are not seen with folate deficiency.

    ii. Inpatient testing (e.g., Schilling test for vitamin B_{12} absorption) is required to determine the nature of the vitamin deficiency in these patients.

3. **Evaluation.** Although the history may be diagnostic in patients with anemia, physical examination (e.g., jaundice from hemolytic anemia) and laboratory testing (e.g., peripheral RBC smear) often provide diagnostic direction.

a. **Physical examination findings**

    i. Adenopathy, hepatomegaly, splenomegaly, neuropathy, or bony tenderness may be present in patients with anemia of various causes.

    ii. Patients with significant volume loss may be orthostatic and have other signs of hypovolemia.

b. **Laboratory studies**

    i. **Stool guaiac.** All patients with anemia should undergo stool guaiac for blood. Other findings depend on the degree of blood loss and the specific cause of anemia.

    ii. **Blood work**

        a) A CBC quantifies the anemia and assesses the white blood cell and platelet counts. The MCV is an important part of the CBC because its results direct further workup. Other tests are indicated as directed by the clinical situation. Much of the subsequent evaluation, such as iron-binding capacity, haptoglobin levels, and bone marrow evaluation, takes place outside the ED.

          1) In patients with a normal MCV, serum iron levels, total iron-binding capacity, reticulocyte counts, haptoglobin levels, a Coombs test, and a peripheral smear should be obtained. Further testing is directed by results of these analyses.

          2) Patients with a low MCV require assessment of serum iron and iron-binding capacity, with ferritin levels and bone marrow analysis indicated if these tests are below normal. Normal iron testing in patients with a low MCV should prompt hemoglobin electrophoresis.

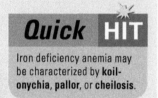

Quick HIT

Iron deficiency anemia may be characterized by **koilonychia, pallor,** or **cheilosis.**

Hematologic and Oncologic Emergencies

        3) Patients with a high MCV should undergo reticulocyte count and assessment of folate and vitamin B_{12} levels.

    b) The reticulocyte count allows assessment of the hematopoietic response to anemia.

    c) A peripheral smear provides morphologic information on the presence of abnormal cells, such as spherocytes or schistocytes, which are RBC fragments indicating mechanical hemolysis.

        1) Heinz bodies, intra-RBC hemoglobin precipitates, may be seen in G6PD-deficient patients.

        2) Patients with hereditary spherocytosis may have splenomegaly and jaundice in addition to characteristic spherocytosis on peripheral RBC smear.

    d) Plasma-free hemoglobin, lactic dehydrogenase, and unconjugated bilirubin levels are elevated in patients with hemolysis.

    e) Haptoglobin levels are decreased in patients with hemolytic anemia, although the acute phase character of haptoglobin may cause a rise initially.

    f) Plasma iron levels, ferritin levels, and transferrin saturation are low and total iron-binding capacity is high in patients with iron deficiency.

    g) Direct Coombs test. This test evaluates RBC surface immunoglobulin or complement and is positive in cases of autoimmune hemolysis. (An indirect Coombs test assesses for free antibodies and is used in the setting of transfusion screening.)

    iii. Urinalysis may reveal a source of occult bleeding.

    iv. Enzyme assay. In patients without previously known disease, the diagnosis of G6PD deficiency is made with an enzymatic assay.

    v. Osmotic fragility test. An osmotic fragility test is necessary to definitively diagnose hereditary spherocytosis.

  c. Diagnostic imaging studies (e.g., CT scan, ultrasound) may be required to delineate occult hemorrhage.

4. Therapy

  a. Blood loss or anemia of chronic disease. In the ED, therapy may include transfusion or vitamin and iron supplementation.

  b. Autoimmune hemolysis

    i. Patients with severe autoimmune hemolysis may require oral prednisone (1 mg/kg/day) or transfusion therapy. Because cross-matching is difficult, transfusion therapy in these patients is complicated and should be undertaken only after hematologic consultation. Splenectomy or immunosuppressive drugs are sometimes required for long-term disease management.

    ii. Treatment of underlying disease (e.g., leukemia, syphilis) and avoidance of precipitating factors often result in improvement or cure of autoimmune hemolysis.

    a) Therapy for drug-induced autoimmune hemolysis is discontinuation of the offending agent.

    b) Patients with cold antibody hemolytic anemia should avoid cold temperatures to prevent hemolysis.

  c. G6PD deficiency anemia. There is no specific therapy for this disorder. Optimal therapy for these individuals consists of prevention of hemolytic episodes by avoidance of oxidant drugs and other precipitating factors.

  d. Hereditary spherocytosis. Therapy is splenectomy, which results in discontinued RBC destruction and prevents anemia.

  e. Aplastic anemia. Therapy involves expectant management (when marrow function is expected to recover) or possible marrow transplant.

  f. Pure red cell aplasia. Patients may respond to immunosuppressive therapy, bone marrow transplantation, or antithymocyte globulin.

  g. Iron deficiency anemia is treated by addressing the underlying disease and attempting to restore body iron levels to normal. Subjective improvement

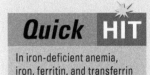

Quick HIT

In iron-deficient anemia, iron, ferritin, and transferrin saturation are low, whereas total iron-binding capacity is high.

Hematologic and Oncologic Emergencies

may be seen within days of institution of iron therapy. The determination of nonresponse (and need for parenteral iron) should be made by hematologists.

    i. **Salts of iron** provide effective oral replacement therapy and are best given in divided doses. Because these medications irritate the gastro-intestinal tract, doses should increase gradually to the recommended 325 mg of ferrous sulfate three times daily. Parenteral iron preparations can be used in the patient who needs more urgent therapy or responds poorly to oral therapy.

    ii. **Ascorbic acid** may increase absorption of oral iron preparations.

  h. **Megaloblastic anemia.** Folate (200 μg orally) or **vitamin B$_{12}$** (1 to 5 μg intramuscularly) may be useful. Long-term therapy is generally indicated.

  5. **Disposition.** All patients with significant anemia require hospital admission. In cases where outpatient management is judged to be reasonable, follow-up is important for continuation of workup and potential definitive therapy (e.g., splenectomy).

D. **Platelet abnormalities**

  1. **Discussion.** Platelet abnormalities may be classified as disorders of quantity (for which transfusion is effective) or disorders of dysfunction (for which transfusion therapy may be futile).

    a. **Decreased platelet production** may be seen in patients with marrow dys-function caused by infiltration, infection, drugs, or radiation.

    b. **Increased platelet destruction** is seen in patients with idiopathic thrombocy-topenic purpura or TTP, hemolytic–uremic syndrome, DIC, or viral infections.

    c. **Splenic sequestration of platelets** can occur in hypothermic patients or in those with hypersplenism (e.g., with portal hypertension).

    d. **Platelet loss** can be seen with hemorrhage or hemodialysis.

    e. **Thrombocytosis**, seen in patients with polycythemia vera, splenectomy, or malignancy, may result in coagulopathy when platelet counts exceed 1 million/mm^3.

  2. **Clinical findings**

    a. **Asymptomatic.** Incidental thrombocytopenia may be found by laboratory testing in asymptomatic patients.

    b. **Hemorrhage.** Patients with significant platelet dysfunction may have some form of mucocutaneous hemorrhage, and extreme platelet disease may result in catastrophic cerebrovascular hemorrhage.

      i. The presence of petechiae, ecchymosis, or purpura may provide clues to the presence of thrombocytopenia.

      ii. Mucocutaneous bleeding is suspicious for platelet abnormality.

    c. **Splenomegaly.** The finding of splenomegaly on abdominal examination may help define the cause.

  3. **Evaluation.** Laboratory assessment includes a hematocrit, platelet count, and coagulation profile. Measurement of the bleeding time to assess platelet func-tion is usually performed in a specialized laboratory. The bleeding time usu-ally becomes abnormal with platelet counts lower than 50,000/mm^3 (normal counts range from 150,000 to 450,000/mm^3).

  4. **Therapy**

    a. Platelet administration is indicated for all patients with platelet levels below 10,000/mm^3 and for many patients with platelet levels below 50,000/mm^3. Administration of platelets may be counterproductive in some patients with hematologic disease (e.g., TTP). Consultation should be obtained before transfusing platelets in such patients.

    b. Other therapies are necessary when thrombocytopenia is caused by platelet destruction. Prednisone is often indicated for patients with TTP, idiopathic thrombocytopenic purpura, or hemolytic–uremic syndrome.

E. **Sickle cell anemia**

  1. **Discussion**

    a. **Incidence.** Approximately 8% of the black population of the United States carries the sickle hemoglobin gene. Most of these patients do not have

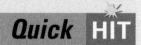

Quick HIT

Thrombocytopenia is also associated with commonly used drugs: nonsteroidal anti-inflammatory drugs, heparin, some antibiotics, dextran, and many others.

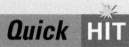

Quick HIT

Pseudothrombocytopenia may be associated with laboratory error introduced by agglutination or platelet adherence to other cells.

Hematologic and Oncologic Emergencies

homozygous disease (i.e., Hb SS, seen in 0.15% of blacks born in this country) but are asymptomatic carriers of sickle cell trait (i.e., Hb SA). Others, although not homozygous for sickle disease, have mixed hemoglobinopathies (e.g., Sβ thalassemia, SC) with phenotypic manifestations varying from nearly asymptomatic to severe sickle disease. Patients with heterozygous disease (Hb Sβ$_{thal}$ or Hb SC) may present to the ED with unknown disease states because these individuals often sickle only under certain circumstances (e.g., high altitude).

b. **Pathogenesis**

　i. The hallmark of sickle cell disease is substitution of valine for glutamic acid on the β-hemoglobin chain. This substitution results in distortion of reduced RBCs into a characteristic sickle shape.

　ii. The sickle-shaped RBCs obstruct capillary blood flow, resulting in a cycle of increased hypoxia and worsening RBC sickling. Recurrent episodes of hypoxia may cause chronic tissue ischemia and resultant organ failure.

　iii. Sickled RBCs are subject to hemolysis, and patients with sickle disease suffer chronic anemia. Hematopoiesis accelerates in an attempt to maintain RBC numbers.

　iv. One of the most important features of sickle cell disease is the increased risk of infection. Hyposplenism (due to repeated ischemic insults) and other immunologic dysfunctions render sickle cell patients especially susceptible to attack from encapsulated organisms (e.g., *Streptococcus pneumoniae*, *Haemophilus influenzae*, *Salmonella* species).

2. **Clinical features**

a. **Vaso-occlusive pain crisis.** RBC sickling and the resultant microvascular occlusion with tissue ischemia are a source of potentially severe pain. The location and type of pain may differ between presentations. Patients with pain crisis typically have low-grade fever, mild leukocytosis, and reticulocytosis as well as the chronic anemia expected for those with sickle cell anemia. There are different types of vaso-occlusive crises, depending on location.

　i. **Chest crisis,** most commonly seen in children with sickle cell anemia, is characterized by chest pain with dyspnea, hyperventilation, or both.

　ii. **Bone crisis** usually involves extremities, but back pain can occur.

　iii. **Joint crisis** may present as monoarticular or oligoarticular pain.

　iv. **Abdominal crisis** usually is manifest by acute and constant abdominal pain without localized tenderness or peritonitis.

b. **Aplastic crisis.** In these patients, there is failure of hematopoiesis to keep pace with ongoing hemolysis.

c. **Sequestration crisis.** Heterozygous patients may develop sequestration, presenting with acute anemia. The anemia is caused by the sudden sequestration of a large portion of circulating RBCs, usually in the spleen, but the liver may also be involved.

d. **Other acute conditions** (see Clinical Pearl 16-2) seen in patients with sickle disease are either more likely to occur or are associated with increased morbidity in these patients.

e. **Chronic conditions**

　i. **Symptomatic anemia** may result from the chronicity of sickle cell disease.

　ii. **Sickle lung disease,** resulting from chronic hypoxia and recurrent infection and infarction, may cause **cor pulmonale** in those older than 30 years of age.

　iii. **Leg ulcers,** resulting from chronic tissue hypoxia and venous stasis, also occur.

　iv. **Cholelithiasis,** due to chronic hemolysis, is also more common.

3. **Differential diagnosis**

a. The primary differential in patients with acute sickle crisis is investigation for presence of precipitating infectious disease. Noninfectious precipitating

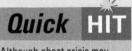

Quick HIT

Although chest crisis may be caused by microvascular occlusion in the thorax, pulmonary infarction and other intrapulmonary disease must be considered.

CLINICAL PEARL   16-2

Acute Conditions Associated with Sickle Cell

1. Approximately 10% of sickle cell patients have a **cerebrovascular accident**. Cerebrovascular accident often occurs in patients younger than 10 years.
2. **Pulmonary infarction** is much more common in patients with sickle cell anemia than in the general population. In addition, there is increased incidence of venous thromboembolism and fat embolism (from bone infarction).
3. Those with sickle cell anemia are no more likely to develop **hyphema** than the general population, but complications are potentially worse in patients with sickle trait or disease.
4. **Priapism** occurs relatively more frequently among those displaying sickle cell anemia.

---

  factors, including hypoxia, stress, dehydration, hemorrhage, fever, acidosis, alcohol intoxication, and pregnancy, should also be considered.

 b. Patients with bony pain may have fractures or osteomyelitis.

 c. Sickle cell patients with chest crisis should be evaluated for other cardiopulmonary disease, including pneumonia, pulmonary embolus, and pulmonary or myocardial infarction.

 d. Although sickle crisis presenting as abdominal pain may mimic surgical abdominal disease, diagnoses of pyelonephritis, biliary tract disease, hepatitis, appendicitis, gynecologic disease, and hepatic or splenic infarction should also be highly suspected.

 e. Joint pain in the setting of sickle cell disease may be due to joint crisis but may also be due to infection, gout, or trauma.

4. **Evaluation**

 a. **History.** Pain crises may be precipitated by acute infection, and crisis patients should be thoroughly evaluated for the presence of encapsulated organisms or other infectious agents. The history should address possible precipitating factors, including potential sites of infection, and whether the patient is taking prophylactic penicillin.

 b. **Physical examination** of patients with sickle cell disease should be thorough to differentiate types of crises and to rule out concurrent disease states.

  i. **Orthopedic examination.** Patients with bone crisis may be expected to have slight local bony tenderness, but presence of warmth or erythema should increase suspicion of skin or deep tissue infection. Significant bony tenderness may signal fractures. Identification of joint effusions is important in patients with sickle cell who display arthralgias. Such effusions require diagnostic drainage.

  ii. **Pulmonary examination,** for respiratory rate and auscultation, is particularly important in patients with chest symptoms and possible pneumonia.

  iii. **Neurologic examination.** Because microvascular deficiencies in sickle cell disease usually involve the central nervous system, careful neurologic examination may unmask the presence of acute stroke caused by sickle cell disease.

  iv. **Abdominal examination**

   a) Sickle cell patients with abdominal crisis must be examined carefully for significant abdominal tenderness and signs of peritonitis, which are usually absent in vaso-occlusive abdominal sickle crisis.

   b) Identification of an enlarged, painful, and tender liver or spleen is critical to making the diagnosis of acute syndromes of sequestration in these organs.

  v. **Extremities.** Nonpitting edema in the extremities is a clue to the presence of dactylitis ("hand-foot syndrome"), which can be the first manifestation of sickle disease.

vi. **Vision.** Evaluation of visual acuity is important in sickle cell patients with visual complaints because they may have proliferative or nonproliferative retinopathy.

c. **Laboratory studies.** For adult patients with acute crisis, ancillary studies have traditionally included a CBC and reticulocyte count, with other tests performed only if indicated. For pediatric patients, most authorities recommend performing routine urinalysis and chest radiograph as well as the CBC and reticulocyte count.

   i. **Blood work**

      a) The CBC is always important in evaluating sickle cell patients in the ED. Hematocrit can drop to 30% below baseline low levels in acute sequestration syndromes and can also be low in aplastic crisis. Comparison to known baseline levels is desirable.

      b) The reticulocyte count is important in ruling out aplastic crisis (in which the reticulocyte count is low) and in differentiation of aplastic from sequestration crises (normal to high reticulocyte count).

   ii. Urinalysis for identification of urinary tract infection is indicated for all children with sickle crisis as well as for adults with abdominal pain.

   iii. Arterial blood gas determination. The threshold for obtaining an arterial blood gas analysis is relatively low in sickle cell patients with chest complaints.

   iv. Blood cultures should be obtained from those sickle cell patients with identified or strongly suspected infection.

   v. Blood chemistries and liver enzyme tests are indicated for crisis patients with abdominal pain. Other tests may be indicated as directed by the clinical situation.

   vi. Arthrocentesis and laboratory evaluation of joint fluid are necessary to rule out infection in patients with joint effusions.

   vii. Cerebrospinal fluid analysis. In the setting of neurologic deficit and negative cranial CT, lumbar puncture should be performed to exclude subarachnoid hemorrhage or infection.

d. **Diagnostic imaging studies**

   i. The presence of any chest symptoms mandates a chest radiograph. Bony pain from sickle crisis, if located in a specific area, is an indication for plain radiography of the involved region to search for fracture or osteomyelitis.

   ii. Ultrasonography may help identify biliary disease and sequestration.

   iii. Emergent cranial CT scan to rule out cerebrovascular accident should be performed on sickle cell patients with neurologic symptoms. Subsequent magnetic resonance imaging or arteriography may be required.

5. **Therapy.** For the majority of sickle cell anemia patients visiting the ED for vaso-occlusive crisis, therapy is based on hydration and analgesia, usually intravenous opioids. If no contraindications, intravenous hydration should be aggressive.

a. **Analgesia.** The chronicity of sickle disease and the inability to confirm crisis pain with bedside or laboratory testing have resulted in an unfortunate pattern of crisis pain undertreatment. Appropriate opioid analgesia should be administered.

   i. **Meperidine should not be administered** to patients with sickle crisis pain. Repeated dosing, which is almost always required in patients with sickle cell anemia, leads to accumulation of the epileptogenic metabolite normeperidine.

   ii. **Oral and injectable nonsteroidal anti-inflammatory drugs** are an option for pain control in patients with sickle cell disease, but precautions for renal effects of these agents should be particularly heeded.

b. Transfusion may be required for refractory pain or pain associated with aplastic crisis. Given the difficulty of diagnosing pulmonary infarction, some hematologists advocate transfusion for all patients with chest crisis.

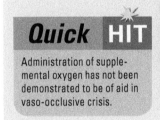

Quick HIT

Administration of supplemental oxygen has not been demonstrated to be of aid in vaso-occlusive crisis.

Hematologic and Oncologic Emergencies

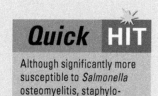

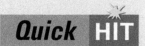

Acetazolamide, used to decrease intraocular pressures, is contraindicated in sickle cell patients because its pH effects promote sickling.

Hematologic and Oncologic Emergencies

c. **Antibiotic therapy**
   i. For patients with infectious complications requiring admission, a reasonable choice for initial empiric therapy is ceftriaxone (1 g in adults, 50 to 75 mg/kg up to 1 g in children). Other agents may be more appropriate depending on the site of infection (e.g., antistaphylococcal agents for osteomyelitis) and other clinical variables. Prompt administration of antibiotics is important.
   ii. Pediatric patients with localized infectious processes not requiring admission should be prescribed antibiotics reliably covering pneumococcus and *H. influenzae* (e.g., amoxicillin–clavulanate). These patients should receive conservative ED return precautions as well as close follow-up.
d. **Management of specific disorders in sickle cell disease**
   i. **Cerebrovascular accident.** Therapy for patients with cerebral infarction includes standard management and simple or partial exchange transfusion with a goal of reducing the overall burden of Hb S to lower than 30%. Similar therapy is used for sickle cell patients with hemorrhagic cerebrovascular accident.
   ii. **Increased intracranial pressure (ICP).** Therapy is similar to the standard therapy except that special care must be made to avoid extreme hypocarbia (i.e., an arterial carbon dioxide tension of less than 24 mm Hg), which can worsen vasospasm, hypoxia, and RBC sickling.
   iii. **Priapism.** Therapy in patients with sickle cell anemia includes hydration and analgesia. Urologic consultation (for corpora aspiration or a shunting procedure) is indicated for patients whose priapism persists beyond 4 to 6 hours.
   iv. **Hyphema.** Early ophthalmologic consultation is indicated for sickle cell patients with hyphema because surgical management is often indicated.
   v. **Acute sequestration syndromes.** Therapy includes transfusion and vigorous hydration to mobilize RBCs.
e. **Management of sickle cell disease in pregnant women.** Other than lowering the transfusion threshold, treatment of sickle crisis in pregnancy does not differ from that in other patients. Be wary of opiate usage just prior to delivery of infant.
6. **Disposition.** Patients with refractory pain, infection, dactylitis, priapism, transfusion requirement, neurologic deficit, pulmonary complications, or sequestration syndromes require admission. Thresholds for both prophylactic antibiotics and admission of pediatric sickle cell patients are lower than those for adults.

F. **DIC**
1. **Discussion.** DIC is a syndrome of consumptive coagulopathy that occurs in the presence of another disease. Widespread activation of the coagulation pathway results in secondary activation of fibrinolysis, with resultant thrombosis, hemorrhage, or both.
   a. **Mechanisms.** Intravascular coagulation is prompted by one of three mechanisms:
      i. Extrinsic procoagulant (e.g., amniotic fluid, snake venom)
      ii. Blood contact with a foreign surface (e.g., grafts, trauma, burns)
      iii. Intrinsic procoagulant (e.g., promyelocytic leukemia)
   b. **Pathogenesis.** After diffuse microcirculatory clot formation, fibrinolysis occurs with a subsequent release of fibrin degradation products, and the body's homeostasis between clot and lysis becomes disrupted.
      i. Circulating plasmin cleaves fibrinogen and further decreases levels of factors V and VIII.
      ii. Fibrin degradation products add to the overall disruption of hemostasis, delaying fibrin polymerization and impairing platelet function.
2. **Clinical features.** In many cases, the most striking clinical feature of DIC is the comorbid disease that prompts its development. Most commonly, DIC is seen

CLINICAL PEARL 16-4

Complications of Tumor Growth

1. **Airway obstruction** may be seen in patients with tumors of the ears, nose, or throat; lymphoma; and metastatic lung carcinoma. Tumor impingement may occur at all levels of the respiratory tract, with upper respiratory tract, ear, nose, and throat tumors causing proximal obstruction and endobronchial lesions restricting airflow distally.

2. **Malignant pericardial effusion** and **tamponade** may be seen after radiation therapy or in patients with breast, ovary, or lung carcinoma. In addition, acute leukemia, Hodgkin lymphoma, or melanoma may present with pericardial disease.

3. **Superior vena cava syndrome** is seen in patients with lymphoma or with oat-cell or squamous-cell lung carcinomas.

4. **Spinal cord compression** may be the first sign of neoplasm, and it is seen in patients with multiple myeloma; lymphomas; and carcinoma of the lung, breast, or prostate.

d. Overwhelming infection, which may occur with opportunistic microbes, is a major cause of death in patients with cancer.

3. **Mechanical complications of tumor growth** may be the first manifestations of cancer, and they often threaten life or limb (see Clinical Pearl 16-4).

B. **Clinical features**

1. **Biochemical derangements**

a. Hypercalcemia, occurring in up to 40% of patients with multiple myeloma and also commonly seen in multiple squamous cancers (especially squamous of lung). May cause back pain, constipation, or altered mental status

b. SIADH is primarily a laboratory diagnosis in patients presenting with inappropriate free water retention.

c. Hyperviscosity syndromes occur when the serum viscosity is greater than five times that of water, and it may be seen when the hematocrit increases beyond 50% to 60%. A leukocrit exceeding 10% may also be associated with significant hyperviscosity.

i. Fatigue, headache, anorexia, and somnolence are early nonspecific symptoms of hyperviscosity.

ii. Localized neurologic deficits, with possible progression to coma, may develop as microthromboses develop in the central nervous system.

d. Adrenal insufficiency, like hyperviscosity, can manifest as altered mental status. Potentially life-threatening cardiovascular involvement with adrenal shock is possible.

e. Tumor lysis syndrome can be characterized by multiple organ failure and death.

2. **Immunologic complications.** Features of thrombocytopenia (from immune-mediated platelet destruction) and anemia in patients with cancer are similar to presenting signs and symptoms of these disorders in other patients.

3. **Mechanical complications**

a. Airway obstruction may be indicated by dyspnea, stridor, nasal flaring, or wheezing.

b. Malignant effusions accumulate over long periods of time and, therefore, may reach significant size (sometimes greater than 500 mL) before causing symptoms characteristic of pericardial fluid accumulation.

c. Superior vena cava syndrome results from tumor restriction of blood flow in the superior vena cava (Figure 16-2). Blood flow obstruction results in elevated venous pressures in the areas drained by the superior vena cava (i.e., arms, neck, face, cerebrum). Symptoms reflect the anatomic distribution of the vein's drainage and include headache, facial or arm edema, and fullness in the neck and face. As the disease progresses, an increase in ICP and syncope may be noted.

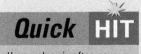

Quick HIT

Hypercalcemia often causes stones (kidney/biliary), bones (bone pain), groans/moans (constipation or abdominal pain), and psychiatric moans (mood swings).

Hematologic and Oncologic Emergencies

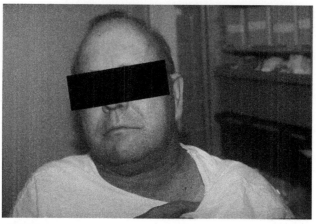

FIGURE
16-2 Patient with superior vena cava syndrome.
(Courtesy of Lawrence B. Stack, MD.)

    d. Spinal cord compression may present as paraparesis, hypoesthesia, or gait disturbance. Paraplegia, marked sensory deficits, urinary incontinence or retention, and loss of rectal sphincter tone usually indicate a more advanced process.

  4. Signs and symptoms of other concurrent diseases. Concurrent disorders occur in patients with cancer with increased frequency because of the malignancy, cancer therapy, or the patient's generalized debilitated state. These include coronary artery disease, hypercoagulability and thrombosis (e.g., Trousseau syndrome of visceral malignancy), intravascular volume depletion; rapidly progressive renal failure from glomerular amyloid deposition may be seen in patients with multiple myeloma or lymphoma; and occult bleeding in cancer patients may be caused by intra-arterial chemotherapy or vomiting (e.g. Mallory-Weiss tears).

C. Differential diagnosis. The long list of tumor-related emergencies implies a similarly extensive list of differential diagnoses. Because oncologic emergencies may affect blood chemistries, organ function, airway patency, and perfusion, the potential of cancer-related illness should be considered in any patient who presents to the ED.

D. Evaluation

  1. Biochemical derangements

    a. Hypercalcemia of malignancy represents a relatively easy diagnostic entity. Calcium levels are readily measured by the hospital laboratory.

      i. Ionized calcium levels should be interpreted in light of pH and serum albumin. Parathyroid hormone levels should be measured.

      ii. An electrocardiogram may demonstrate a shortened QT interval in patients with hypercalcemia.

    b. SIADH is evaluated by laboratory analysis of serum and urine sodium and urine-specific gravity. Physical examination clues may point toward intracerebral or intrapulmonary processes in patients with SIADH and no known tumor.

      i. The primary abnormalities in SIADH are hyponatremia and urine that contains a high sodium level (greater than 30 mEq/L) and is not optimally concentrated.

      ii. Normal renal, adrenal, and thyroid function must be demonstrated before the diagnosis of SIADH is established.

    c. Hyperviscosity syndromes may be difficult to diagnose clinically because presenting symptoms can be vague. Laboratory analysis is usually diagnostic.

      i. A CBC reveals elevated hematocrit and microscopic Rouleau formation. Sometimes, the clue to the diagnosis of hyperviscosity comes with laboratory reporting that the blood is "too thick" to run tests.

      ii. Neurologic examination may reveal focal deficits.

      iii. Funduscopy should be performed to search for "sausage-link" retinal vasculature, hemorrhages, or exudates.

   d. Adrenal insufficiency is suspected based on either electrolyte analysis or the clinical appearance of a patient with potential adrenal dysfunction. Because treatment is empiric, response to therapy may aid in making the diagnosis.

      i. Primary laboratory abnormalities are hypoglycemia, hyponatremia, hyperkalemia, and eosinophilia.

      ii. Physical examination for cardiovascular stability is important in patients with adrenal insufficiency; hypotension causes hemodynamic collapse.

   e. Tumor lysis syndrome. The diagnosis may be made based on the history and recent cancer therapy or steroids. Some of these patients may not have a known history of neoplasm. Laboratory analysis helps make the definitive diagnosis.

      i. Hyperkalemia occurring in tumor lysis syndrome may also cause peaked T-wave electrocardiogram changes and prolonged QRS complexes.

      ii. Hyperuricemia can be found in patients with tumor lysis. Uric acid levels should be checked on all patients who are candidates for this diagnosis.

      iii. Hyperphosphatemia may cause dangerous hypocalcemia.

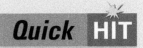

Quick HIT

In tumor lysis syndrome, hyperkalemia can cause cardiac derangements and should be treated immediately, although other metabolic abnormalities can also be life-threatening.

2. **Immunologic complications**

   a. Infection. The frequency and severity of infection increase with absolute neutrophil count lower than 1000/mm³. Evaluation of febrile neutropenic patients involves empiric antibiotics, radiography, body fluid analysis, and culturing to detect the site of infection.

   b. Immune-mediated thrombocytopenia may be suggested by the presence of petechiae on physical examination.

   c. Anemia. Patients report fatigue, and the physical examination may reveal skin or palpebral conjunctival pallor. The CBC is diagnostic, but optimal interpretation requires comparison with a known hemoglobin baseline.

3. **Mechanical complications**

   a. Airway obstruction. Portable chest radiography is usually performed because of potential patient instability. Fiberoptic laryngoscopy may be used for airway visualization.

   b. Malignant pericardial effusion and tamponade present with similar physical findings as do other causes of pericardial tamponade. Beck triad of hypotension, venous distention, and muffled heart tones is a late finding.

      i. Echocardiography is the best tool for evaluation of pericardial fluid but may not be available in the ED.

      ii. Pericardiocentesis is indicated in patients with hemodynamic compromise and is both diagnostic and therapeutic.

   c. Superior vena cava syndrome, in its advanced stages, may be associated with papilledema caused by increased ICP.

      i. Early findings are neck and upper thoracic venous distention, facial plethora and telangiectasia, and mild edema of the face and arms.

      ii. A palpable supraclavicular mass may be identified.

      iii. A chest radiograph often demonstrates mediastinal or lung abnormality.

   d. Spinal cord compression may present as acute urinary retention. Patients with this or any other neurologic complaint suggestive of cord compression (e.g., loss of perirectal sensation) should undergo examination of reflexes, gait, sensorimotor function, and sphincter tone to further evaluate for signs of acute cord compression. A sensory level or distal flaccid paralysis may be seen. Patients with suspected cord compression require further consultation, often including emergent CT scan, magnetic resonance imaging, or myelographic imaging.

E. **Therapy**

1. **Biochemical derangements**

   a. Hypercalcemia associated with cancer usually improves with saline infusion and possibly intravenous furosemide. Hemodialysis or peritoneal dialysis is reserved for patients who do not respond to more conservative measures. Bisphosphonates and glucocorticoids are usually initiated in the inpatient setting.

  b. SIADH. Treatment focuses on free water restriction and, in cases of cardiac or neurologic toxicity, includes infusion of 100 to 250 mL of 3% saline solution.

  c. Symptomatic hyperviscosity syndrome in patients with a hematocrit greater than 60% is treated with hydration and phlebotomy (of 1 to 2 U) with saline and RBC replacement.

  d. Adrenal insufficiency and shock. Primary therapy is the administration of intravenous hydrocortisone along with volume resuscitation. This dose may be repeated every 6 to 8 hours. Occasionally, higher doses or pressors may be necessary. If the diagnosis of adrenal insufficiency is unclear, treatment can proceed using dexamethasone while performing an adrenocorticotropic hormone stimulation test.

  e. Tumor lysis syndrome. Ideally, therapy is preventive, but the ED physician can effectively address many of the abnormalities resulting from lysis.

    i. Vigorous hydration, with careful attention to renal function, is a cornerstone of tumor lysis syndrome treatment.

    ii. Urinary alkalinization (to pH greater than 7) and allopurinol are recommended to address increased uric acid levels caused by tumor lysis.

    iii. Careful monitoring of calcium levels is important, especially for patients receiving bicarbonate for urinary alkalinization.

2. **Immunologic complications**

  a. Infection. Antibiotic therapy should be tailored toward any known sources of infection based on physical exam and laboratory evaluation. Without a clear source of infection, broad-spectrum antibiotics should be administered with the primary goal to administer appropriate antibiotics as early as possible.

  b. Immune-mediated thrombocytopenia may require transfusion, but transfused platelets also are likely susceptible to destruction. Hematology consultation is recommended before platelet transfusion in these patients.

  c. Indications for transfusion in anemia are not significantly different in patients with cancer as compared with other individuals.

3. **Mechanical complications**

  a. Airway obstruction is treated by establishment of a secure airway. Those patients with true airway emergencies require intubation in the ED. Other oncologic patients with airway compromise may require surgical tracheostomy.

  b. Malignant pericardial effusion and tamponade are treated with fluid resuscitation and pericardiocentesis.

  c. Superior vena cava syndrome, when accompanied by papilledema, should be treated with furosemide and methylprednisolone to reduce the ICP pending definitive mediastinal radiotherapy.

  d. Spinal cord compression is a true emergency, and it is amenable to rapid therapy in the ED. Patients should receive dexamethasone while awaiting definitive radiographic, radiotherapeutic, or operative intervention. Emergency surgical decompression or radiotherapy can prevent irreversible neurologic impairment.

4. **Concurrent disorders.** Patients with cancer are known to have increased frequency of thrombotic disease, but the dangers of anticoagulation in this group may prompt mechanical (i.e., filter placement) rather than pharmacologic therapy. Early nephrology consultation is indicated in patients with tumor lysis syndrome and potential renal insufficiency because hemodialysis may be helpful.

F. **Disposition.** Admission is the rule for patients with oncologic emergencies.

17

TRAUMATIC EMERGENCIES

William Gossman

I. INTRODUCTION

Trauma is the leading cause of mortality in the first four decades of life. It accounts for approximately 60 to 80 million injuries and 10 million disabilities per year.

II. GENERAL APPROACH TO THE TRAUMA PATIENT

A. **Introduction.** Quick evaluation and treatment is the key to survival in the trauma patient. Death from trauma may occur within minutes from injuries such as subdural and epidural hematomas, hemopneumothorax, tension pneumothorax, pericardial tamponade, ruptured spleen, lacerations of the liver, pelvic fractures, and aortic disruption.

B. **Primary survey.** The primary survey consists of the "**ABCs**" (see Clinical Pearl 17-1).

C. **Patient history.** Whenever possible, an **AMPLE** history (*a*llergies, *m*edications, *p*ast medical history, *l*ast meal, and *e*vents surrounding the injury and its mechanism) should be obtained from the patient and prehospital personnel. X-rays (chest and pelvis) and lab tests are now ordered (complete blood count, basic metabolic panel, pregnancy test, type and screen, and prothrombin time/international normalized ratio).

D. **Secondary survey.** This is a head-to-toe complete physical exam, examining each region systematically. During the primary or secondary survey, a focused assessment sonography in trauma (FAST) exam can be done in 2 minutes to risk stratify the trauma patient.

III. TRAUMATIC SHOCK

A. **Discussion.** Hemorrhage is the most common cause of shock in trauma. Less frequently, cardiogenic and neurogenic shock will be seen (see Clinical Pearl 17-2).

1. **Cardiogenic shock.** Myocardial dysfunction may occur due to **pericardial tamponade**, **tension pneumothorax**, **air embolism**, **myocardial contusion**, or an acute **myocardial infarction**.

2. **Neurogenic shock** may be seen with **spinal cord injury** with loss of sympathetic tone.

B. Clinical features

1. **Hypovolemic shock.** In adults, the blood volume is 7% of the body weight (5 L in a 70-kg person); in children, it is 8% of body weight, or 80 mL/kg.

2. **Cardiogenic shock.** Decreased cardiac output due to muscle damage or ischemia

3. **Neurogenic shock.** Hypotension, bradycardia, and warm well-perfused extremities due to a cervical or high thoracic spine injury

C. Treatment

1. **Fluid resuscitation**

   a. **Intravenous fluids.** Initial fluid resuscitation in an adult is no more than 2 L of lactated Ringer or normal saline. In a child, 20 mL/kg is infused as a bolus and may be repeated twice.

   b. **Blood transfusion.** Blood should be fully typed and cross-matched. In a critical patient, type-specific or O− blood (O+ in males) may be given quickly.

   i. In an adult patient who fails to respond to approximately 2,000 mL of crystalloid infusion, blood should be transfused.

   ii. In a child, the initial transfusion is 10 mL/kg of packed red blood cells.

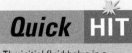

Quick **HIT**

Assessment, treatment, and disposition must occur quickly to decrease mortality in the trauma patient (the "**golden hour**").

Quick **HIT**

AMPLE history = *a*llergies, *m*edications, *p*ast medical history, *l*ast meal, and *e*vents surrounding the injury and its mechanism.

Quick **HIT**

Shock is the inadequate oxygenation of tissues caused by decreased perfusion (hypoperfusion).

Quick **HIT**

The initial fluid bolus in a child is 20 mL/kg.

Quick **HIT**

Blood should be started if a hypotensive trauma patient does not respond to 2 L of crystalloid.

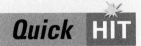

Traumatic Emergencies

CLINICAL PEARL 17-1

Primary Trauma Survey

1. **A—airway and cervical spine control.** The patency of the airway is assessed, with cervical spine immobilized. The presence of a cervical spine injury should be assumed until proven otherwise.
2. **B—breathing and ventilation.** The chest is auscultated and inspected, and the quality, depth, and rate of respirations are noted.
3. **C—circulation and hemorrhage control.** Capillary refill, pulses, and the color of the skin should be assessed. Active hemorrhages should be identified and treated with direct pressure or surgical repair. Two large-bore (14- to 16-gauge) intravenous catheters are inserted and intravenous fluids (lactated Ringer or normal saline) started. Place the patient on a cardiac monitor and a pulse oximeter.
4. **D—disability.** A rapid **neurologic assessment** is performed, assessing the **pupils** for size, equality, and reactivity, and **a Glasgow coma scale**.
5. **E—exposure.** The patient should be completely undressed then warm blankets applied to prevent hypothermia.

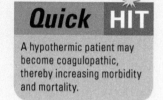

Quick HIT

A hypothermic patient may become coagulopathic, thereby increasing morbidity and mortality.

2. **Early surgical intervention** should be considered for patients who fail to respond to fluid resuscitation.
D. **Disposition.** Patients who present in shock should be admitted to an intensive care unit (ICU), transferred to the operating room, or transferred to a facility that can provide a higher level care.

IV. HEAD INJURIES

A. **Discussion.** Head injuries are responsible for 50% of trauma deaths.
B. **Clinical features**
  1. **Diffuse brain injuries** include concussion and diffuse axonal injuries.
    a. **Concussion** is as a transient loss of consciousness or other neurologic function that lasts for a few minutes occurring immediately after blunt head trauma.
    b. **Diffuse axonal injury** is secondary to shearing or tearing of nerve fibers and is characterized by coma in the absence of a focal lesion. The mortality rate ranges from 35% to 50%, and autonomic dysfunction (i.e., increased BP, increased temperature, sweating) may be seen.
  2. **Focal lesions** include subarachnoid hemorrhage, epidural hemorrhage, subdural hematoma, and cerebral contusion.
    a. **Subarachnoid hemorrhage** (Figure 17-1C) is the most common site of bleeding after head trauma.
    b. **Subdural hematoma** (Figure 17-1B) is a collection of blood lying between the dura and the arachnoid mater. It results from the tearing of the bridging veins traversing the subdural space.

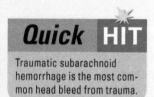

Quick HIT

Traumatic subarachnoid hemorrhage is the most common head bleed from trauma.

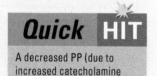

Quick HIT

A decreased PP (due to increased catecholamine release) is one of the early signs of shock.

CLINICAL PEARL 17-2

1. **Class I hemorrhage (15% [750 mL] blood loss).** Normal: pulse, blood pressure (BP), pulse pressure (PP) (systolic–diastolic pressure), respiratory rate (RR), urine output >30 mL/hour, and mental status (MS)
2. **Class II hemorrhage (15% to 30% [800 to 1,500 mL] blood loss).** Pulse >120, BP normal, PP decreased, RR 20 to 30, urine output 20 to 30 mL/hour, and an anxious MS
3. **Class III hemorrhage (30% to 40% [1,500 to 2,000 mL] blood loss).** Pulse 120 to 140, BP decreased, PP decreased, RR 30 to 40, urine output 5 to 15 mL/hour, and confused MS
4. **Class IV hemorrhage (>40% [>2,000 mL] blood loss).** Pulse >140, BP decreased, PP decreased, RR >35, urine output negligible, confused MS

Traumatic Emergencies

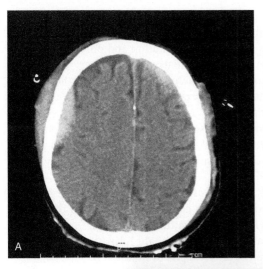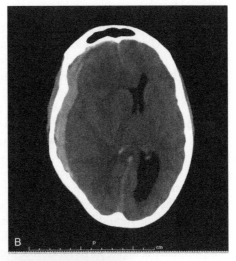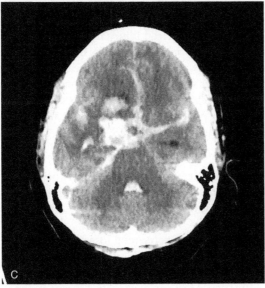

17-1 **(A) CT brain showing epidural hematoma. (B) Subdural hematoma with midline shift. (C) Extensive subarachnoid hemorrhage extending into ventricle.**

(Used by permission of Martin Huecker, MD.)

  c. **Epidural hematoma** (Figure 17-1A) results from tearing of a dural artery (usually the middle meningeal artery).
   i. Suspected with a skull fractures involving the temporal bone where the middle meningeal artery passes between the dura and the skull
   ii. It is characterized by a brief initial period of unconsciousness, a lucid interval lasting minutes to hours, and subsequent deterioration in neurologic status secondary to increasing intracranial pressure (ICP).
C. **Evaluation.** A computed tomography (CT) scan of the head is the test of choice and should be performed on any patient with loss of consciousness, altered MS, intoxication, or an abnormal neurologic exam.
D. **Treatment**
 1. **Initial stabilization.** The ABCs must be ensured.
  a. **Fluid resuscitation.** If a patient with a head injury is hypotensive, volume resuscitation must be initiated first. Intravenous fluids must be adequate to maintain BP while avoiding overhydration if increased ICP is suspected.
  b. **Adequate oxygen and glucose levels** must be maintained.

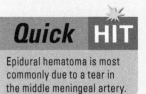
Quick **HIT**

Epidural hematoma is most commonly due to a tear in the middle meningeal artery.

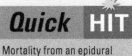
Quick **HIT**

Mortality from an epidural hematoma decreases if the patient is alert on presentation.

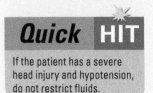
Quick **HIT**

If the patient has a severe head injury and hypotension, do not restrict fluids.

Traumatic Emergencies

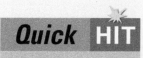

Quick HIT

Phenytoin is the drug of choice for seizures, but it may inhibit brain recovery.

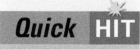

Quick HIT

Patients should have a responsible adult with them if they are being discharged.

Quick HIT

Patients on anticoagulants require special considerations. With an international normalized ratio above 3, admission should be considered. If the patient is to be discharged, a repeat CT at 4 hours from arrival should be obtained prior to discharge.

Quick HIT

Spinal shock is a cord injury resulting in flaccidity and areflexia.

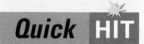

Quick HIT

Neurogenic shock is characterized by hypotension, bradycardia, and warm well-perfused extremities.

2. Lowering the ICP
   a. **Hyperventilation.** If the patient has a severe head injury, hyperventilation ($PaCO_2$ 30 to 35 mm Hg) may be used in moderation and only for a short period of time while other treatments are initiated.
   b. **Additional treatments** for increased ICP include elevation of the head of the bed, sedating the patient, and administration of mannitol (1 g/kg of a 20% solution) or hypertonic saline.
3. **Treatment of seizures.** Seizures are treated with **phenytoin** (1 g infused at 50 mg/min for adults; approximately 15 mg/kg at 0.5 to 1 mg/kg/min, not to exceed 50 mg/min, for children) or **levetiracetam** (500 mg intravenously) with or without **benzodiazepines**.
4. **Treatment of scalp wounds.** Scalp wounds are copiously irrigated. Pressure should be applied to control bleeding (which can be extensive), and the wound should be closed in a single layer with sutures or staples.
5. **Emergent neurosurgical consultation** should be sought for patients with lateralizing signs, large focal mass lesions, or any signs of herniation.

E. Disposition
   1. **Discharge.** Patients with a minor head injury, and no loss of consciousness, may be discharged home. Head injury instructions should be reviewed with the patient and a family member, spouse, or friend. The patient and caretaker should be advised to watch for persistent headache, vomiting, dizziness, alterations in MS, or other signs of deteriorating neurologic function.
   2. **Admission.** Patients with loss of consciousness or unreliable follow-up are admitted to the hospital for 24-hour observation. Patients with severe head injury require admission to an ICU.

V. SPINAL INJURIES

A. **Discussion.** Motor vehicle collisions account for the largest number of spinal cord injuries, followed by falls, firearm injuries, and recreational injuries. Ten percent of patients with head or facial injuries have associated cervical spine injuries.

B. Clinical features
   1. **Complete cord injuries** involve total loss of motor and sensory function below the lesion.
   2. **Incomplete cord injuries** carry a better prognosis than complete injuries for some recovery of function. Most can be classified in one of the three following clinical syndromes: Anterior, Brown-Séquard, and Central (see Clinical Pearl 17-3).
   3. **Spinal shock** is the immediate neurologic condition seen after spinal cord injury, and it is characterized by flaccidity and areflexia. As spinal shock resolves (days to weeks), function may return or spasticity replaces the flaccidity initially present.
   4. **Neurogenic shock** is associated with cervical or high thoracic injuries causing impairment of the descending sympathetic pathways. It is characterized by hypotension (due to loss of vasomotor tone); bradycardia (secondary to unopposed vagal tone to the heart); and warm, well-perfused skin.

CLINICAL PEARL 17-3

Incomplete Cord Injuries

1. **Anterior cord syndrome** follows a cervical flexion injury that compresses the anterior spinal cord and injures the anterior spinal artery. Motor paralysis, decreased sensation (including loss of pain and temperature sensation), and preservation of posterior column function (e.g., position sense, light touch, vibratory sensation) distal to the trauma characterize this lesion.
2. **Brown-Séquard syndrome**, or hemisection of the cord, is usually the result of penetrating injuries or lateral mass fractures. It presents as paralysis and loss of gross proprioception and vibration on the same side as the lesion and as loss of pain and temperature sense on the contralateral side.
3. **Central cord syndrome** follows a hyperextension injury. The ligamentum flavum buckles into the cord, resulting in a concussion of the most central portions of the cord (central portions of the pyramidal and spinothalamic tracts). Neurologic deficits of the upper extremities are greater than those of the lower extremities, and scattered sensory losses are seen.

C. **Assessment.** The spine should be palpated, while the patient is kept immobilized, to assess for tenderness or deformity of the spine. Complete neurologic and rectal exam are required.

D. **Diagnostic imaging studies.** CT scan of the cervical spine is the standard of care for patients requiring radiographic evaluation after trauma.

E. **Treatment**
1. **Spinal immobilization** should be maintained with a cervical collar until spinal injury has been ruled out. Spine boards should be removed as soon as possible to prevent skin breakdown and limit pain.
2. **Neurosurgical consultation** should be obtained for patients with known or suspected spinal cord injuries as well as for any unstable spinal fractures.

F. **Disposition.** Any patient with significant spinal injury should be managed at a regional trauma center.

VI. PENETRATING AND BLUNT NECK TRAUMA

A. **Discussion.** Injuries that violate the platysma are considered penetrating neck injuries. For the purposes of injury management, the neck is divided into three zones. Zone I is the inferior aspect of the cricoid cartilage to the thoracic outlet. Zone II extends from the cricoid cartilage to the angle of the mandible. Zone III is from the angle of the mandible to the base of the skull.

B. **Clinical features.** Categories of neck injuries include the following:
1. **Laryngotracheal (airway) injuries** are caused by direct blunt trauma, sudden acceleration or deceleration forces, increased intratracheal pressure against a closed glottis, or penetrating injuries. They may include fracture of the thyroid cartilage, disruption of the arytenoid cartilage, dislocation of the cricothyroid joint, and thyrotracheal separation, all of which result in airway compromise. Signs include dyspnea, stridor, hemoptysis, dysphonia, subcutaneous emphysema, and pain.
2. **Vascular injuries** may result from direct blunt trauma, stretching of the vessels, basilar skull fractures, or penetrating injuries. Hematomas, bruits, or obvious bleeding may be observed. Complications include airway compromise secondary to bleeding or expanding hematoma, hemorrhage, air embolus, and thrombus formation in the carotid arteries, which can lead to cerebral ischemia and neurologic deficits.
3. **Neurologic injuries** include injuries to the brachial plexus; cervical plexus; and the glossopharyngeal, vagus, spinal accessory, and hypoglossal nerves.

C. **Diagnostic studies (Figure 17-2)**
1. **Zone I injuries.** Patients require an emergent CT angiogram to evaluate the aorta and the innominate, carotid, and subclavian vasculature. The patient also requires evaluation of the esophagus (esophagram) and trachea (bronchoscopy).

Quick HIT

A patient who has a normal MS and who has no complaint of pain, neurologic deficit, tenderness on examination, or distracting injury may be clinically cleared.

Quick HIT

Injury to spinal cord segments C3 through C5 may lead to phrenic nerve damage and subsequent diaphragmatic paralysis.

Quick HIT

An injury that penetrates the platysma muscle is considered a penetrating neck injury.

Quick HIT

Dyspnea, stridor, hemoptysis, dysphonia, subcutaneous emphysema, and pain are indicators of laryngeal injury.

Quick HIT

Regional motor and sensory deficits may be seen, and Horner syndrome (i.e., ptosis, miosis, and anhydrosis) is seen with injury to the cervical sympathetic chain.

Traumatic Emergencies

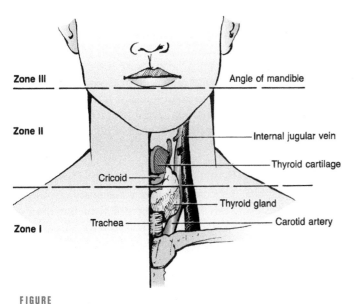

FIGURE
17-2 **Zones I, II, and III in the neck.**

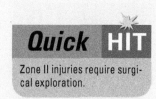

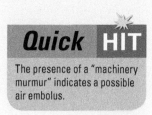

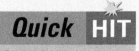

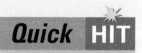

2. **Zone II injuries.** Patients are usually taken to the operating room for exploratory neck surgery. If this is not done, a CT angiogram, esophagram, and bronchoscopy are done.

3. **Zone III injuries.** Patients require an angiogram and careful inspection of the oropharynx.

4. **Vertebral artery injuries.** A vertebral artery angiogram should be obtained if penetrating or blunt trauma has occurred near these vessels.

D. **Treatment**

1. **Airway control.** Blind nasotracheal intubation should be avoided if massive facial trauma exists or if the patient is apneic. Orotracheal intubation should be accomplished with inline stabilization of the cervical spine.

2. **Immobilization of the neck.** If a cervical spine injury cannot be ruled out, the neck should be immobilized.

3. **Bleeding control**

   a. **Direct pressure** is used to control bleeding.

   b. **Occlusive dressings** should be maintained over major bleeding sites to avoid **air embolus**. If a stable patient suddenly becomes tachypneic, tachycardic, and hypotensive, an air embolus must be considered. A "machinery murmur" may be auscultated. The patient should be placed in the Trendelenburg position in the left lateral decubitus position.

4. **Establishing intravenous access.** Placement of central lines in proximity to an injury should be avoided if there is a possibility of vascular disruption.

E. **Disposition.** Patients with superficial wounds and no evidence of cervical spine injury may be discharged. All other patients should be admitted for diagnostic studies, observation, or operative intervention.

VII. THORACIC TRAUMA

A. **Discussion.** Chest injuries account for 25% of trauma deaths. Approximately 15% of traumatic chest injuries require operative intervention; the remaining 85% can be managed in the emergency department. The **cardiac (anterior) box** is the most worrisome region. The boundaries are the sternomanubrial angle (superiorly), lower ribs (inferiorly), and the right and left nipples (lateral).

B. **Clinical features**

1. **Simple pneumothorax** is a collection of air in the pleural space that does not communicate with the external chest wall. Findings include decreased breath sounds and hyperresonance on the affected side, dyspnea, and chest pain. Chest wall injury may or may not be present.

2. **Open pneumothorax.** "Sucking chest wound" is a defect in the chest wall. If the wound is greater than two-thirds of the diameter of the trachea, air may enter the chest through the wound rather than through the normal airway, causing collapse of the ipsilateral lung and ineffective respiration.

3. **Tension pneumothorax** is a continuous accumulation of air in pleural space with no available exit. This increased intrapleural pressure leads to mediastinal shift and compression of the contralateral lung and great vessels, resulting in deceased cardiac filling, decreased cardiac output, and severe respiratory compromise. Findings include dyspnea, agitation, cyanosis, tachypnea, subcutaneous emphysema, hypotension, tachycardia, increased jugular venous pressure, decreased breath sounds, hyperresonance, tracheal shift to the uninvolved side, and increased resistance to ventilation.

4. **Hemothorax** occurs when there is blood found in the chest cavity. It may be secondary to lung injury or bleeding from intercostal or internal mammary vessels. **Massive hemothorax** is defined as blood loss of greater than 1,500 mL into the chest cavity. Decreased breath sounds or dullness may be found on the affected side.

5. Flail chest is when two or more ribs are broken in two or more places. There is a paradoxic inward motion of the flail segment with inspiration and outward movement on expiration. Crepitus and abnormal chest wall motion may be present. This paradoxical chest wall motion, underlying pulmonary contusion, and significant pain lead to hypoxia and hypercapnia.

6. **Pulmonary contusion** is a parenchymal lung injury that results in interstitial edema and capillary damage. Patients present with dyspnea, tachypnea, tachycardia, hypoxia, and chest pain. Opacifications may be seen immediately on chest radiograph and always within 6 hours. If opacifications persist on the chest radiograph for longer than 48 hours, a **pulmonary laceration** should be suspected.

7. **Tracheobronchial injuries** result in labored or noisy breathing, subcutaneous emphysema, and hemoptysis. Most blunt injuries to the bronchus occur within 2.5 cm of the carina and are due to a deceleration mechanism. Persistence of a large air leak or pneumothorax after placement of a chest tube for pneumothorax should raise the suspicion for a major bronchial tear.

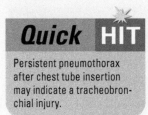

Persistent pneumothorax after chest tube insertion may indicate a tracheobronchial injury.

8. **Cardiac contusion** should be suspected if a patient has sustained blunt trauma to the chest. The patient may complain of chest wall or retrosternal pain. Various atrial and ventricular dysrhythmias, conduction disturbances, altered cardiac wall motion, and decreased cardiac output may be present. The electrocardiogram may be normal, and the most commonly encountered rhythm is sinus tachycardia. Permanent sequelae are uncommon after cardiac contusion.

9. **Pericardial tamponade** may occur after blunt or penetrating trauma to the chest. Bleeding into the nondistensible pericardial sac increases intrapericardial volume and pressure, leading to decreased cardiac output. **Beck triad** may be seen and consists of increased central venous pressure (jugular venous distention), decreased BP, and muffled heart tones. **Electrical alternans** (alternating morphology and amplitude of the QRS complex) and diffuse low voltage (short QRS complexes) may be found on the electrocardiogram. Removal of even small amounts of fluid (20 to 30 mL) can lead to significant improvement in patients with acute pericardial tamponade.

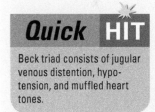

Beck triad consists of jugular venous distention, hypotension, and muffled heart tones.

10. **Traumatic rupture of the aorta** may be caused by bending, shearing, or torsional forces on the aorta (see Clinical Pearl 17-4). The most common area of injury of the aorta is just distal to the ligamentum arteriosum. The descending aorta is relatively fixed by the ligamentum arteriosum and the intercostal arteries as compared to the relatively mobile ascending aorta. An intact adventitial layer may contain the hematoma and allow the patient to survive until arrival at the hospital.

    a. **Causes.** Traumatic rupture of the aorta is caused by deceleration of greater than 30 mph, a fall from greater than 30 feet, or sudden compression of the chest (car falling on chest).

    b. **Symptoms.** The patient may have minimal symptoms and no apparent chest wall injury. A minority of patients will have retrosternal or intrascapular pain, dyspnea, stridor, or dysphagia.

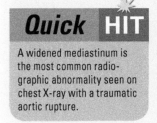

A widened mediastinum is the most common radiographic abnormality seen on chest X-ray with a traumatic aortic rupture.

11. **Diaphragmatic injury** may follow either blunt or penetrating trauma. It must be ruled out in all patients with thoracoabdominal penetrating injuries.

CLINICAL PEARL 17-4

Radiographic Findings of Traumatic Rupture of the Aorta

1. Widened mediastinum
2. Obscured aortic knob
3. Obliteration of the aortopulmonary window (the space between the pulmonary artery and the aorta)
4. Presence of an apical pleural cap
5. Deviation of the trachea or esophagus
6. Fracture of the first or second rib
7. Elevation and rightward displacement of the right mainstem bronchus
8. Depression of the left mainstem bronchus
9. Widening of the paravertebral stripe

Traumatic Emergencies

The patient may present with respiratory distress, and a chest radiograph may show viscera or a nasogastric tube in the chest.

12. **Rib fractures** mandate a search for other injuries and are primarily of concern because of the structures that the ribs cover. Pain with breathing may impair ventilation secondary to splinting.

C. **Diagnostic imaging studies**

1. **Blunt chest trauma** patients should have a chest X-ray followed by a chest CT angiogram if indicated.

2. **Penetrating chest injury.** All patients with penetrating injury to the chest should have a chest radiograph performed. If negative, an expiratory film or CT of the chest can be done. A pneumothorax may be more evident with the lung in expiration. If all films are negative, the patient should have a CT of the chest or repeat chest radiograph in 4 to 6 hours.

D. **Treatment**

1. **Pneumothorax and hemopneumothorax** are treated with a tube thoracostomy.

   a. **Chest tube placement** is at the third or fourth intercostal space, anterior axillary line on the affected side. The tube size does not matter in treating hemothorax versus pneumothorax.

   b. **Indications for open thoracotomy**

      i. Initial blood loss through the chest tube of 1,500 mL

      ii. Ongoing blood loss of approximately 300 mL/hour

      iii. Persistent hypotension after adequate blood replacement

      iv. Radiographic evidence of increased hemothorax despite functioning chest tubes

      v. Worsening of the patient's clinical condition

2. **Tension pneumothorax** may be treated initially with insertion of a 14-gauge angiocatheter at the second intercostal space in the midclavicular line to relieve the tension followed quickly by a chest tube.

3. **Suspected pericardial tamponade.** Pericardiocentesis may be performed while awaiting formal thoracotomy.

E. **Disposition.** Patients with stab wounds who are responsible and who have no evidence of intrathoracic penetration on a repeat chest X-ray after 4 to 6 hours may be discharged home. Most patients with thoracic trauma require admission to a monitored bed, ICU, or operating suite for further care.

VIII. ABDOMINAL TRAUMA

A. **Discussion.** The primary goal with abdominal trauma is determining whether the patient requires emergent operative intervention, not identifying the specific abdominal injury (see Clinical Pearl 17-5).

1. A rapid ultrasound examination (FAST) is sensitive and highly specific in diagnosing hemoperitoneum (Figure 17-3).

B. **Specific organ injuries**

1. The **duodenum** can be injured following frontal impact or penetrating injuries. Duodenal injury may be suspected if there is blood on nasogastric aspirate, retroperitoneal air, or elevated lavage enzymes.

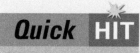

Quick HIT

The presence of subcutaneous air or a deep sulcus sign on the chest X-ray indicates a pneumothorax even if the lung fields appear normal.

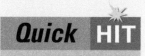

Quick HIT

A pneumothorax may be better seen with an expiratory chest X-ray.

Traumatic Emergencies

CLINICAL PEARL 17-5

Indications for Emergent Operative Management

1. Shock or hemodynamic instability with ongoing blood loss
2. Peritoneal irritation
3. Retained instrument (e.g., knife blade, impaled object) causing trauma
4. Evisceration
5. Transabdominal missile injury
6. Free air
7. Gross blood on nasogastric or rectal examination

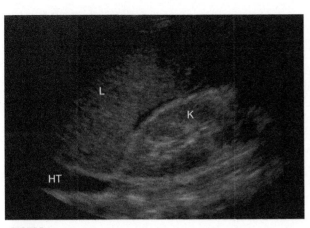 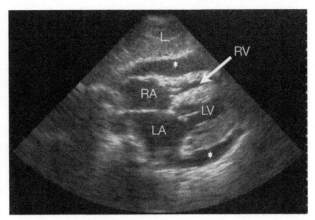

FIGURE
17-3 Focused Assessment with Sonography for Trauma (FAST) scan. (A) *HT,* hemothorax; *K,* kidney; *L,* liver. Note clear fluid in Morison's Pouch between liver and kidney. (B) *RA,* right atrium; *L,* lung; *LA,* left atrium; *LV,* left ventricle; *RV,* right ventricle; (*), fluid (blood) in pericardial sac.

    2. **Pancreatic injuries** occur from a direct epigastric blow (e.g., handlebar injury) that compresses the organ against the vertebral bodies.

    3. **Hepatic injuries** are common because it is a large solid organ and is relatively immobile. Liver injury should be suspected in patients with right lower rib fractures or right upper quadrant tenderness or in patients who are hypotensive after abdominal trauma. Although many liver lacerations can be managed nonoperatively, liver injuries may involve major venous or arterial damage with massive bleeding and high mortality.

    4. **The spleen** is the most common intra-abdominal organ injured from blunt trauma.

  C. **Evaluation**

    1. **Blunt abdominal trauma.** The FAST exam is the initial test of choice. If it is negative or equivocal, and the suspicion is high for a significant injury, an abdominal CT scan with intravenous contrast can be done.

    2. **Penetrating injury** evaluation depends on the mechanism (e.g., stab wound or gunshot wound), the location of the injury, the pathway of the implement, and the patient's clinical presentation.

      a. **Stab wounds**

        i. **Stab wounds of the anterior abdomen** can be evaluated by local wound exploration, FAST exam, or CT.

        ii. Patients with **stab wounds of the back and flank** should have a FAST scan performed. If the FAST scan is negative, CT scan with intravenous, and possibly oral and rectal contrast, is recommended.

      b. **Gunshot wounds** that penetrate the abdomen require operative intervention because the majority of these injuries cause damage that requires surgical repair.

  D. **Treatment**

    1. **Resuscitation.** Patients with abdominal trauma require the standard trauma resuscitative measures.

    2. **Antibiotic therapy.** Patients with suspected bowel injury require preoperative antibiotics to cover aerobes and anaerobes, pending operative findings.

  E. **Disposition** of the patient depends on the extent of the injury sustained. Patients with stab wounds not penetrating the peritoneum may be safely discharged home after local wound care. Patients with a minor mechanism of blunt trauma, reliable examinations, and no evidence of injury may also be discharged home with instructions to return if there is any abdominal pain. Most other patients require admission for observation and treatment as dictated by their injuries.

IX. PELVIC TRAUMA

  A. **Discussion.** Pelvic trauma most commonly results from motor vehicle collisions (especially those involving pedestrians) or falls from heights. Lateral compression accounts for 70% of fractures, whereas anteroposterior compression (15%) and vertical shear (15%) make up the rest.

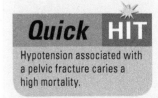

Quick HIT

Hypotension associated with a pelvic fracture caries a high mortality.

Traumatic Emergencies

B. Evaluation
  1. Secondary survey
     a. **Pelvic examination.** Anteroposterior + lateral compression and palpation over the symphysis pubis is required.
     b. **Genitourinary examination.** The presence of blood at the urinary meatus and any scrotal or perineal hematomas should be noted. Female patients should have a vaginal examination.
     c. **Rectal examination.** On rectal examination, the physician should note the presence of gross blood, the position of the prostate, sphincter tone, and any bony abnormality.
     d. **Extremities** should be examined for distal pulses, sensation, dislocation, and any leg length discrepancy.
  2. **Diagnostic imaging studies**
     a. **Radiography.** A standard anteroposterior view of the pelvis is necessary.
     b. **CT** scanning of the pelvis can better demonstrate acetabular disruption, the sacroiliac joint, and the amount of rotation of the pelvis as well as nonbony injuries.
     c. **Angiography** may be performed in patients who continue to bleed despite efforts to terminate hemorrhaging. Angiography allows localization of arterial bleeding sites and, possibly, transcatheter embolization of smaller arteries.
     d. **Retrograde urethrography and cystography** are indicated for patients with penetrating pelvic trauma, pelvic fracture, and/or abnormalities present on physical exam.
C. **Treatment.** The major life threat with pelvic fractures is hemorrhage.
  1. **Resuscitation.** Patients with pelvic trauma should have all the standard resuscitative measures initiated. Intravenous catheters should not be placed in the lower extremities if there is possible proximal venous disruption.
  2. A **pelvic binder** is applied before transport of the patient. This helps compress the pelvis and tamponade venous bleeding, stabilize pelvic fractures, and improve bony alignment.
  3. **Early orthopedic consultation** should be obtained, and transfer to a trauma center should be done quickly.
  4. **Operative intervention** may be required but entails the risk of increased bleeding from disruption of the tamponade effect of the peritoneum on pelvic bleeding.

X. GENITOURINARY TRAUMA

A. **Discussion.** Genitourinary trauma should be suspected in patients who have sustained high-speed deceleration injuries, blunt trauma to the back or flank, lower rib fractures, high falls, and penetrating injuries.
B. **Clinical features.** Signs include flank tenderness, flank hematoma, fractures of the transverse processes of the vertebrae, and hematuria.
  1. **Kidney injuries**
     a. **Renal contusion** (Figure 17-4A) involves parenchymal ecchymoses, subcapsular hematomas, and small lacerations. Hematuria is usually present, and the intravenous pyelogram shows normal function. Contusions account for approximately 90% of renal injuries.
     b. **Renal lacerations** may involve either the cortex or the pelvicaliceal system (Figure 17-4B).
     c. **Renal fracture** ("shattered kidney") involves complete disruption of the parenchyma from the collecting system (Figure 17-4C). The patient is unstable secondary to blood loss.
     d. **Renal pedicle injury** (Figure 17-4D) results from penetrating trauma or deceleration from high speeds. Injuries include lacerations and thromboses of the renal arteries and veins.
  2. **Ureters.** Traumatic injury to the ureters is rare. Most penetrating ureteral injuries are in the upper third of the ureter.

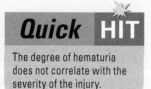

Quick HIT

Continued movement of a patient with a pelvic fractures increases pain and bleeding.

Quick HIT

The degree of hematuria does not correlate with the severity of the injury.

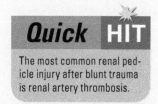

Quick HIT

The most common renal pedicle injury after blunt trauma is renal artery thrombosis.

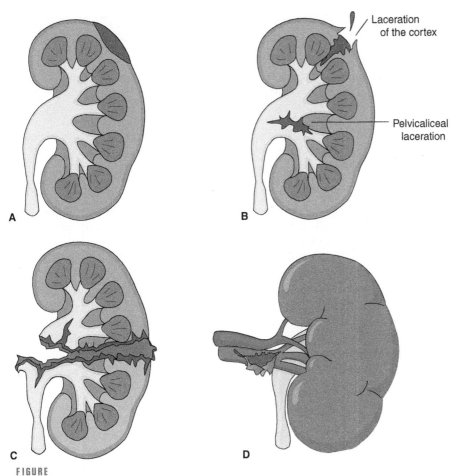

FIGURE 17-4 (A) Renal contusion. (B) Renal lacerations. (C) Renal fracture. (D) Renal pedicle injury.

3. **Bladder** injuries are the second most common traumatic genitourinary injuries. They are most commonly seen after blunt trauma and pelvic fractures and usually are associated with a distended bladder (which elevates the bladder from its protected position in the pelvis).

a. **An intraperitoneal bladder rupture** is a tear typically found in the fundus or posterior wall of the bladder. (The peritoneal surface of the bladder is the weakest area of the bladder wall and therefore most likely to rupture.) The tear allows opening into the peritoneum and spillage of urine into the peritoneal cavity (Figure 17-5).

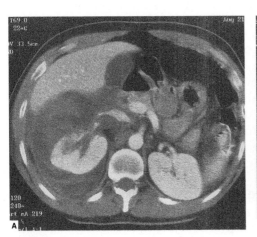
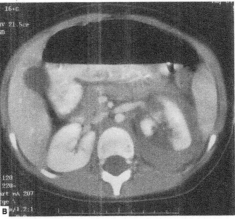

FIGURE 17-5 Intraperitoneal bladder. (A) Rupture. (B) Spillage of urine into the peritoneal cavity.

Traumatic Emergencies

> **CLINICAL PEARL 17-6**
>
> ### Anterior and Posterior Urethra
> 1. The **anterior urethra** consists of the bulbous and penile urethra. Anterior urethral injuries are associated with direct trauma to the urethra, such as with straddle injuries or fractured penis. Blood at the urinary meatus and perineal hematoma are usually seen.
> 2. The **posterior urethra** consists of the membranous and prostatic urethra. Posterior urethral injuries are typically associated with pelvic fractures. Examination reveals perineal hematoma, a high-riding prostate with a boggy consistency, and blood at the urinary meatus.

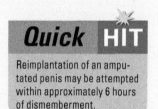

> **Quick HIT**
>
> Reimplantation of an amputated penis may be attempted within approximately 6 hours of dismemberment.

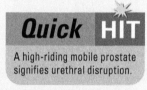

> **Quick HIT**
>
> A high-riding mobile prostate signifies urethral disruption.

> **Quick HIT**
>
> If a urethral injury is suspected, a retrograde urethrogram is performed before urinary catheterization to avoid converting a partial urethral disruption into a complete disruption.

      b. **An extraperitoneal bladder rupture** is a tear outside of the peritoneum that allows urine to spill into the perivesicular space but not into the peritoneum.

   4. **Urethra.** Urethral injuries are uncommon.

      a. **Men.** In men, the urethra is divided by the urogenital diaphragm into the anterior and posterior urethra (see Clinical Pearl 17-6).

      b. **Women.** In women, urethral injuries are not common and are associated with pelvic fracture and perineal injury.

   5. **Penis.** Penile injuries range from simple lacerations to amputation. Penile fracture occurs when an erect penis is subjected to a direct blow, with tearing of the tunica albuginea.

   6. **Testicles.** Testicular injuries include contusions, lacerations, rupture, and dislocation, usually as a result of a fall or direct blow.

C. Evaluation

   1. **Secondary survey.** The pelvis and perineum should be carefully inspected for instability, hematomas, or lacerations. The rectum should be examined, noting sensation, tone, position, and quality of the prostate. The **scrotum and penis** are inspected for hematoma, tenderness, and blood at the urethral meatus.

   2. **Diagnostic imaging studies.** The workup of patients with blunt trauma and microscopic hematuria is controversial. If hematuria fails to clear or is associated with shock, further workup is required.

      a. **Radiography.** Radiologic studies generally proceed in a caudad to cephalad direction.

         i. **A pelvic X-ray** is obtained early followed by a lumbar spine X-ray (looking for a transverse process fracture) if indicated.

        ii. When blood is noted at the urinary meatus, a **retrograde urethrogram** is performed by instilling radiopaque material into the distal urethra and obtaining a radiograph to visualize the urethra.

        iii. **Cystography** is performed after the urethrogram by instilling 350 mL of contrast into the bladder through a Foley catheter by gravity.

      b. An **abdominal CT scan** with contrast should be performed in cases of suspected renal trauma. An abdominal CT scan can show the retroperitoneal space, hematomas, renal disruption, and vascular injuries.

D. Treatment

   1. **General care**

      a. **Consultation.** Early urologic consultations should be sought.

      b. **Antibiotic therapy.** Patients with rectal or vaginal lacerations should receive intravenous antibiotics. Use of antibiotics in other genitourinary injuries depends on the location of injury, if an operation is required, whether urine has extravasated, and if a penetrating injury occurred.

   2. **Specific care**

      a. **Renal injuries**

         i. **Renal contusions** are treated conservatively by following serial hematocrits and urinalyses.

        ii. **Renal laceration, rupture, and pedicle injury.** Minor renal lacerations generally heal without sequelae. Hemodynamic instability of the patient secondary to a serious renal laceration may prompt surgical exploration.

b. **Urethral injuries.** Partial anterior and posterior urethral lacerations may be managed with an indwelling urinary catheter (fluoroscopically placed) or suprapubic cystostomy.

E. **Disposition.** Most patients, except those with very superficial external genitourinary injuries (who have no difficulty urinating), should be admitted to the hospital for observation or surgical intervention.

XI. PEDIATRIC TRAUMA (SEE ALSO CHAPTER 15)

A. **Discussion.** Trauma accounts for approximately one-half of deaths in the pediatric age group. The initial assessment of children proceeds as with the adult, first completing a primary survey and then the secondary survey (see Clinical Pearl 17-7).

B. **Clinical features**

1. **Shock** can be rapidly fatal to a child. Children have extensive compensatory capabilities, and a drop in BP is a late and ominous sign, not occurring until there has been 25% to 30% of blood volume loss.

   a. **Tachycardia** is the primary response to hypovolemia in children. Tachycardia may also be associated with pain and anxiety in children.

   b. **Tachypnea.** RR may also be increased to compensate for metabolic acidosis secondary to decreased tissue perfusion.

   c. **Delayed capillary refill.** Capillary refill may be delayed (longer than 2 seconds) if there is decreased perfusion and shock.

2. **Head injury** is common in the pediatric population and accounts for approximately 50% of accidental deaths, with motor vehicle accidents being the leading cause.

   a. **Scalp lacerations** may cause extensive blood loss in children, and pressure should be applied to control bleeding.

   b. Most **skull fractures** in children are **linear** and may have no associated symptoms except local tenderness. **Depressed skull fractures** usually result from direct blunt trauma and may be open. **Basilar skull fractures** include fractures in the basal portion of the frontal, temporal, and occipital bones, and ethmoid and sphenoid fractures. Findings are the same as those seen in the adult.

   c. **Epidural and subdural hematomas** are relatively uncommon and occur more frequently in older children. Diagnosis and management principles are the same in child as in adults. Approximately 75% of these children continue to have seizures.

3. **Spinal cord injury** is uncommon in children, accounting for approximately 5% of all spinal cord injuries seen.

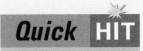

Quick HIT

Complete anterior and posterior urethral injuries require surgical repair.

Quick HIT

Children may cry from fear as well as pain, and they may be less able to localize their pain than adults.

Quick HIT

The Broselow tape is a great resource when treating injured children.

Quick HIT

Early recognition of hypovolemia to prevent shock cannot be overly stressed.

Quick HIT

Head injury is the leading cause of trauma deaths in children.

Quick HIT

Fractures are seen in only approximately 50% of pediatric patients with epidural hemorrhages.

Quick HIT

More children than adults, though, may have spinal cord injury without radiographic abnormality.

CLINICAL PEARL 17-7

Differences between Children and Adult Trauma Victims

1. A child's head occupies a relatively larger proportion of body surface area than an adult's. Bony sutures fuse by 18 to 24 months. A child's brain has a larger proportion of unmyelinated fibers, making it more susceptible to shear injury.
2. Children have shorter necks with less muscle support and more cartilage.
3. The **larynx is more cephalad and anterior**, located at approximately C3–C4 in the infant (C4–C5 in the adult). In children younger than 8 years, the subglottic area at the cricoid ring is the narrowest part of the upper airway (in adults, it is at the level of the vocal cords). It is this area that is the limiting factor in determining endotracheal tube size.
4. The **chest is much more compliant** with less bony structure in the chest wall, more cartilage, less overlying protective muscle mass, and a more horizontally placed and distensible diaphragm.
5. The **mediastinum is more mobile** and more susceptible to a tension pneumothorax.
6. The **abdominal wall is thinner with less protective muscle and fat**. The liver, spleen, and bladder (which is an intraperitoneal structure in children) are all more susceptible to injury.
7. Children have a **higher proportion of body surface area to body mass** and are more subject to heat loss and hypothermia.

Traumatic Emergencies

C. Evaluation
1. **Primary and secondary survey.** The evaluation of the pediatric trauma patient should proceed in a systematic fashion as in adults.
2. **Diagnostic imaging studies**
   a. **CT** is the preferred imaging modality in moderate and severe injuries. Due to the cancer risks from excessive radiation, judicious use should be the rule. The "pan-scan" philosophy in all trauma cases is potentially dangerous.
   b. **Ultrasonography** is a valuable screening tool for abdominal and thoracic injuries.
D. Treatment
1. **Initial stabilization**
   a. **Fluid resuscitation.** Children become hypothermic quickly, and this could negatively affect outcome. Warming lights, blankets, and warmed intravenous fluids should be used in all cases.
      i. Normal saline or Ringer lactate (20 mL/kg bolus over 10 minutes) is the initial fluid of choice. If the patient fails to respond, a repeat bolus of 20 mL/kg may be given.
      ii. If there is no response to crystalloid, packed red blood cells (RBCs) are given at 10 mL/kg.
   b. **Airway**
      i. **Rapid sequence induction** (see Chapter 1.III.B.3) should be done when intubating a trauma patient.
         a) **Atropine** is given (0.02 mg/kg, minimum dose 0.1 mg) to prevent bradycardia secondary to vagal stimulation.
         b) **Neuromuscular blockade**
            1) A defasciculating dose of **a nondepolarizing paralytic is not required in young children.**
            2) The dose of **succinylcholine** is higher in children (2 mg/kg) as opposed to adults and children (1 to 1.5 mg/kg) older than 10 to 12 years.
      ii. **Endotracheal intubation.** Endotracheal tube size may be estimated using the following formula: $(16 + \text{age in years}) \div 4$. Uncuffed endotracheal tubes are used in patients younger than 6 to 8 years.
2. **Management principles** for chest, abdomen, and head injuries are the same in children as in adults.
E. **Disposition.** Children with minor head injury and no loss of consciousness, normal neurologic examination, and a reliable caretaker may be discharged. Many children with isolated orthopedic injuries may also be treated and discharged home. Patients with any other significant injury require admission to a general pediatric floor or to an ICU; some patients may require transfer to a pediatric trauma center.

XII. TRAUMA IN PREGNANCY

A. **Discussion.** Treatment of the pregnant trauma patient proceeds along the same line as treatment of the nonpregnant patient, with some additional significant differences based on anatomic and physiologic changes during pregnancy (see Clinical Pearl 17-8). The most important factor in determining fetal outcome is the status of the mother; optimally treating the mother provides the best treatment for the fetus.
B. **Clinical features**
1. **Abruptio placentae,** separation of the placenta from the uterine wall, is the most common cause of fetal death after trauma. There may be little evidence of external abdominal trauma. It should be suspected in patients who have sustained deceleration injuries as well as direct trauma to the abdomen. Disseminated intravascular coagulation may develop after abruption secondary to release of placental thromboplastin or myometrial plasminogen activator. Findings may include:
   a. Abdominal pain
   b. Uterine tenderness
   c. Tetanic contractions
   d. Amniotic fluid leak
   e. Enlarging uterus

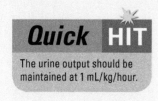

Quick HIT

The urine output should be maintained at 1 mL/kg/hour.

Traumatic Emergencies

CLINICAL PEARL 17-8

Physiologic Changes in Pregnancy

1. **Cardiovascular changes**
   a. **Cardiac output increases** by the 10th week of pregnancy by 1 to 1.5 L/min.
   b. **Heart rate increases** by approximately 20 beats.
   c. **Systolic and diastolic BP are lower** in the first and second trimesters, reaching approximately normal levels by term. **Profound hypotension**, secondary to the gravid uterus compressing the inferior vena cava and decreasing preload, may be seen when the pregnant patient is in the supine position.
2. **Hematologic changes**
   a. **Physiologic anemia.** Pregnant patients have a greater increase in plasma volume than in RBC mass, resulting in a physiologic anemia.
   b. The **WBC count is increased**.
   c. A **hypercoagulable state** exists due to increased clotting factors, venous stasis, and increased loss of protein S and C in the urine.
3. **Pulmonary changes**
   a. There is a **decreased oxygen reserve** secondary to decreased functional residual capacity and increased oxygen consumption. The diaphragm is elevated as uterine size increases.
   b. **Increased risk of aspiration can occur** due to decreased gastric motility and gastric emptying.
4. **Renal changes. Blood urea nitrogen and creatinine are decreased** by approximately 50% secondary to increased glomerular filtration rate.

---

  f. Evidence of fetal distress (noted on fetal heart monitoring)
  g. Vaginal bleeding
 2. **Uterine rupture** results from significant forces causing an increase in intrauterine pressure. Maternal shock, abdominal pain, peritoneal signs, and fetal parts outside of the uterus may be found.
 3. **Fetomaternal hemorrhage**, or passage of fetal RBCs into the normally separate maternal circulation, can occur after relatively minor trauma. In Rh-negative mothers, it can lead to development of maternal antibodies against Rh-positive fetal RBCs and to subsequent hemolysis of fetal RBCs.
  a. **Rho(D) immune globulin** can prevent this isoimmunization if administered within 72 hours of maternal exposure to fetal cells. The usual dose is 300 μg for every 30 mL of fetal blood found in the maternal circulation.
  b. The **Kleihauer-Betke test** can measure the amount of fetal–maternal hemorrhage in milliliters and should be used in suspected cases of massive fetomaternal hemorrhage. In pregnancies of less than 16 weeks' duration, the fetal blood volume, and therefore fetomaternal hemorrhage, would not be expected to exceed 30 mL.

C. **Evaluation**
 1. **Primary and secondary surveys** are done in a standard fashion.
  a. **Fetal monitoring** for at least 4 hours should be performed in all pregnant trauma patients. **Evidence of fetal distress** (late decelerations or loss of beat-to-beat variability on fetal monitor) may be an **early sign of maternal distress**. As blood is shunted away from nonessential organs in the mother, uterine blood flow decreases, affecting the fetus before signs of maternal hypotension are seen.
  b. **Pelvic examination** is done to assess for the presence of blood, amniotic fluid, cervical dilatation, effacement, and presenting fetal parts.
  c. **Abdominal examination** should assess for uterine size (with estimate of gestational age/viability), uterine tenderness, and contractions.
 2. **Diagnostic imaging studies.** Indicated **radiographic studies** should be obtained as mandated by the condition of the mother, shielding the abdomen when possible.
 3. **Early obstetric consultation** should be sought.

D. **Treatment.** The pregnant patient is treated the same as the nonpregnant patient, with the following additions:
 1. Unless spinal injury is suspected, the pregnant patient with a fetus of greater than 20 weeks' gestational age should be **positioned on her left side**. Alternatively, the

Traumatic Emergencies

backboard can be tilted, or the gravid uterus can be manually displaced off the vena cava.

2. Given the greater circulating blood volume of the pregnant patient, a **greater volume of fluid resuscitation is required**, especially if there is any evidence of fetal distress or maternal hypovolemia.

3. **Tetanus prophylaxis** with either tetanus–diphtheria toxoid or tetanus immunoglobulin may be given as indicated.

E. **Disposition.** Patients beyond 20 weeks' gestation should undergo fetal heart monitoring for at least 4 hours. Patients should go to the operating room or ICU as dictated by their injuries.

XIII. BURNS

A. **Discussion.** Death rates are higher in children younger than 4 years of age and in adults older than 65 years of age.

1. **Classification of burns**
   a. **First-degree burn** involves the epidermis and is characterized by erythema, edema, pain, and the absence of blistering. Sunburn is an example of a first-degree burn.
   b. **Second-degree burn** involves the epidermis and dermis. These burns are characterized by blisters and pain.
   c. **Third-degree burns** are full-thickness burns and involve the epidermis, dermis, and subcutaneous fat. The skin is charred, leathery, and insensate.
   d. **Fourth-degree burns** are those involving structures underlying the skin, including fascia, bone, and muscle.

2. **Size of the burn** is expressed as a percentage of body surface area. Estimating the percentage of burn area is important in determining the amount of fluid resuscitation the patient needs (see Clinical Pearl 17-9).

3. **Inhalation burns**, which may be associated with carbon monoxide poisoning, noxious gases, or thermal injury to the airways, may be suspected if burns occurred in an enclosed space, involved the face, singed nasal hairs, or caused carbonaceous sputum. The **half-life of carbon monoxide** is approximately 4 to 5 hours at room air, 90 minutes on 100% oxygen, and 20 minutes on hyperbaric oxygen at three atmospheres.

B. **Evaluation.** Burn patients should be evaluated as trauma patients until the presence of other injuries has been fully assessed. Efforts should be made to **avoid contamination** of the burn.

1. **Primary and secondary surveys** should be completed on patients with major burns.
   a. Burns should be evaluated for depth and size.
   b. The **eyes** should be closely examined for corneal burns.
   c. **Peripheral pulses**, **perfusion**, and **sensation** should be carefully evaluated, especially at points distal to circumferential burns.

2. **Patient history.** A history of the burn should include where the burn occurred, timing of the burn, exposure to gases and chemicals, falls, and any explosions or other trauma.

3. **Laboratory studies** may include a complete blood count; serum electrolyte panel; blood urea nitrogen, creatinine, and glucose levels; arterial blood gas

---

CLINICAL PEARL 17-9

Estimating Size of Burn

1. The **"rule of nines"** divides the body surface area into areas of approximately 9% each. In children, the head accounts for a larger percentage of body surface area, whereas the legs account for a smaller percentage (Figure 17-6).
2. The **"rule of palms"** approximates that the palm size of the patient estimates 1% of the patient's body surface area. Adding up the number of palm areas gives the approximate percentage of body surface area burned.
3. A **Lund-Browder burn diagram** provides for burn estimates adjusted for age.

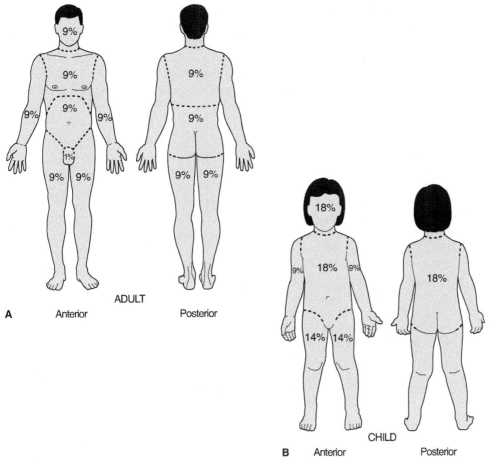

FIGURE 17-6 Approximate burn surface area: (A) adult and (B) child.
(From Jenkins B, Van Kleunen JP, et al. *Step-Up to USMLE Step 2 CK*. 3rd ed. Baltimore: Lippincott Williams & Wilkins; 2014.)

determinations; carbon monoxide level; creatine phosphokinase level; urinalysis; urinary myoglobin; toxicology screen; and ethanol level. Laboratory work is determined by the extent and circumstances of the burn.

4. **Diagnostic imaging studies.** A **chest radiograph** should be obtained but may initially appear normal.

5. **Fiberoptic bronchoscopy** can evaluate the larger airways in patients with suspected inhalation injury.

C. **Treatment**

1. **Transport.** The burn should be covered with sterile sheets, except for small burns, which may be covered with cool cloths.

2. **Initial burn treatment**

   a. The burning process should be terminated by removing the patient from the burn environment and removing all burning clothing.

   b. The patient should be appropriately immobilized and a trauma assessment performed.

   c. Patients with possibility of inhalation injury should have **100% oxygen administered** and their airway should be assessed. **Early intubation** should be considered for patients with possible airway compromise.

   d. Hypothermia should be avoided.

3. **Fluid resuscitation.** Lactated Ringer or normal saline is given at a rate of 4 mL/kg/% total body surface area burned. The first half of fluids should be administered in the first 8 hours from the time of the burn, with the remainder of fluids given over the following 16 hours. Children generally require this amount of fluid in addition to normal maintenance fluids. To assess for

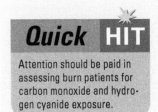

***Quick* HIT**

Attention should be paid in assessing burn patients for carbon monoxide and hydrogen cyanide exposure.

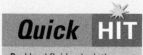

adequacy of fluid resuscitation, urinary output should be monitored (30 to 50 mL/hour in adults or 1 mL/kg/hour in children).

4. **Cleansing, debridement, and application of topical antibiotics.** Burn wounds are gently cleansed, and devitalized tissue is debrided. Once evaluated at the definitive treatment center, the burn may be covered with a topical antibiotic ointment (e.g., silver sulfadiazine). Some centers prefer bacitracin for facial burns.

5. **Tetanus immunization** depending on the extent of the burn and the patient's immunization history

6. Patients with greater than approximately 20% body surface area burn are prone to **ileus** and should have a **nasogastric tube** inserted.

7. **Escharotomy** may be required for circumferential burns to the extremities or chest.

8. **Intravenous antibiotics** are generally not employed initially.

9. **Analgesia** should be administered carefully, monitoring cardiovascular response.

D. **Disposition** depends on the extent of the burn, age of the patient, location of the burn, comorbid factors, and associated injuries, as well as factors such as patient's ability to care for the wound, safety for the patient, and capabilities of the hospital to which the patient initially presents.

1. **Admission (see Clinical Pearl 17-10)**

2. **Burn center treatment** is recommended for burns of greater than 25% in healthy patients aged 10 to 50 years, burns involving greater than 20% in patients younger than 10 years or older than 50 years, or full-thickness burns involving greater than 10% of the total body surface area.

3. **Discharge.** Patients with burns covering less than 15% of the total body surface area in healthy adults or less than 10% in children and older adults, and those not meeting any other criteria for admission may be treated locally and referred for close follow-up.

CLINICAL PEARL   17-10

Patients Who Meet Any of the Following Criteria Should Be Admitted

1. Healthy adults with partial-thickness burns affecting more than 15% of the body surface area or full-thickness burns affecting more than 5% of the total body surface area
2. Young children and older adults with partial-thickness burns affecting more than 10% of the body surface area or full-thickness burns affecting more than 3% of the body surface area
3. Patients with burns involving the face, hands, perineum, or feet
4. Patients with circumferential burns or those covering major joints
5. Patients with electrical or chemical burns
6. Patients with burns associated with inhalation injury or trauma
7. Immunocompromised patients
8. Patients with burns associated with child abuse

ORTHOPEDIC EMERGENCIES

18

Royce Coleman

I. INTRODUCTION

Orthopedic emergencies are acute medical problems involving the abnormal form or function of the extremities, spine, or associated structures. Orthopedic emergencies are common in the emergency department (ED) and can be a threat to long-term limb function.

A. Types of orthopedic emergencies

1. **Muscle contusion (bruise).** A muscle contusion is extravasation of blood into the muscle tissue due to direct trauma. Initially, the bruised muscle will be swollen and tender, and the overlying skin will appear red or blue (ecchymosis). As the blood is resorbed, the skin changes in color from purple to greenish yellow.

2. **Strain.** Muscle strains injuries are classified by the extent of muscle fiber injury that results when the muscle is either excessively stretched or when the muscle is forcibly contracted against resistance.

   a. **First-degree muscle strain** is a minor stretching injury of the muscle fibers that is characterized by muscle spasm, mild swelling, local tenderness, and a slight decrease in function.

   b. **Second-degree muscle strain** is a partial tearing of the muscle fibers that is characterized by moderate swelling, ecchymosis, and decreased functional strength.

   c. **Third-degree muscle strain** is a complete disruption of the muscle that is characterized by swelling, ecchymosis, decreased strength, and a palpable "bulge" caused by the retracted unattached muscle belly. Third-degree muscle strains can lead to significant long-term disability but fortunately are not as common as first- and second-degree strains.

3. **Sprain.** Sprains are injuries to joint ligaments that result from a forced abnormal motion of the joint.

   a. **First-degree sprains** are characterized by mild hemorrhage and swelling, minimal point tenderness, and no abnormal joint motion (i.e., the joint is stable).

   b. **Second-degree sprains**, which occur when the ligaments are partially torn, result in moderate hemorrhage and swelling, tenderness, painful motion, loss of function, and minor joint laxity.

   c. **Third-degree sprains** occur when the joint ligaments are completely disrupted. Third-degree sprains may initially appear similar to second-degree sprains, but the patient will have severe joint instability after the swelling subsides.

4. **Dislocation.** A joint is dislocated when the opposing articular surfaces of the bones are no longer in contact. **Subluxation** is an incomplete dislocation (i.e., the articular surfaces are in partial contact).

5. **Fracture.** A fracture is the disruption of the bony cortex. The broken bone bleeds into the surrounding tissue, resulting in pain, swelling, and deformity.

   a. **Descriptive terms.** Important details include the following: the affected bone, fracture location, whether the fracture is open or closed, whether

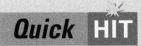

Quick HIT

Third-degree strains require immobilization and early follow-up for potential surgical repair.

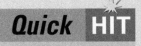

Quick HIT

In order for a dislocation or subluxation to occur, the joint ligaments must be disrupted; therefore, dislocations and subluxations are characterized by swelling, pain, and tenderness around the joint.

Orthopedic Emergencies

419

intra-articular extension has occurred, the type of fracture line, description of bone fragments (if present), whether the fracture is complete or incomplete, neurovascular status, and the position or alignment of the bone segments.

    i. An **open fracture** occurs when the skin overlying the fracture is not intact either due to direct trauma or a fragment of bone that penetrates the skin. A subtle open fracture can occur when a bone fragment pierces the skin and then withdraws, leaving only a small puncture wound. Therefore, any fracture with an overlying skin wound should be suspected of being open. A **closed fracture** occurs when the skin and soft tissue overlying the fracture are intact.

    ii. An **intra-articular fracture** is a fracture that extends into the joint surfaces.

    iii. The fracture line may be **spiral**, **oblique**, or **transverse** (Figure 18-1). Fractures in children are often described as **buckle (torus)**, **greenstick**, or **complete** fractures (Figure 18-2). A fracture can also be described as a **compression**, **avulsion (chip)**, or **comminuted (shattered)** fracture.

    iv. The bone segments may be in contact with each other or separated by a measurable distance (usually stated in millimeters). The bone segments may be completely **displaced** (i.e., lying next to each other instead of end to end), **partially displaced** (i.e., offset from each other by a measured amount), or **nondisplaced**.

    v. The **angulation** of the two bone segments is described by both the **direction of the angle** (e.g., radial, dorsal, anterior, lateral) and by the **degree of the angle** formed by the two bone segments.

b. **Special fractures**

    i. **Pathologic fractures** occur when a relatively minor force is applied to diseased or otherwise weakened bone.

    ii. **Stress fractures** are caused by the repetitive application of a minor force to a bone, usually a long bone in the lower extremities. Stress fractures are commonly seen in military personnel (march fracture) and athletes (e.g., joggers, dancers).

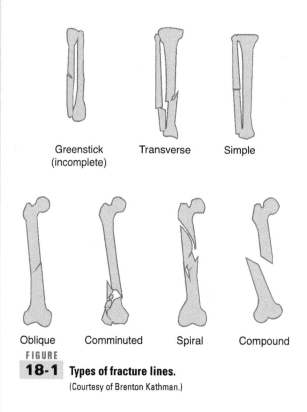

Greenstick (incomplete)   Transverse   Simple

Oblique   Comminuted   Spiral   Compound

FIGURE 18-1 **Types of fracture lines.**
(Courtesy of Brenton Kathman.)

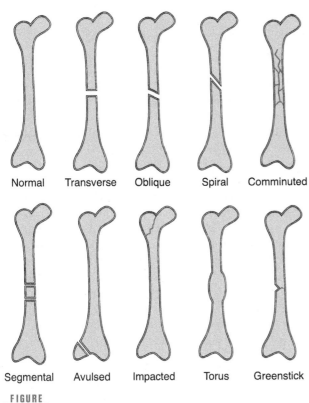

18-2 **Children's fractures.**
(Courtesy of Brenton Kathman.)

      iii. Salter-Harris fractures (Figure 18-3) involve the epiphyseal plate
      (i.e., the growth plate) and are common in children.
B. Diagnosis of orthopedic emergencies. Many orthopedic emergencies can be
   diagnosed by a careful patient history and a thorough physical examination. The
   emergency physician uses the history and physical examination to discern the
   potential type and degree of injury and to choose the appropriate radiographic
   image that will verify the suspected diagnosis.
   1. Patient history
     a. Patient age. The patient's age may give some indication of the type of injury,
     (e.g., Salter-Harris fractures only occur in young patients, whereas hip frac-
     tures are more common in the elderly).

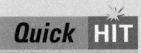

Damage to the epiphyseal
plate may destroy its ability
to form new bone, resulting
in malformations as the child
grows.

Orthopedic Emergencies

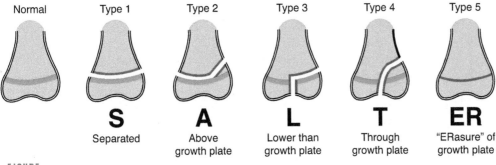

18-3 Salter-Harris classification of epiphyseal fractures. Note that type III and IV injuries are
intra-articular fractures. Type V injuries are crush injuries.
(Courtesy of Brenton Kathman.)

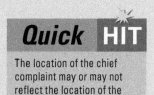

b. **Chief complaint.** Patients with orthopedic emergencies typically present with one or more of the following complaints: **pain, swelling, redness, deformity, or diminished function.**

c. **Mechanism of injury**

   i. The mechanism of injury (i.e., how the injury occurred) is important for predicting the type of injury. For example, if the physician does not know the mechanism of injury, it may be difficult to reach a diagnosis in a young child with normal radiographs who refuses to use his or her right arm. However, if the physician knows that the child had been recently pulled by that arm, the probable diagnosis (subluxation of the radial head) becomes readily apparent.

   ii. The mechanism of injury also aids in determining which radiographic views to obtain, especially when the patient is unable to cooperate, has referred pain, or has a distracting injury. For example, a patient who complains of acute shoulder pain after an injury may have a normal routine shoulder radiograph. However, if the mechanism of injury suggests posterior dislocation, then an additional view of the shoulder can be obtained to confirm this diagnosis.

d. **Preexisting illnesses or conditions.** The physician should inquire about illnesses and conditions that may negatively impact the healing process (e.g., diabetes, heart disease, steroid therapy, and cancer chemotherapy).

2. **Physical examination**

a. **Inspection.** The suspected area of injury should be inspected for swelling, discoloration, deformity, abrasions, puncture wounds, and lacerations.

   i. Orthopedic injuries (including fractures) may have few or no obvious visible abnormalities, especially in children.

   ii. Muscle contusions and severe sprains may result in localized swelling that is similar to the swelling seen with fractures. Radiographs are frequently needed to differentiate sprains and fractures.

b. **Palpation** of the entire extremity may reveal point tenderness, subtle deformities (e.g., a "step off"), or bony crepitus. The area distal and proximal to the pain location should be systematically palpated. Complete palpation is important for two reasons:

   i. The patient may be unaware of a second injury because of the pain of the primary injury.

   ii. If radiographs are ordered prior to complete palpation, radiographs of the correct bone may not be obtained.

c. **Range of motion assessment.** When possible, each joint proximal and distal to the injury should be assessed for both passive and active range of motion. The degree of flexion, extension, and pain should be noted. This examination of the function of the joint may need to be repeated on the contralateral (unaffected) joint to discern subtle abnormalities.

d. **Neurologic examination.** Nerve injury can result in either sensory or motor deficits. Sensation distal to the injury should be identified before any manipulation of the extremity takes place. Muscles that are innervated by the major nerves of the extremity should be examined for motor function.

e. **Arterial blood flow assessment.** Some orthopedic emergencies (e.g., knee dislocation, fracture or dislocation of the ankle, supracondylar fracture of the elbow in children) are commonly associated with vascular (arterial) injuries. The earlier circulatory compromise is identified and addressed, the less likely it is that permanent injury will result.

3. **Radiography**

a. **Views**

   i. **Standard.** The area to be examined radiographically should be based on the history and physical examination findings. Frequently, imaging the joint above and the joint below a suspected fracture is indicated to detect associated fractures or dislocations. Most extremity radiographs include an **anteroposterior view**, a **lateral view**, and an **oblique view.**

ii. **Special.** Some fractures are only visible using special radiographic views. Some common orthopedic emergencies that require special views include acromioclavicular separation, fracture of the carpal navicular, posterior shoulder dislocation, and sternoclavicular dislocation. Children may need comparison views of the unaffected extremity to detect epiphyseal plate injuries.

b. **Findings**

i. In the case of **stress fractures**, the initial radiographs may be normal. However, the presence of new bone growth or bone resorption (which causes the fracture line to become visible) on radiographs taken 2 to 3 weeks later may suggest the fracture. If a fracture is highly suspected but the radiograph is normal, treatment for the fracture should be initiated.

ii. The normal growth plate appears as a transverse, radiolucent line at the end of the bone. The growth plate can be easily confused with a transverse fracture.

C. **Basic management of orthopedic emergencies**

1. **Sprains.** Because ligaments lack a robust blood supply, a sprain may require up to 8 weeks to heal. Physicians should take care to avoid dismissing the injury as "only a sprain," as such statements give the patient the unrealistic expectation of a rapid and complete recovery.

a. **First- and second-degree sprains.** Initial treatment entails **RICE**—*r*est, *i*mmobilization, *c*ompression and cold packs, and *e*levation—and **analgesics** or **anti-inflammatory agents.** First- and second-degree sprains usually do not result in long-term sequelae.

b. **Third-degree sprains.** Urgent orthopedic consultation should be obtained for patients with third-degree sprains, which can lead to permanently diminished joint function. These sprains are sometimes immobilized in circumferential casts for several weeks or **may require surgical repair.**

2. **Fractures and dislocations**

a. **Stabilization of the patient.** Although orthopedic emergencies are seldom life-threatening, concurrent life-threatening injuries may be present. Therefore, **airway, breathing, and circulation** (the **ABCs**) should be assessed first and appropriate measures taken. Generally, in multiple trauma patients, airway, head, thorax, and abdominal injuries are treated before orthopedic injuries, although some orthopedic injuries (e.g., pelvic fractures of midshaft femur fracture) can significantly contribute to hemodynamic instability.

b. **Reduction of swelling.** Swelling occurs early after a fracture or dislocation and can increase the patient's pain and delay the application of definitive immobilization.

i. Elevation of the extremity and application of cold compresses are effective measures for preventing the progression of swelling.

ii. Potentially constricting jewelry on the injured extremity should be removed in anticipation of extremity swelling.

c. **Temporary immobilization.** The suspected fracture or dislocation should be immobilized early in the ED visit. Immobilization reduces the patient's pain, diminishes the potential for damage to the neurovascular bundle, and reduces swelling and bleeding. Additionally, stabilization and immobilization facilitates patient transport, expedites the radiographic examination, and, in the case of fractures, reduces the chance of a sharp bone fragment puncturing the skin and converting a closed fracture to an open fracture.

i. For **fractures**, temporary immobilization is accomplished by **splinting** across the fracture and the joints proximal and distal to the fracture.

ii. For **dislocations**, the joint may be immobilized using a **splint** or **sling.**

d. **Pain control.** Most patients with fractures or dislocations will be become increasingly comfortable when the extremity is sufficiently immobilized.

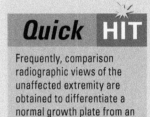

Quick HIT

Frequently, comparison radiographic views of the unaffected extremity are obtained to differentiate a normal growth plate from an injured one.

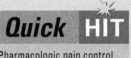

Quick HIT

Pharmacologic pain control is commonly required and has a positive impact on the patient's experience.

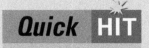

Quick HIT

For patients in whom the physician anticipates general anesthesia in the near term, only parenteral analgesics should be given in the ED.

Orthopedic Emergencies

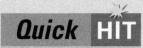

Not all fractures require reduction—the decision to reduce a fracture depends on variables such as the age of the patient, the involved bone, the location and type of fracture, and the amount of deformity.

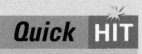

When there is gross deformity and no palpable distal pulse, emergent reduction is indicated to restore circulation to the limb.

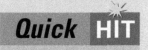

A neurovascular examination should also be performed and documented following reduction.

e. **Reduction** is the process of restoring the bone or joint to its normal anatomic configuration. Early reduction decreases pain, may restore circulatory or nerve function, and prevents the progression of swelling.
   i. Generally, a radiograph of the bone or joint is obtained prior to the reduction of the fracture or dislocation.
   ii. Analgesics and sedatives are usually required for most reductions, which are generally accomplished by applying slow, steady, longitudinal traction.
   iii. A postreduction radiograph is always needed to document the success of the procedure, to determine if additional injuries are present, and to assess the need for additional treatment.
f. **Postreduction immobilization.** Reduced fractures and reduced dislocations must be immobilized before the patient is released from the ED (see Clinical Pearl 18-1).
g. **Disposition**
   i. **Hospital admission.** Patients at high risk for serious complications (see VII) and those with open fractures, fractures that require open reduction or internal fixation, hip fractures, or severe hand infections may require admission to the hospital or to the operating room.
   ii. **Discharge.** Most patients with orthopedic emergencies can be treated in the ED and then discharged with follow-up plans. Prior to discharging the patient, the physician should see that the following general measures have been taken:
      a) The patient should be provided with **discharge instructions.** The patient should be advised to:
         1) Keep the extremity elevated at all times.
         2) Alert a physician if excessive swelling, decreased sensation, discoloration, or increased pain in the digits is observed following the application of a splint.
      b) If the patient cannot walk or if the patient should not bear weight on a lower extremity, then arrangements for **crutches** or a **walker** (and instructions for their use) should be provided.
      c) **Pain control** should be addressed for all patients.
      d) Every patient with a dislocation or a fracture requires **follow-up with an orthopedist or a physician skilled in fracture care.** For most orthopedic emergencies, the emergency physician should contact the follow-up physician to arrange an appointment and discuss a discharge plan appropriate to the injury. For simple fractures and reduced dislocations, the patient should usually be seen within 10 days. For a patient with a more complex injury that may require surgical repair, the patient should be seen sooner.

CLINICAL PEARL 18-1

Immobilization

1. **Splints** or **circumferential casts** are usually used to immobilize **fractures.** Splinting is less likely than circumferential casting to lead to pressure sores, circulatory compromise, and neurapraxia. After the swelling has decreased, a circumferential cast can be applied.
   a. Patients with fractures that are not prone to complications and have only minimal swelling may be treated in the ED with circumferential casting.
   b. Splints are usually made from plaster of Paris or fiberglass. Water causes an exothermic chemical reaction, which causes the material to harden over several minutes. During this process, the splint is molded along one side of the extremity, which is held in the appropriate position. Padding is placed between the skin and splint, and the splint is secured to the extremity with an elastic bandage wrapped circumferentially around the extremity and splint.
2. **Immobilization dressings.** In addition to splints, several dressings are commonly used in the ED. Examples include the **shoulder sling, sling and swath, and knee immobilizer.**

II. HAND AND WRIST INJURIES

Injuries and infections of the wrist and hand result in over 6 million visits to the ED each year.

A. **Descriptive terms**
  1. **Location.** The terms **radial, ulnar, palmar (volar), and dorsal** are used to describe the location of the hand injury.
  2. **Digits.** The digits can be numbered or named: **I (thumb), II (index finger), III (long finger), IV (ring finger), and V (little finger).**
  3. **Joints.** The joints are the **distal interphalangeal (DIP), proximal interphalangeal (PIP), metacarpophalangeal (MCP), and carpometacarpal.**

B. **Diagnosis**
  1. **Patient history.** Important aspects of the history include hand dominance (right-handed versus left-handed), details of the mechanism of injury, the position of the hand at the time of injury (e.g., fist, fingers extended), the timing and nature of all symptoms, the patient's occupation, previous hand deficits, and the patient's medical history.
  2. **Physical examination**
      a. **Inspection.** Abnormal flexion or extension of individual digits when the hand is at rest should be noted, as should swelling, scars, amputations, and discolorations.
      b. **Palpation** of the entire hand and wrist should be performed to determine deformity or point tenderness (see Clinical Pearl 18-2).
      c. **Tendon function assessment.** Each muscle–tendon group is tested individually by determining strength and pain against resistance as well as pain with active and passive motion. When the tendon is completely ruptured, there is no movement; with partial ruptures, intact motion may exist but pain and decreased strength are present.
          i. The deep flexor tendons are assessed by having the patient flex each finger at the DIP joint while the examiner keeps the PIP and MCP joints of all the patient's fingers in extension.
          ii. The superficial flexor tendons are assessed in a similar fashion by having the patient flex each PIP joint while the examiner keeps the patient's other fingers in extension.
          iii. The individual extensor tendons are assessed by having the patient extend all digits. The thumb should be extended and abducted (away from the palm) against resistance.
      d. **Wrist function assessment.** Wrist function is examined by having the patient flex the wrist, extend the wrist, and deviate the wrist to the radial and ulnar side against resistance.
      e. **Neurologic examination**
          i. **Motor function**
              a) Because the median nerve innervates the abductor pollicis brevis, this nerve can be tested by having the patient abduct the thumb against resistance.
              b) The ulnar nerve innervates the hypothenar muscles, the thumb adductor, and the intrinsic interosseous muscles of the hand. This nerve can be tested by determining the strength of the index and little fingers when the patient is instructed to abduct the fingers against resistance.

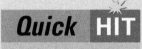

Quick HIT

When inspecting a tendon for injury through an open wound, the position of the hand and fingers must be the same as they were at the time of injury.

Orthopedic Emergencies

CLINICAL PEARL 18-2

Navicular Fracture

The navicular bone lies in the anatomist's snuff-box; palpation for tenderness is necessary to detect fractures of the navicular bone, which are often occult and not visible radiographically. This is a commonly missed fracture and evaluation for this injury should be documented.

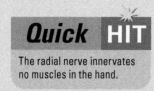

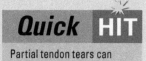

       c) The radial nerve is injured if the patient cannot **extend** the wrist against resistance (wristdrop).

   ii. **Sensation**

       a) Both the radial and ulnar aspect of each digit (digital nerves) should be tested using 5-mm two-point touch.

       b) All three nerves to the hand should be assessed by determining sensation at the dorsal web space between the thumb and index finger (radial nerve), the tip of the long finger (median nerve), and the tip of the little finger (ulnar nerve). Light touch should be used to test sensation in the dorsal aspect of the fingers and hand because this area is less sensitive than the palmar aspect.

  f. **Arterial blood flow assessment.** The color, warmth, and nail bed capillary refill time should be examined in each finger. Both radial and ulnar pulses should be palpated.

C. Treatment

  1. **Wounds** that penetrate the skin frequently damage tendons, nerves, vessels, and joint capsules. Deep sutures should never be placed in the hand by ED personnel (except to repair extensor tendons). Elevation, splinting, and close follow-up are important components in the care of hand wounds.

  2. **Tendon injuries.** Although some complete extensor tendon ruptures can be repaired in the ED, flexor tendon injuries should never be repaired in the ED and always require orthopedic consultation.

D. Specific injuries

  1. **Hand**

    a. **Infections**

      i. **Paronychia** is the most common hand infection and presents as swelling, erythema, pain, and tenderness around the base of the nail. The causative organism is usually *Staphylococcus* or *Streptococcus*. Following appropriate anesthesia, drainage is performed by inserting a scalpel blade between the nail and the nail fold. Antibiotics are controversial.

      ii. **Felon** is an extremely painful infection of the pulp tissue in the tip of a digit. The causative organism is usually *Staphylococcus*, and the major symptom is pain and swelling of the fingertip. Felons should be drained by making an incision along one lateral aspect of the fingertip then separating the septum of the fingertip by blunt dissection; close follow-up is necessary and antibiotics are commonly prescribed.

      iii. **Tenosynovitis** usually occurs along a flexor tendon and is characterized by tenderness over the tendon, swelling of one finger, pain on passive extension, and a flexed resting position of the finger. If detected early, a trail of high-dose intravenous antibiotics is indicated, but frequently, surgical drainage is required.

      iv. **Cellulitis** of the hand typically requires hospital admission, appropriate intravenous antibiotics immobilization, and elevation.

      v. **Septic arthritis** of any digital joint or of the carpometacarpal joint can occur. Treatment entails irrigation and drainage in the operating room.

    b. **Tendon injuries**

      i. **Mallet finger** is caused by detachment of the extensor tendon from the distal phalanx. The patient usually complains of pain at the DIP joint and is unable to fully extend the affected finger. The radiograph of the finger may appear normal, or there may be a small avulsion fracture at the base of the distal phalanx. Unless accompanied by a fracture, mallet finger is treated with a dorsal splint that prevents flexion of the PIP for 6 weeks. If it is accompanied by a large avulsion fracture, surgical pinning may be required.

ii. **Boutonniere deformity**, a disruption of the extensor hood apparatus near the PIP, can be easily overlooked. In the ED, it is treated with a dorsal splint with the PIP in full extension or slight flexion. This injury requires close follow-up.

c. **Trauma**

i. **Fingertip amputations** are common injuries that require copious irrigation and careful debridement in the ED. If the distal phalanx is not exposed, the digit can be dressed and the patient referred to a hand surgeon for definitive care within a few days.

ii. **Finger sprains**

a) Collateral ligament sprains of the MCP, PIP, and DIP are common. Lateral stress should be applied to the extended joint to determine the amount of laxity and the degree of sprain. All sprains should be splinted for several weeks or until the follow-up examination.

b) Third-degree sprains that cannot be reduced in the ED frequently require surgical repair. "Gamekeeper's thumb" ("skier's thumb") is a serious injury that is caused by disruption of the ulnar collateral ligament of the MCP joint of the thumb. These injuries require splinting and close follow-up.

c) The most significant carpometacarpal joint sprain involves the first metacarpal joint. These sprains are caused by hyperextension, and the joint may be dislocated. Severe sprains require operative treatment.

iii. **Finger dislocations.** Dislocations of the DIP and PIP joints are usually easily reduced using longitudinal traction following digital block anesthesia. Reductions of MCP dislocations can be extremely difficult and may require surgery. All reduced dislocations should be splinted for several weeks or until the follow-up examination.

iv. **Finger fractures**

a) **Phalanx fractures**

1) **Distal phalanx** fractures are usually treated with a protective splint, leaving all joints free. Subungual hematomas are common and should be drained to alleviate pain. Associated nail bed injuries should be repaired. As discussed in II.D.1.b.i, some fractures associated with mallet finger require surgery.

2) **Middle and proximal phalanx** fractures that are not displaced can be splinted and the patient referred a hand specialist or orthopedist. Fractures that are displaced may require surgical pinning after reduction.

b) **Metacarpal fractures** usually occur at the distal neck rather than at the head, shaft, or proximal base. All metacarpal fractures can be treated with an ulnar gutter splint in the ED prior to referral.

1) **Distal neck fractures.** The most common distal neck fracture is "boxer's fracture" (i.e., fracture of the neck of the fifth metacarpal). Distal fractures of the fourth or fifth metacarpal require reduction if the angulation is greater than 30 degrees.

2) **Head, shaft, or base fractures** require early follow-up.

v. **High-pressure injection injuries** are discussed in Chapter 19.V.E.

2. **Wrist injuries**

a. **Carpal dislocations (Figure 18-4)**

i. **Anterior (volar) lunate dislocation** is the most common carpal dislocation. The lunate appears rotated on the lateral radiograph.

ii. **Posterior perilunate dislocation** is also common. The capitate is dorsally dislocated in relation to the lunate.

b. **Carpal fractures** may occur when a patient falls on an outstretched hand. Because carpal fractures can be radiographically occult, any patient with

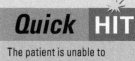

Quick HIT

The patient is unable to grasp items between the thumb and index finger.

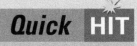

Quick HIT

Distal fractures of the second or third metacarpal require reduction if the angulation is greater than 15 degrees.

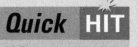

Quick HIT

Initially, there may be only mild swelling and tingling, but high-pressure injuries (despite their initial near-normal appearance) require immediate consultation by a hand surgeon.

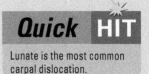

Quick HIT

Lunate is the most common carpal dislocation.

Orthopedic Emergencies

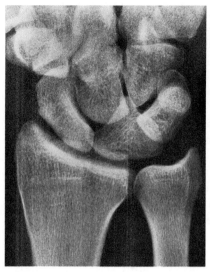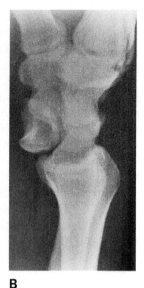

A   **B**

FIGURE
18-4 Lunate and perilunate dislocation.

significant signs or symptoms of a wrist fracture should be treated with a
thumb spica splint and referred to an orthopedic surgeon.

  i. The **scaphoid (navicular)**, **triquetrum**, and **lunate** are the most
    commonly fractured carpal bones (Figure 18-5).

  ii. **Distal radius** fractures with significant displacement are usually reduced
    in the ED.

    a) **Colles fracture** is a fracture of the distal radius in which the distal
      radius fracture fragment is dorsally displaced, producing a character-
      istic "dinner fork" deformity.

    b) **Smith fracture** is a fracture of the distal radius characterized by volar dis-
      placement (i.e., it is a reversed Colles fracture) of the fracture fragment.

c. **Carpal tunnel syndrome** is caused by inflammation of the carpal canal,
resulting in compression of the median nerve.

  i. **Etiology.** Carpal tunnel syndrome is usually a result of repetitive wrist
    flexion.

  ii. **Clinical signs.** Patients usually complain of paresthesia ("pins and needles")
    in the index finger, long finger, and radial aspect of the ring finger.

  iii. **Treatment.** Emergency treatment consists of a volar wrist splint,
    nonsteroidal anti-inflammatory drugs, and referral to a hand specialist.

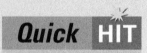

Quick **HIT**

The paresthesia is exacerbated by tapping the volar
wrist (Tinel sign) or by holding the wrist in the flexed
position (Phalen sign).

Orthopedic Emergencies

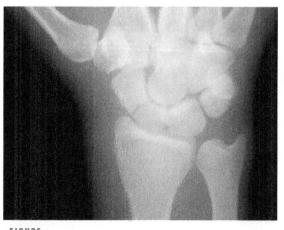

FIGURE
18-5 Scaphoid fracture.

(Courtesy of Colleen Campbell, MD; from Greenberg MI, et al.
Greenberg's Text-Atlas of Emergency Medicine. Philadelphia:
Lippincott Williams & Wilkins; 2005.)

III. FOREARM, ELBOW, UPPER ARM, AND SHOULDER INJURIES

A. **Forearm.** Forearm shaft fractures of the ulna or radius frequently occur together and are usually displaced; therefore, after finding a fracture in one forearm bone, the other bone should be closely scrutinized for fracture. Careful examination for swelling, deformity, and point tenderness is required; however, most closed forearm fractures do not result in nerve or vascular injury.

1. **"Nightstick" fractures** are nondisplaced midshaft fractures of the ulna often caused by a direct blow to the forearm. These fractures are treated with a long arm splint and close follow-up.

2. **Monteggia fracture–dislocation** is a fracture of the proximal ulna and a dislocation of the radial head at the elbow. Adults with this injury are treated with open reduction and internal fixation. Children are treated with closed reduction and immobilization.

3. **Galeazzi fracture** (fracture of the distal radial shaft) is often associated with a distal radioulnar joint dislocation near the wrist; it is often thought of as **reverse Monteggia fracture.** The anteroposterior radiograph may show only slight widening of radioulnar space. On the lateral view, the ulna is displaced dorsally. This injury is treated with open reduction and internal fixation.

4. **Radial shaft fractures.** In adults, displaced fractures of the radial shaft typically require open reduction and internal (or external) fixation. In children, displaced fractures can sometimes be treated with closed reduction.

B. **Elbow**

1. **Subluxation of the radial head (nursemaids' elbow)** is seen only in children younger than 7 years and is caused by the application of sudden traction to a pronated hand (i.e., by pulling the child by the hand). The child presents in apparently no pain but keeps the affected arm pronated and in slight flexion. Treatment is by either passive supination or extension of the forearm; a "click" can be felt over the radial head as the subluxation is reduced.

2. **Elbow dislocations** are usually posterior and occur following a fall on an outstretched arm.

   a. Because **neurovascular complications** (most commonly, ulnar nerve and brachial artery injuries) are associated with up to 21% of elbow dislocations, the function of the ulnar, radial, and median nerves and the presence of the radial and ulnar pulses should be assessed. Associated fractures should be sought.

   b. **Treatment.** Reduction is accomplished by traction and countertraction after adequate sedation. After reduction, the neurovascular examination is performed again and the arm splinted in 90-degree flexion. Cylindrical casts should not be used.

C. **Upper arm**

1. **Distal humerus fractures** are usually supracondylar in children and intercondylar (intra-articular) in adults.

   a. **Complications.** These fractures often cause severe swelling; injuries to the median, ulnar, and radial nerves; transection of the brachial artery; and Volkmann's ischemic contracture (compartment syndrome; see VII).

   b. **Treatment** for displaced fractures normally consists of open reduction and internal fixation and hospital admission for neurovascular observation.

2. **Proximal humerus fractures** can occur at the anatomic neck, surgical neck, greater tuberosity, lesser tuberosity, or shaft.

   a. **Complications.** Anatomic neck fractures can result in vascular compromise to the humeral head, leading to necrosis of the articular segment. Significantly displaced surgical neck fractures and shaft fractures may have associated brachial plexus and vascular injuries.

   b. **Treatment.** If neurovascular injuries are not present, these fractures are immobilized in the ED with a sling and swath, and the patient is referred for follow-up.

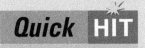

Within a few minutes of successful reduction, the child will use the affected arm normally. Immobilization after reduction is usually not required.

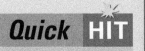

Hemarthrosis, characterized by a posterior "fat pad" sign on the lateral radiograph, may be the only evidence of a nondisplaced fracture.

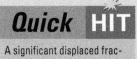

A significant displaced fracture of the greater tuberosity implies concomitant rotator cuff injury.

Orthopedic Emergencies

CLINICAL PEARL | **18-3**

Classification of Acromioclavicular Joint Injuries

1. **Type I** injuries are characterized by a minor ligament sprain. Patients have joint tenderness but no disruption of the joint.
2. **Type II** injuries consist of one ruptured ligament and slight widening of the acromioclavicular joint. There may be a slight step-off deformity that becomes apparent following comparison with the opposite acromioclavicular joint.
3. **Type III** injuries are characterized by rupture of all acromioclavicular ligaments and significant widening of the joint.

D. **Shoulder**
  1. **Acromioclavicular joint injuries (shoulder separations)** are common.
    a. **Classification.** Shoulder separations are classified according to the amount of ligament disruption (see Clinical Pearl 18-3).
    b. **Treatment** of all three grades of injury consists of rest, ice, analgesics, and immobilization with a simple sling. In addition, some type III injuries may require open reduction and repair.
  2. **Glenohumeral dislocations**
    a. **Anterior dislocations**, in which the humeral head is displaced anterior to the glenoid and inferior to the coracoid, are the most common type of glenohumeral dislocation (Figure 18-6). A flattening deformity of the lateral aspect of the shoulder can be seen, and the humeral head can usually be palpated anteriorly.
      i. **Complications.** Anterior dislocation is frequently associated with a greater tuberosity fracture, humeral head fracture, rotator cuff tear, disruption of the axillary artery, and transient axillary nerve injury.
      ii. **Treatment.** Many reduction techniques have been described and are used in the ED. Because this injury has a recurrence rate of up to 90%, patients are treated with a sling following reduction and referred to an orthopedist for follow-up care.
    b. **Posterior dislocations** often occur as a result of a fall or during an epileptic seizure. Posterior dislocations are frequently not clinically recognized, and a lateral shoulder or "scapula Y" radiograph may be required to make the diagnosis.
  3. **Clavicle fractures** are the most common fractures of childhood. The mechanism of injury is usually a blow to the shoulder, and most fractures occur in

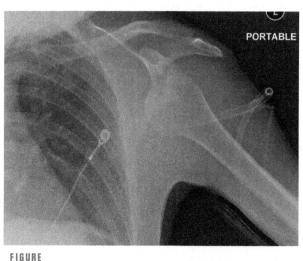

FIGURE
18-6 Anterior glenohumeral shoulder dislocation.
(Used by permission of Martin Huecker, MD.)

Orthopedic Emergencies

the middle third. Therefore, the clavicle should be inspected and palpated along its entire length in every patient with a suspected shoulder injury. Most clavicle fractures heal within 6 weeks without complications.
  a. Nondisplaced fractures require only immobilization with a sling.
  b. Displaced fractures do not need immediate reduction and only require treatment with a sling.

IV. PELVIS, HIP, AND FEMUR INJURIES

A. **Pelvis. Pelvic fractures** commonly result from blunt trauma sustained during motor vehicle collisions or falls from a significant height. All multiple trauma patients should be initially suspected of having a pelvis fracture. Fractures that result in a widened pubic symphysis are unstable.
  1. **Diagnosis.** Most pelvic fractures are suggested by mechanism of injury and physical examination findings (e.g., pain on palpation).
  2. **Associated injuries and complications**
    a. Common associated injuries include intra-abdominal organ injuries, femur fractures, bladder and urethral injuries, nerve root injuries, and vaginal injuries.
    b. The pelvis is extremely vascular; therefore, hemorrhage is a major cause of death in patients with pelvic trauma. Retroperitoneal bleeding is very common, and up to 6 L of blood can be accommodated in the retroperitoneal space.
  3. **Treatment** consists of resuscitation with intravenous fluids and blood products, immobilization of the pelvis, and a careful search for concomitant injuries. Orthopedic consultation is required. Stable, nondisplaced fractures require only bed rest. Other pelvic fractures may require open reduction and fixation.

B. **Hip**
  1. **Hip dislocations** are posterior in 90% of patients and occur when force is applied to the anterior of the flexed knee.
    a. **Complications.** Acetabulum fractures and femur fractures often occur with hip dislocations.
    b. **Treatment** consists of closed reduction under general anesthesia. Ideally, hip dislocations are treated within 6 hours of the injury.
  2. **Slipped capital femoral epiphysis** may occur bilaterally and is seen most often in boys between the ages of 10 and 16 years. The cause is unknown; symptoms include the gradual onset of groin discomfort following activity, knee pain, hip stiffness, and limping. The slightly posterior displaced epiphyseal plate is visible on a lateral radiograph. Treatment entails weight-bearing restrictions and referral to an orthopedist for definitive diagnosis and treatment.
  3. **Septic arthritis** is discussed in Chapter 10.

C. **Femur**
  1. **Intertrochanteric fractures** are most often seen in elderly patients following a fall or motor vehicle collision. Movement of the hip or weight-bearing produces severe pain. Surgical fixation by an orthopedic surgeon is required.
  2. **Subtrochanteric fractures** are usually caused by a fall or motor vehicle collision. Signs and symptoms are similar to those seen with intertrochanteric fractures, but these fractures can cause severe hemorrhage and large amounts of blood can accumulate in the thigh. Orthopedic consultation should be obtained for definitive treatment.
  3. **Femoral shaft fractures** usually occur in young adults following a fall or motor vehicle collision. The leg should be splinted in the ED using a traction device that applies a sling to the ankle and foot. The patient requires hospitalization, fracture reduction, and surgical insertion of an intramedullary rod.

V. KNEE INJURIES

A. **Diagnosis.** The injured knee should always be compared with the noninjured knee. The patient's gait, degree of active flexion, and degree of active extension should be noted, along with the presence of skin trauma or swelling.
  1. **Abduction and adduction stress testing** should be performed by applying lateral stress to the knee while the patient holds it in 30-degree flexion. By comparing

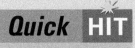

Quick HIT

Rectal examination occasionally reveals superior displacement of the prostate (indicative of urologic injury) or blood in the rectum (indicative of intra-abdominal injury).

Quick HIT

The leg is shortened, internally rotated, and adducted with a posterior hip dislocation.

Quick HIT

Dislocation of the hip can disrupt the blood vessels between the acetabulum and the femur, causing avascular necrosis of the femoral head. Sciatic nerve injury is also a common complication.

Quick HIT

The leg is shortened, adducted, and externally rotated with a intertrochanteric femur fracture.

Quick HIT

In patients with an acute knee injury, it may be difficult to appreciate joint laxity as a result of hemarthrosis and pain.

Orthopedic Emergencies

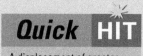

the degree of laxity of the injured knee to the noninjured knee, the degree of injury (if any) to the medial and lateral collateral ligaments can be measured.

2. **Lachman test.** To perform Lachman test, the examiner stabilizes the femur in his or her left hand and uses his or her right hand to grasp the posterior aspect of the lower leg below the knee. While the knee is flexed to 20 degrees, the examiner applies anterior force with his or her right hand to pull the lower leg forward.

B. **Specific injuries**
   1. **Meniscus injuries** usually produce hemarthrosis, a clicking sound with movement, or locking of joint on partial flexion. If a meniscus injury is suspected, orthopedic follow-up should be obtained.
   2. **Sprains.** Ligament injuries typically produce hemarthrosis unless the knee capsule is completely disrupted. Minimal ligament injuries that appear stable can be treated with a knee splint, ice packs, elevation, and ambulation as tolerated. More severe injuries require an orthopedic consultation for definitive management.
   3. **Dislocations**

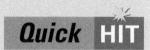

   a. **Tibia–femur dislocations** are common, and spontaneous reductions occur frequently. Suspicion of this injury is important because of the associated risk of injury to the ligaments, popliteal artery, and peroneal nerve. Early reduction and orthopedic consultation are required, and an arteriogram is customarily obtained.
   b. **Lateral dislocation** of the patella is usually evident on physical examination.
   4. **Fractures** can result from a direct blow to the patella. Nondisplaced, simple patella fractures are treated by immobilization. A comminuted or displaced fracture may require open reduction and fixation.

VI. LOWER LEG, ANKLE, AND FOOT INJURIES

A. **Lower leg**
   1. **Tibial plateau fractures** most commonly occur through the superior aspect of the lateral condyles but may also affect the medial tibia condyles. These fractures can be difficult to detect by physical examination and radiography.
      a. Nondepressed fractures can be treated with immobilization and restricted weight bearing.
      b. Depressed fractures require open reduction and elevation of the bony segment.
   2. **Tibial shaft fractures** are common in children and usually result from the application of a twisting force. The fibula is usually fractured also. These fractures require reduction, immobilization, and follow-up with an orthopedist. Compartment syndrome of the anterior compartment of the lower leg is a common complication of tibial shaft fractures (see VII.A).

B. **Ankle**
   1. **Sprains.** Ankle sprains most often involve the lateral collateral ligaments and result from the application of an inversion force. The sprain can be graded using the clinical impression of the amount of ligament injury as a basis.
   2. **Dislocations.** Ankle dislocations usually have concomitant malleolar fractures. The ankle should be reduced with in-line traction and immobilized. Orthopedic consultation is required.
   3. **Fractures.** Malleolar fractures usually occur when the ankle is forcibly adducted and may be accompanied by avulsion fractures of both the medial and lateral malleolus (i.e., the tibia and fibula, respectively). A malleolar fracture is treated by either closed reduction and immobilization or by open reduction and fixation, depending on the type and severity of the fracture.

C. **Foot**
   1. **Calcaneal fractures** are the most common type of tarsal bone fracture. The mechanism of injury is usually a fall from a height. These fractures are often associated with other injuries to the lower extremity or to the spine. Orthopedic consultation is usually required to reduce these difficult fractures.

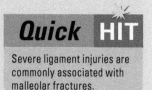

Orthopedic Emergencies

2. **Metatarsal fractures.** Avulsion fractures of the base of the fifth metatarsal are the most common type of metatarsal fracture. The mechanism of injury is plantar flexion and inversion; patients often say they "slipped while walking." Treatment consists of restriction of weight bearing and follow-up.

3. **Phalanx fractures** are common and usually result from a direct blow to the toe. Treatment consists of reduction of the fracture by traction following digital anesthesia. The digit is then immobilized by "buddy taping" the broken toe to the adjacent toe or applying a walking cast.

VII. COMPLICATIONS OF ORTHOPEDIC INJURIES

A. **Compartment syndromes** are extremely serious complications of orthopedic injuries that, without early recognition and treatment, can result in permanent disability.

1. **Pathogenesis.** Compartment syndromes occur when tissue pressures greater than 20 mm Hg in closed compartments compromise the capillary blood flow, leading to muscle and nerve ischemia and necrosis. Compartment syndromes are caused by either a decrease in compartment size (usually due to constrictive casts or burn eschars) or an increase in compartment contents (usually due to hemorrhage or edema). Palpation of the compartment may not reveal swelling.

2. **Clinical features** include muscle pain at rest that is exacerbated by movement and muscle tenderness. Later, hypesthesia of the area innervated by the ischemic nerve may occur. A diminished distal pulse is a late finding that occurs after muscle necrosis.

3. **Diagnosis.** Compartment syndromes can be difficult to diagnose early. Suspicion of the compartment syndrome must be based on pain location and knowledge of the recent injury.

   a. **Differential diagnoses** for a painful extremity include compartment syndrome, fracture, muscle strain, muscle contusion, venous thrombosis, and cellulitis.

   b. **Definitive diagnosis** is provided by inserting an 18-gauge needle into the compartment tissue and measuring the pressure using an electronic monitor or mercury manometer.

4. **Treatment.** A pressure greater than 30 mm Hg usually requires **emergency fasciotomy** in the operating room. This procedure is performed by making longitudinal skin and fascia incisions to free the contents of the compartment and to decrease the pressure.

B. **Osteomyelitis** may occur in a patient with an open fracture or following surgery to repair the fracture. The following precautions are usually taken to prevent osteomyelitis in patients with open fractures:

1. **Prophylactic antibiotics** (e.g., a parenteral cephalosporin and an aminoglycoside) are administered in the ED.

2. **Careful irrigation** and **debridement** are performed in the operating room.

C. **Pulmonary fat embolus** results when a bone marrow fat particle reaches the venous circulation, leading to respiratory compromise. When it occurs, this complication usually develops within a few days of fracturing a long bone.

D. **Avascular necrosis** of the bone segment can occur and may necessitate prosthetic replacement.

E. **Nonunion** occurs when a fracture does not heal.

F. **Malunion** occurs when a fracture heals with a deformity.

G. **Joint stiffness** or **traumatic arthritis** may occur following a fracture.

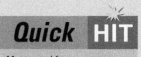

Metatarsal fractures are often misdiagnosed when local tenderness is attributed to an ankle sprain.

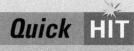

Severe pain (out of proportion to exam) may be the only finding early in the course of compartment syndrome.

Quick **HIT**

Commonly affected areas include the forearm (usually from supracondylar humerus fractures), hand and thigh (usually from crush injuries), and the lower leg (usually from tibial fractures).

Orthopedic Emergencies

I. STAGES OF WOUND HEALING (TABLE 19-1)

II. EVALUATION OF WOUNDS IN THE EMERGENCY DEPARTMENT

The goals of wound care in the emergency department (ED) are to **prevent infection, restore function,** and **restore physical integrity.**

A. **Examination of the wound** allows the physician to assess the level of care required. Attention to the area of injury, and its underlying structures, guides the physician in deciding whether the wound can be treated in the ED or requires a surgeon.

B. **History of present injury**

1. **Contamination of the wound.** Wounds with high concentrations of bacterial contamination (e.g., by feces, saliva, or organic matter) need extensive debridement and irrigation. Some of these wounds may have such extensive contamination that they will require delayed closure.

2. **Age of injury.** The **golden period of wound care** is generally considered to be less than 6 to 8 hours following injury. Between 8 and 12 hours, some wounds can be closed without significant additional risk of infection. It is best to not close wound that are greater than 16 hours unless there is a cosmetic issue. In contrast, in a heavily contaminated wound of the foot, closure may not be safe in as little as 3 hours postinjury.

3. **Extent of injury.** Inspect all wounds for injuries to deep structures like tendon, nerves, and blood vessels. Pull wounds open and debride so the entire wound can be seen.

4. **Past medical history**
   a. **Past medical history.** Diabetes, immunosuppression (e.g., caused by steroids, AIDS, cancer treatment), and alcoholism are examples of conditions that affect wound healing. These conditions lead to slower healing and higher infection rates. In the presence of such conditions, sutures should be left in longer and prophylactic antibiotics should be considered.
   b. **Age of the patient.** Patients younger than 2 years and older than 50 years have higher rates of infection.
   c. **Smoking status.** Tobacco use decreases peripheral blood flow and increases the risk of other vascular injury.
   d. **Nutritional status.** Patients with severe nutritional deprivation have slower wound healing and higher infection rates. Supplemental nutrition may be necessary for these individuals.
   e. **Medications.** Steroids and immunosuppressive medications may slow healing and increase infection rates. Aspirin, antiplatelet agents, and warfarin may cause accumulation of blood in wounds that are primarily closed, causing swelling and possible infection.
   f. **Tetanus immunization.** Tetanus is a potentially fatal disease that is highly preventable. All patients with wounds should be questioned as to their immunization status.

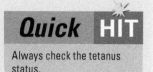

Quick HIT

Every attempt should be made to rule out foreign bodies and document the search as foreign body retention is a common medical-legal issue.

Quick HIT

Facial wounds can generally be closed up to 12 to 24 hours following injury because the higher vascularity of the face leads to lower infection rates than in wounds occurring to the rest of the body.

Quick HIT

Always check the tetanus status.

TABLE 19-1	Stages of Wound Healing
Immediate response to tissue injury	• Vasoconstriction and tissue contraction occur. • Platelets aggregate, and clotting cascade is activated. • Once hemostasis is complete, the release of vasoactive amines causes capillary dilation and an exudate forms.
Inflammatory phase	• Granulocytes and lymphocytes accumulate to control growth of bacteria and prevent infection. • Immunoglobulins contribute to control of infection. • Macrophages phagocytize debris, encourage collagen deposition, and stimulate neovascularization.
Epithelialization	• Within 12 hours of injury, cells of the stratum germinative are activated, and within 24 hours, initial epithelialization may be complete.
Neovascularization	• New blood vessels form and bring nutrients and oxygen to the healing wound. • Neovascularization begins at day 3 and peaks at day 7. • By day 21, the process is complete and the new blood vessels withdraw as the tissue matures.
Collagen synthesis	• Fibrocytes initially lay down disorganized pattern of collagen. • Over months to years, the matrix is remodeled to form organized meshwork of collagen.
Wound contraction	• Myofibroblasts are responsible for wound contraction, in which the initial scar contracts to a smaller size.

C. **General inspection**
  1. **Description of wounds.** Document length, depth, ability to visualize the base, and shape (stellate, linear, jagged, flap). The entire wound should be visualized. If it is covered by matted blood or hair, gently clean if off.
  2. **Functionality of wounded area.** The initial inspection is used to evaluate functioning of the area as well as distal functioning. Attention to neurologic function (i.e., sensation, reflexes, strength) prior to the use of local anesthesia is important. Muscle movement and tendon function should be evaluated through the entire range of motion. Vascular integrity should be evaluated (i.e., temperature, color, capillary refill, pulses).

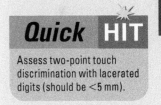

Quick HIT

Assess two-point touch discrimination with lacerated digits (should be <5 mm).

III. WOUND CARE
  A. **Skin cleansing and wound preparation.** Cleanse the skin to remove debris and decrease the bacterial count of the surrounding skin.
  1. The area surrounding the wound must be cleansed to remove blood and other debris. Mild cleansing or scrubbing can usually be accomplished prior to administering local anesthesia. Skin preparation is essential if the anesthesia method involves injecting through the skin (field blocks).
  2. Wound care is often based on common practice rather than research. For example, hydrogen peroxide is still used by some medical professionals even though it is a poor antimicrobial solution with significant tissue toxicity.
  3. Several solutions are available for skin cleansing. A skin-cleansing solution should be fast-acting and have a broad spectrum of antimicrobial activity. These requirements must be weighed against the solution's toxicity to wound tissues. Povidone–iodine and chlorhexidine are the two most commonly used skin preparation solutions.
    a. **Povidone–iodine solutions.** Povidone–iodine is a potent germicidal solution. It has broad-spectrum coverage and is fast-acting. However, it is toxic to open tissues. Toxicity reduces the immune response, thereby increasing risk of infection. It is an excellent skin cleanser but should not be used inside of wounds.

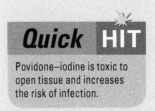

Quick HIT

Povidone–iodine is toxic to open tissue and increases the risk of infection.

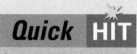

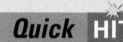

b. **Chlorhexidine.** This has reasonable bactericidal activity, but its antiviral activity is not well understood. It is toxic to wound tissue, and contact with open wounds should be avoided.

c. **Hydrogen peroxide.** Because of its poor antimicrobial activity and significant wound toxicity, this solution should not be used for skin preparation or wound irrigation. Hydrogen peroxide may be used to dissolve dried blood and matted hair (e.g., on the scalp). Care should be taken to keep the solution away from wound tissues.

d. **Alcohols** have poor antimicrobial activity and are toxic to tissues. Alcohols can cause significant pain when used around open wounds and are not good skin preparation solutions.

4. Shaving the area around the wound is not recommended because it increases the risk of infection.

   a. If hair removal is necessary to visualize the wound, the hair should be clipped with scissors.

   b. Eyebrows should never be clipped or shaved.

B. **Anesthesia.** After a neurovascular examination has been completed and documented, it is essential that the area of the wound be adequately anesthetized to allow pain-free examination, cleansing, debridement, irrigation, and closure.

1. **Pain associated with the injection.** For both regional and local anesthesia, several factors affect the level of pain associated with injection of the anesthetic (see Clinical Pearl 19-1).

2. **Regional anesthesia** is the preferred method of anesthesia in most cases when wound treatment is necessary. Regional blocks allow injection of anesthetic agents away from the injury site, which can be quite sensitive, and they allow for longer anesthesia. In addition, more than one wound can be repaired from a single injection site.

   a. Wounds of the fingers, hands, feet, toes, ears, face, and mouth are appropriate for regional blocks. These small areas often have important landmarks. Local anesthesia can distort landmarks and cause tissues to swell, making them more difficult to examine, debride, irrigate, and close.

   b. The injection of anesthesia is usually done with a 27- or 30-gauge needle.

3. **Local anesthesia**

   a. **Injected local anesthesia** is the most commonly used method of local anesthesia; it is the simplest, fastest, and most effective for nearly all wounds. There are two basic approaches:

      i. **Parallel margin infiltration (field block).** Anesthesia is injected through the **intact skin** next to the wound. If local anesthesia is injected through intact skin, the skin must be cleansed prior to injection to help prevent skin bacteria from being carried subcutaneously.

      ii. Anesthesia may be injected through **exposed subcutaneous tissue** of the wound edge. Injecting through the exposed wound tissue causes less pain but may carry contaminants in the wound to deeper tissues.

   b. **Topical local anesthesia** is associated with high patient satisfaction because there is no pain associated with injection of anesthesia.

      i. **Agents**

         a) TAC, a mixture of **tetracaine, adrenaline (epinephrine), and cocaine liquid,** has been used for topical wound anesthesia. Results are

CLINICAL PEARL 19-1

Factors affecting level of pain associated with injection include:

1. **Rate of injection** (a slow injection is less painful)
2. **Size of the needle** (a smaller needle is less painful; anything less than a 27 gauge doesn't decrease pain)
3. **Location of the injection** (intradermal is more painful, subdermal is less painful)
4. **Temperature of the injected agent** (warm is less painful)
5. **Presence or absence of buffering lidocaine prior to injection** (buffering the anesthetic decreases pain)

somewhat mixed, but TAC appears to provide good wound anesthesia for most patients. **Potential risks** of using TAC include increased incidence of infection and wound edge necrosis, although proponents of TAC believe this risk to be minimal.

    b) **LET or LAT,** a mixture of **lidocaine, epinephrine (adrenaline), and tetracaine,** is a possible alternative to TAC. This compound offers pain control similar to that provided by TAC but is associated with fewer toxic effects.

  ii. **Administration**

    a) Both compounds are formulated by the hospital pharmacy and should be applied 20 minutes prior to initiating wound care.

    b) Neither TAC nor LET should be used on wounds involving areas of distal vascularity (e.g., ears, tip of nose, penis, or digits) because of the constrictive properties of epinephrine and cocaine.

4. **Anesthetic agents**

  a. **Esters.** Procaine, tetracaine, chloroprocaine, benzocaine, and cocaine (not for injection) are examples of esters. Most of these are not used except as topical agents.

  b. **Amides.** Lidocaine, bupivacaine, and mepivacaine are all examples of amide-type anesthetics and are preferred over ester-based anesthetics.

    i. **Lidocaine** and **bupivacaine** are the two most commonly used local anesthetics. Lidocaine has a fast onset of action and a duration of action of 20 to 60 minutes. Bupivacaine has a slower onset of action than lidocaine but is effective about four times longer.

    ii. Some allergic reactions may be caused by preservatives present in both amide- and ester-type agents. Lidocaine that is used for intravenous administration does not contain these preservatives and may be used if the patient is allergic only to the preservatives.

  c. **Antihistamines.** Diphenhydramine is an amide antihistamine that provides some local anesthesia when infiltrated near a wound.

  d. **Epinephrine.** Epinephrine added to an anesthetic agent prolongs the agent's activity. The vasoconstrictive action of the epinephrine reduces local wound bleeding. Agents with epinephrine are still avoided in areas of limited distal vascularity.

C. **Inspection and exploration**

1. **General comments**

  a. The wound must be **adequately anesthetized** before inspection and exploration can take place. A **bloodless field** must be obtained by applying a local tourniquet (i.e., a Penrose drain) around a digit or by using an extremity pneumatic tourniquet.

  b. The wound edges should be **pulled apart with instruments so that the entire wound can be adequately examined.** It is very important that the bottom of the wound be visualized. The entire wound should be examined for tracts that may lead to other areas of injury.

2. **Location of the wound.** Vascularity of the wound, stress on the wound, and the bacterial skin count are related to the location of the wound on the body.

  a. **Vascularity** is one of the most important factors that determine the likelihood of a wound becoming infected. Areas of high vascularity (e.g., face) generally have lower infection rates. Areas with low vascularity (e.g., hands and feet) have higher infection rates.

  b. **Bacterial skin count** also contributes to the infection potential. Moist areas (e.g., axillae, perineum) have high bacterial skin counts. Careful preparation of wounds in these areas is imperative.

  c. **Stress on the wound** is a factor in determining scar size. Wounds that are parallel to the lines of tension in the body leave smaller scars than those perpendicular to these lines (Figure 19-1).

3. **Underlying structures.** When examining a wound, the physician should consider the surrounding anatomy and any possible injury to underlying

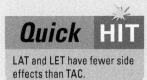
Quick HIT

LAT and LET have fewer side effects than TAC.

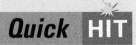
Quick HIT

Success of anesthesia is made evident by blanching of the area around the wound.

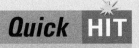
Quick HIT

Because epinephrine may weaken the defenses of the wound, increasing the risk of infection, epinephrine should be avoided in wounds that are contaminated or have a high infection potential.

Quick HIT

An extremity tourniquet may be inflated for up to 2 hours without risk of causing tissue injury.

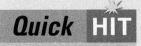
Quick HIT

If necessary, the wound should be extended surgically to allow a complete examination.

Wound Emergencies

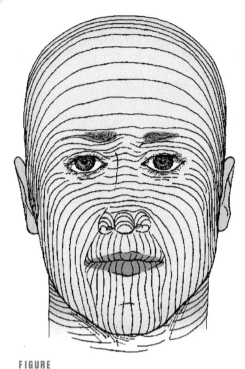

FIGURE 19-1 Skin tension lines of the face. Incisions or lacerations parallel to these lines are less likely to create widened scars than those that are perpendicular to them.

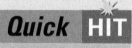

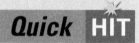

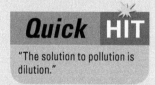

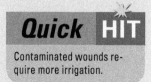

structures, such as tendons, joints, nerves, vascular structures, bone, and organs. It may be necessary to extend the wound surgically to obtain adequate visualization of all underlying structures.

4. **Foreign bodies.** All foreign bodies must be removed from a wound.
   a. The incidence of infection dramatically increases when foreign bodies are left in a wound. In general, 10^6 bacteria per gram of wound tissue cause infection. Occasionally, a wound contains so many foreign bodies that it is necessary to take the patient to the operating room for wound cleansing and foreign body removal.
   b. In some situations, radiographic studies may be necessary to locate foreign objects. Radiographic studies should not be used in place of good wound inspection and exploration but rather as an adjunct.
      i. Metal, gravel, and some glass may be visualized using ordinary radiographs.
      ii. Wood, plastic, and other less dense objects may be visualized with computed tomography or ultrasound.

D. **Debridement** is the removal of devitalized and heavily contaminated tissue from the wound. Clots from the initial coagulum require removal as well. Devitalized tissue acts much like a foreign body. Any tissue that has lost its blood supply becomes a source of infection. If a wound has significant devitalized or contaminated tissue, surgical consult may be necessary. Upon completion of the debridement process, all tissues in the wound should look healthy and have a good blood supply.

E. **Irrigation.** High pressure irrigation—rather than soaking—is the method used to decrease the bacterial count of a wound.
   1. The solutions most commonly used for irrigation are sterile normal saline and nonionic detergents, but tap water is acceptable.
   2. Irrigation should be high volume (200 to 2,000 mL, depending on the size and contamination of the wound) and high pressure (7 psi). This can be accomplished by using an 18- or 19-gauge intravenous catheter on a 35-mL syringe. Most wounds require at least 200 to 500 mL of irrigating solution.

TABLE **19-2**	Laceration Repair Guidelines	
Location	**Closure Material**	**Sutures in Place For**
Face	6-0 nylon or polypropylene; may use fast-absorbing gut to avoid removal in anxious children	3–5 days
Scalp	5-0 polypropylene or staples	7 days
Intraoral	5-0 fast-absorbing gut, chromic gut for deep layers	Absorbable
Upper extremities	4-0, 5-0 polypropylene	7 days
Lower extremities	4-0, 5-0 polypropylene	8–10 days
Joint	5-0 polypropylene	10–14 days

IV. WOUND CLOSURE

A. **Categories of wound closure (Table 19-2)**
  1. **Primary closure** is closure using sutures, tapes, staples, or adhesives. It can be performed on wounds with low infection potential.
  2. **Secondary closure (intention).** Smaller wounds that have a high infection potential are left open and allowed to heal by granulation and reepithelialization. This is called secondary closure. These wounds still require proper wound care (i.e., inspection, exploration, debridement, irrigation).
  3. **Tertiary closure (delayed primary closure).** Wounds that have a high infection potential and are quite large may be best treated by delayed primary closure. Following proper wound care, the wound may be packed with saline gauze mesh and covered. If the wound does not show any signs of infection after 4 or 5 days of daily dressing changes, it may be closed using percutaneous sutures or tapes. The wound may need to be revised (i.e., trimming of the wound edges until tissue with a good vascular supply is reached). Proper wound care should be repeated prior to closure.

B. **Sutures**
  1. **General comments**
    a. The purpose of sutures is to restore physical integrity and function. Although the patient may come to the ED to "get stitches," the emergency physician should focus on proper wound care. It does little good to close a wound only to have it become infected later or to close a wound and leave an underlying structure damaged and nonfunctional.
    b. Sutures need to be placed to adequately close the wound and provide even tension in the wound. The suture itself may invoke an inflammatory response that weakens resistance to infection. As few sutures as possible should be used to adequately close the wound and provide even tension.
  2. **Suture types**
    a. **Absorbable.** Sutures that lose their tensile strength in 60 days or less are considered absorbable. Types include synthetic absorbable sutures (Vicryl [Ethicon, Somerville, NJ], PDS [Ethicon]), plain gut (collagen), chromic gut, and rapidly absorbable gut.
    b. **Nonabsorbable.** These sutures are usually made of polymer nylon (Prolene [Ethicon]). Sutures made from silk are rarely used.
      i. **Monofilament sutures** (nylon, Prolene) are most often used.
      ii. **Multifilament sutures**, made of polymers such as nylon, may be used because of their ease of handling. There is some concern that a multifilament suture may wick fluid and contaminants from the surface of the skin into the wound, increasing the risk of infection.
  3. **Suture placement**
    a. **Percutaneous suturing** is the most common method of suturing, in which the needle and suture enter through the skin at the edge of the wound.

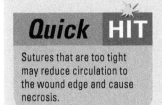

Quick **HIT**

Sutures that are too tight may reduce circulation to the wound edge and cause necrosis.

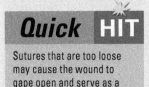

Quick **HIT**

Sutures that are too loose may cause the wound to gape open and serve as a portal of entry for infection.

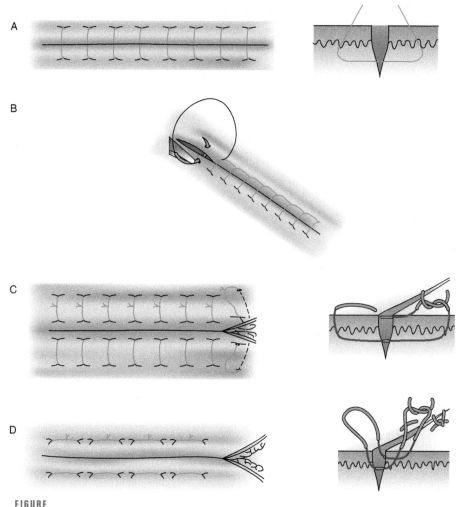

FIGURE 19-2 Types of wound closures: (A) simple interrupted suture, (B) running suture, (C) vertical mattress suture, and (D) horizontal mattress suture.
(From Jarrell BE, Kavic SM. *NMS Surgery*. 6th ed. Baltimore: Wolters Kluwer; 2016.)

Sutures can be continuous (running) or interrupted. Interrupted sutures are most commonly used. The sutures should be placed evenly and provide even closure and tension on the wound. There are several methods of percutaneous suture placement (Figure 19-2).

b. **Dermal (subcuticular) suturing.** In this method of wound closure, the sutures are placed just below the surface of the skin. Except at the ends of the wound, the sutures do not enter through the skin. When the wound is closed, only the ends of the suture are visible. If absorbable suture is used, no suture may be visible. Dermal sutures can be used in clean wounds but should be avoided in contaminated wounds.

C. **Staples.** In areas where scars are less likely to show (e.g., the scalp), staples provide a fast and inexpensive method of skin closure. The staple invokes very little inflammatory response. The wound is held securely closed by the strength of the staple, with only a minimal amount of material below the skin surface.

1. Compared with suturing, positioning the wound edges is more difficult using staples, and the staple punctures are larger.

2. Because of their ease of use, there may be a temptation to rush through proper wound care and proceed directly to stapling. This defeats the purpose of good wound care.

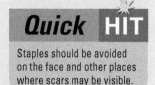

Quick **HIT**

Staples should be avoided on the face and other places where scars may be visible.

D. **Tapes.** Tapes (i.e., Steri-Strips [3M, Saint Paul, MN]) are a fast, painless method of skin closure. They have the lowest rate of infection. As with other methods of closure, proper wound care must be performed prior to their use.

1. The skin must be dry, and tincture of benzoin (or Mastisol [Eloquest Healthcare, Ferndale, MI]) is generally applied to help the tapes adhere better. Care should be taken to keep tincture of benzoin from coming in contact with the wound because it is quite toxic to wound tissues.

2. Tapes can be used on areas of the skin that have relatively low skin tension and are not over areas of motion (i.e., joints).

E. **Adhesives.** Several wound adhesives are available. These may prevent some of the problems that occur with sutures and staples, and studies have shown that the wound infection rate and the appearance are as good or better.

V. CARE OF SPECIFIC WOUND TYPES

A. **Closed-fist injuries.** These wounds are generally associated with young men and alcohol consumption.

1. **Characteristics.** Closed-fist injuries often involve the fist coming in contact with the teeth of another individual. Because the patient is often intoxicated, these wounds may receive delayed care. The laceration is over the metacarpophalangeal joint and extends into the joint.

2. **Therapy.** Inspection, exploration, debridement, and irrigation usually must be done in the operating room. All of these wounds should be radiographed. Intravenous antibiotics that cover gram-positive, gram-negative, and anaerobes should be administered. Splinting is very important to prevent infection. These wounds are not sutured closed. Most of these patients will need to be admitted for close follow-up and continued antibiotics.

B. **Bite wounds**

1. **Characteristics**

a. A total of 80% to 90% of bite wounds result from dog bites, 5% to 10% from cat bites, 2% to 3% from human bites, and 2% to 3% from other animals (e.g., rats, hamsters).

b. Cat bites have the highest infection rate, followed by human bites and then dog bites. Most bite wounds have mixed-flora inoculum; *Streptococcus* and *Staphylococcus* species are common.

2. **Therapy**

a. Wound inspection, exploration, debridement, and irrigation are necessary. Radiographs may be required to rule out fractures and the existence of retained foreign bodies.

b. Suturing may be considered at other locations. Delayed primary closure may be advisable to reduce the potential for infection.

c. Antibiotics should be prescribed for most bite wounds. Penicillin and a cephalosporin are recommended. If the patient is allergic to penicillin and is not pregnant, erythromycin or tetracycline may be used.

d. Follow-up should take place in 12 to 24 hours and again in 36 to 72 hours. The patient may need to be evaluated at 5 and 7 days as well. Bite wounds should be considered tetanus-prone wounds. Rabies should also be considered in patients with animal bite wounds (see Chapter 6.III.D).

C. **Puncture wounds**

1. **Characteristics.** Most puncture wounds occur to the feet. If the puncture occurred through a rubber-soled shoe, *Pseudomonas aeruginosa* infections are possible.

2. **Therapy.** Puncture wounds should be opened, inspected, debrided, and left open. Soaking puncture wounds is not an adequate treatment, and performing high-pressure irrigation is not indicated. Prophylactic antibiotics are usually not required, unless the patient was wearing rubber-soled shoes at the time of injury. In this case, a quinolone may be prescribed. Frequent follow-up visits (on days 1, 3, 5, and 7) to watch for infection are necessary.

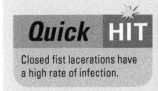
Closed fist lacerations have a high rate of infection.

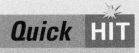
Pasteurella multocida is a common pathogen of cat bites and some dog bites. It is very sensitive to ordinary penicillin but not sensitive to penicillinase-resistant penicillins.

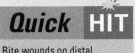
Bite wounds on distal extremities should not be sutured closed.

Wound Emergencies

D. **Fingertip injuries**
1. **Digital tip avulsion**
   a. **Characteristics.** Tip avulsion often occurs as a result of slamming fingers in doors or by accidentally cutting oneself with a saw or sharp knife. If the bone is not exposed and only skin and soft tissue are missing, these wounds often heal by secondary intention (i.e., secondary closure).
   b. **Therapy.** Some hand surgeons may attempt skin grafts. Regardless of the final treatment, these wounds need proper wound care. Digital block with a long-acting anesthetic (e.g., bupivacaine) is indicated. If healing by secondary intention is preferred, these wounds can be covered with antibiotic ointment and petroleum jelly–impregnated gauze and then bandaged. Regular examinations to watch for infection are important.
2. **Digital tip amputation with exposed bone.** Treatment of these injuries depends on the level at which the finger is amputated. If the tip is amputated and bone is exposed, shortening of the bone and movement of a viable flap over the finger may be indicated. If the finger is amputated at the distal interphalangeal joint or proximal to the distal interphalangeal joint, replantation may be indicated.
3. **Nail bed injuries**
   a. **Characteristics.** Nail bed injuries are common and usually result from hitting the fingertip with a hammer or slamming the finger in a door.
   b. **Therapy**
      i. The presence of a subungual hematoma affecting 25% or more of the nail bed may warrant removal of the nail and examination of the nail matrix. Lacerations of the nail bed often require suturing with absorbable suture.
      ii. When history indicates that enough force may have been present to fracture the distal phalanx, radiographs should be obtained. Approximately 50% of nail bed injuries are associated with distal phalanx fractures. These fractures may require a surgical consultation and stabilization of the fracture with Kirschner wires.
E. **High-pressure injection injuries**
1. **Characteristics.** These injuries are often caused by paint, grease, or air guns. They involve injection of air and other materials under the skin and along vascular and tendon sheaths. The opening to these injuries (i.e., injection site) may be quite small. The patient may not initially complain of pain, but swelling, pain, and severe infection in deep tissues usually develop within a few hours of injury.
2. **Therapy.** Pain control, splinting, and intravenous antibiotics are indicated while waiting for consultation.

VI. FOLLOW-UP CARE
A. **Wound care**
1. Most wounds benefit from being covered with antibiotic ointment to prevent them from drying out. Antibiotic ointments have been shown to improve healing and decrease infection. If there is risk of the dressing adhering to the wound, a petroleum jelly–impregnated porous gauze may be indicated. The dressing should then be covered with an absorbent layer to collect exudate from the wound.
2. The first dressings are usually left in place for 24 to 48 hours. After the first dressing change, they should be changed every 24 hours. After 48 hours, the wound is usually sealed and resistant to new infection. A light washing with sterile saline helps to remove accumulated debris from the surface of the wound, allowing for inspection of the wound for infection and reapplication of antibiotic ointment and fresh dressings.
B. **Medications**
1. **Pain control** should be considered for all patients. This is easily forgotten while the patient is still in the ED and the wound is still anesthetized.

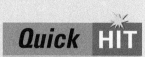

Quick HIT

A hand surgery consultation is usually required for distal fingertip amputations.

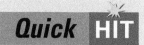

Quick HIT

Subungual hematomas affecting less than 25% of the nail bed may be drained through the nail.

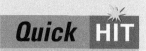

Quick HIT

Immediate surgical consultation with exploration is always indicated for air gun injuries.

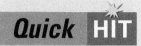

Quick HIT

Bandaging should be firm enough to hold the dressing in place but not so tight that it restricts circulation.

CLINICAL PEARL 19-2

Wound Care Instructions

1. The patient should be told whether he or she is permitted to take a shower or bath. In most cases, showering is permissible, but activities that involve submerging the wound in water (e.g., baths, soaking in a hot tub, swimming) should be avoided for the first 1 to 3 days.
2. The patient should also be told how long to keep the wound immobile and elevated and when to have the sutures or staples removed (Table 19-3).
3. Patients should know when, where, why, and with whom they should seek follow-up care. The name, address, and phone number of the person the patient is to see should be provided, and if possible, a follow-up appointment should be made prior to the patient leaving the ED.
   a. Wounds that carry a high risk of infection should be referred for close follow-up. Many of these wounds should be seen in 1, 3, 5, and 7 days.
   b. Patients should be instructed to return to the ED if their condition worsens acutely.

Nonsteroidal anti-inflammatory drugs and narcotics are often prescribed. It is common for local anesthesia to wear off while the inflammatory response is increasing, causing the patient to wake up in pain in the middle of the night.

2. **Antibiotics.** Patients with wounds that are at high risk of infection (e.g., bites, heavily contaminated wounds) should be *considered* for prophylactic antibiotics.

C. **Discharge instructions**

1. **Signs of infection** should be explained: redness, increasing pain, swelling, purulent discharge from the wound, red streaks moving up the extremity, and fever.
2. **Care for the wound** should be explained (i.e., dressing changes, pain control, follow-up appointments). Discharge instructions can be a valuable tool for providing adequate wound care follow-up (see Clinical Pearl 19-2).

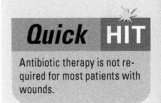

Quick HIT

Antibiotic therapy is not required for most patients with wounds.

Wound Emergencies

TABLE 19-3	Guidelines for Suture Removal
Location	**Days Following Closure**
Face	3–5
Scalp	7–10
Trunk	7–10
Arms and legs	10–14
Joints	14

Some sutures may be removed earlier if the wound can be reinforced with tape closure. Patients with conditions causing immunocompromise (e.g., steroid therapy, AIDS) or who have demonstrated slow healing previously may need to have sutures left in place longer.

I. APPROACH TO THE PATIENT

A. **Initial stabilization.** As with any other patient in the emergency department (ED), initial stabilization of the poisoned patient involves assessment of airway, breathing, and circulation (the ABCs).

1. **Airway.** Check for the presence of a gag reflex and assess the need for intubation, initially and serially, over the period of observation. Causes of airway compromise include:

   a. Posterior displacement of the tongue (e.g., from central nervous system [CNS] and respiratory depressants)

   b. Oropharyngeal mucosal injury or edema (e.g., from caustic ingestions)

   c. Angioedema (e.g., from angiotensin-converting enzyme inhibitors)

   d. Trauma

2. **Breathing.** Assess the adequacy of oxygenation and ventilation with pulse oximetry and arterial blood gas (ABG) determinations. Breathing may be compromised by any of the following:

   a. **Hypoventilation** (e.g., from CNS or respiratory depressants, peripheral muscle toxins)

   b. **Aspiration** (e.g., from CNS or respiratory depressants, peripheral muscle toxins)

   c. **Pulmonary edema** (e.g., from inhalational injuries, heroin, salicylates)

3. **Circulation.** Assess the heart rate and rhythm, the blood pressure, and the adequacy of perfusion. Circulation may be compromised by a multitude of medications and toxins.

B. **Patient history (see Clinical Pearl 20-1).** The patient may not be cooperative or may be unable to give an accurate history of ingestion or exposure. Other sources of information include family members, friends, coworkers, rescue personnel, the patient's physician or pharmacist, and old hospital records.

CLINICAL PEARL 20-1

Questions to ask include the following:

1. **What?**

   a. What drugs is the patient taking?

   b. What drugs or chemicals are available to the patient?

   c. What chemicals or toxins is the patient exposed to at work?

   d. What (e.g., pill bottles, chemical containers, drug paraphernalia) was present at the scene?

   e. What events have occurred since the ingestion or exposure?

2. **How much?**

   a. How much of the drug or chemical was initially available?

   b. How much of the drug or chemical is remaining in the bottle or container?

3. **When?**

   a. When was the patient last observed to be at his or her baseline?

   b. When did the patient ingest or become exposed to the drug, chemical, or toxin?

C. **Physical examination**
  1. **Vital signs** should be assessed and managed as appropriate.
  2. **Neurologic findings.** During the neurologic examination, the level of consciousness, pupil size, and reactivity should be assessed, and focal neurologic abnormalities should be noted.
  3. **"Toxidromes"** are physical signs of toxicologic syndromes that may aid in the diagnosis (see Clinical Pearl 20-2).
  4. **Other findings.** Evidence of trauma (e.g., head trauma) or a medical disorder (e.g., hypo- or hyperglycemia, hypothyroidism) should be sought.
D. **Administration of the "coma cocktail"**
  1. **Thiamine.** Malnutrition or alcoholism predisposes the patient to thiamine deficiency. Patients suspected of having **Wernicke-Korsakoff syndrome** (see Chapter 8.I.E.1) should receive thiamine, 1 g intravenously. To prevent the development of Wernicke-Korsakoff syndrome in alcoholic patients, thiamine (100 mg intravenously) should be administered as proximate in time to dextrose as possible.
  2. **Dextrose.** As is the case with any patient with an altered mental status, the serum glucose should be assessed by rapid bedside testing. **Hypoglycemia** is treated with intravenous dextrose.
  3. **Naloxone.** If an opioid toxidrome exists, or the patient's mental status is consistent with **opiate ingestion**, an initial dose of naloxone (0.01 mg/kg intravenously) is administered.
      a. Doses as high as 10 mg or more may be required to reverse respiratory depression, and patients who have ingested certain types of synthetic opioids may require large or repeated doses of naloxone.

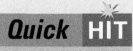

Quick HIT

The "coma cocktail" consists of a group of antidotes that may be of value, both diagnostically and therapeutically, during the initial assessment and treatment of patients with altered mental status.

CLINICAL PEARL | **20-2**

Toxidromes

1. **Sympathomimetic "toxidrome"**
   a. Hyperthermia
   b. Tachycardia
   c. Hypertension
   d. Dilated pupils
   e. Warm, moist skin
   f. Altered mental status (e.g., agitation, hallucinations, combativeness) and seizures
2. **Cholinergic "toxidrome"**
   a. Profuse salivation
   b. Bradycardia or tachycardia
   c. Pinpoint pupils
   d. Diaphoresis
   e. Excessive bronchial secretions and bronchospasm
   f. Hyperactive bowel sounds
   g. Urinary or fecal incontinence (or both)
   h. Muscle fasciculations and weakness
   i. Altered mental status and seizures
3. **Anticholinergic "toxidrome"**
   a. Hyperthermia ("hot as Hades")
   b. Tachycardia
   c. Hypertension
   d. Hot, flushed, dry skin ("red as a beet")
   e. Dilated pupils ("blind as a bat")
   f. Dry mucous membranes ("dry as a bone")
   g. Diminished bowel sounds
   h. Urinary retention
   i. Altered mental status (e.g., agitation, hallucinations) and seizures ("mad as a hatter")
4. **Opioid "toxidrome"**
   a. Pinpoint pupils
   b. Respiratory depression
   c. Altered mental status (e.g., obtundation)

Toxicologic Emergencies

b. Administration of naloxone may precipitate withdrawal in patients with physiologic dependence to an opiate. Therefore, a lower dose such as 0.1 mg can be attempted initially to look for response.

4. **Flumazenil**, a benzodiazepine antagonist, is capable of reversing **benzodiazepine-induced CNS depression.** The dose is 0.5 mg (to a maximum dose of 5 mg) administered by slow intravenous push. Flumazenil has a half-life of 57 minutes, so resedation after administration may occur within 1 to 2 hours and repeat doses may be required. Flumazenil has limited applicability due to numerous risks.

a. **Adverse effects** include seizures, arrhythmias, induction of benzodiazepine withdrawal, and increased intracranial pressure in patients with head trauma.

b. **Contraindications** to the use of flumazenil include:

i. Co-ingestion of seizure-inducing agents, especially cyclic antidepressants

ii. The presence of a seizure disorder that is being therapeutically suppressed with benzodiazepines

iii. A history of chronic benzodiazepine use, suspected benzodiazepine dependence, or potential benzodiazepine withdrawal

iv. Evidence on physical examination of anticholinergic or sympathomimetic "toxidromes"

E. **Gastric decontamination procedures**

1. **Activated charcoal** decreases the systemic absorption of many drugs and should be administered once airway patency has been assured. The initial dose is generally 1 g/kg.

2. **Gastric lavage**, in general, has no advantage over activated charcoal in terms of preventing the absorption of toxins. Gastric lavage is appropriate in certain situations and should be considered early in the presentation but only when the airway is secure. Consider gastric lavage for:

a. Large, life-threatening ingestions of medications or toxins for which there is no antidote or which impair gastrointestinal motility

b. Life-threatening ingestions of medications or toxins that are not adsorbed to activated charcoal

3. **Whole-bowel irrigation.** Administration of polyethylene glycol solutions at appropriate rates (2 L/hour in adults and 0.5 L/hour in children) speeds the transit of substances through the gastrointestinal tract, thus decreasing their systemic absorption. Unlike cathartics (e.g., magnesium sulfate), whole-bowel irrigation is not associated with any adverse concomitant fluid/electrolyte shifts. Decontamination by whole-bowel irrigation may be of benefit in several cases, once a patent airway has been secured:

a. Life-threatening ingestions of sustained-release drugs

b. Life-threatening ingestions of medications or toxins that are not adsorbed by activated charcoal

c. Ingestion of drug vials, bags, or packets

F. **Laboratory and diagnostic studies.** There are several quick studies that can help isolate the toxicologic agent.

1. **Laboratory studies**

a. **Urinary fluorescence.** When urine in a plastic container is exposed to ultraviolet light, fluorescence may indicate the presence of fluorescein, a marker for **ethylene glycol**, in the urine.

b. **Urinalysis.** The presence of crystals, specifically calcium oxalate, may help confirm **ethylene glycol** ingestion.

c. **Blood color.** Blood that is chocolate brown in color has at least a 15% **methemoglobin** concentration.

d. **Toxicology screens.** Screening capabilities vary among laboratories.

i. **Urine benzodiazepine screens.** False-negative results may occur with benzodiazepines that are not metabolized to oxazepam (e.g., clonazepam, alprazolam) or in the presence of oxaprozin, a nonsteroidal anti-inflammatory drug.

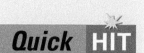

Quick HIT

There are a few substances that are not adsorbed, or are poorly adsorbed, by activated charcoal: alcohols, lithium, iron, lead, hydrocarbons, and caustics. Furthermore, in the case of a caustic ingestion, administration of charcoal will limit endoscopic evaluation of mucosal injury.

Toxicologic Emergencies

    ii. **Urine opiate screens** assay for morphine and codeine.
- a) False-positive results may occur if the patient has ingested foods containing a high concentration of poppy seeds.
- b) Fentanyl and its analogs are not detected on most urine opiate screens, causing false-negative results after their use.

    iii. **Quantitative serum drug levels** are certainly more helpful than qualitative urine testing in directing clinical emergency management in the following situations:
- a) Acetaminophen overdose
- b) Salicylate overdose
- c) Theophylline overdose
- d) Lithium overdose
- e) Lead poisoning
- f) Carbon monoxide poisoning
- g) Methemoglobinemia
- h) Alcohol toxicity
- i) Digoxin toxicity

2. **Diagnostic studies**
  a. **Electrocardiography.** An electrocardiogram (ECG) is an easy way to evaluate drug-induced rhythm disturbances, conduction abnormalities, and axis changes.
  b. **Radiography.** The radiopacity of tablets or capsules in the stomach depends on several variables, including the size of the patient, the arrangement of pills (i.e., bezoars), the presence of air around or in the pill, the presence of an enteric coating, and the time since ingestion. The following are often radiopaque:
    i. Halogenated hydrocarbons
    ii. Iron-containing preparations
    iii. Potassium preparations
    iv. Iodinated compounds
    v. Heroin or cocaine packets

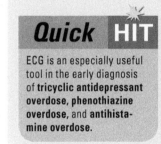

Quick HIT

ECG is an especially useful tool in the early diagnosis of **tricyclic antidepressant overdose, phenothiazine overdose,** and **antihistamine overdose.**

II. OVER-THE-COUNTER DRUGS

A. **Acetaminophen toxicity**

1. **Discussion.** Acetaminophen is a commonly used analgesic and antipyretic, available in various formulations, including sustained-release preparations.
  a. **Pharmacokinetics.** The **recommended maximum dose** is 4 g/day in adults and 90 mg/kg/day in children.
    i. **Absorption and distribution.** Acetaminophen is well absorbed and widely distributed. Peak serum levels occur within 4 hours of an overdose.
    ii. **Metabolism**
- a) In therapeutic doses, 90% of the dose is conjugated to glucuronide or sulfate. Approximately 5% is metabolized by the **cytochrome P-450 system** to a toxic intermediate, NAPQI, which is detoxified by conjugation to glutathione.
- b) The **half-life** is 2 to 3 hours and longer in patients with hepatic dysfunction.

  b. **Pathophysiology.** The **toxic dose** is 140 mg/kg as a single ingestion.
    i. **Mechanism.** In overdose, excess acetaminophen is metabolized via the cytochrome P-450 system to NAPQI. Depletion of glutathione to less than 30% of normal allows the accumulation of NAPQI and other toxic metabolites, leading to hepatic cell death. Renal toxicity and pancreatitis may occur.
    ii. **Predisposing factors.** If the patient has reduced glutathione stores (such as occurs with malnutrition or chronic alcoholism) or an enhanced ability to form NAPQI through cytochrome P-450 enzyme induction (as occurs with antiepileptic therapy or chronic ethanol abuse), the patient may be at increased risk for toxicity.

CLINICAL PEARL 20-3

Acetaminophen Toxicity

1. **Initial stage (0 to 24 hours).** Gastrointestinal symptoms (e.g., nausea, vomiting, anorexia) may be present, but patients at this stage are often asymptomatic.
2. **Latent stage (24 to 48 hours).** A subclinical increase in hepatic aminotransferases and bilirubin occurs during this stage.
3. **Hepatic stage (3 to 4 days).** This stage is characterized by progressive hepatic failure, manifested as right upper quadrant pain, vomiting, jaundice, encephalopathy, coagulopathy, hypoglycemia, metabolic acidosis, and renal failure.
4. **Recovery stage (4 days to 2 weeks).** The recovery stage is characterized by resolution of hepatic dysfunction.

---

2. **Clinical features.** Acetaminophen toxicity occurs in four stages (see Clinical Pearl 20-3).
3. **Differential diagnoses.** During the initial stage, acetaminophen toxicity may mimic **gastritis** or **gastroenteritis**. Other hepatotoxic insults (e.g., **iron toxicity**, **mushroom toxicity**, **pancreatitis**, **renal failure**, and **sepsis**) should also be considered.
4. **Evaluation**
   a. **Serum acetaminophen levels**
      i. **Timing.** A serum acetaminophen level should be drawn **4 hours postingestion**.
         a) If the time of ingestion is unknown, a level should be drawn immediately and again in 4 hours, and the presence of developing liver dysfunction assessed. The decision to treat should be made based on the initial lab testing and clinical scenario.
         b) If a sustained-release preparation has been ingested, a level should be drawn at 4 and 8 hours postingestion to assess the development of toxic levels.
      ii. **Interpretation.** The **Rumack-Matthew nomogram** assesses the degree of toxicity. It is based on a single ingestion of regular-release acetaminophen and a serum level drawn at a known time since ingestion. The level at which treatment is required is approximately 150 μg/mL at 4 hours.

b. **Liver function tests**, including the aspartate aminotransferase, alanine aminotransferase, prothrombin time (PT), and bilirubin level, should be ordered. Elevated aspartate aminotransferase and alanine aminotransferase are often the first detectable sign of toxicity.

c. **Glucose, blood urea nitrogen (BUN), and creatinine levels; a serum electrolyte panel; ABG determinations; and a pregnancy test** (in women) are indicated.

5. **Therapy**

   a. **Initial stabilization** includes airway management and cardiovascular resuscitation, including assessment of hemorrhage.

   b. **Gastric decontamination. Activated charcoal** should be administered.

   c. **Antidote treatment. N-acetylcysteine**, a glutathione precursor, repletes glutathione stores and enhances conjugation of toxic NAPQI to glutathione. N-acetylcysteine should be administered within 8 hours of ingestion for maximum benefit.

      i. **Indications.** N-acetylcysteine is indicated in the following situations:

         a) Ingestions with potential toxicity

         b) Late presentations with potential or ongoing toxicity

         c) Chronic overdose and evidence of ongoing hepatic damage (e.g., elevated aminotransferases, elevated PT, vomiting)

      ii. **Dosage**

         a) **Oral.** The current protocol is a loading dose of 140 mg/kg, followed by 70 mg/kg every 4 hours for 17 doses.

         b) **Intravenous.** The N-acetylcysteine dose is 300 mg/kg intravenously.

6. **Disposition**

   a. **Discharge.** Patients with nontoxic levels who present at a known time after a single ingestion of acetaminophen may be safely discharged.

   b. **Admission.** The following patients should be considered for admission for N-acetylcysteine therapy:

      i. Patients with known toxicity or potentially toxic levels

      ii. Patients who have laboratory evidence of ongoing hepatic damage

      iii. Patients with an unknown time of ingestion and symptoms consistent with toxicity

      iv. Patients who present at an unknown time postingestion who still have measurable acetaminophen levels

      v. Patients with significant gastrointestinal symptoms

   c. **Referrals.** Poor prognostic indicators include acidemia, encephalopathy, PT elevation, and creatinine elevation.

B. **Salicylate toxicity**

1. **Discussion.** Acetylsalicylic acid, or aspirin, is contained in analgesics, cold preparations, and topical liniments. Preparations vary in their concentration of salicylate.

   a. **Pharmacokinetics**

      i. **Absorption.** Acetylsalicylic acid is a weak acid. Due to the low stomach pH, the non-ionized form is easily absorbed in the stomach. Small intestinal absorption is also rapid due to large surface area and increase in solubility in the alkaline environment.

         a) Enteric-coated preparations are more slowly absorbed, causing delayed serum levels.

         b) In large ingestions, the dose may precipitate as a bezoar in the stomach that slowly leaches acetylsalicylate, prolonging absorption.

      ii. **Distribution.** Most of the drug (50% to 80%) is protein-bound. Hypoalbuminemia and serum acidemia increase salicylate penetration of tissues.

      iii. **Metabolism and elimination.** In therapeutic doses, 80% of acetylsalicylate is conjugated in the liver. In large doses or chronic dosing, hepatic enzymes become saturated. Renal excretion is dependent on an alkaline

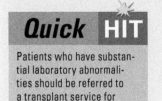

Quick HIT

Patients who have substantial laboratory abnormalities should be referred to a transplant service for consultation.

Toxicologic Emergencies

urinary pH, adequate serum potassium, normal hepatic and renal function, and the size of the dose.

b. **Pathophysiology.** The **toxic dose** is approximately **160 mg/kg**. The **lethal dose** in adults is approximately **480 mg/kg**.

   i. **Mixed respiratory alkalosis–metabolic acidosis.** Salicylate initially stimulates the respiratory center, causing hyperventilation and respiratory alkalosis.

      a) The serum ionized calcium level decreases. Renal excretion of potassium, sodium, and bicarbonate occurs.

      b) In addition, salicylate interferes with the tricarboxylic acid cycle, uncouples oxidative phosphorylation, and limits adenosine triphosphate production, causing lactate generation. Fatty acids are metabolized, generating ketone bodies.

   ii. **Hypoglycemia.** Oxygen consumption and glucose utilization increase. Heat production increases, and hypoglycemia occurs, especially in the CNS. In children poisoned by salicylate, metabolic acidosis and hypoglycemia predominate.

   iii. **Noncardiogenic pulmonary edema (NCPE)** and **direct hepatic toxicity** may also occur.

2. **Clinical features**

   a. **Vital signs.** Tachypnea, hyperpnea, tachycardia, and mild to moderate hyperthermia may be seen.

   b. **Acid–base status.** Initially, a mixed respiratory alkalosis–metabolic acidosis may be present. Of note, any patient with a metabolic acidosis will typically compensate with a respiratory alkalosis. Salicylate toxicity induces a primary respiratory alkalosis due to CNS stimulation.

   c. **Fluid and electrolyte status.** Altered serum glucose is common, and cerebrospinal fluid glucose levels may be low despite a normal serum glucose. Serum sodium, potassium, and calcium levels may be low. An anion-gap metabolic acidosis is often present. Mild to moderate dehydration (secondary to vomiting) and insensible losses from tachypnea and perspiration contribute to the fluid and electrolyte derangement.

   d. **Gastrointestinal symptoms.** The patient may experience abdominal pain, nausea, vomiting, and blood-tinged emesis.

   e. **CNS signs and symptoms.** Tinnitus, hearing loss, lethargy, asterixis, hallucinations, seizures, altered mental status, and coma may occur.

   f. **Cardiovascular signs.** NCPE may be seen in older patients; in patients with chronic ingestions; or in conjunction with metabolic acidosis, neurologic symptoms, and high serum salicylate levels.

3. **Differential diagnoses**

   a. Sepsis, pneumonia, pulmonary edema, gastritis, CNS depressant ingestion, and electrolyte abnormalities, especially hypoglycemia in pediatric patients, must be ruled out.

   b. Chronic toxicity is most common in geriatric patients and may be misdiagnosed as fever of unknown origin, pneumonia, pulmonary edema, dehydration, or a change in mental status.

4. **Evaluation**

   a. **General laboratory studies**

      i. **Electrolyte** and **ABG determinations** to assess the acid–base status

      ii. **Glucose, calcium, BUN,** and **creatinine levels** should be assessed.

      iii. A **complete blood count** should be sent.

      iv. **Liver function tests** should be sent and the **PT** assessed.

      v. The **urinary pH** should be assessed.

      vi. A **pregnancy test** is indicated for women of childbearing age.

   b. **Serum salicylate levels.** Toxicity occurs at levels exceeding 25 mg/dL. However, toxicity correlates poorly with levels. Evaluation using the **Done nomogram** is no longer recommended. Peak levels can occur well over 6 hours postingestion.

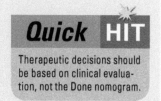

Quick HIT

A respiratory acidosis may indicate co-ingestion of CNS or respiratory depressants or impending respiratory failure.

Quick HIT

Therapeutic decisions should be based on clinical evaluation, not the Done nomogram.

5. **Therapy** is directed by the severity of the clinical signs and the progression of toxicity.
   a. **Initial stabilization**
      i. Airway management, mechanical ventilation, and cardiovascular resuscitation may be necessary. In patients with respiratory failure, great care should be taken when employing sedation with mechanical ventilation. Sedation-induced respiratory depression may cause a precipitous rise in the carbon dioxide tension (PCO_2), a decrease in the pH, sudden tissue penetration of salicylate, and death.
      ii. Electrolyte imbalances (e.g., hypoglycemia, hypokalemia, hypocalcemia) must be corrected, and acidosis treated aggressively with sodium bicarbonate.
   b. **Gastric decontamination**
      i. **Gastric lavage** may be indicated for patients who present early after a lethal ingestion, especially if they have ingested a sustained-release preparation.
      ii. **Activated charcoal** binds acetylsalicylate well. It is administered in a 10:1 ratio for maximal adsorption. Multiple-dose activated charcoal should be administered to enhance gastrointestinal elimination of salicylate.
      iii. **Whole-bowel irrigation** has not been proven to be of benefit in increasing the clearance of salicylate. It may decrease absorption in patients who have large overdoses or who have ingested enteric-coated preparations.
   c. **Elimination enhancement**
      i. **Urinary alkalinization** greatly enhances the renal excretion of salicylate and should be undertaken when the serum level is greater than 35 mg/dL or whenever clinical manifestations are present. By increasing the urine pH to 8, the amount of ionized salicylate in the tubules increases and is "trapped" (i.e., it cannot be reabsorbed).
         a) Alkalinization may be achieved with an intravenous loading bolus of **sodium bicarbonate** (1 to 2 mEq/kg), followed by 3 ampules (132 mEq) of sodium bicarbonate in 1 L of 5% dextrose in water (D_5W) to run at 1.5 to 2 times maintenance.
         b) **Hypokalemia must be corrected in order to achieve adequate alkalinization.**
      ii. **Hemodialysis** removes salicylate and corrects electrolyte abnormalities. Indications include severe and uncorrectable acidemia, fluid overload and pulmonary edema, cardiac or renal compromise, altered mental status, seizures, and coma. Serum salicylate levels that exceed 100 mg/dL (in acute ingestions) or 60 to 80 mg/dL (in chronic ingestions) are also an indication for hemodialysis, but the patient's clinical status should always direct treatment, and hemodialysis at lower serum levels should be instituted when appropriate.
      iii. **Charcoal hemoperfusion** provides better salicylate clearance but does not correct the metabolic abnormalities associated with poisoning.
6. **Disposition**
   a. **Discharge.** Patients who receive activated charcoal and remain asymptomatic can be considered for discharge after 6 to 8 hours. However, absorption is not predictable, especially with significant ingestions.
   b. **Admission.** All patients who have toxic levels, are symptomatic, or develop symptoms during observation in the ED should be admitted to a monitored setting.

III. PRESCRIPTION DRUGS
A. **Drugs used in the treatment of psychiatric disorders**
   1. **Benzodiazepine overdose.** Benzodiazepines are used in the treatment of anxiety disorders, insomnia, and pain disorders, and as muscle relaxants.
      a. **Discussion**
         i. **Toxicity.** Benzodiazepines are a common ingestant in overdoses; however, deaths caused by benzodiazepine ingestion alone are very rare.

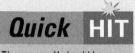

Quick HIT

The serum pH should be maintained at 7.45 to 7.50 to maximize protein binding of salicylate and minimize tissue penetration.

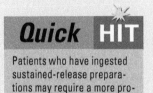

Quick HIT

Patients who have ingested sustained-release preparations may require a more prolonged period of observation.

Toxicologic Emergencies

Deaths, when they occur, are usually secondary to benzodiazepines taken in combination with other depressant substances.

ii. **Mechanism of action.** All benzodiazepines exert varying sedative, hypnotic, amnestic, anxiolytic, anticonvulsant, and muscle relaxant properties, secondary to their potentiation of the inhibitory effect of γ-aminobutyric acid (GABA), the major inhibitory neurotransmitter in the CNS.

    a) The benzodiazepine binds to the CNS benzodiazepine receptor, inducing a conformational change, facilitating the binding of GABA to the GABA receptor.

    b) GABA binding enhances chloride channel opening in the neuron, and the resultant influx of chloride into the neuron hyperpolarizes the cell. As a result, excitatory activity is inhibited in the hyperpolarized cell.

b. **Clinical features.** CNS depression is the hallmark of overdose. Findings may include:

    i. Dizziness, depression, apathy

    ii. Drowsiness, stupor, ataxia

    iii. Hypotonia or motor retardation

    iv. Low-grade coma

    v. Profound coma, hypotension, respiratory depression, or hypothermia (very rare)

c. **Differential diagnoses** include **head trauma, stroke, hypoglycemia or other metabolic abnormalities, and carbon monoxide poisoning.**

d. **Evaluation**

    i. **Physical examination.** The ABCs should be assessed and evidence of trauma sought.

    ii. **Laboratory studies**

        a) **Rapid bedside testing** of glucose should be performed.

        b) A **pregnancy test** is indicated for women of childbearing age.

        c) An **ethanol level** should be obtained to check for concurrent ethanol ingestion.

        d) **Urine drug screening** may help to confirm the diagnosis or suggest other drugs that could be contributing to the patient's altered mental status, but emergency management should not necessarily wait for, or be changed by, these results.

        e) **Quantitative serum levels of benzodiazepines** have no usefulness in the emergency management of patients with benzodiazepine overdose.

    iii. **Diagnostic studies.** An ECG should be obtained.

e. **Therapy.** Most patients require only supportive care and observation.

    i. **Supportive measures.** Most patients with benzodiazepine overdose become arousable within 12 to 36 hours when treated supportively.

        a) A **patent airway** must be ensured, and aspiration precautions must be in place.

        b) **Activated charcoal** and **intravenous fluids** should be administered.

    ii. **Antidote treatment** with **flumazenil** (see I.D.4) can be considered in select cases. Flumazenil inhibits effects of benzodiazepines by competitively binding to the benzodiazepine receptor.

        a) Because the half-life of flumazenil is less than that of many benzodiazepines, resedation may occur.

f. **Disposition**

    i. **Discharge** from the ED after a period of several hours of observation is appropriate for patients who are awake and who have ingested only benzodiazepines.

    ii. **Admission.** Indications for inpatient admission include:

        a) Profound CNS or respiratory depression

        b) Evidence of concomitant drug ingestion

        c) The use of flumazenil

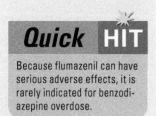

Quick HIT

Because flumazenil can have serious adverse effects, it is rarely indicated for benzodiazepine overdose.

2. **Lithium toxicity.** Lithium's primary use is in the treatment of manic-depressive disorders.
    a. **Discussion**
        i. **Toxicity.** Lithium has a narrow toxic:therapeutic ratio. Chronic lithium poisoning is associated with higher morbidity and mortality rates than acute lithium poisoning.
        ii. **Pathophysiology.** Lithium poisoning most often occurs as the result of altered drug pharmacokinetics, leading to chronic toxicity. Many drugs affect lithium metabolism.
    b. **Clinical features**
        i. **CNS signs** are the most common. Tremors, fasciculations, and movement disorders can be present in mild poisonings. In severe poisonings, stupor, coma, seizures, and a prolonged encephalopathy can be present.
        ii. **Renal signs** are also common. Lithium compromises the ability of the kidneys to concentrate the urine, leading to transient diuresis, nephrogenic diabetes insipidus, and renal tubular acidosis. Dehydration and high urine output are clinical signs of renal involvement.
        iii. **Other signs**
            a) **Cardiopulmonary signs** may be present but are rare.
            b) **Gastrointestinal symptoms** (e.g., nausea, vomiting, diarrhea) are common but are usually not life-threatening.
            c) **Endocrine signs** include those of hypothyroidism.
    c. **Differential diagnoses** include **head trauma, encephalitis, acute schizophrenia or psychosis, parkinsonism, and primary hypothyroidism.**
    d. **Evaluation**
        i. **Laboratory studies**
            a) A **serum lithium level, glucose level, serum electrolyte panel, BUN and creatinine level, urinalysis, and thyroid function tests** should be obtained for all patients with suspected lithium toxicity.
            b) If diabetes insipidus is suspected, **urinary electrolytes** should be obtained.
        ii. **Other studies.** If encephalopathy is suspected, a computed tomography (CT) scan of the head and lumbar puncture should be considered.
    e. **Therapy**
        i. **Gastric decontamination. Gastric lavage** and **whole-bowel irrigation** should be considered. Lithium does not bind to charcoal.
        ii. **Elimination enhancement**
            a) **Intravenous saline** should be administered to replace and maintain sodium and water balance. Sodium facilitates the elimination of lithium. A Foley catheter should be inserted to monitor fluid status.
            b) **Hemodialysis** is the most effective method of eliminating systemic lithium. Hemodialysis should be considered in patients who meet any of the following criteria:
                1) Chronic poisoning with clinical signs
                2) Lithium level greater than 4 mEq/L with clinical signs
                3) Persistent electrolyte disorders or renal dysfunction
    f. **Disposition**
        i. **Admission** is indicated for:
            a) All symptomatic patients
            b) All patients with a serum lithium level greater than 2 mEq/L
        ii. **Referral.** Psychiatric consult may be warranted for suicidal patients.
3. **Tricyclic antidepressant overdose** remains a common cause of death by intentional overdose of a prescription medication.
    a. **Discussion**
        i. **Mechanism of action.** Tricyclic antidepressants prevent the reuptake of synaptic neurotransmitters (e.g., norepinephrine, serotonin). In addition to improving mood, these drugs have class Ia antiarrhythmic effects.

ii. **Pathophysiology.** Death is predominantly caused by dysrhythmias and cardiovascular compromise. The newer antidepressant agents (e.g., selective serotonin reuptake inhibitors, clozapine) have less toxicity.

b. **Clinical features**

i. Most antidepressants have an **anticholinergic effect**, characterized by xerostomia, dry skin, blurred vision, mydriasis, urinary retention, and delirium. Agitation and myoclonic jerks are also common findings.

ii. In severe poisonings, hypotension, seizures, respiratory depression, and cardiac dysrhythmias are classic findings.

c. **Differential diagnoses** include **myocardial infarction (MI), hyperkalemia, sympathomimetic abuse, and alcohol withdrawal.**

d. **Evaluation**

i. **Diagnostic studies.** Special attention should be paid to the **ECG.** Sinus tachycardia and a prolonged QRS interval (longer than 0.1 second) are the most concerning.

ii. **Laboratory studies** include an ABG determination in ill-appearing patients, a serum electrolyte panel, and a glucose level.

e. **Therapy**

i. **Initial stabilization.** Standard advanced cardiac life support (ACLS) protocols should be employed.

ii. **Treatment of dysrhythmias and hypotension**

a) **Sodium bicarbonate.** Bolus therapy should precede a continuous infusion (three ampules in 1 L of D_5W at a rate of 250 mL/hour).

b) **Hyperventilation** to an arterial pH between 7.45 and 7.50 (if bicarbonate is unavailable)

c) **Lidocaine** or **phenytoin** can be administered if dysrhythmias persist. Avoid Na-channel blocking agents such as class Ia antiarrhythmics (e.g., procainamide, quinidine).

d) **Intravenous norepinephrine** may be indicated for patients with life-threatening hypotension.

iii. **Treatment of seizures and agitation.** If seizures are present, **diazepam**, a benzodiazepine, is the first-line drug. The dose is 5 mg in adults and 0.1 to 0.5 mg/kg in children, administered intravenously. Most seizures are short-lived.

iv. **Gastric decontamination.** Charcoal (1 mg/kg) should be administered.

f. **Disposition.** All patients with known or suspected cyclic antidepressant overdose should undergo cardiac monitoring for at least 6 to 8 hours.

i. **Discharge.** Asymptomatic patients with a normal cardiac rhythm and normal cardiac conduction intervals at the end of the observation period can be transferred to a psychiatric facility or discharged home.

ii. **Admission.** Patients with symptoms or cardiac conduction abnormalities should be admitted to an intensive care unit (ICU).

iii. **Referral.** All patients with intentional overdoses should be referred for psychiatric evaluation.

4. **Antipsychotic overdose.** Antipsychotic drugs include phenothiazines, thioxanthenes, and butyrophenone.

a. **Discussion**

i. **Toxicity.** Although generally considered to have a high toxic:therapeutic ratio, antipsychotic medications vary considerably. Haloperidol is associated with a low rate of life-threatening events, whereas thioridazine is associated with a higher rate of life-threatening events. Atypical antipsychotics such as quetiapine and ziprasidone often result in more mild toxidromes.

ii. **Pathophysiology.** Certain antipsychotic medications (e.g., thioridazine, mesoridazine) can cause cardiac dysrhythmias and hypotension similar to that caused by tricyclic antidepressant overdose.

b. **Clinical features**
   i. **Neurologic features** of overdose include **sedation and depressed mental status, seizures, movement disorders, and neuroleptic malignant syndrome** (NMS; see Chapter 9.VIII). **Dystonic reactions** are a side effect of certain drugs (in particular antipsychotics and antiemetics) thought to be caused by CNS dopamine blockade; they are most commonly associated with haloperidol.
   ii. **Cardiovascular features** include hypotension and cardiac dysrhythmias. QTc prolongation is very common with atypical antipsychotic medications.
   iii. **Anticholinergic features.** Most antipsychotics have anticholinergic properties.

c. **Differential diagnoses** include an **acute psychotic episode, cyclic antidepressant overdose, sepsis, meningitis, and seizures.** In patients exhibiting dystonic reactions, **cerebrovascular accident, psychogenic catatonia, tetanus, parkinsonism, and strychnine poisoning** should be considered.

d. **Evaluation**
   i. **Glucose, BUN, creatinine, and creatinine phosphokinase levels** should be obtained for all patients.
   ii. **Special studies** may be appropriate depending on the patient's clinical presentation:
      a) **Dystonic reactions.** In patients with prolonged dystonic reactions, **urinalysis** and a **serum electrolyte panel** should also be considered. A **diagnostic challenge with an anticholinergic agent** (e.g., diphenhydramine, 0.5 to 1 mg intravenously or intramuscularly, or benztropine, 1 to 2 mg intravenously or intramuscularly) should resolve symptoms within 1 hour.
      b) **NMS.** In patients with signs of NMS, a septic workup should be considered.
   iii. A **CT scan** of the head may be warranted.

e. **Therapy**
   i. **Initial stabilization.** Standard ACLS protocols should be carried out.
   ii. **Treatment of dysrhythmias and hypotension** is the same as that for dysrhythmias caused by cyclic antidepressant overdose (see III.A.3.e.ii).
   iii. **Treatment of seizures** is with intravenous benzodiazepines.
   iv. **Treatment of dystonic reactions.** Dystonic reactions are treated with diphenhydramine (25 to 50 mg orally every 6 to 8 hours in adults, 5 mg/kg/day in children in divided doses) or benztropine (1 to 2 mg/day) for 24 to 48 hours to prevent recurrence of the dystonic reaction.
   v. **Treatment of NMS** entails the administration of a benzodiazepine, bromocriptine (2.5 mg orally twice daily), or dantrolene (0.8 mg/kg orally or intravenously every 6 hours) and vigorous hydration to prevent rhabdomyolysis.

f. **Disposition**
   i. **Discharge.** Asymptomatic patients can be discharged if asymptomatic after observation for 4 to 6 hours.
   ii. **Admission** is indicated for patients with signs of toxicity more than 4 to 6 hours after acute overdose.

B. **Drugs used in the treatment of cardiovascular disorders.** Medications used for the treatment of hypertension, cardiac dysrhythmias, and angina are a common cause of toxicity and morbidity in overdose.

1. **β-Adrenergic antagonist (β blocker) overdose.** β Blockers are class II antiarrhythmics used for the treatment of hypertension, angina, dysrhythmias, thyrotoxicosis, migraines, and glaucoma.

   a. **Discussion**
      i. **Pharmacokinetics.** Most agents are rapidly absorbed from the gastrointestinal tract.
      ii. **Pathophysiology.** In overdose, β blockers cause cardiovascular and CNS effects. Symptoms occur within hours, and the half-life is prolonged.

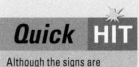

Toxicologic Emergencies

Cardiotoxicity varies, depending on the agent's degree of β agonist activity, membrane depressant effects, and lipid solubility.

a) **β_1 Antagonists** decrease the sinus rate, contractility, conduction, and renin release.

b) **β_2 Antagonists** increase bronchial smooth muscle contraction and may precipitate bronchoconstriction in patients with asthma. In addition, they alter insulin release and triglyceride metabolism, especially in patients with insulin-dependent diabetes mellitus.

c) **Partial agonists** increase the heart rate and smooth muscle tone.

d) **Agents that have membrane depressant effects** decrease sodium influx, prolonging depolarization, and calcium release, depressing myocardial contractility and electrical conduction.

e) **Lipid-soluble agents** cause more CNS depression, seizures, and apnea.

b. **Clinical features**

i. **Cardiovascular features** include bradycardia, conduction abnormalities, hypotension, and pulmonary edema. Partial agonists may cause hypertension and tachycardia.

ii. **Neurologic features** include lethargy, dilated pupils, coma, and seizures.

iii. **Other features** include hypoglycemia and bronchospasm.

c. **Differential diagnoses** include **calcium channel blocker overdose, digitalis toxicity, primary cardiac disease, sedative-hypnotic overdose, stroke, and hypoglycemia.**

d. **Evaluation.** An ECG and chest radiograph should be obtained. Appropriate laboratory studies include a serum glucose level, serum electrolyte panel, ABG determination, and cardiac enzyme studies.

e. **Therapy**

i. **Initial stabilization** involves airway management, cardiovascular resuscitation, and continuous cardiac monitoring.

a) **Hypotension** is treated with intravenous fluid boluses, epinephrine or norepinephrine infusion, and glucagon. These agents have a high lethality in overdose, and some patients may require aortic balloon pump placement to maintain hemodynamic stability sufficient for adequate perfusion during the acute period of toxicity.

b) **Bradycardia** is treated with atropine or isoproterenol infusion. Temporary transvenous pacemaker placement should be considered for patients with refractory bradycardia.

c) **Seizures** are treated with benzodiazepines.

d) **Bronchospasm** is treated with β_2 agonists.

ii. **Gastric decontamination**

a) **Gastric lavage** is indicated if the patient presents early enough in the course of the poisoning.

b) **Activated charcoal** should be administered.

c) **Whole-bowel irrigation** may be appropriate for patients with massive ingestions or those who have ingested a long-acting preparation.

iii. **Antidote treatment**

a) **Glucagon** is a non–β-adrenergic receptor agonist that increases intracellular cyclic adenosine monophosphate synthesis, enhancing contractility by increasing calcium influx.

1) **Indications** include hemodynamic compromise.

2) **Dosage.** The dosage for adults is 3 to 5 mg administered as an intravenous bolus, followed by an infusion titrated to normalization of vital signs. Large doses should be mixed in a normal saline diluent.

b) **Insulin infusion and intravenous dextrose** is used in most severe cases of beta blocker overdose. Evidence is mixed, but this therapy has low likelihood of patient harm.

c) **Lipid emulsion** can be attempted in hemodynamically unstable patients and has, in many cases, led to return of spontaneous circulation after arrest.

f. **Disposition**

    i. **Discharge.** Patients who receive activated charcoal and are observed to be asymptomatic with a normal ECG after 4 to 6 hours may be discharged.

    ii. **Admission** to a cardiac monitoring unit is indicated for all symptomatic patients and considered in those who have ingested sustained-release or long-acting preparations.

2. **Calcium channel antagonist overdose.** Calcium channel blockers are class IV antiarrhythmics, used in the treatment of hypertension, dysrhythmias, angina, migraine, and subarachnoid hemorrhage with cerebral vasospasm. In overdose, calcium channel antagonists carry high morbidity and mortality.

a. **Discussion**

    i. **Pharmacokinetics.** Calcium channel blockers are well absorbed and highly protein bound. With regular-release formulas, the onset of action occurs within 1 hour. Sustained-release preparations have a delayed onset of action.

    ii. **Mechanism of action.** These agents inhibit calcium influx across voltage-dependent slow channels, decreasing sinoatrial and atrioventricular (AV) node conduction. They prevent calcium influx across fast channels during the plateau phase of contraction, decreasing contractility and causing smooth muscle relaxation.

b. **Clinical features**

    i. **Cardiovascular features** include conduction delays and blocks, myocardial depression, reduced cardiac output, vasodilation, and hypotension.

    ii. **Neurologic features** include dizziness, coma, apnea, and seizures.

    iii. **Other features** include metabolic acidosis and, possibly, hyperglycemia.

c. **Differential diagnoses** include **β blocker overdose, digitalis toxicity, primary cardiac abnormalities, sedative-hypnotic overdose, and stroke**.

d. **Evaluation.** Appropriate studies include an ECG, a chest radiograph, ABG determinations, serum electrolyte panel, and cardiac enzyme levels.

e. **Therapy**

    i. **Initial stabilization** involves airway management, cardiovascular resuscitation, and continuous cardiac monitoring. Hypotension and bradycardia often respond to intravenous administration of calcium and glucagon (see III.B.2.e.iii.a to b) other approaches include the following:

        a) **Hypotension** can be treated with intravenous fluid boluses or epinephrine or norepinephrine infusion (see III.B.1.e.ia).

        b) **Bradycardia** can be treated with atropine. Temporary transvenous pacemaker placement may be necessary.

    ii. **Gastric decontamination**

        a) **Gastric lavage** may be indicated for early presentations.

        b) **Activated charcoal** is effective.

        c) **Whole-bowel irrigation** should be considered for patients who have ingested a sustained-release preparation.

    iii. **Antidote treatment**

        a) **Calcium** overcomes the toxicity of calcium channel blockers by entering the cell through other channels, enhancing contractility. It is administered as 10 mL of **10% calcium chloride** or 30 mL of **calcium gluconate** (both have roughly the same elemental calcium content). Repeat boluses are administered every 15 to 20 minutes, for a total of four to five doses. CaCl should ideally be infused through a central line due to severe vein irritation and pain.

        b) **Glucagon** is administered as a 5-mg bolus intravenously every 5 minutes until vital signs stabilize and then as an infusion at a rate of 5 mg/hour. Large doses should be diluted in normal saline.

        c) **Amrinone** may be used in refractory cases to enhance contractility.

        d) **Lipid** emulsion therapy has also been effective in case series of calcium channel antagonist toxicity.

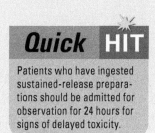

f. Disposition
   i. **Discharge.** Patients who receive activated charcoal and remain asymptomatic with a normal ECG for 6 hours (after ingesting a regular-release formula) may be discharged.
   ii. **Admission.** All symptomatic patients, including those with AV conduction abnormalities, should be admitted to a cardiac care setting.
3. **Digitalis toxicity.** Digoxin is the most common digitalis preparation in the United States. Cardiac glycoside–containing plants include oleander, foxglove, and lily of the valley and may cause digitalis toxicity if ingested.
   a. Discussion
      i. **Pharmacokinetics.** Digoxin is fairly well absorbed from the gastrointestinal tract and is widely distributed to muscle tissue.
      ii. Pathophysiology
          a) **Mechanism.** Digoxin affects the ATPase-dependent sodium–potassium pump, allowing potassium efflux from the cell and sodium and calcium influx into the cell. This may result in hyperkalemia, increased automaticity, and impaired conduction.
          b) **Predisposing factors** to enhanced toxicity include advanced age, hepatic or renal disease, electrolyte abnormalities, and preexisting cardiac disease.
   b. Clinical features
      i. **Acute toxicity.** The onset of symptoms may be delayed as long as 6 hours.
         a) **Cardiovascular features** include tachydysrhythmias with all grades of AV block, bradycardia, depressed contractility, and decreased cardiac output.
         b) **Gastrointestinal symptoms** include anorexia, nausea, vomiting, and abdominal pain.
         c) **Neurologic symptoms** include confusion, headache, hallucinations, and visual disturbances (e.g., abnormal color perception, yellow halos).
      ii. **Chronic toxicity.** Electrolyte abnormalities and renal insufficiency predispose to cardiovascular abnormalities (e.g., dysrhythmias, especially accelerated atrial or junctional tachycardia with all grades of AV block; ventricular automaticity; and extrasystoles) as well as malaise, anorexia, nausea, vomiting, blurred vision, and confusion.
      iii. **Acute on chronic toxicity** appears clinically similar to acute toxicity.
   c. **Differential diagnoses** include **calcium channel blocker or β blocker overdose, primary cardiac abnormalities, stroke, and electrolyte abnormalities.**
   d. Evaluation
      i. Laboratory studies
         a) **Serum digoxin levels** are unpredictable. In acute overdose, levels under 6 hours can be significantly elevated despite minor signs of toxicity. Serious toxicity occurs at serum digoxin levels of 10 to 15 ng/mL, but dysrhythmias may occur at lower levels.
         b) **Serum electrolytes.** Hyperkalemia (a serum potassium level greater than 5 to 5.5 mEq/L) indicates serious toxicity. Calcium and magnesium levels should also be assessed.
         c) **BUN, creatinine, and cardiac enzyme levels** should also be ordered.
      ii. **Diagnostic studies.** An ECG and **chest radiograph** can be obtained.
   e. Therapy
      i. **Initial stabilization** involves airway management, cardiovascular resuscitation, and continuous cardiac monitoring. Electrolyte imbalances should be corrected carefully, especially K+, which can rise subsequently.
      ii. **Gastric decontamination.** Gastric lavage (for early presentations) and the administration of activated charcoal are indicated.
      iii. **Antidote treatment** is with digoxin-specific antibodies, which consist of Fab fragments that bind digoxin, removing it from cardiac receptors

and reversing toxicity. Indications include significant dysrhythmias and elevated potassium.

    iv. **Calcium** therapy for hyperkalemia in the setting of digitalis toxicity is controversial due to possibility of inducing a rigid myocardium.

  f. **Disposition**

    i. **Discharge.** Patients who receive activated charcoal and remain asymptomatic with normal digoxin and potassium levels 6 hours postingestion may be discharged.

    ii. **Admission** to a cardiac monitoring unit is indicated for elevated digoxin levels or symptomatic patients, including those with ECG abnormalities.

4. **Clonidine toxicity.** Clonidine is used for the treatment of hypertension and as adjunctive therapy in the treatment of opiate withdrawal. It is available in oral and transdermal preparations.

  a. **Discussion**

    i. **Pharmacokinetics.** Clonidine is well absorbed from the gastrointestinal tract and widely distributed in the body. Clonidine is capable of penetrating the blood–brain barrier. The onset of action is within 1 hour.

    ii. **Mechanism of action.** Clonidine is a centrally acting α_2 agonist that decreases peripheral sympathetic stimulation, decreasing norepinephrine activity and lowering systemic vascular resistance, heart rate, and cardiac output.

    iii. **Pathophysiology.** Hypotension induced by α_2 agonist activity. The drug also possesses opiate-like CNS depressant activity.

  b. **Clinical features**

    i. **Cardiovascular features** include bradycardia and hypotension. Early paradoxical hypertension may occur transiently.

    ii. **Neurologic features** include miosis, sedation, coma, hypotonia, hyporeflexia, respiratory depression, and apnea.

  c. **Differential diagnoses.** Consider **β blocker or calcium channel blocker overdose, narcotic or sedative-hypnotic overdose, stroke, head injury, and hypoglycemia.**

  d. **Evaluation.** An ECG, ABG determination, chest radiograph, glucose level, and serum electrolyte panel should be obtained.

  e. **Therapy**

    i. **Initial stabilization** includes airway management, cardiovascular resuscitation, and continuous cardiac monitoring.

      a) **Early hypertensive symptoms** may be treated with nitroprusside infusion.

      b) **Hypotension** may be treated with intravenous fluid boluses or dopamine infusion.

      c) **Bradycardia** may be treated with atropine.

    ii. **Gastric decontamination** is with **activated charcoal.**

    iii. **Antidote treatment. Naloxone** may be of benefit in reversing CNS depression. It has been reported to alleviate respiratory toxicity to a certain degree.

  f. **Disposition**

    i. **Discharge.** Patients who receive activated charcoal and are asymptomatic after 6 hours of observation may be discharged.

    ii. **Admission.** Symptomatic patients must be admitted to a cardiac monitoring setting.

IV. DRUGS OF ABUSE

A. **Opiate overdose.** Heroin is the most commonly abused illicit opioid. Although its popularity has been declining since its height of popularity in the 1970s and 1980s, it has seen a recent resurgence in popularity.

  1. **Discussion**

    a. Opioids can be ingested, insufflated, smoked, or intravenously injected.

b. **Pathophysiology.** Deaths from opiate abuse usually result from respiratory depression. Newer, synthetic agents can cause other life-threatening events (e.g., meperidine metabolites and dextromethorphan can cause seizures; propoxyphene can cause seizures and cardiac dysrhythmias).

2. **Clinical features**
    a. **Symptoms.** Patients usually have depressed mental status.
    b. **Physical examination findings** include pinpoint pupils and depressed respiratory drive. Frothy sputum, rhonchi, and rales are suggestive of NCPE, which has been reported in heroin users. Chest wall rigidity is a sign of an idiosyncratic reaction to fentanyl derivatives.

3. **Differential diagnoses** include **organophosphate poisoning, pontine hemorrhage, and clonidine overdose.**

4. **Evaluation**
    a. **Response to naloxone.** Opioid intoxication may be diagnosed by its response to naloxone (an opiate antagonist).
    b. A **drug screen** may be helpful, but certain opioids (e.g., newer, synthetic agents such as fentanyl) may not show up on routine drug screens.
    c. **ABG determinations** and a **chest radiograph** may be helpful in patients with suspected NCPE.

5. **Therapy**
    a. **Initial stabilization.** ACLS protocols should be followed as indicated. Careful attention should be given to maintaining the airway. If the patient does not have an adequate respiratory drive, 100% oxygen should be administered by mechanical or assisted ventilation.
    b. **Naloxone** should be administered intravenously (1 to 2 mg every 2 to 3 minutes) until a total dose of 10 mg is reached or the desired effect is achieved. In patients with a known addiction to opiates, a lower dose of naloxone can be used to avoid withdrawal (0.1 mg every 2 to 3 minutes until the desired effect is achieved).
    c. **Antiarrhythmic agents.** Class Ia antiarrhythmic agents should be avoided in patients with propoxyphene-induced dysrhythmias.
    d. **Oxygen** should be used for patients with heroin-induced NCPE. Mechanical ventilation and positive end-expiratory pressure should be considered.
    e. **Neuromuscular paralysis and respiratory support** are indicated for patients with fentanyl-induced chest wall rigidity.

6. **Disposition**
    a. **Discharge.** Known heroin abusers who respond to naloxone therapy can be discharged after 4 to 6 hours of observation, when it is certain that respiratory depression will not recur.
    b. **Admission**
        i. Patients who overdose on sustained-release opioids (e.g., methadone) should be admitted; consider the ICU.
        ii. Patients who suffered a life-threatening, opioid-induced period of hypoxia should be admitted for observation.
    c. **Referral.** All patients with opium toxicity should receive drug counseling. In addition, referral to a detoxification program should be offered.

B. **Amphetamines and cocaine** are sympathomimetic agents that cause stimulation of the CNS. These drugs are among the most popular drugs of abuse, especially methamphetamine ("crystal meth").

1. **Discussion**
    a. Amphetamines and cocaine can be smoked, injected, nasally insufflated, and ingested.
    b. **Pathophysiology.** Death can be caused by cardiac dysrhythmias, MI, cerebrovascular accident, hyperthermia, and renal failure.

2. **Clinical features**
    a. **Symptoms.** Patients may be euphoric, anxious, paranoid, or agitated. They usually present to the ED with more than one complaint, the most common being chest pain.

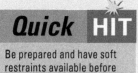

Quick HIT

Be prepared and have soft restraints available before titration of naloxone to help protect the patient and staff members when the patient "suddenly" wakes up.

  b. Physical examination findings. In significant poisonings, various life-threatening presentations can manifest.

    i. Neurologic findings

      a) Seizures can occur. These are usually self-limited and brief. Status epilepticus may be a manifestation of a secondary pathologic process (e.g., intracerebral hemorrhage, co-ingestion).

      b) Focal findings on neurologic examination suggest cerebrovascular accident.

      c) A **"wash-out" syndrome** (i.e., depressed mental status, lethargy, and obtundation) has been described with chronic use or after prolonged binging. Patients usually recover spontaneously with supportive care only.

    ii. Cardiopulmonary findings

      a) Dysrhythmias, hypotension or hypertension, and signs of MI are reflective of cardiotoxicity.

      b) Asthma or reactive airway disease can be precipitated by smoking "crack" (an alkaloidal cocaine) or "crank" (an amphetamine).

    iii. Profound hyperthermia (greater than 105°F) can occur.

 3. Differential diagnoses include **CNS infection, pheochromocytoma, thyroid storm, vasculitis, and hypoglycemia.**

 4. Evaluation

  a. Laboratory studies include cardiac enzyme levels, a complete blood count, a serum electrolyte panel, BUN and creatinine levels, liver function tests, coagulation studies, glucose levels, and an ABG determination.

  b. Diagnostic studies. A chest radiograph and head CT scan should be considered. An ECG should be performed.

  c. Other studies. A lumbar puncture should be considered if infection or subarachnoid hemorrhage is suspected.

 5. Therapy

  a. Initial stabilization. ACLS protocols should be implemented if warranted. **Benzodiazepines** are the mainstay of therapy.

  b. Treatment of cardiotoxicity

    i. Patients with evidence of MI should be treated with nitrates, anticoagulants, and emergency cardiac catheterization as indicated.

    ii. Patients with significant hypertension can be treated with calcium channel blockers, although benzodiazepines are first line.

    iii. Class Ia antiarrhythmics (due to sodium channel blockade) and β blockers (due to unopposed alpha stimulation) should be avoided.

  c. Treatment of bronchospasm. Patients with bronchospasm should be treated with bronchodilators and steroids.

  d. Treatment of intracranial hemorrhage. Patients with evidence of intracranial hemorrhage require emergent neurosurgical consultation.

  e. Treatment of hyperthermia must be aggressive. The core temperature should be reduced to below 104°F as rapidly as possible.

    i. Ice baths or constant water misting with intense fanning are used for treating hyperthermia.

    ii. Sedation or neuromuscular paralysis can be employed.

    iii. Phenothiazines should be avoided.

  f. Treatment of rhabdomyolysis must also be aggressive (see Chapter 9.VII.B).

 6. Disposition

  a. Discharge. Patients who are asymptomatic and show no evidence of end-organ damage at 6 hours may be discharged.

  b. Admission. Patients who are symptomatic and show end-organ toxicity require admission. Patients with cardiac or neurologic toxicity require ICU admission.

  c. Referral. All patients should be offered drug counseling and the opportunity to enroll in a detoxification program.

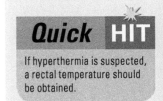

Quick HIT

If hyperthermia is suspected, a rectal temperature should be obtained.

Toxicologic Emergencies

C. **Hallucinogens**
1. **Discussion.** Many drugs or compounds have hallucinogenic properties, and certain substances are sought out and consumed for these properties. Synthetic hallucinogens include lysergic acid diethylamide, 3,4-methylenedioxyamphetamine (MDMA), and N,N-dimethyltryptamine. Naturally occurring hallucinogens include psilocybin, peyote, and myristicin.
   a. **Mechanism of action.** The exact mechanism of action has not been elucidated for most hallucinogens. It is thought that hallucinogens interact with serotonin and dopamine mechanisms in the CNS.
   b. **Toxicity.** The effect and toxicity of various hallucinogens are highly variable. Although most drugs of abuse that are consumed primarily for their hallucinogenic properties have low intrinsic toxicity, patients suffer morbidity and mortality from actions that they perform while intoxicated (e.g., driving).
2. **Clinical features**
   a. **Symptoms.** Patients experiencing a "bad trip" will often complain of **anxiety, paranoia, and unusual thought processes**. Most patients who are under the influence of hallucinogens have a **"sense of self"** and are therefore oriented and coherent.
   b. **Signs.** Certain hallucinogenic agents can have various side effects.
      i. **Hyperthermia** has been associated with synthetic hallucinogens with amphetamine-like properties (e.g., synthetic stimulants, MDMA).
      ii. **Anticholinergic effects** have been associated with other agents (e.g., psilocybin, myristicin) causing dry mouth, mydriasis, tachycardia, flushed skin, and delirium.
3. **Differential diagnoses** include **acute psychosis, conversion disorder, encephalitis, neurosyphilis, and dementia**.
4. **Evaluation.** Most hallucinogenic agents will not be apparent on routine "drugs of abuse" screens performed through the ED. Urinalysis and creatine phosphokinase, BUN, and creatinine levels should be considered in patients with protracted symptoms to rule out rhabdomyolysis.
5. **Therapy**
   a. Most patients have stable vital signs. These patients usually require only reassurance and seclusion in a nonthreatening environment. Anxiolytics (e.g., diazepam, 2.5 mg intravenously or orally, titrated to effect) can also be administered.
   b. Patients with evidence of rhabdomyolysis or hyperthermia require aggressive therapy (see IV.B.5.e to f).
6. **Disposition**
   a. **Discharge.** Asymptomatic patients may be discharged after 4 to 6 hours of observation.
   b. **Admission.** Patients with evidence of hyperthermia, anticholinergic delirium, rhabdomyolysis, or persistent symptoms after a 4- to 6-hour observation period should be admitted.
   c. **Referral.** All patients should be offered drug abuse counseling and the opportunity to enroll in a detoxification program.

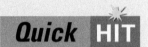

Quick HIT

Phencyclidine is one hallucinogenic agent (although usually not consumed primarily for its hallucinogenic properties) in which patients lose this "sense of self."

V. ALCOHOLS

The metabolites of many alcohols cause morbidity and mortality. An alcohol ingestion causing clinical toxicity should be suspected when an anion gap metabolic acidosis and osmolal gap are present. However, a normal osmolal gap does not exclude a toxic alcohol ingestion.
A. **Ethylene glycol** is used as a coolant and in antifreeze solutions (see Clinical Pearl 20-4). The **lethal ingested dose** can be a very small amount even in an adult.
   1. **Discussion.** Ethylene glycol is absorbed rapidly from the gastrointestinal tract. It is sequentially oxidized in the liver to **glycoaldehyde, glycolate, and glyoxylate**, producing an elevated reduced nicotinamide adenine dinucleotide:nicotinamide adenine dinucleotide ratio and lactic acidosis.

CLINICAL PEARL 20-4

Effects of Ethylene Glycol Metabolites

1. **CNS euphoria, intoxication, and depression** result from ethylene glycol.
2. **Myocardial depression** is caused by glyoxylate.
3. **Acute tubular necrosis** results from calcium oxalate crystal deposition and direct toxicity.
4. An **anion gap acidosis** is caused by glycolate, glyoxylate, and lactate.
5. **Hypocalcemia** occurs secondary to calcium oxalate crystal formation and deposition.

2. **Clinical features.** Ethylene glycol and its metabolites cause CNS effects that approximate acute ethanol intoxication. There are generally three stages of toxicity from ethylene glycol ingestion (see Clinical Pearl 20-5).
3. **Differential diagnoses** include **ingestion of another type of toxic alcohol or a CNS depressant, head injury, stroke, pulmonary edema, sepsis, and acute renal failure.**
4. **Evaluation**
   a. **Laboratory studies**
      i. **Ethylene glycol, methanol, and ethanol levels** should be ordered.
      ii. An **ABG determination, serum osmolality (less necessary if sending quantitative ethylene glycol and methanol levels), serum electrolyte panel, calcium, and BUN and creatinine levels** should be obtained.
      iii. **Urine** should be examined for **calcium oxalate crystals**. Although insensitive, **fluorescence** can be present when exposed to ultraviolet light.
   b. **Diagnostic studies**
      i. An **ECG** should be evaluated for prolonged QT intervals, suggestive of hypocalcemia.
      ii. A **chest radiograph** should be evaluated for pulmonary edema.
5. **Therapy (see Clinical Pearl 20-6)**
   a. **Initial stabilization** entails airway management, mechanical ventilation, and cardiovascular resuscitation. Acidosis should be corrected by administering intravenous sodium bicarbonate. Electrolyte imbalances should be corrected, and calcium repleted.
   b. **Elimination enhancement. Fomepizole** is first-line therapy for ethylene glycol toxicity. **Hemodialysis** is still an option if fomepizole is unavailable or patient is not responding to therapy: profound metabolic acidosis, deteriorating vital signs, crystalluria, renal compromise, and pulmonary edema.

B. **Methanol** is used in solvents, antifreeze, windshield washer fluid, canned heat, paints, paint removers, and varnishes.
   1. **Discussion.** Methanol is rapidly absorbed from the gastrointestinal tract and the skin; it may also be inhaled. It is sequentially oxidized in the liver to **formaldehyde** and **formate**, producing an elevated nicotinamide adenine dinucleotide:nicotinamide adenine dinucleotide ratio and lactic acidosis. These metabolites concentrate in the vitreous humor and optic nerve, causing ocular toxicity.
      a. **CNS depression** and an **osmolal gap** are caused by methanol.
      b. **Ocular toxicity** and an **anion gap acidosis** are caused by formate.

CLINICAL PEARL 20-5

Three Stages of Ethylene Glycol Ingestion

1. **Stage I** (1 to 12 hours postingestion) is characterized by CNS depression, cerebral edema, coma, and seizures. Myoclonic jerking, nausea, and vomiting may occur. At this stage, metabolic acidosis is beginning to develop.
2. **Stage II** (12 to 24 hours postingestion) is characterized by tachycardia, tachypnea, and mild hypertension, followed by the development of congestive heart failure and circulatory collapse.
3. **Stage III** (24 to 72 hours postingestion) is characterized by acute tubular necrosis, oliguria, and acute renal failure.

> **CLINICAL PEARL** 20-6
>
> ### Antidote Treatment
>
> 1. **Fomepizole** may be given intravenously and slows formation of toxic products of ethylene glycol metabolism.
> 2. **Ethanol** competitively inhibits the metabolism of ethylene glycol to its harmful metabolites.
>   a. **Indications.** When fomepizole is unavailable and transfer to a tertiary care center is not feasible
> 3. **Cofactors** aid in the detoxification of ethylene glycol's metabolites and include:
>   a. **Pyridoxine** (50 mg every 6 hours intravenously)
>   b. **Thiamine** (100 mg every 6 hours intravenously)

2. **Clinical features.** Methanol causes CNS effects similar to those caused by ethanol. Symptoms and signs of toxicity may be delayed hours to days.
   a. **CNS features** include euphoria, intoxication, headache, vertigo, lethargy, confusion, seizures, and coma.
   b. **Ocular features** include blurred vision; decreased visual acuity; classically, a "snowstorm" effect; dilated, minimally responsive pupils; retinal edema; and hyperemia of the optic disk.
   c. **Gastrointestinal features** include nausea, vomiting, abdominal pain, and symptoms of pancreatitis.
   d. **Renal features.** Myoglobinuria and acute renal failure have been reported.
3. **Differential diagnoses** include **ethanol or another toxic alcohol ingestion, CNS depressant ingestion, head injury, stroke, and other causes of acute retinopathy.**
4. **Evaluation**
   a. **Ethylene glycol, methanol, and ethanol levels** should be obtained.
   b. **An ABG determination, serum osmolality, serum electrolyte panel, and BUN and creatinine levels** should be obtained. A **urinalysis** should be ordered to assess myoglobin.
   c. **Visual acuity** should be evaluated.
5. **Therapy**
   a. **Initial stabilization** includes airway management, mechanical ventilation, and cardiovascular resuscitation. Electrolyte imbalances should be corrected, and the patient should be monitored for the development of hypoglycemia and myoglobinuria.
   b. **Elimination enhancement. Hemodialysis** is indicated if fomepizole is not available. Hemodialysis can be considered in patients with profound metabolic acidosis, deteriorating vital signs, visual impairment, or renal failure.
   c. **Antidote treatment**
      i. **Fomepizole** may be given intravenously and may be more advantageous in some patients.
      ii. **Folate,** a cofactor, aids in the detoxification of formate. **Folic or folinic acid** (50 to 77 mg) is administered intravenously every 4 hours.
      iii. **Ethanol** competitively inhibits further metabolism of methanol to its harmful metabolites.
C. **Isopropyl alcohol (isopropanol)** is used as a solvent and a disinfectant and is a component of rubbing alcohol, many skin and hair products, and window cleaning solutions.
   1. **Discussion.** Isopropanol is rapidly absorbed from the gastrointestinal tract. Dermal absorption may also occur. Isopropyl alcohol is metabolized to **acetone.**
      a. **CNS depression** is caused by isopropanol and acetone.
      b. **Cardiovascular collapse** may occur after the ingestion of large quantities of isopropanol.
      c. **Mild acidosis** may occur due to acetate and formate.

2. **Clinical features.** Isopropyl alcohol has twice the CNS depressant effects of ethanol. Acetone may be smelled on the patient's breath.
   a. **CNS features** include euphoria, intoxication, dizziness, incoordination, headache, confusion, and coma.
   b. **Gastrointestinal features** include early abdominal pain, nausea, and vomiting.
   c. **Cardiovascular features** include hypotension, tachycardia, and respiratory depression.
   d. **Other features.** Acute tubular necrosis, hepatic dysfunction, hemolytic anemia, and myoglobinuria have been reported.
3. **Differential diagnoses include ethanol or another toxic alcohol ingestion, acetone ingestion, CNS depressant ingestion, head injury, stroke, and other causes of ketoacidosis or electrolyte abnormalities.**
4. **Evaluation.** Isopropanol ingestion should be suspected in a patient with ketosis and acidosis. Isopropanol, acetone, and ethanol levels and the serum osmolality should be obtained. Serum electrolytes and BUN and creatinine levels should be assessed.
5. **Therapy**
   a. **Initial stabilization** entails airway management, mechanical ventilation (if necessary), cardiovascular resuscitation, intravenous fluid hydration, and supportive care. Most ingestions can be managed successfully with appropriate supportive care.
   b. **Elimination enhancement.** Hemodialysis is rarely recommended.

VI. CARBON MONOXIDE

A. **Discussion.** Carbon monoxide is an odorless, colorless, tasteless gas produced during the incomplete combustion of carbon-containing compounds.

B. **Clinical features.** Carbon monoxide affects the tissues with the highest oxygen requirements (e.g., CNS tissue, myocardium).
   1. With **mild exposures,** headache, nausea, and malaise predominate. The physical examination is often unremarkable.
   2. With **significant exposures,** symptoms include chest pain, impaired mental status, syncope, and coma. The examination may reveal a decreased level of consciousness, focal neurologic signs, hypotension, and dysrhythmias. "Cherry red" skin and bright red venous blood are suggestive of carbon monoxide poisoning, but these signs are infrequently noted and are more often a postmortem finding.

C. **Differential diagnoses** include **head trauma,** drug or chemical **intoxication** (especially **cyanide** or **hydrogen sulfide exposure**), and **infection** (especially **meningitis** or **encephalitis**).

D. **Evaluation**
   1. **Carboxyhemoglobin level.** Diagnosis is made by obtaining a carboxyhemoglobin level. The amount of carboxyhemoglobin is measured with a q-wavelength spectrophotometer (co-oximeter). Pulse oximetry and standard ABG testing often will not detect carbon dioxide poisoning.
   2. **Pregnancy testing; creatinine phosphokinase, BUN, and creatine levels; urinalysis; a serum electrolyte panel; an ECG; and a head CT scan** may be helpful in making the diagnosis and determining treatment protocols.

E. **Therapy**
   1. **Initial stabilization.** ACLS protocols should be followed as warranted. The administration of **oxygen at the highest possible concentration** is the cornerstone of management (i.e., 100% oxygen via a tight-fitting face mask). Treatment should continue until all symptoms resolve or the carbon monoxide level is reduced to below 5%.
   2. **Hyperbaric oxygen therapy** to enhance carbon monoxide elimination is used in the treatment of severe toxicity. Indications for hyperbaric treatment include loss of consciousness or altered mental status and an initial carboxyhemoglobin level of greater than 25% (or 20% in pregnancy).

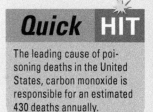

Quick HIT

The leading cause of poisoning deaths in the United States, carbon monoxide is responsible for an estimated 430 deaths annually.

Toxicologic Emergencies

F. **Disposition**
1. **Discharge.** Patients who are asymptomatic or become asymptomatic within 4 to 6 hours of observation and treatment, and who have normal examination findings and a normal ECG, may be discharged home.
2. **Admission.** All other patients should be admitted. Patients with ECG changes, a history of chest pain, or depressed mental status should be admitted to the ICU.

VII. ANTICHOLINERGICS

A. **Discussion**
1. **Causes of anticholinergic poisoning.** Various drugs and plants can cause anticholinergic poisoning.
   a. **Drugs** with anticholinergic properties include antihistamines; benztropine; phenothiazines; cyclic antidepressants; over-the-counter sleep medications; atropine ophthalmic drops; and scopolamine, a drug that has been used to incapacitate and take advantage of unwary victims.
   b. **Plants.** *Datura stramonium* (jimsonweed), ingested to induce a hallucinogenic experience, may also cause a severe anticholinergic reaction.
2. **Pharmacokinetics.** Most preparations are well absorbed from the gastrointestinal tract, have large volumes of distribution, and are largely protein-bound. Many of these substances delay gastric emptying, prolonging drug absorption and causing delayed onset of symptoms.
3. **Pathophysiology.** These agents inhibit the muscarinic effects of acetylcholine at central and peripheral cholinergic receptors. Hyperthermia, resulting from increased muscle tone and inhibited perspiration, is centrally and peripherally mediated.

B. **Clinical features.** The anticholinergic "toxidrome" is described in Clinical Pearl 20-2.

C. **Differential diagnoses.** Consider ingestions of **hallucinogens or sympathomimetic agents, hypertensive crisis, sepsis, CNS hemorrhage, or psychosis.**

D. **Evaluation**
1. Quantitative serum levels are of no therapeutic value in the emergency setting. Many over-the-counter preparations of antihistamines contain analgesics and antipyretics, so **acetaminophen** and **salicylate levels** should be obtained.
2. A **glucose level**, a **serum electrolyte panel**, and an **ABG determination** should be ordered. If rhabdomyolysis is suspected, **creatinine phosphokinase** and **urine myoglobin levels** should be ordered. An **ECG** should be obtained to assess conduction abnormalities.

E. **Therapy**
1. **Initial stabilization** involves airway management, cardiovascular resuscitation, and continuous cardiac monitoring.
   a. Hyperthermia must be treated aggressively with rapid cooling measures.
   b. Agitation, hallucinations, and seizures are treated with benzodiazepines.
   c. Ventricular dysrhythmias may be treated with lidocaine. Class Ia antiarrhythmics should be avoided. If the ECG reveals a prolonged QRS complex, sodium bicarbonate should be administered to alkalinize the serum to a pH of 7.45 to 7.55.
2. **Gastric decontamination** consists of the administration of **activated charcoal**. The drug may persist in the stomach due to impaired gastric emptying.
3. **Antidote treatment. Physostigmine salicylate** is a tertiary amine that reversibly binds cholinesterase enzyme, inactivating it, and enhancing cholinergic tone. It acts at muscarinic and nicotinic receptors and crosses the blood–brain barrier, reversing CNS toxicity.
   a. **Adverse effects** of physostigmine include bradycardia, asystole, seizures, and bronchoconstriction.
   b. **Indications** include severe agitation not responsive to other measures.
   c. **Absolute contraindications** include evidence of ingestion of drugs with class Ia–like cardiotoxic effects, including cyclic antidepressants.

F. **Disposition**
1. **Discharge.** Asymptomatic patients who receive activated charcoal and are observed for 6 hours to have no change in temperature or pulse rate over serial measurements, and no anticholinergic signs, may be safely discharged.

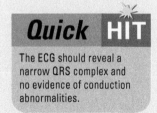

Quick HIT

The ECG should reveal a narrow QRS complex and no evidence of conduction abnormalities.

2. **Admission.** Patients with significant toxicity, those who require heavy doses of benzodiazepines for sedation, or those who receive physostigmine should be admitted to a monitored setting.

VIII. INDUSTRIAL CHEMICALS

A. **Organophosphates** and **carbamates** are cholinesterase-inhibiting insecticides, available for use in both industrial and home settings.

1. **Organophosphates**

a. **Discussion.** Organophosphates are carbon-containing molecules derived from phosphorous acid. The phosphate group is responsible for the molecule's binding and toxicity.

i. These agents are absorbed through dermal, conjunctival, gastrointestinal, and pulmonary surfaces. Symptoms occur minutes to hours post exposure. Fat-soluble organophosphates may accumulate in fat, producing delayed or prolonged symptoms.

ii. The organophosphate forms a complex with acetylcholinesterase. Without treatment, the enzyme is "aged" and destroyed, preventing the breakdown of acetylcholine. There is a wide variability in an individual's "normal" acetylcholinesterase activity. Generally, symptoms occur when the acetylcholinesterase activity is less than 50% of baseline, indicative of acute poisoning.

iii. Acetylcholine accumulates, stimulates, and exhausts cholinergic receptors. Cholinergic excess occurs in the parasympathetic system, in the preganglionic synapses of the sympathetic system, and at the neuromuscular junction. Sites of toxicity include:

a) **Muscarinic sites** (i.e., postganglionic parasympathetic synapses)

b) **Nicotinic sites** (i.e., autonomic ganglia, somatic neuromuscular endplates)

c) **CNS sites**

b. **Clinical features.** Patients often exhibit a garlic-like or petroleum-like odor. NCPE, hyperthermia, and hepatotoxicity may also occur (see Clinical Pearl 20-7).

c. **Differential diagnoses**

i. **Ingestion of or exposure to carbamates or short-acting cholinesterase inhibitors** (e.g., pyridostigmine and some ophthalmic preparations used to treat glaucoma, such as demecarium and echothiophate) should be considered.

ii. **CNS depressant ingestions, head injury, stroke, pulmonary edema, sepsis, and severe gastroenteritis** may be ruled out.

d. **Evaluation**

i. **General studies.** An ABG determination should be made, and the need for mechanical ventilation assessed. A glucose level, complete blood count, electrolyte panel, BUN and creatinine levels, and liver function tests should be ordered. The ECG should be assessed for dysrhythmias.

ii. **Confirmatory studies**

a) **Erythrocyte (true) cholinesterase** is found in nervous tissue and on erythrocytes. This level most accurately reflects cholinesterase activity in nervous tissues.

b) **Plasma (pseudo) cholinesterase** is produced in the liver and circulated in the plasma. This level is more labile and less specific than the true cholinesterase level and is affected by liver disease, cirrhosis, malnutrition, chronic inflammation, and morphine or codeine administration.

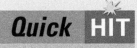

Quick HIT

Toxicity is graded according to the percentage of acetylcholinesterase activity: mild toxicity = 20% to 50%, moderate toxicity = 10% to 20%, and severe toxicity = less than 10%.

Toxicologic Emergencies

CLINICAL PEARL 20-7

Other signs and symptoms of organophosphate intoxication are classified as:

1. **Muscarinic** (e.g., salivation, lacrimation, urination, defecation, gastrointestinal cramping, emesis, bronchospasm, bronchorrhea, sweating, and miosis)

2. **Nicotinic** (e.g., muscle fasciculations, cramping, weakness, paralysis, areflexia, tachycardia, hypertension, pallor, and hyperglycemia)

3. **CNS** (e.g., restlessness, agitation, headache, drowsiness, confusion, ataxia, delirium, seizures, and coma)

e. **Therapy**
   i. **Initial stabilization** involves airway management (including endotracheal intubation, mechanical ventilation, vigorous suctioning, and the administration of supplemental oxygen as necessary), cardiovascular resuscitation, and treatment of ventricular arrhythmias. Seizures are treated with benzodiazepines.
   ii. **Decontamination**
      a) **Gastric decontamination.** Gastric lavage may be indicated if the patient presents early after ingestion. Activated charcoal should be administered in most cases.
      b) **Dermal decontamination.** Contaminated clothing should be removed and placed in plastic bags for disposal. Skin, hair, and nails should be washed with soap and water, and the conjunctivae should be irrigated.
         1) Wash water and irrigation fluids must be disposed of separately.
         2) Health care workers must wear protective clothing, masks, and rubber gloves to prevent secondary exposure and toxicity.
   iii. **Antidote treatment**
      a) **Atropine** antagonizes the effects of acetylcholine. It reverses muscarinic effects and penetrates the CNS to alleviate effects at central cholinergic receptors.
         1) **Indications.** Atropine should be administered as soon as evidence of cholinergic excess is apparent. Tachycardia is not a contraindication to atropine administration. Heart rate may actually decrease as bronchial secretions dry and oxygenation improves.
         2) **Dosage.** The initial dose in adults is 2 to 4 mg intravenously, and in children, 0.05 mg/kg intravenously. This dose may be doubled every 5 to 10 minutes.
      b) **Pralidoxime (2-PAM)** attacks the phosphorylated acetylcholinesterase, freeing the enzyme. It acts at nicotinic and muscarinic sites and may relieve CNS toxicity.
         1) **Indications.** Pralidoxime should be administered as soon as evidence of cholinergic excess is apparent or if organophosphate poisoning is suspected, preferably within 24 hours. Late presentation does not preclude its use.
         2) **Dosage.** The adult dose is 1 g administered intravenously (20 to 40 mg/kg, up to a total dose of 2 g in children). This dose may be repeated or continuous infusion may be used.

f. **Disposition**
   i. **Discharge.** Patients with inconsequential exposures who have been monitored for 6 to 8 hours and who have no cholinergic symptoms may be discharged.
   ii. **Admission.** Patients who are symptomatic or who have received atropine, pralidoxime, or both should be admitted to an ICU. Patients with ingestions or exposures to fat-soluble organophosphates should be admitted and monitored for delayed onset of toxicity.

2. **Carbamates**
   a. **Discussion.** Carbamate insecticides cause cholinergic symptoms, but CNS toxicity is thought to be minimal because these chemicals do not penetrate the blood–brain barrier to a great extent.
      i. Carbamates are readily absorbed after dermal, gastrointestinal, and pulmonary exposure.
      ii. Carbamates prevent the normal breakdown of acetylcholine, causing cholinergic excess. However, their bond to acetylcholinesterase spontaneously hydrolyzes, and therefore symptoms are usually less severe and less prolonged (as compared with those of organophosphate toxicity).
   b. **Clinical features:** Carbamate-induced cholinergic toxicity consists of muscarinic and nicotinic symptoms, but CNS toxicity is generally less than that of organophosphates.
   c. **Differential diagnoses** include **ingestion of organophosphates or other cholinesterase inhibitors** (e.g., physostigmine, pyridostigmine), CNS

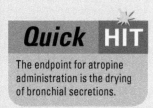

Quick HIT

The endpoint for atropine administration is the drying of bronchial secretions.

depressant ingestion, head injury, stroke, pulmonary edema, cardiogenic shock, sepsis, and severe gastroenteritis.

d. **Evaluation** should proceed as for organophosphates (see VIII.A.1.d). True and pseudocholinesterase levels should be obtained.

e. **Therapy** entails airway management, stabilization, and decontamination. Antidote treatment is with atropine. The administration of pralidoxime in cases of carbamate poisoning is controversial but may improve respiratory function and may also be administered.

f. **Disposition**

   i. **Discharge.** Patients with inconsequential exposures who are monitored for 6 hours and show no signs of cholinergic excess may be discharged.

   ii. **Admission.** Symptomatic patients and patients who have been treated with atropine, pralidoxime, or both should be admitted to an ICU.

B. **Hydrocarbons** are a diverse group of organic compounds with a wide range of toxicity. In addition, hydrocarbons are often used as a solvent for other chemicals, which can have their own intrinsic toxicity.

1. **Discussion**

   a. **Incidence.** Children younger than 5 years have the highest incidence of reported exposure requiring hospital admission.

   b. **Pathophysiology.** Toxicity occurs mainly in three organ systems:

      i. **Lung toxicity** is caused by aspiration and leads to respiratory failure. Aspiration is most likely with hydrocarbons of low viscosity and high volatility. The lungs are the organ most often affected in acute exposures.

      ii. **Cardiac toxicity** produces dysrhythmias.

      iii. **CNS toxicity** produces lethargy, stupor, coma, and seizures.

2. **Clinical features**

   a. **Patient history.** A history of coughing, grunting, gasping, or vomiting strongly suggests aspiration.

   b. **Physical examination findings** may include tachypnea, stridor, cyanosis, rales, respiratory distress, irregular heart rate, and CNS depression.

      i. CNS and cardiac signs usually occur within 1 hour of intoxication.

      ii. Pulmonary signs and symptoms usually become apparent later.

3. **Differential diagnoses** include **child abuse, salicylate toxicity, caustic ingestion, cardiogenic pulmonary edema, or secondary poisonings** (e.g., from pesticides containing hydrocarbons as a solvent).

4. **Evaluation** is with continuous cardiac monitoring and pulse oximetry. An ABG determination, electrolyte panel, and chest radiograph may also be considered.

5. **Therapy.** Aggressive supportive care is the mainstay of treatment.

   a. **Initial stabilization** is according to ACLS protocols. Cardiopulmonary resuscitation may be necessary.

      i. In cases of severe respiratory distress and persistent hypoxia, consider intubation, positive end-expiratory pressure, and extracorporeal membrane oxygenation.

      ii. Epinephrine should be avoided because of the theoretical risk of catecholamine sensitization of the heart, leading to ventricular dysrhythmias.

   b. **Gastric decontamination** is a **relative contraindication** because decontamination procedures may increase the chance of aspiration. Decontamination should be considered in cases of toxic co-ingestions or when hydrocarbons have been ingested in association with camphor, heavy metals, toluene, benzene, pesticides, carbon tetrachloride, methylene chloride, or other halogenated hydrocarbons.

6. **Disposition**

   a. **Discharge.** Patients who are asymptomatic after 4 to 6 hours of observation and who have normal physical examination findings, normal results on room air ABG determinations or pulse oximetry, and a normal chest radiograph may be discharged home with a responsible party.

   b. **Admission.** Symptomatic patients must be admitted. Patients who have significant persistent hypoxia should be admitted to an ICU.

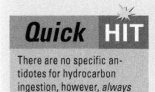

Quick HIT

There are no specific antidotes for hydrocarbon ingestion, however, *always* consider the possibility of co-ingestion.

21 ENVIRONMENTAL EMERGENCIES

Joseph Bales • Melissa Platt

I. INTRODUCTION

This chapter deals with the diagnosis and treatment of illness and injury related to nature's dangerous forces, including wildlife. Also discussed in this chapter are the special problems encountered when the sick or injured patient is located far from civilization—the subspecialty of wilderness medicine.

II. COLD-RELATED ILLNESS AND INJURY

When people interact with cold environments and are unable to protect themselves properly, injuries may result. These injuries may be generalized (e.g., hypothermia) or localized (e.g., frostbite). Both types of injuries may occur at temperatures above and below freezing.

A. Hypothermia
   1. Discussion
      a. **Definitions.** Hypothermia is a decrease in core body temperature to 35°C (95°F) or below often preventing the body from normal function.
         i. **Primary hypothermia (accidental hypothermia)** refers to a reduction in core body temperature, usually from exposure to a cold environment without adequate protection. It can occur in healthy people.
         ii. **Secondary hypothermia** often occurs as a complication in patients with a systemic disease that compromises the body's thermoregulatory mechanisms (e.g., an endocrine disorder).
      b. **Risk factors** include (see Clinical Pearl 21-1):
         i. Increased heat loss owing to extreme cold, insufficient clothing or shelter, infancy (infants have a high surface-to-body ratio), or old age (altered mental status/dementia)
         ii. Decreased heat production (old age, medications, disease)
         iii. Impaired thermoregulation (illness)
         iv. Other factors such as human error, abnormal behavioral responses to cold weather, ethanol abuse, and race (blacks are at higher risk)
      c. **Pathophysiology.** The pathophysiologic changes that occur in hypothermic patients depend on the severity of the temperature reduction, the underlying cause, and the patient's preexisting medical condition. The body functions optimally when its core temperature is maintained within 1°C (1.8°F) of its normal value, and any deviation from this narrow range affects all organ systems.
         i. **Cardiovascular responses**
            a) As the body cools, initial tachycardia is followed by bradycardia, at core body temperatures below 30°C (86°F), resulting from decreased spontaneous depolarization of the pacemaker cells. This bradycardia is resistant to treatment with atropine. If tachycardia is present in a significantly hypothermic patient, then hypovolemia, hypoglycemia, drugs, or other conditions must be ruled out.
            b) **Systemic vascular resistance** increases initially; however, when the core temperature drops below 24°C (75°F), systemic vascular resistance decreases.

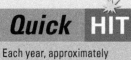

Quick HIT

Each year, approximately 1,300 people in the United States die of exposure to cold.

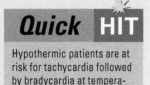

Quick HIT

Hypothermic patients are at risk for tachycardia followed by bradycardia at temperatures below 30°C (86°F).

CLINICAL PEARL **21-1**

1. **Mechanisms of heat transfer.** Normal heat loss of the human body occurs through five mechanisms:
   a. **Radiation** is heat transfer by electromagnetic waves. It accounts for 55% to 65% of heat loss in a person at rest in cool climates. The amount of heat lost depends on the temperature gradient between the body surface and the environment.
   b. **Conduction** is the transfer of heat energy from warmer to cooler objects by direct physical contact. It normally accounts for less than 3% of heat loss; however, if the person is in direct contact with cold surfaces or water, heat loss may increase up to 32 times the normal amount.
   c. **Convection** is heat transfer to air and water vapor molecules circulating around the body. It accounts for 10% of heat loss; greater heat loss occurs with wind blowing against the skin surface. As ambient temperature rises, the amount of heat dissipated by convection becomes minimal.
   d. **Evaporation** is conversion from a liquid to a gas, with a loss of energy of 0.58 kcal/mL of water evaporated. Insensible water loss from the skin and lungs normally accounts for 25% of heat loss. At ambient temperatures above body temperature, evaporative heat loss becomes the primary means of dissipating heat, exceeding radiation.
   e. **Respiration.** Warming the inspired air accounts for 2% to 9% of heat loss; this percentage varies with the temperature of the ambient air.
2. **Summary.** Considering these mechanisms, it can be said that a person would lose the most heat on a cold, windy, dry day in contact with a cool surface while perspiring and wearing few protective items of clothing.

    c) Most types of atrial and ventricular dysrhythmias are seen in patients with moderate and severe hypothermia, from 28°C to 32°C (82°F to 90°F) and below 24°C (82°F).
        1) **Electrocardiogram (ECG) changes** occur. The cardiac cycle is prolonged typically most affecting the QT interval. Osborne waves may appear after QRS complex. Varying degrees of AV block may occur (Figure 21-1).
        2) **Atrial fibrillation** is seen commonly at core temperatures below 32°C (90°F) and usually converts spontaneously on rewarming.
        3) **Ventricular fibrillation** and **asystole** can occur spontaneously when the core temperature drops below 25°C (77°F), and the patient is often resistant to defibrillation attempts until the body temperature is raised above 30°C (86°F).

ii. **Respiratory responses**
    a) The initial response to hypothermia is an increase in respiratory rate; as body temperature declines and the medullary respiratory center becomes depressed, there is a progressive decrease in minute ventilation proportional to the decreasing metabolic rate.
    b) Even though carbon dioxide production is decreased in hypothermia, the patient often develops a respiratory acidosis due to decreased ventilation.
    c) Airway protective reflexes are depressed, resulting in a cold-induced bronchorrhea. This may lead to atelectasis, bronchopneumonia, aspiration pneumonia, and postwarming pulmonary edema.

iii. **Central nervous system (CNS) responses**
    a) Hypothermia progressively decreases CNS function. Significant brain electroencephalogram slowing begins below 33.5°C (92°F). Below 20°C (68°F), the electroencephalogram demonstrates no brain activity. The alteration in mental status may lead to maladaptive behavior that worsens the patient's condition (e.g., removing the clothes in freezing conditions).
    b) Hypothermia protects the brain from the effects of ischemia. When core body temperatures drop below 20°C (68°F), total circulatory arrest may be tolerated for longer than 1 hour with no neurologic sequelae following rewarming.

Quick HIT

Patients with hypothermia should not be declared dead until they have been rewarmed and their brain activity has been reevaluated.

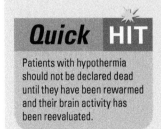

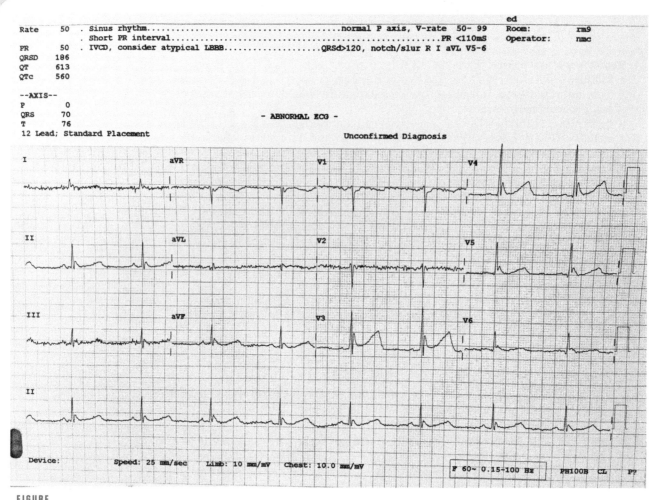

```
                                                              ed
Rate    50   . Sinus rhythm...........................normal P axis, V-rate  50- 99   Room:        rm9
             . Short PR interval................................PR <110mS   Operator:    nmc
PR      50   . IVCD, consider atypical LBBB.............QRSd>120, notch/slur R I aVL V5-6
QRSD   186
QT     613
QTc    560

--AXIS--
P        0
QRS     70                         - ABNORMAL ECG -
T       76
12 Lead; Standard Placement              Unconfirmed Diagnosis
```

I   aVR   V1   V4

II   aVL   V2   V5

III   aVF   V3   V6

II

Device: Speed: 25 mm/sec   Limb: 10 mm/mV   Chest: 10.0 mm/mV   F 60~ 0.15-100 Hz   PH100B CL   P?

FIGURE 21-1 Prototypical electrocardiogram in hypothermia may show bradycardia and Osborne waves.

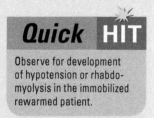

Quick HIT

Observe for development of hypotension or rhabdomyolysis in the immobilized rewarmed patient.

c) The reflexes initially are hyperreflexic, but when the core body temperature decreases to below 32°C (90°F), they become hyporeflexic, with the knee-jerk the last reflex to disappear (at temperatures below 26°C (79°F).

iv. **Renal responses**

a) Exposure to cold induces a diuresis despite a decrease in glomerular filtration rate and renal blood flow. The production of a large volume of dilute urine (up to three times normal) results principally from the vasoconstriction and a blunted response to antidiuretic hormone. As a result, when the hypothermic patient is warmed, hypovolemia occurs, contributing to "rewarming shock."

b) Prolonged immobilization and decreased perfusion may lead to rhabdomyolysis.

v. **Hematologic responses**

a) Hypothermia impairs coagulation; thus, despite normal prothrombin time and partial thromboplastin time values, clinical coagulopathy may be present. This coagulopathy most often resolves when the patient is rewarmed, although rare cases of disseminated intravascular coagulation have been reported.

b) Hypothermia induces hepatosplenic sequestration and bone marrow suppression, which decreases leukocyte and platelet counts. This also reverses with warming.

c) Blood viscosity increases by 2% for every 1°C drop in temperature. Hemoconcentration develops, additive to the cold diuresis.

          d) The oxyhemoglobin curve shifts to the left, diminishing the release of oxygen to tissue.

      vi. **Gastrointestinal responses.** Complications of hypothermia may include ileus, pancreatitis, and gastric stress ulcers. Hepatic function is reduced, which can lead to increased levels of lactate, drugs, and toxins in the blood.

2. Clinical features

    a. The history may be difficult due to unresponsiveness but may be gathered from bystanders or emergency medical services.

    b. **Signs** other than core temperature below 35°C (95°F) (see Clinical Pearl 21-2)

      i. In wilderness travel, the onset of hypothermia often is slow and subtle; some early signs are mood changes, unusual behavior, and impaired judgment.

      ii. In general, the presenting signs and symptoms of hypothermic patients reflect decreased function of most organ systems (see II.A). The patient may demonstrate hypotension with bradycardia, initial tachypnea followed by slowed respirations progressing to hypoventilation, ileus, and a depressed level of consciousness. Shivering may be present or absent. Skin changes may include frostbite, erythema, pallor, cyanosis, edema, and other changes.

3. Differential diagnoses or comorbidities include thyroid deficiency, stroke, myocardial infarction, infection, drugs, and other causes of a depressed body temperature.

4. Evaluation. Accurate diagnosis and early treatment are important. The diagnosis of hypothermia can be made once an accurate core temperature is measured. Determining the cause or causes can be more difficult, especially if the patient is unable to communicate. Underlying medical problems must be identified and addressed.

    a. **Core temperature** is best determined by measuring the esophageal or rectal temperature. Oral or tympanic temperatures are an unreliable and often inaccurate measure of core temperature.

    b. **Laboratory studies**

      i. Specific laboratory tests should be ordered to confirm the diagnosis of hypothermia and to identify any possible underlying cause. A thorough evaluation is required and includes a complete blood count (CBC), electrolytes, arterial blood gas (ABG) determination, liver function tests, coagulation studies, urinalysis, total creatinine kinase, and toxicology screening if possible. Additional tests useful outside the emergency department (ED) may include endocrine evaluation (cortisol, thyroid) and sputum and blood cultures.

      ii. **Serum pH determination.** The evaluation of arterial and venous blood samples in the hypothermic patient is controversial. Reliable prediction of acid–base status in the clinical setting is not possible; one study

---

CLINICAL PEARL   **21-2**

Classification of Hypothermia

Hypothermic patients can be divided into three groups based on core temperature:

1. **Severe hypothermia: core temperature below 28°C (82°F).** All endocrinologic and autonomic nervous system mechanisms for heat conservation fail. Survival can be rare despite aggressive medical treatment.

2. **Moderate hypothermia: core temperature between 32°C and 28°C (90°F and 82°F).** Heat loss is minimized by vasoconstriction, but the body is too cold to shiver. (Shivering is synchronized muscle group contractions that produce heat.)

3. **Mild hypothermia: core temperature above 32°C (90°F).** Shivering plays a significant role in rewarming, and vasoconstriction, decreased perspiration, and nonshivering basal and endocrinologic heat production help retain body warmth.

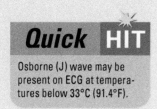

showed that 25% of hypothermic patients were alkalotic and 30% were acidotic. Most authors agree that correction of ABG parameters is unnecessary and potentially harmful.

c. **Diagnostic tests.** ECG findings in hypothermia may include an Osborne (J) wave if the core temperature is below 33°C (91.4°F). The J wave is seen at the junction of the QRS complex and ST segment, which are upright in the aVL, aVF, and left precordial leads. The size of the J wave increases as the temperature decreases; it is diagnostic but not prognostic. Bradycardia, cardiac cycle prolongation, heart block, and atrial fibrillation also can be seen in varying degrees.

d. **Imaging studies.** If a traumatic mechanism is suspected or known, radiologic examination is appropriate. Chest radiograph can be useful when trying to determine infectious versus traumatic etiology. In a patient with a persistent altered level of consciousness, a brain computed tomography scan may be appropriate.

5. **Therapy**
   a. **Prehospital management.** The basic prehospital treatment protocol is rescue, evaluate, insulate, resuscitate, and transport.
      i. **Rescue.** Make sure the site is safe or remove patients from site. If the site is unsafe, rescue should proceed only if the benefits outweigh the risks.
      ii. **Evaluate.** Obtain a brief history and perform a physical examination. Assessment, stabilization, and management of airway, breathing, and circulation (ABCs) should be done without delay.
      iii. **Insulate.** The prime directive in prehospital treatment of the hypothermic patient is the prevention of additional heat loss. However, rescuers at the scene often are hampered by the cold environment, limited supplies, and lack of shelter. The patient's wet clothing should be removed and the patient should be placed in dry, warm sheets (passive warming).
      iv. **Resuscitation**
         a) **Cardiopulmonary resuscitation** should be administered to hypothermic patients in cardiac arrest if survival is considered possible. At core temperatures below 30°C (86°F), the heart may be refractory to pharmacologic interventions and defibrillation.
         b) Warm humidified oxygen and warm intravenous fluids should be administered as soon as possible to prevent further cooling.
         c) If initial attempts at cardioversion are not successful, continue cardiopulmonary resuscitation, warm the patient, and repeat defibrillation attempts with every 2°C to 4°C rise in temperature.
      v. **Transport.** The patient should be transported to a medical center.
   b. **ED management.** Resuscitation efforts should be continued as described for prehospital. Thermal stabilization should continue as well as maintenance of tissue oxygenation through adequate circulation and ventilation. ECG monitoring to detect cardiac arrhythmias and accurate core temperature evaluation are required to monitor the severity of hypothermia and the response to treatment.
      i. It is important to determine whether the hypothermia is primary or secondary and to treat the underlying medical problems when identified.
      ii. **Supportive care**
         a) Patients with an altered mental status should have their glucose checked and may receive intravenous naloxone, glucose, and thiamine.
         b) The hypothermic patient is typically dehydrated and may develop hypotension and hypoglycemia as warmed; therefore, warm (40°C to 42°C) intravenous fluid boluses should be given.
      iii. **Rewarming methods.** The dictum "You are not dead until you are warm and dead" is based on past experience with patients who have

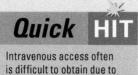

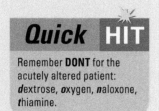

been successfully resuscitated despite being unresponsive, stiff, and cold on initial presentation.

    a) Patients with mild hypothermia typically have an intact shiver reflex; if shelter and passive external rewarming are provided, endogenous heat production will enable these patients to rewarm gradually on their own.

    b) Patients with moderate or severe hypothermia often are unable to rewarm their bodies using passive external rewarming alone. Therefore, the physician may employ active rewarming techniques using exogenous heat sources. The active techniques may be external or internal (core), with the choice of technique being controversial.

        1) Active external warming directly exposes the body to an exogenous heat source, such as warm baths, hot water bottles, heat lamps, heating blankets/pads, or other heat source.

        2) Active core rewarming may be used in patients with moderate to severe hypothermia, especially in those with unstable cardiac arrhythmias. Techniques include:

            (a) Heated, humidified oxygen by way of a face mask or endotracheal tube

            (b) Warmed intravenous fluids

            (c) Warm fluid lavage via intragastric (using oral or nasogastric tubes), bladder (Foley catheter), and peritoneal or thoracic (using chest tubes or Foley catheters inserted into the abdominal or chest cavities)

            (d) Extracorporeal warming (the most rapid method). Methods of extracorporeal rewarming include hemodialysis, arteriovenous or venovenous extracorporeal warming, and cardiopulmonary bypass. The latter is the treatment of choice for the cardiac arrest patient who is severely hypothermic.

6. Disposition. The patient with severe hypothermia may appear clinically dead; however, in the appropriate setting, resuscitative efforts should continue until the patient's core temperature reaches a level (32°C or 90°F) that would allow accurate determination of response to resuscitation.

    a. Discharge. Victims of mild hypothermia who are rewarmed to a normal temperature without complications may be discharged.

    b. Admission. Survivors of severe or moderate hypothermia should be admitted to a monitored bed in an intensive care unit for close observation.

B. Frostbite and other localized cold injuries may occur in the absence of generalized hypothermia.

    1. Discussion

        a. Areas at risk. The areas of the body most likely to suffer localized cold injury are those most exposed to cold and farthest away from the body's core, such as the feet, hands, nose, and ears.

        b. Severity. Several factors influence the severity of localized cold injury, including the conducting surface (wet surfaces), ambient temperature, wind speed, and the physiologic condition of the patient.

        c. Types of localized cold injuries

            i. Nonfreezing cold injury can be divided into two groups on the basis of exposure to dry or wet cold environments:

                a) Chilblain (perniosis) describes skin that has been exposed chronically to cold, dry air (e.g., mountain climbers).

                b) Trench foot (immersion foot) is caused by prolonged exposure to wet, cold conditions (Figure 21-2). The name is derived from the fact that soldiers exposed to harsh conditions often developed this condition; it is now often seen in homeless patients.

            ii. Freezing cold injury. Frostbite occurs when a body surface comes in contact with cold, resulting in tissue freezing. The depth of freezing is related to the duration and intensity of the cold exposure. Clinical Pearl 21-3 describes the degrees of frostbite.

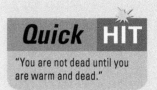

Quick HIT

"You are not dead until you are warm and dead."

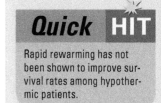

Quick HIT

Rapid rewarming has not been shown to improve survival rates among hypothermic patients.

Environmental Emergencies

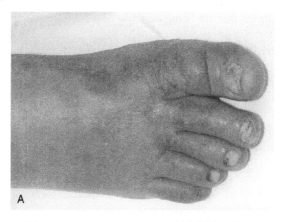
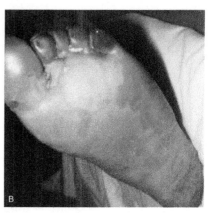
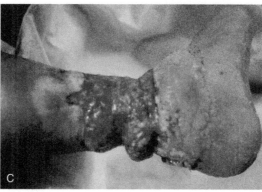

FIGURE
21-2 **Trench foot.**

(Courtesy of Robert G. Hendrickson, MD; from Greenberg MI, et al. *Greenberg's Text-Atlas of Emergency Medicine.* Philadelphia: Lippincott Williams & Wilkins; 2005.)

2. **Clinical features**
   a. **Chilblain.** The skin has small, erythematous, superficial ulcerations, plaques, nodules, and vesicles over exposed areas, which are pruritic and hypersensitive. The skin lesions appear 12 to 14 hours after exposure to cold.
   b. **Trench foot** resembles superficial burns (hyperemia, pain, edema, vesiculation) and can be very debilitating. Severe cases can progress to liquefaction gangrene.
   c. **Frostbite**
      i. **Symptoms** are related to the severity of the injury. True frostbite always results in damaged skin after rewarming. Most patients will report coldness and numbness of the involved skin initially but during rewarming will complain of extreme pain. Usually, the severity of the injury defines the extent of neuropathologic damage, and a wide variety of symptoms occur.
      ii. **Physical examination** of the skin reveals the degrees of injury. Historically, four levels of injury have been described (see Clinical Pearl 21-4).

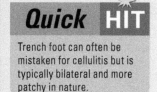

Quick HIT

Trench foot can often be mistaken for cellulitis but is typically bilateral and more patchy in nature.

CLINICAL PEARL 21-3

Four Pathologic Phases of Frostbite
1. **Prefreeze phase.** Chilling causes vasospasm and transendothelial plasma leakage. The tissue temperature ranges from 3°C to 10°C (37°F to 50°F).
2. **Freeze–thaw phase.** Actual tissue ice crystals form. Owing to underlying radiation of heat energy, the skin must be supercooled to −4°C (24.8°F) to freeze.
3. **Vascular stasis phase.** Because of the freezing injury to the overlying skin, blood vessels are damaged, and plasma leakage, coagulation, and shunting occur.
4. **Late ischemic phase.** Arteriovenous shunting, thrombosis, and ischemia lead to gangrene and autonomic dysfunction.

CLINICAL PEARL 21-4

Levels of Frostbite Injury

1. **First-degree injury:** numbness and erythema of skin, with a firm white or yellow plaque in the area of injury
2. **Second-degree injury:** superficial skin vesiculation, with clear or milky fluid within the blisters, surrounded by edema and erythema
3. **Third-degree injury:** deeper blister formation, with purple, blood-containing fluid, and injury extending into the deep dermis layers
4. **Fourth-degree injury:** involves tissue below the dermis, with muscle and bone involvement, causing mummification of the digit or extremity

3. **Differential diagnoses** for localized cold injuries include burns, chemical irritation, tissue damage, infections, trauma, vascular compromise, and cutaneous manifestation of systemic disease. Often, the patient's history makes the diagnosis simple.

4. **Evaluation.** If cold injury alone is strongly suspected, no specific tests are necessary. If the diagnosis is uncertain, tests to eliminate differential diagnoses should be obtained.

5. **Therapy**
   a. **Chilblain.** Management is supportive and consists of gentle rewarming, use of local skin moisturizers, and avoidance of cold conditions. Most cases heal well with proper care. The victim is prone to recurrence from similar exposure.
   b. **Trench foot.** Treatment includes local skin care, elevation, rest, and avoidance of wet, cold conditions. Prognosis is better than for frostbite, although these injuries often are clinically indistinguishable initially. Most cases heal well with proper care, although progression to gangrene is possible.
   c. **Frostbite.** The treatment of frostbite is directed at saving as many cells as possible in the skin and underlying tissue.
      i. **Prehospital management** consists of rapid transportation to a medical center, with the involved extremity wrapped in loose and dry clothing, elevated, and protected from trauma and further freezing. It is important to prevent refreezing injuries as it can cause severe cellular damage.
      ii. **ED management.** Initially, it is difficult to predict the extent of frostbite damage. Only a few patients arrive with tissue still frozen. With rapid rewarming, there is almost immediate hyperemia, even in severe injuries. The initial treatment of all four frostbite levels is identical, and so initial distinctions are artificial.
         a) Systemic hypothermia should be corrected as first priority.
         b) Rapid rewarming should be started immediately after the patient has been stabilized. Rapid rewarming is accomplished by immersing the affected body part in a gently circulating warm water bath; the water temperature should be 40°C to 42°C (104°F to 108°F). Higher temperatures may produce a burn wound, and lower temperatures are less beneficial for tissue survival.
            1) Rewarming should continue until the skin is soft, pliable, and erythematous at the affected part's most distal aspect.
            2) Avoid excessive movement or massage as movement when still frozen can cause more damage.
            3) After rewarming, edema appears within several hours, and blisters in 6 to 24 hours. Over the next several weeks, demarcation, eschar, and mummification occur.
         c) Parenteral analgesics are required to manage the significant pain associated with rewarming.
         d) Other considerations include tetanus prophylaxis, debridement of white blisters (hemorrhagic blisters should be left intact), aloe vera cream, elevation, prophylactic antibiotics, and daily hydrotherapy.

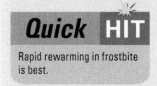

Quick HIT

Rapid rewarming in frostbite is best.

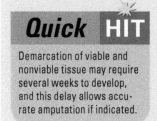

Quick HIT

Demarcation of viable and nonviable tissue may require several weeks to develop, and this delay allows accurate amputation if indicated.

Environmental Emergencies

6. **Disposition.** Most patients with frostbite will require admission to the hospital for further evaluation and treatment. All patients with potential for significant skin damage should be admitted and observed.

III. HEAT-RELATED ILLNESS

A. **Introduction.** Humans have a reasonable ability to tolerate environmental heat stress, but in certain conditions, heat illness may occur.

1. **Physiology of temperature regulation.** Regulation of human body temperature is complex, involving the thermosensors (located in the skin and centrally in the preoptic anterior hypothalamus), the thermoregulatory effectors (sweating and peripheral vasodilatation), and the brain. The basal metabolism consumes 50 to 60 kcal/hour/m^2; in the absence of cooling mechanisms, this rate of consumption would result in a 1.1°C (2°F)-per-hour increase in body temperature.

2. **Factors contributing to increased heat production**
   a. **Hyperthyroidism**
   b. **Drugs** (e.g., haloperidol, alcohol)
   c. **Increased activity level.** Heat production may be increased up to 20 times by strenuous exertion.
   d. **Hot weather.** Environmental heat adds to the heat load, interfering with the dissipation of heat through the four mechanisms of conduction, convection, evaporation, and radiation.

3. **Adaptations to heat**
   a. **Evaporation** is the most effective method of heat loss when environmental temperature is at or above body temperature.
   b. **Acclimatization** is the physiologic adaptation that occurs in a normal person after 7 to 14 days of exposure to work in a hot environment. This is characterized by an earlier onset of sweating, increased sweat volume with lowered sweat electrolyte concentrations, and hormonal changes. In trained marathon runners, temperatures as high as 42°C (107.6°F) have been recorded without ill effects.

4. **Predisposing factors to heat illness**
   a. Hot environment
   b. Lack of behavior modification (not drinking enough fluids, not seeking shade)
   c. Extremes of age
   d. Drugs
   e. Occupation
   f. Lack of acclimatization
   g. Sweat gland abnormalities
   h. Psychological factors

5. **Categories of heat illness.** Heat illness may be divided into four categories: minor heat illness, heat exhaustion, heat stroke, and unusual heat disorders.

B. **Minor heat illness**
1. **Discussion.** Most cases of minor heat illness occur within the first several days of exposure in a hot environment.
2. **Clinical features**
   a. **Heat cramps** are brief, often severe muscular cramps that typically affect muscles heavily used by workers or athletes who are sweating profusely in hot environments. The cramps usually occur after the activity has ceased, while the person is relaxing, possibly resulting from salt deficiency (after sweating).
   b. **Heat syncope** is related to the vasodilation that occurs in people (particularly elderly) exposed to hot conditions. The vasodilation of cutaneous vessels results in relative hypovolemia of the thoracic blood vessels, decreased central venous return, a drop in cardiac output, and decreased cerebral perfusion. The dehydrated person is at high risk for syncope.
3. **Differential diagnoses.** Congestive heart failure, deep venous thrombosis, and lymphedema must be ruled out in cases of heat edema. Syncope has a wide differential, and other serious causes should be excluded.

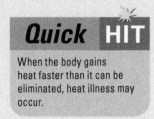

Quick HIT

When the body gains heat faster than it can be eliminated, heat illness may occur.

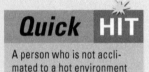

Quick HIT

A person who is not acclimated to a hot environment may develop heat edema, cramps, syncope, and tetany.

4. Evaluation
   a. An accurate history should be obtained, including the length of exposure to heat, type of work or activity, intake of water or food, salt intake, and events surrounding the onset of symptoms.
   b. **Studies.** In patients with severe heat cramps or syncope, analysis of serum electrolytes and a CBC may be required to guide therapy. ECG may be important as well in cases of injury.

5. Therapy
   a. **Heat cramps** are treated with rest and replacement of the deficient salt with an oral salt solution or may require intravenous isotonic saline (0.9% sodium chloride). Most patients respond rapidly to treatment.
   b. **Heat syncope** usually resolves when the person faints and assumes a supine position. Because the patient may be dehydrated, intravenous rehydration is often indicated. Persons at risk for heat syncope should be informed of preventive measures such as moving frequently, flexing leg muscles while standing, and sitting or lying down whenever early symptoms (e.g., vertigo, nausea, weakness) appear.

6. **Disposition.** The minor heat illnesses are easily treated, and most are preventable through patient education and ensuring adequate fluid and salt replacement.

C. Heat exhaustion
1. **Discussion.** Heat exhaustion is a clinical syndrome characterized by volume depletion in patients exposed to heat stress. Most cases of heat exhaustion occur because of mixed salt and water depletion after inadequate fluid and salt replacement in persons in a hot environment.
2. **Clinical features.** The signs and symptoms of heat exhaustion are variable.
   a. **Symptoms.** Early complaints of fatigue and vague malaise may progress to weakness, vertigo, nausea and vomiting, and headache.
   b. **Physical examination findings.** With significant dehydration, signs may include muscle cramps, orthostatic syncope, tachycardia, hyperventilation, and hypotension. Body temperature is normal or slightly elevated. Sweating may be profuse. Signs of severe CNS damage are absent, with mental function essentially intact.
3. **Differential diagnoses** include cerebrovascular accident, drug ingestion, exacerbation of preexisting medical illness, viral syndromes, psychological factors, infection, and heat stroke.
4. **Evaluation**
   a. A history and physical examination should lead to an accurate diagnosis.
   b. **Laboratory studies.** In mild cases, no laboratory studies are needed. In moderate to severe cases, a CBC, a serum electrolyte panel, and hepatic function panel may be helpful in identifying hypernatremia, hyponatremia, hemoconcentration, or hepatic damage. Blood urea nitrogen/creatinine and urine specific gravity values aid in determining the level of dehydration.
5. **Therapy.** If any doubt exists about the severity of the heat illness, the patient should be treated aggressively for possible heat stroke.
   a. **Cool environment.** The patient with an elevated body temperature should be cooled using a room-temperature water mist spray and fan to aid in evaporation. Cool packs placed on the neck, axilla, and groin speed cooling.
   b. **Correction of volume and electrolyte imbalances.** Usually, symptoms resolve rapidly with intravenous and oral hydration.
      i. The type and volume of fluid should be determined by the patient's condition.
      ii. The free water deficit in the hypernatremic patient should be replaced slowly over 48 hours to prevent cerebral edema. Severely hyponatremic patients should also be handled carefully and slowly corrected.
6. **Disposition**
   a. **Discharge.** In young, healthy patients who respond rapidly to treatment, no additional testing is required; these patients may be discharged with education about preventive techniques.

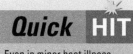

Quick HIT

Even in minor heat illness, patients with complicating illnesses, unstable vital signs, or abnormal mental status should be admitted and evaluated further.

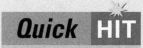

Quick HIT

Heat exhaustion may progress to heat stroke if untreated; the symptoms are similar in the early stages.

Environmental Emergencies

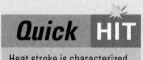

Quick HIT

Heat stroke is characterized by hyperpyrexia (core body temperature higher than 40°C or 105°F) plus neurologic symptoms

b. **Admission.** Older patients, particularly those with cardiovascular disease or serious illness, require more careful fluid and electrolyte replacement and may need admission. Extremely young patients may also need extended intravenous fluid therapy.

D. **Heat stroke**

1. **Discussion.** A true medical emergency, heat stroke is life-threatening and often fatal.

   a. **Definition.** Heat stroke is characterized by hyperpyrexia (core body temperature higher than 40°C or 105°F) and neurologic symptoms.

   b. **Pathophysiology.** In heat stroke, the homeostatic thermoregulatory mechanisms fail to work effectively, and the body is unable to maintain proper temperature. This failure results in elevation of body temperature to extreme levels (over 40°C, or 105°F), which produces multisystem damage, organ dysfunction, and sometimes death. Clinical Pearl 21-5 details the risk factors of heat stroke:

      i. **CNS system dysfunction** is a hallmark of heat stroke.

      ii. **Other systemic effects** include cerebral edema, circulatory/cardiac failure, and hepatic damage.

   c. **Forms of heat stroke**

      i. **Classic heat stroke** occurs in conditions of high ambient heat and humidity. The victims are often poor, elderly, and living in poorly ventilated homes. Frequently, these patients suffer from psychiatric and medical conditions that predispose them to heat illness, especially if they are taking medications that impair cooling. Sweating is absent in 84% to 100% of classic heat stroke patients.

      ii. **Exertional heat stroke** occurs in previously healthy young people who have exercised or exerted themselves strenuously. In these patients, the endogenous heat production is too high relative to the hot environment and the body's cooling mechanisms are overwhelmed, causing the body temperature to increase to dangerously high levels. Patients are at increased risk for rhabdomyolysis and acute renal failure, owing to heavy exercise and muscular exertion.

2. **Clinical features**

   a. **Symptoms.** Prodromal symptoms are nonspecific and include weakness, nausea, vomiting, vertigo, headache, and anorexia. Later, more serious symptoms include confusion, drowsiness, disorientation, ataxia, and psychiatric symptoms; these CNS symptoms eventually progress to coma and possibly death.

   b. **Physical examination findings**

      i. **Sweating** may persist in early heat stroke but is often absent later due to failure of compensatory mechanisms to work properly and/or lack of free water.

CLINICAL PEARL 21-5

Risk Factors for Heat Stroke

1. **Age.** Infants and the elderly are at increased risk. Infants have poorly developed compensatory mechanisms, whereas the elderly are at increased risk owing to disease, polypharmacy, and a decreased ability to escape hot environments.
2. **Occupation** (e.g., roofers, military personnel)
3. **Hot, humid environment**
4. **Alcohol abuse**
5. **Medication side effects**
6. **Sweat gland abnormalities**
7. **Obesity**
8. **Psychological factors**
9. **Certain diseases** (e.g., scleroderma, diabetes)
10. **Socioeconomic factors** (e.g., lack of a fan or air conditioning)

    ii. **Seizures** occur in 75% of victims.

    iii. **Varied pupil size** may be found.

    iv. **Cardiovascular** findings include tachycardia, an elevated cardiac index, and low peripheral vascular resistance.

    v. **Pancreatic and hepatic damage** are often present, resulting in blood sugar and coagulation abnormalities.

    vi. **Urine** may be dark brown from concentration, myoglobinuria, red blood cells, or acute oliguric renal failure.

    vii. **Respiratory alkalosis** from hyperventilation may be severe and may produce tetany.

    viii. **Lactic acidosis** is often present and is used as a predictor of mortality.

3. **Differential diagnoses** include meningitis, encephalitis, sepsis, cerebrovascular accident, thyroid storm, drug-induced heat illness (i.e., anticholinergic poisoning), typhus, and delirium tremens.

4. **Evaluation**

    a. **History and physical examination** are vital for diagnosis. Information from witnesses or prehospital personnel is critical if the patient has a severe CNS abnormality.

    b. **Laboratory studies** should include a CBC, serum electrolyte panel, blood and urine cultures if sepsis is suspected, coagulation studies, liver and pancreatic tests, and lactate, total creatinine kinase, and urinalysis. Lumbar puncture is required in any uncertain case to rule out meningitis and encephalitis.

    c. **Diagnostic tests** include ECG, electroencephalogram (75% of heat stroke victims have seizures), and radiologic tests should be considered.

5. **Therapy**

    a. **Prehospital management.** Treatment of heat stroke requires immediate cooling. The patient should be removed from the hot environment and, during transport to the hospital, should be unclothed and fanned, and the skin kept wet with tepid water.

    b. **ED management**

        i. **Stabilization.** Attention must be paid to the patient's ABCs. Intubation may be indicated for altered patients, and circulatory support may require central venous monitoring.

        ii. **Monitoring** of the core temperature, urine output, and cardiac rhythm is important.

        iii. **Supportive care.** Glucose (*d*extrose), *o*xygen, *n*aloxone, and *t*hiamine (**DONT** treatment) may need to be administered to unresponsive patients.

        iv. **Cooling techniques** vary, but optimally, cooling includes disrobing the patient, sponging or misting with room-temperature water, and circulating air over the patient using fans.

        v. **Antipyretics** (e.g., aspirin, acetaminophen) are contraindicated. They are ineffective in heat stroke victims and may worsen liver or kidney function.

        vi. **Treatment of complications**

            a) **Shivering** may be treated with chlorpromazine or diazepam.

            b) **Rhabdomyolysis** is treated with aggressive fluid support which may be helped later by mannitol, alkalinization of the urine, and dialysis.

            c) **Acid–base and electrolyte disturbances** should be treated appropriately.

6. **Disposition.** All patients with heat stroke should be hospitalized and closely monitored for complications. Consultation with specialists may be required to deal with organ failure or damage.

7. **Prevention** of heat stroke is very important; people at risk should be educated about preventive measures. Activity should be restricted in hot, humid conditions.

E. **Unusual causes of hyperthermia**

1. **Malignant hyperthermia.** Certain patients with a rare genetic predisposition who undergo general anesthesia may rapidly develop severe hyperthermia, muscular rigidity, and acidosis. Malignant hyperthermia is caused by

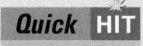

The initial core temperature does not correlate well with outcome; patients with heat stroke may arrive at the hospital with only a minimally elevated temperature.

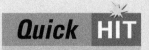

When the core temperature reaches 39°C (102°F), the cooling efforts should be slowed to prevent hypothermic overshoot.

Environmental Emergencies

inappropriate intracellular calcium release. Treatment includes dantrolene (which lowers myoplasmic calcium), cooling, and supportive measures.

2. **Neuroleptic malignant syndrome.** This rare syndrome is induced by antipsychotic medications (e.g., haloperidol) and manifests as muscular rigidity, severe dyskinesia, dystonia, hyperthermia, dyspnea, tachycardia, and urinary incontinence. The mechanism involves dopamine receptor blockade in the brain. Haloperidol also suppresses thirst, which exacerbates the problem. Treatment includes supportive and cooling measures, with possible medications including dantrolene, amantadine, bromocriptine, and benzodiazepines.

3. **Drug overdose.** Overdose of anticholinergic medications and sympathomimetic agents such as amphetamines may cause fatal hyperpyrexia.

4. **Cerebrovascular accident.** Ischemic or hemorrhagic strokes involving the thermoregulatory centers in the brain can cause elevation of body temperature and should be considered in the differential diagnosis of hyperthermia.

IV. INHALATION INJURIES

A. **Discussion.** Inhalation injuries and fatalities are caused by heat, flames, altered gas levels (low oxygen, high carbon dioxide and carbon monoxide), direct irritation and damage to the respiratory tract, indirect injuries, and smoke.

1. **Heat-related inhalation injuries.** Breathing heated air may cause damage to the respiratory tract. Air temperatures of 93°C (200°F) could be tolerated for 30 minutes, but temperatures of 250°C (480°F) will be tolerated for only 3 minutes, with death more likely with longer exposures.

2. **Smoke-related inhalation injuries.** Fire is the most common cause of exposure to toxic inhalants. Smoke contains a large variety of substances that may cause injury or death when inhaled. Many products of combustion may be inhaled:
   a. **Simple asphyxiants** include dust, ash, and nontoxic carbon particles.
   b. **Pulmonary irritants** include hydrogen chloride, phosgene, and other toxins. Inhalation may result in laryngospasm, bronchospasm, and pulmonary epithelium damage and may possibly lead to noncardiogenic pulmonary edema.
   c. **Chemical asphyxiants** result in tissue anoxia despite a normal PaO_2.

3. **Altered gas level–related inhalation injuries.** Hydrogen cyanide, hydrogen sulfide, carbon monoxide, and agents that produce methemoglobinemia interfere with oxygen delivery and utilization.
   a. **Carbon monoxide poisoning** is the most common toxicologic cause of death and fire-related mortality (see Chapter 20.VI).
   b. **Hypoxia.** In open wilderness fires, hypoxia is rare due to the constant fresh air available. However, in a closed burning space (e.g., house), the oxygen level may be quite low and toxic gases may accumulate.

B. **Clinical features.** Most victims have coughing and upper airway irritation. Patients with more severe exposures have stridor, worsening dyspnea and hypoxia, headache, confusion, and seizures. Clinical Pearl 21-6 explains the clinical features of several inhalation disorders.

C. **Evaluation**

1. **History.** Knowledge of the circumstances, products burned, location, odors at the fire, and symptoms of other victims can provide important clues. It is important to focus on the mechanism of injury and, if possible, to identify the inhalation agents because specific toxins may require specific antidotes and treatment.

2. **Laboratory and diagnostic studies**
   a. If the history and physical examination suggest toxic exposure, specific tests such as an ABG with carboxyhemoglobin, chest radiograph, and toxicology screens should be considered. Elevated serum lactate is highly predictive of cyanide toxicity if clinical suspicion is high.
   b. In patients with subacute complications due to prolonged exposure, pulmonary edema, or thermal injury, serial ABGs and chest radiographs may be indicated.

Environmental Emergencies

CLINICAL PEARL 21-6

Features of Inhalation Disorders

1. **Smoke inhalation.** Simple irritants found in smoke often cause a cough and upper airway irritation. Symptoms often resolve spontaneously without specific treatment.
2. **Airway burns.** Signs of potential airway burns include facial and upper chest burns, singed facial or nasal hair, black carbonaceous particles in the airway, and local erythema and swelling of the upper airway.
3. **Pulmonary signs.** Pulmonary irritants such as hydrogen chloride may cause significant burning and stinging to the eyes, mucous membranes, nasal passage, and lower respiratory tract. Bronchospasm may result and, if severe chemical burning occurs, stridor and pulmonary edema may be seen.
4. **Chemical asphyxiation.** Chemical asphyxiants cause varying degrees of symptoms depending on the amount and duration of exposure. Carbon monoxide, hydrogen cyanide, and hydrogen sulfide poisoning symptoms range from a mild headache and nausea to severe headache, psychiatric disturbance, seizures, coma, and death.

D. Therapy
  1. Prehospital management
    a. **Removal from the scene.** The victim should be removed from the fire and smoke while paying attention to scene safety. All burned or exposed clothes should be removed. An adequate airway must be ensured, and supplemental 100% oxygen should be provided.
    b. **Stabilization** of the patient is with standard prehospital protocols. Spine protection must be ensured. Initial treatment for burns, cuts, and other coexisting trauma can be provided.
  2. **ED management.** Airway, breathing, and circulatory support should be continued, and intravenous access obtained.
    a. **Minor bronchospasm and airway irritation.** Patients may require supportive care only.
    b. **Simple asphyxiant exposure.** Patients may require only administration of oxygen and observation for complete resolution of symptoms.
    c. **Thermal burns to the airway.** Patients likely require intubation, which should be performed before stridor or compromise occurs.
    d. **Bronchospasm.** Patients should be treated with nebulized bronchodilators and close observation.
    e. **Stridor** indicates that thermal injury to the vocal cords has occurred. Intubation should be performed to prevent obstruction as a result of swelling.
    f. **Noncardiogenic pulmonary edema.** Patients may require continuous positive airway pressure or positive end-expiratory pressure.
    g. **Altered level of consciousness.** Patients require standard treatment and evaluation.
    h. Specific chemical asphyxiates
      i. **Carbon monoxide poisoning** is discussed in Chapter 20.VI.E.
      ii. **Hydrogen cyanide poisoning.** Hydroxocobalamin is first-line therapy. Cyanide binds tightly to the ferric (Fe^{3+}) cytochrome complex and blocks the cytochrome oxidase system. The hydroxocobalamin (a vitamin B_{12} precursor) has a cobalt moiety that complexes with cyanide to form cyanocobalamin which is then eliminated in the urine. The second-line standard antidote kit contains amyl nitrite, sodium nitrite, and sodium thiosulfate. 4-Dimethylaminophenol may be used in conjunction with hydroxocobalamin.
      iii. **Hydrogen sulfide poisoning.** Hydrogen sulfide inhalation may result in poisoning similar to hydrogen cyanide poisoning, except that the cytochrome oxidase system is reversibly blocked. Standard resuscitation techniques are usually sufficient to reverse hydrogen sulfide toxicity; in severe cases, amyl and sodium nitrite or 4-dimethylaminophenol may

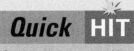

Quick HIT

Care must be taken to avoid exposure to potentially toxic chemicals on the patient's clothes and body.

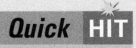

Quick HIT

A definitive airway (intubation) should be achieved *before* any signs of airway compromise.

Environmental Emergencies

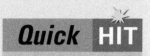

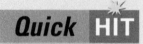

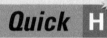

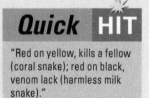

be used as with hydrogen sulfide poisoning. Sodium thiosulfate is not used in the treatment of hydrogen sulfide poisoning.

 iv. **Mixed inhalations.** In patients with mixed inhalations (prolonged smoke exposure likely resulting in cyanide and carbon monoxide poisoning), treatment with nitrites should be avoided because they form methemoglobin, which may further reduce tissue oxygen delivery. Hydroxocobalamin can be given and a carboxyhemoglobin level obtained.

 a) If the carboxyhemoglobin level is low and the patient has persistent acidosis or unstable vital signs, hydroxocobalamin may be given.

 b) If the carboxyhemoglobin level is high, the patient should be transferred to a hyperbaric oxygen facility.

E. Disposition

 1. **Discharge.** Patients with resolution of symptoms and who are not at risk for toxic inhalation may be discharged.

 2. **Admission**

 a. Any patient who is persistently symptomatic (cough, dyspnea, bronchospasm) requires admission to the hospital, close observation, and treatment of complications.

 b. Inhaled chemicals may result in delayed pulmonary or systemic complications, prolonged observation (over 6 hours) or admission may be necessary.

 c. Most smoke inhalations involve uncertain combustion products that may result in delayed effects.

V. VENOMOUS SNAKEBITES

A. Discussion. Venomous snakes inhabit all states with the exceptions of Maine, Alaska, and Hawaii. In addition, exotic venomous snakes are kept in zoos and private collections throughout the United States. Therefore, the potential for bites by venomous snakes exists everywhere.

 1. **Incidence.** Each year in the United States, over 8,000 victims of venomous snakebites are recorded; 5 or 6 die each year.

 2. **Identification of snakes.** If possible, the type of snake responsible for the snakebite should be identified to determine whether the snake is venomous and the type of venom injected.

 a. **Venomous snakes** may be classified as crotalids (pit vipers), elapids, or colubrids. Most venomous snakes in the United States are pit vipers.

 i. **Crotalids or pit vipers** are classified in three groups in the United States: the rattlesnake, the water moccasin ("cottonmouth"), and the copperhead. Characteristics of pit vipers include:

 a) Small "pit" indentation between the snake's eye and nostril

 b) Vertical slit pupils

 c) Arrowhead-shaped head

 d) A single caudal row of plates from the anal plate to one-third of the way from the tail (nonpoisonous snakes have two rows of plates)

 e) May have "rattles" on the tail (in rattlesnakes)

 f) Movable front fangs

 ii. **Elapids** are snakes with fixed front fangs (e.g., coral snakes). Coral snakes are small and shy and have red and black bands that are wider than the interspaced yellow rings; the red band is surrounded by yellow bands.

 iii. **Colubrids** have hind fangs. None are native to the United States, although they are found in exotic collections.

 b. **Harmless snakes** have round eyes, oval heads, two rows of plates near the anal plate, and no pit.

 3. **Pathogenesis.** Many venomous snakes have long, sharp hollow fangs.

 a. **Crotalid venom** is composed of a mixture of enzymes, polypeptides, and glycoproteins that, when injected, causes tissue destruction, hemolysis, nerve damage, capillary damage, and breakdown of the host cells and coagulation factors.

 b. **Coral snake venom**, composed of a strong neurotoxin and several enzymes, causes systemic neurologic symptoms but very little local tissue damage.

B. Clinical features

 1. Severity of symptoms is related to:

  a. Amount of venom released

  b. Type of snake (strength of venom varies)

  c. Age and size of snake

  d. Age and size of victim

  e. Prior health of victim

  f. Location of the bite (bites to the head and trunk are three times as dangerous as bites to the extremity)

  g. Treatment time and type received

 2. Local effects

  a. Oozing nonclotting blood at site of bite indicates envenomization.

  b. Immediate severe pain out of proportion to the wound suggests pit viper envenomation.

  c. Numbness may occur following envenomation by coral snakes.

  d. Local swelling occurs within several hours. Edema, cyanosis, hemorrhagic blebs, and lymphangitis may occur and may spread progressively.

 3. Systemic effects

  a. Shock and hypotension

  b. Compartment syndrome (see Chapter 18.VII)

  c. Fluid shift

  d. Hemolysis

  e. Coagulopathies

  f. Petechiae and bleeding

  g. Pulmonary edema

  h. Neurotoxicity, seizures, altered mental status (especially with coral snake and Mojave rattlesnake)

C. Differential diagnoses. Most snakebites are a memorable experiences, but some victims are unable to recall the event. Unless obvious signs and symptoms of venomous snakebite are present, consideration should be given to a "dry bite" without venom, other animal or insect bites, local trauma with cellulitis or other infection, and systemic illness.

D. Evaluation

 1. Snake identification. Efforts should be made to safely retrieve and identify the snake.

 2. Laboratory studies. For severely symptomatic victims, the tests ordered should include a CBC with platelet count; blood urea nitrogen, creatinine, and electrolyte levels; coagulation profile; urinalysis; and blood type and cross match.

 3. Diagnostic tests and imaging studies. An ECG and appropriate radiographs, including chest radiographs, are indicated.

E. Therapy

 1. Prehospital management

  a. **Transport.** The victim should go rapidly to a hospital. Attempts should be made to calm the patient to prevent the spread of venom. If possible, the patient should be carried, with the site of the bite immobilized and placed in a dependent position.

  b. The use of ice, incision and suction, tourniquets, electrical shock, and administration of antivenin should be avoided by prehospital providers. Hospital management is best, hence the saying, "A set of car keys is the best first aid for snakebite."

 2. ED management

  a. **Stabilization.** Management of the patient's ABCs, with fluid resuscitation for shock and hypotension, should be initiated.

  b. **Examination.** The patient should be examined carefully to determine the extent of injury. Mark the skin to identify the rate of spread of erythema

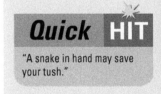

Quick **HIT**

"A snake in hand may save your tush."

and swelling, observing closely for the development of compartment syndrome. Monitor for systemic signs such as hypotension, pulmonary edema, coagulopathy, and neurologic disturbances.

c. **Prophylaxis.** Tetanus toxoid should be administered as needed. The use of prophylactic broad-spectrum antibiotics is recommended by many authorities, but studies supporting the administration of antibiotics are rare.

d. **Debridement.** The site of injury should be cleansed and debrided.

e. **Antivenin** is the definitive treatment for snake envenomation. Antivenin is historically an equine antibody solution that binds and neutralizes the harmful components of snake venom. CroFab (BTG International Inc., West Conshohocken, PA) is a newer ovine antibody solution used for crotalid bites in the United States.

   i. **Indications.** Antivenin administration is indicated for significant envenomations. There is a four-grade classification system used to evaluate severity of envenomation: from grade I (minimal symptoms, no antivenin required) to grade IV (very severe, with rapid swelling, ecchymosis, CNS symptoms, convulsions, and shock). Grades II and III typically have administration of antivenin in order to prevent progression.

   ii. **Administration.** Antivenin should be administered within 4 hours if possible. After 12 hours, the risk–benefit ratio is questionable. Examples of usual dose ranges are 2 to 4 vials for grade II envenomation and 15 or more vials for grade IV envenomation.

   iii. **Adverse reactions** can range from mild urticaria to severe anaphylaxis; however, CroFab has a much lower side effect profile than previously used horse serum and is even used in minor envenomations.

   iv. **Contraindications.** Antivenin should not be administered if the patient is definitely sensitive to serum and the pit viper bite is within grade I or II. However, if it is a severe grade III or IV bite, lack of antivenin therapy could be fatal.

F. **Disposition.** All patients with serious snakebite envenomations should be hospitalized for continued care and observation. If the snakebite is minor, and no systemic effects or significant local findings are found, and no other toxin is present (i.e., alcohol) the patient can be discharged home with close observation.

VI. INSECT AND ARACHNID BITES AND STINGS

A. **Introduction.** Problems caused by the bites and stings of insects and arachnids include primary toxicity from envenomation, local infection, immediate hypersensitivity to the venom, delayed hypersensitivity, and transmission of infectious diseases.

B. **Black widow spider bites**
   1. **Discussion**
      a. The black widow spider (*Latrodectus mactans*) is found throughout the United States (except Alaska). It lives in protected locations such as woodpiles, basements, and garages.
      b. **Description.** Both male and female are venomous, but only the female can envenomate a human. The female is twice as large as the male, with a body about 1 cm long, and a total length, including legs, of 3 cm. The body is glossy black with the classic "hourglass" red shape located on the central abdomen.
      c. **Pathogenesis.** The most toxic component of the venom is a neurotoxin that causes depletion of acetylcholine from nerve terminals, leading to diffuse muscle spasm.
      d. **Risk for severe reaction.** Small children and infants are at increased risk for severe reaction because of their small body size. Adults with preexisting illness also are at greater risk.
   2. **Clinical features**
      a. **Symptoms**
         i. **Local.** A sharp pinprick may be felt from the spider's bite, but often, the bite is not remembered by the victim. A dull and crampy pain, warmth, or numbness develops around the bite and slowly spreads.

  ii. **Systemic** symptoms include dizziness, nausea, headache, itching, increased salivation, and weakness. Intense pain from abdominal muscle cramps may simulate an acute abdomen. Upper extremity bites may cause chest wall cramps that simulate an acute infarction or other serious disorder. Symptoms begin to resolve after several hours.

 b. **Physical examination findings** may include severe muscle spasm, ptosis, edema, hypertension, and fever.

3. **Differential diagnoses** include bites of other insects or animals and puncture wounds. Systemic symptoms can mimic an acute abdomen or serious chest pain etiology, dystonic reactions, tetanus, strychnine poisoning, or hypocalcemia.

4. **Evaluation.** The history may not reveal the bite; a thorough examination and wide differential should be maintained.

 a. **Laboratory studies.** All patients with serious symptoms require a CBC, serum electrolyte panel, blood urea nitrogen and creatinine levels, clotting studies, and urinalysis.

 b. **Diagnostic tests** include local imaging, chest radiograph, and an ECG.

5. **Therapy**

 a. **Prehospital management** may include placing ice on the bite wound to reduce swelling and symptoms. If safety permits, the spider should be brought to the hospital.

 b. **ED management**

  i. **Stabilization.** The patient's vital signs should be monitored, and life support measures should be instituted as indicated.

  ii. Local cleansing of the bite and tetanus prophylaxis are required.

  iii. Muscle relaxants and analgesics are used to treat pain and muscle spasm with controversial use of a slow intravenous calcium infusion.

  iv. **Antivenin** should be administered to very old and very young victims, pregnant women, patients with preexisting illness, and seriously symptomatic victims. Adverse reactions include horse serum sensitivity, which can cause serum sickness, anaphylaxis, and even death.

   a) **Horse serum sensitivity.** The patient should be asked about a history of sensitivity or previous reaction to horse serum.

6. **Disposition.** All patients with serious signs and symptoms require admission to the hospital and close observation. If asymptomatic after 2 hours, the patient may be sent home with instructions to return to the ED if any symptoms develop.

C. **Brown recluse spider bites**

1. **Discussion.** The brown recluse spider (*Loxosceles reclusa*) is located predominantly in the South Central United States. It is brown and smaller than the black widow (about 2 cm in overall length) and usually has a violin-shaped mark on the back of the cephalothorax.

2. **Clinical features**

 a. **Local effects.** The initial bite may feel sharp, or it may cause little or no pain. Pain gradually develops after 1 to 2 hours. An erythematous area surrounded by a white area of vasoconstriction may appear. A central dark-red blister or bleb with a "bull's-eye" appearance may form. The lesion slowly grows in size, with rupture of the bleb and formation of an ulcer after several days. A black eschar then forms over a large tissue defect (Figure 21-3). Pain can be severe.

 b. **Systemic effects.** Although local destruction of skin and subcutaneous tissue is the hallmark of the brown recluse bite, the victim may also develop chills, fever, malaise, nausea, and vomiting. Children, and rarely adults, may develop intravascular hemolysis, hemorrhage, disseminated intravascular coagulation, thrombocytopenia, renal failure, and death.

3. **Differential diagnoses** include other insect bites, puncture wounds, local infection, foreign body, and cutaneous manifestation of infectious or systemic disease.

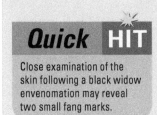

Quick HIT

Close examination of the skin following a black widow envenomation may reveal two small fang marks.

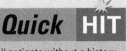

Quick HIT

All patients without a history of horse serum sensitivity or previous reaction should be tested for sensitivity with a dilute intradermal injection of serum.

Environmental Emergencies

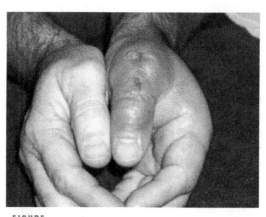

FIGURE 21-3 Brown recluse bite with swelling and necrosis of surrounding tissue.

4. Evaluation
   a. **History and physical examination** lead to suspicion or confirmation. Observation and repeated examination over several days may be needed to confirm the diagnosis. Early diagnosis is difficult without a positive identification of the spider.
   b. **Laboratory tests.** CBC, electrolytes, urinalysis, coagulation studies, and cardiac monitoring are indicated if the patient has signs of systemic involvement or a confirmed bite with symptoms. Type and cross-match and transfusion of blood may be required for patients with severe hemolysis.
5. **Therapy.** Treatment of the brown recluse bite is controversial, but local supportive care and careful cleansing with soap and water are important. Tetanus prophylaxis should be administered as needed. Vital signs and urinary output should be closely monitored.
   a. **Medications.** Analgesia and muscle relaxers are keys to proper therapy. Others with varying degrees of success include steroids, antihistamines, antivenin, dapsone, and antibiotics.
   b. **Wound management** is a mainstay of treatment, although excision of the wound has not been shown to improve outcomes.
6. **Disposition**
   a. **Discharge.** If no symptoms are present and suspicion of a brown recluse bite is low, outpatient management is acceptable.
   b. **Admission.** All patients with signs of envenomation should be admitted to the hospital and monitored closely for hemolysis or other complications.
D. **Scorpion stings**
   1. **Discussion.** The scorpion is a nocturnal arachnid found in the Southwestern United States. It has a stinger in its tail with two venom glands. Most species are relatively harmless, and their sting usually causes a localized reaction such as occurs with a bee sting. However, the bark scorpion (*Centruroides sculpturatus*) has a neurotoxin in its venom that can cause a severe reaction. This dangerous scorpion is found on trees in Arizona and New Mexico.
   2. **Clinical features**
      a. **Local effects.** The symptoms from the *C. sculpturatus* scorpion sting include immediate severe pain at the sting site, swelling, and, later, numbness. The injured area is hypersensitive, and the involved extremity may be paralyzed.
      b. **Systemic effects.** The neurotoxin is strongly cholinergic and can cause excessive salivation, blurred vision, muscular spasms, hypertension, and respiratory difficulties.
   3. **Differential diagnoses** include snakebite, puncture wound or other trauma, insect or spider bite, or drug intoxication.
   4. **Evaluation.** Typically, the offending scorpion is seen or assumed by history; if safety allows the scorpion to be brought in, this is best. Due to wide range of symptoms and quick progression, thorough history and physical are necessary.

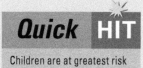

Quick **HIT**

Children are at greatest risk for complications of scorpion envenomation, and they may develop respiratory compromise within 30 minutes.

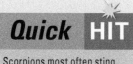

Quick **HIT**

Scorpions most often sting the extremities, especially the feet after hiding in victim's shoes.

5. **Therapy**
   a. **Prehospital management** includes rapid transportation of the patient, application of an ice pack to the sting site, and safe transport of the scorpion for identification. If severe symptoms occur, life support measures should be initiated.
   b. **ED management**
      i. **Antivenin** should be administered in all cases of severe envenomation.
      ii. **Ventilatory support** may be required, with intubation and oxygen for patients with severe systemic response or anaphylaxis.
      iii. **Atropine** may be required to counteract the cholinergic effects; the dose is titrated to relieve the cholinergic signs.
      iv. **Benzodiazepines** may be used for seizures and muscle spasms.
6. **Disposition.** All victims should be observed for 24 hours, especially children. Symptomatic patients should be transferred to the intensive care unit if symptoms are severe.

E. *Hymenoptera* **stings**
   1. **Discussion**
      a. *Hymenoptera* include honeybees, wasps, hornets, yellow jackets, fire ants, and harvester ants.
      b. Identification of the offending insect can be difficult.
   2. **Pathogenesis.** The venom injected may contain histamine, serotonin, amines, phospholipase, hyaluronidase, and other substances; the components vary with the insect type. Toxic reactions to *Hymenoptera* insect stings are quite common in the United States, and types are discussed in Clinical Pearl 21-7.
   3. **Differential diagnoses** include infection, local trauma, foreign body, and skin disorder. Few patients forget a painful sting, but identification of the exact insect may be difficult. If anaphylaxis is present, the history may be impossible to obtain; in such cases, the skin should be carefully searched for sting sites.
   4. **Evaluation.** If moderate or severe symptoms are present, a CBC, electrolytes, ABG, chest radiograph, and ECG should be obtained. Cardiac monitoring and close observation are indicated.
   5. **Therapy**
      a. **Local reactions.** If a stinger is present in the wound, it should be scraped out (not squeezed). The wound should be thoroughly washed and ice packs placed. Oral antihistamines and analgesics should be administered to relieve discomfort. For moderate swelling, elevation and use of oral steroids for several days are indicated.

CLINICAL PEARL 21-7

Five Types of Reaction to *Hymenoptera* Stings

1. **Local reaction** consists of significant edema, pain, and erythema at the sting site. If the sting site is around the mouth or throat, airway obstruction may occur. Some insects can sting repeatedly and cause local tissue damage, blisters, and severe pain.
2. **Toxic reaction.** If there are 10 or more stings, a systemic reaction may develop because of the large toxin load. Vomiting, dizziness, syncope, edema, and diarrhea may develop. Multiple stings may result in convulsions and death. Africanized bees ("killer bees") that are now in the Southern United States actually have weaker envenomations than other bees, but they may cause more illness and death because the victim is stung many times.
3. **Anaphylactic reaction** is the major cause of death associated with bee or wasp stings. The allergen component of single or multiple stings may cause an antigen–antibody, immunoglobulin E–mediated systemic anaphylactic reaction. Histamine, slow-reacting substance of anaphylaxis, and other factors are released that within minutes produce generalized urticaria, pruritus, dry cough, and wheezing. Severe symptoms include dyspnea, bronchospasm, cyanosis, cramps, nausea and vomiting, laryngeal stridor, hypotension, shock, loss of consciousness, and death.
4. **Delayed reaction** consists of serum sickness–like symptoms of headache, malaise, generalized pruritus, fever, and polyarthritis. These symptoms appear 10 to 15 days after a sting.
5. **Unusual reaction.** Rare reactions include encephalopathy, vasculitis, neuritis, and autonomic dysfunction.

b. **Anaphylactic reactions** are treated with local care, intravenous fluids, anti-histamines, and steroids.
   i. If life-threatening symptoms occur, epinephrine should be administered.
   ii. Albuterol nebulizer treatments are indicated in bronchospasm. If severe airway compromise exists, endotracheal intubation may be indicated.
   iii. Hypotensive patients require large volumes of intravenous fluids and may need vasopressors.

6. **Disposition**
   a. **Discharge.** Patients with minor local reactions may be treated symptomatically and discharged.
   b. **Admission.** Any patient with a systemic reaction should be treated, observed closely, and admitted for continued symptoms. Patients with anaphylactic reactions require intensive care monitoring in the hospital.
   c. **Long-term management** is indicated for patients with serious reactions to *Hymenoptera* stings. The patient should be referred to an immunologist for desensitization.

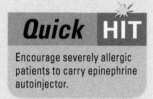

Quick HIT

Encourage severely allergic patients to carry epinephrine autoinjector.

MEDICOLEGAL CONSIDERATIONS

Peter Van Ligten

I. INTRODUCTION

The American legal system allows those who feel they have been wronged to argue their cases in court.

A. **Criminal versus civil law**

1. **Criminal law.** A **crime** is a wrong committed against the public or the public good. For an action to be a crime, there must be both an intent to commit the illegal act as well as the commission of the act itself. A **criminal action** is brought by the government against the wrongdoer to seek a sanction (e.g., a monetary fine or incarceration). The crime victim is not a party to the criminal action and usually does not receive any compensation for resulting losses or injuries. Seldom is criminality an issue in treating patients. As long as the patient consents to medical care, charges such as assault (i.e., confrontation causing reasonable apprehension of unpermitted personal contact) or battery (i.e., unpermitted personal contact) rarely occur.

2. **Civil law.** Civil cases **(torts)** involve wrongs committed against private parties. When a patient or family member is angered by an interaction with a health care provider, he or she may bring a lawsuit against the physician and hospital. The remedy sought in a civil action is usually monetary compensation for the injured party. Although many claims can be made in a lawsuit, the most frequent tort is that of **negligence**.

B. **Medical negligence** is the failure to follow acceptable standards of care in a way that results in injury to the patient. Medical negligence is the most common claim in a malpractice lawsuit (see Clinical Pearl 22-1).

1. **Avoiding malpractice.** Excessive diagnostic testing will not reduce the likelihood of being sued (see Clinical Pearl 22-2).

II. INFORMED CONSENT

The concept of informed consent was laid down in 1914 by Justice Cardozo in *Schloendorff v New York Hospital:* "Every human being of adult years and sound mind has a right to determine what shall be done to his body; a surgeon who performs an operation without his patient's consent commits an assault for which he is liable in damages."

A. **Emergency implied consent** applies in all true emergencies. A true emergency exists when there is an immediate threat to life or limb. In this situation, the physician should perform what a "reasonably prudent person" would want done under the same circumstances and document the rationale for the procedure in the patient's chart.

B. **Informed consent** is required for all nonemergency procedures and should be in writing. Even in the busiest of emergency departments (EDs), fewer than 5% of all patients represent true life or limb emergencies.

1. **Adults.** The patient must:
   a. **Give consent voluntarily** (not under duress or financial inducement).
   b. **Be informed.** The patient must:
      i. Understand the nature of the procedure
      ii. Understand the risks and benefits of the procedure

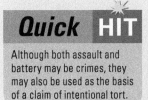

Quick **HIT**

Although both assault and battery may be crimes, they may also be used as the basis of a claim of intentional tort.

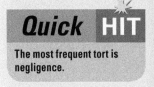

Quick **HIT**

The most frequent tort is negligence.

Medicolegal Considerations

CLINICAL PEARL 22-1

1. **Elements of negligence.** In order to bring a successful lawsuit on the tort of negligence, four elements must be proven:
   a. **Duty to treat.** A physician has a duty to treat the patient if a doctor–patient relationship is established. For the purposes of emergency medicine, all patients, regardless of their ability to pay, establish a physician–patient relationship by presenting themselves to the ED; therefore, the physician must render care.
   b. **Breach of duty.** To prove this element of negligence, the law requires that a physician's actions must be demonstrated to be below the acceptable standard of care.
      i. The standard of care is established by an expert's testimony. It is not necessarily defined by information in reference books nor is it established by common local practice, cost-cutting guidelines, hospital protocols, or policies.
      ii. If a plaintiff's attorney can produce an expert that is willing to testify that the defendant's practice is below the standard of care in his or her opinion, the case will move forward. Defense hinges on producing appropriate experts to testify that documentation of the case reflects the level of care someone in the same field of medicine would provide under similar circumstances. Some states have limited experts to those board-certified in the field of emergency medicine with a minimum number of years of direct clinical practice.
   c. **Injury.** The patient must have suffered an injury as a result of the physician's breach of duty. Injuries are defined differently by lawyers than by physicians. Although the patient may appear healthy, injuries such as pain and suffering, loss of consortium (inability to have sexual intercourse), loss of wages, and mental anguish have been claimed.
   d. **Proximate cause.** The injury must be a direct result of either the physician's action or his or her failure to act or diagnose a condition that led to the injuries.

      iii. Understand the alternatives to the procedure
      iv. Have the opportunity to ask questions and receive answers to them
    c. **Be competent.** The patient must:
      i. Display normal mental capacity
      ii. Not be under the influence of drugs or alcohol
      iii. Not be cognitively impaired as a result of injury or illness
2. **Minors.** The child's legal guardian (if not the mother or father) must be identified. The adult consenting must meet all of the criteria outlined in II.B.1. In the following situations, it may not be necessary to obtain the consent of the minor's guardian, although rules vary from state to state:
   a. **Emancipated minors** live on their own and are responsible for their own expenses. Military personnel are usually considered emancipated minors.
   b. **Minors who request treatment of pregnancy or sexually transmitted infections.** Some states allow a minor to consent for examination and treatment of suspected sexually transmitted disease or pregnancy because these situations may be embarrassing and without medical treatment could result in illness or injury to others.

CLINICAL PEARL 22-2

Physicians can do much to reduce lawsuits by:
1. **Practicing good medicine.** This is the primary way of preventing malpractice suits.
2. **Communicating well.** The physician should attempt to allay anger and minimize unreasonable expectations on the part of patients and family. Patients will be less likely to sue if they believe that the physician genuinely cares about them.
3. **Documenting thoroughly.** Accurate documentation of all assessments, care rendered, and discussions with patients regarding treatment options is essential. If a patient is refusing recommendations or is being noncompliant, these facts should be noted as well.

C. **Refusal** is the right of a competent adult to not give consent and thereby forego recommended treatment or evaluation.

1. **Adults.** In order to refuse, the adult must meet all of the requirements outlined for consent in II.B.1. The patient's medical record should document that the patient:
   a. Is alert and oriented
   b. Has normal mental capacity
   c. Is not under the influence of alcohol or drugs
   d. Has received an explanation of the proposed procedure, its alternatives, and the risks and benefits of both the procedure and the alternatives
   e. Understands that refusing may lead to death or permanent loss of health
   f. Was invited to return at any time to have the procedure done
   g. Was offered all other reasonable treatments (e.g., oral antibiotics given in a situation where intravenous antibiotics are indicated)

2. **Minors.** Exceptions to the rules of consent include the following when a parent or guardian refuses treatment on behalf of a child:
   a. If the physician believes that the refusal of treatment by the parent or guardian would seriously jeopardize the child's health, then a court order can be sought to compel treatment. For example, if the parents of a child with suspected meningitis refuse a lumbar puncture and antibiotics, the child should be held in the ED and risk management called to initiate a request to a judge for court-ordered treatment.
   b. If the physician believes the child is a victim of abuse or neglect, then evaluation and treatment should occur and the appropriate investigating agency notified.

III. PATIENT CONFIDENTIALITY AND REPORTABLE CONDITIONS

A. **Patient confidentiality.** The physician has a legal and moral duty to hold what a patient discloses to him or her, or what is discovered through examination or medical testing, to be confidential. This information should not be disclosed to anyone, even well-meaning family members, the patient's insurance company, or other caregivers, without the patient's consent. The following are examples of situations where it is inappropriate to provide information regarding the patient's condition without consent from the patient:

1. A family member requests information regarding the patient's diagnosis.
2. An insurance company requests information regarding the presenting complaint of the patient.
3. An employer inquires about an employee's injuries or ability to return to work.
4. The media requests information on hospitalized "newsworthy" patients.
5. An outside hospital requests release of the patient's medical records.
6. An attorney "just wants to talk about a case."

B. **Reportable conditions.** Although the physician–patient relationship is held in highest scrutiny of confidentiality, society has recognized that sometimes a greater duty is owed to the public than to the patient. Many states have specific statutes mandating physicians to report certain conditions that would provide for the greater good to society, despite violating a patient's confidentiality (see Clinical Pearl 22-3).

IV. INVOLUNTARY HOLDS

A patient may have his or her right to leave the hospital suspended under certain conditions.

A. **Mental illness.** A patient who, as a result of mental illness, is unable to care for him- or herself, or poses a danger to him- or herself or others, may be placed on a psychiatric hold. In some jurisdictions, the ability to place this type of hold is granted to medical personnel, police agencies, social workers, and mental health agencies. Laws may differ from county to county as well as from state to state. The intent of this law is to provide psychiatric treatment to the patient; it usually does not give the physician consent to treat medical problems.

B. **Inebriation.** A patient who, as a result of alcohol intoxication, is unable to understand the elements of consent or refusal may be placed on an inebriation hold.

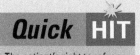

The patient's right to refuse treatment remains his or her own unless superseded by a life-threatening emergency or a court order to treat.

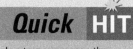

In a true emergency, the concept of emergency implied consent still applies.

Medicolegal Considerations

Medicolegal Considerations

CLINICAL PEARL 22-3

Although statutes vary among states, most require that a physician violate patient confidentiality in the following situations:

1. **Threats.** If a patient makes a threat of violence against a specific person, then the physician must ensure that the person is contacted and warned. The person notified, the specific warning, and the date and time must be recorded in the medical record of the patient who made the threat.
2. **Domestic violence.** Reporting of domestic violence is mandatory in most states. This mandate requires the physician to prepare a written report of injuries sustained as a result of the action of any member of the patient's household, even if the patient does not want to file a police report or seek help.
3. **Sexual assault.** In most states, clear written documentation, usually on a standardized reporting form, is required for victims of alleged sexual assault. Samples obtained from the patient must be labeled and handled as a "chain of evidence" (i.e., each person handling the evidence sample must sign for its receipt until the sample is received at a crime laboratory). Occasionally, the physician may also be asked to obtain hair or blood samples from the alleged perpetrator, and similar chain of evidence procedures apply.
4. **Child abuse.** A physician who suspects that a child has been the victim of physical abuse, sexual assault, or neglect is required to notify the appropriate investigating agency (e.g., the police or Social Welfare Services). The child must be protected from further harm, which may require separating the child from his or her parents and preventing the parents from removing the child from the ED.
5. **Elder abuse.** Like child abuse and domestic violence, the mistreatment or abandonment of an incapacitated elder may require reporting to police, Adult Protective Services, or an elder ombudsman. If a physician believes that a patient has been mistreated in a skilled nursing facility, state law may also require that the incident be reported to the state licensing agency that oversees nursing homes.
6. **Wounds**
   a. **Weapon-inflicted.** Some states require that a physician notify the police immediately of patients with wounds believed to be inflicted by a weapon. The intent of this law is to aid in the investigation of crimes.
   b. **Animal bite wounds.** In some states, bite wounds may have to be reported to local health authorities or animal control agencies. The physician may also be obligated to report the harboring of illegal animals, such as exotic snakes.
7. **Public health issues.** Most states require certain types of illnesses to be reported to public health authorities for investigation and follow-up. Laws vary from state to state, and local health departments should be consulted for requirements. Examples of some of the more common situations that require reporting include:
   a. **Communicable diseases**
      i. Sexually transmitted infections
      ii. HIV and AIDS
      iii. Hepatitis, especially in food handlers
      iv. Childhood diseases (e.g., measles, meningitis)
      v. Unusual infections (e.g., rabies, Hantavirus infection)
   b. **Food poisoning outbreaks**
      i. Staphylococcal food poisoning
      ii. Shellfish-related food poisoning
      iii. Botulism
   c. **Pesticide exposure.** California has extensive regulations requiring physicians to report all cases, no matter how minor, of pesticide-related illness. Surveillance of farm workers is required for many products used in agriculture.
   d. **Disorders that lead to lapse of consciousness** (e.g., epilepsy). Often, it is necessary to notify the health department, which may secondarily release the information to the department of motor vehicles or other mandated licensing authorities. Some states may allow the physician to report directly to the department of motor vehicles.
8. **Impaired physicians.** Some states require a physician to protect the public good if he or she believes a physician is too impaired to treat patients but continues to do so. It is advisable to contact local hospital counsel to determine the exact reporting requirements. Knowledge of physician incompetence and failure to report it may make a fellow physician liable for tort action by an injured party and possible sanction by the state medical licensing board.

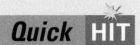

Quick HIT

In the absence of a specific reporting statute, the physician must not disclose a confidential statement by a patient stating that he or she committed a crime.

Quick HIT

The intent of bite reporting laws is to prevent other citizens from being bitten and to control the spread of rabies and other diseases spread by animal vectors.

Even if local statutes do not specifically address this issue, an emergency physician may document in the medical record that the patient is a danger to him- or herself or others as a result of inebriation and that it is necessary to restrain the patient until such a time that sobriety is obtained. When the patient is sober, medical care should again be offered. If the patient refuses once sober, notation of all the elements of refusal and an invitation to return should be documented in the medical record.

C. **Inability to care for self.** Some patients may be unable to care for themselves as a result of their medical illness. Statutes may call for the reporting of elder abuse or abandonment in such cases. The patient should be treated under the concept of emergency implied consent.

1. An application for a guardian if the patient may need to be presented before a judge to best serve the patient's needs. Social service agencies within the hospital can assist the physician in such an application. Admission or nursing home placement may be necessary in the interim.

2. The patient's guardian has the right to consent or refuse for the patient.

D. **Police holds.** A police officer may place in his or her custody any person suspected of a crime. That person might be brought to an ED for medical clearance prior to incarceration.

1. The person under arrest has the same rights of consent and refusal as anyone else.

2. Frequently, in an attempt to be manipulative, an individual under arrest will refuse treatment. If the patient refuses to be seen, the treating physician should note that the patient refused examination and treatment, and instruct the police to return the patient to the ED if the patient changes his or her mind regarding treatment.

E. **Requests for blood samples.** In most states, as a condition of operating a motor vehicle, the operator waives his or her right to refuse blood or breath testing for alcohol. Police may bring a person to the ED and request an alcohol or drug test. The patient need not be under arrest for a request to be made.

1. The physician's first priority should be stabilization and treatment of the patient's medical condition. Once the patient is stabilized, police requests should be honored.

2. In some states, the law even allows noninjurious restraint of the patient to obtain the sample. However, a physician cannot be compelled to perform an act that he or she believes would result in injury to him- or herself, the staff, or the patient. Good judgment in these cases will balance the issue of patient safety against the need of society to prosecute drunken drivers.

V. PATIENT TRANSFER LAWS

In response to an epidemic of hospitals refusing to treat or stabilize uninsured emergency patients, Congress passed the first "antidumping" law in 1986. This law was strengthened further, in a second congressional act, in 1989. Violation of these laws carries a fine of $50,000 per occurrence, which is not covered under a physician's malpractice insurance. The Health Care Finance Administration may also suspend or revoke an involved physician's and hospital's Medicare reimbursement privileges. A single alleged violation allows Health Care Finance Administration to inspect all transfers to search for other violations. Emergency physicians are often in the middle of these potential transfer law violations, so a thorough understanding of these laws is crucial to the practice of emergency medicine.

A. **Consolidated Omnibus Budget Reconciliation Act/Emergency Medical Treatment and Active Labor Act (EMTALA).** These acts provide every person with a medical emergency or active labor (defined by the presence of contractions) the right to be examined and stabilized prior to transfer. The requirements of these laws are as follows:

1. Any person who enters the hospital property (including hospital-owned clinics and ambulances as well as the ED) is entitled to medical evaluation and stabilization.

2. A screening medical examination must be performed to determine if an emergency medical condition exists. An emergency medical condition is defined as

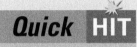

Quick HIT

All of the elements of consent and refusal, the patient's mental state, the advice to the patient and law enforcement officer, and the officer's department and badge number should be documented.

Medicolegal Considerations

a condition that "without immediate treatment could place the health of the patient in serious danger or cause significant impairment of a bodily function or organ; or in the case of a pregnant woman, could cause harm to the woman or unborn child."

3. Stabilization of the emergency medical condition must occur prior to transfer. Stabilization is not clearly defined, but the court will find the physician at fault if any deterioration in the patient's medical condition occurs during transfer.

4. Transfer of unstable patients may occur only if all six of the following conditions are met:
   a. The physician signs a certificate stating that the medical benefits of transfer outweigh the risks of remaining at the treating hospital.
   b. The patient or guardian gives consent to transfer.
   c. The transferring hospital and physician have provided all medical treatment to minimize the risks of transfer.
   d. The receiving physician and facility agree to accept the patient in transfer.
   e. All medical records, laboratory results, and radiographs are sent with the patient.
   f. The transfer is carried out with appropriate and qualified personnel and equipment (e.g., ambulance, aeromedical, or other specialized units).

B. **Omnibus Budget Reconciliation Act.** Additional refinements to Consolidated Omnibus Budget Reconciliation Act include the following:
   1. It is inappropriate to inquire regarding the patient's ability to pay or the patient's insurance status until after the screening medical examination occurs.
   2. When requested to do so by an emergency physician who identifies an unstable condition, on-call specialists have a duty to respond to the ED and treat the patient.
      a. The on-call physician must attend the patient physically.
      b. The emergency physician who is forced to transfer a patient because the on-call physician failed to respond may be protected from liability. Excellent documentation by the emergency physician of attempts to contact the on-call physician and the nature of phone conversations with the on-call physician is vital.
   3. Hospitals with specialized facilities (e.g., burn units, trauma centers, tertiary pediatric centers, high-risk obstetric units, intensive care units) may not refuse a transfer if bed space is available.
   4. A special "whistle-blower" regulation calls for hospitals to report other hospitals that have transferred a patient to them in violation of these laws.

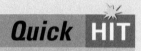

Quick HIT

The emergency physician transferring the patient is responsible for the medical care of the patient while in transit, unless care is transferred to a transporting physician.

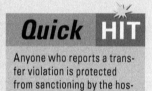

Quick HIT

Anyone who reports a transfer violation is protected from sanctioning by the hospital or medical staff.

Medicolegal Considerations

INDEX

Page numbers followed by *f, t,* and *b* indicate figures, tables, and boxed material, respectively.

A

ABCs. *See* Airway patency, breathing, and circulation
Abdomen, in pediatric patients, 333
Abdominal angina, 134
Abdominal aortic aneurysm, 134–135
Abdominal crisis, 391
Abdominal pain, 107–111, 109*b*
Abdominal processes, 26–27
Abdominal trauma, 408–409, 408*b*, 409*f*
Abduction and adduction stress testing, 431
Abortion, 317–319, 317*b*
Abruptio placentae, 319–321, 414
Abscess
    anorectal, 126–127
    brain, 163–164, 164*t*
    cutaneous, 269–270
    dental, 300–301
    intermuscular, 126
    intersphincteric, 126
    ischiorectal, 126
    parapharyngeal, 299
    perianal, 126–127
    peritonsillar, 297–298, 297*f*, 343, 349
    retropharyngeal, 299–300, 343, 349
    subdiaphragmatic, 26
    supralevator, 126
    tubo-ovarian, 329
Absence seizures, 223, 374–375
Accelerated idioventricular tachycardia, 48
Accelerated junctional rhythm, 47
Acetaminophen toxicity, 447–449, 448*b*, 448*f*
Acetone, 464
Acetone breath, 197
Acetylcholinesterase, 467
N-Acetylcysteine, 449
Acetylsalicylic acid. *See* Salicylate
Achilles tendinitis, 251
Acid–base imbalance, 192–195, 192*b*, 195*t*
Acid burns, of eyes, 287–288
Acidosis. *See also* Ketoacidosis
    lactic, 194, 200–201, 200*b*
    metabolic, 192*b*, 194–195, 195*b*
    respiratory, 192–193, 192*b*
ACLS protocols. *See* Advanced cardiac life support
    protocols
Acoustic schwannomas, 221
Acromioclavicular joint injuries, 429–430, 430*b*
Activated charcoal, 446
Acute arterial occlusion, 77–79, 78*f*
Acute esophageal perforation, 26
Acute interstitial nephritis, 141
Acute intravascular hemolysis, 382
Acute kidney injury (AKI), 141–143, 142*t*
Acute laryngitis, 173
Acute respiratory distress syndrome. *See* Noncardio-
    genic pulmonary edema
Acute respiratory failure, 84–85
Acute sequestration syndromes, 394
Acute tubular necrosis, 141
Acute valvular incompetence, 36
Acyanotic congenital heart disease, 354
Adenomyosis, 329*b*
Adenopathy, 167
Adenosine, 20, 44*t*
Adenovirus, 345
Adhesives, 441

Adrenal crisis, 204–205
Adrenal insufficiency, 204–205, 396–397, 399–400
β-Adrenergic antagonist overdose, 455–457
Advanced cardiac life support (ACLS) protocols, 1
    for bradycardia, 22*f*
    for pulseless dysrhythmias, 20*f*
    for tachycardias, 21*f*
AED. *See* Automatic external defibrillator
Aeromonas hydrophila, 176–177
Agonal gasps, 10
AIDS
    clinical features of, 156–159, 158*f*, 159*f*
    differential diagnoses for, 159
    discussion of, 156, 157*b*
    disposition of, 161
    evaluation of, 159–160
    mycobacterial pulmonary disease in, 102–103,
        103*b*
    therapy for, 160–161
AIDS dementia complex, 158
AIDS psychosis, 158
Air exchange, 3
Airway
    assessment of, 1–3
    bleeding and, 380
    interventions for, 3–9, 4*t*–7*t*, 9*t*
    obstruction of, 397, 397*b*, 400
    in pediatric patients, 331
Airway adjuncts
    assessment for, 2
    maneuvers and devices for, 3–4
Airway patency, breathing, and circulation (ABCs),
    1–2
    for acute respiratory failure, 85
    for altered mental status, 207
    for anaphylaxis, 233
    for hemoptysis, 92–93
    in pediatric patients, 331
    for pulmonary embolism, 96–97
    for stroke, 217
    for toxicologic emergencies, 444
AKI. *See* Acute kidney injury
Akinetic seizures, 374–375
Alcohol abuse
    abdominal pain and, 108
    acute pancreatitis and, 128
    with alcoholic ketoacidosis, 200
    anemia and, 387
Alcoholic ketoacidosis, 199–200
Alimentary hypoglycemia, 196
Alkalosis
    metabolic, 192*b*, 195
    respiratory, 192*b*, 193–194
Allopurinol therapy, 139
ALTE. *See* Apparent life-threatening event
Altered gas level–related inhalation injuries, 482
Altered mental status
    diagnostic studies for, 211
    discussion of, 206
    disposition of, 211
    laboratory studies for, 210–211
    neurologic examination of, 208–210, 208*t*, 209*t*,
        210*b*, 210*f*
    physical examination of, 207–208
    stabilization of, 207
Alveolar fractures, simple, 303

Amaurosis fugax, 275
Amebiasis, 179
Amides, 437
Aminocaproic acid, 384
ε-Aminocaproic acid, 386
Amiodarone, 20
Ammonia level, hepatitis and, 128
Amphetamines, 460–461
AMPLE history, 491
Amputations, fingertip, 427
Amrinone, 457
Anal fissures, 126
Anaphylactoid reactions, 230
Anaphylaxis
    clinical features of, 230–231, 231*t*
    differential diagnoses for, 231, 231*b*
    discussion of, 230
    disposition of, 233
    evaluation of, 231–232, 232*t*
    prevention of, 233
    therapy for, 232–233
Anemia
    asymptomatic, 383
    clinical features of, 387–388
    discussion of, 386–387, 387*b*
    evaluation of, 388–389
    microangiopathic hemolytic, 387, 395
    sickle cell. *See* Sickle cell anemia
    therapy for, 389–390
Angina, 28–32, 30*f*–31*f*, 31*t*
Angioedema, 233–235, 235*f*
Angle closure glaucoma, 273–274, 274*b*
Anion gap, 194, 195*t*, 201
Anion gap acidosis, 463, 463*b*
Ankle–brachial index, 77, 77*t*
Ankle injuries, 432
Ankylosing spondylitis, 244, 251, 253
Anogenitorectal syndrome, 145
Anorectal abscesses, 126–127
Anorectal disorders, 125–127, 125*b*
Anorectal fistulae, 127
Anorectal gonorrhea, 166
Anorexia nervosa, 307–308
Anoscopy, 124
Antemortem evaluation, 338
Anterior cord syndrome, 404*b*
Anterior uveitis, 274–275
Anticholinergic poisoning, 466–467
Anticholinergic toxidrome, 445*b*
Antihistamines, 233, 235, 437
Antipsychotic overdose, 454–455
Antivenin, 486–489
Antrum fractures, 303
Anuria, 141
Anxiety disorders, 308–309, 308*t*
Aorta, traumatic rupture of, 407
Aortic dissection, 26, 56
Aortic regurgitation, 56–57
Aortic stenosis, 53, 55–56
Aortic valve disease, 55–57
Apache II or III criteria, 130
Apathetic thyrotoxicosis, 202
Apical abscesses, 300–301
Aplastic anemia, 387–389
Aplastic crisis, 391
Apneustic breathing, 208

497

Apparent life-threatening event (ALTE), 338–339
Appendicitis, 131–132, 312–313
 in pediatric patients, 372–373
Arachnid bites, 486–489
Areflexia (atonic) bladder, 141
Arm
 forearm. *See* Forearm injuries
 upper arm. *See* Upper arm injuries
Arterial insufficiency, chronic, 76–77, 77t
Arterial occlusion, acute, 77–79, 78f
Arteriovenous malformation, 214
Arthritis
 monarticular. *See* Monarticular arthritis
 neck pain with, 236–237
 polyarticular. *See* Polyarticular arthritis
 septic, 244–249, 427
 transient, 358
 traumatic, 433
Arthrocentesis, 247–248, 248t, 253
Ascariasis, 178
Ascending cholangitis, 130–131
Ascorbic acid, 138
Aseptic meningitis, 359
Aspiration prevention, 3
Aspirin. *See* Salicylate
Assisted ventilation, 10–11. *See also* Mechanical
 ventilation
 in pediatric patients, 334
Asthma, 86–88, 86t
Asymptomatic anemia, 383
Asymptomatic hyperuricemia, 245
Asystole, resuscitation with, 18, 20f
Ataxic breathing, 208
Atheroemboli, 77
Atherosclerotic disease, 216
Athlete's foot, 263
Athlete's heart syndrome, 69
Atonic seizures, 223
Atrial fibrillation, 18–19, 21f, 42, 45, 109
Atrial flutter, 19, 21f, 42, 43t–44t, 45f
Atrophic vaginitis, 327
Atropine, 5, 22, 44t, 468
Atypical pneumonia, 99
Auditory canal, 288
Auscultation, 109b, 133
Auspitz sign, 260
Austin Flint murmur, 57
Autoimmune hemolysis, 387, 389
Automatic external defibrillator (AED), 13
Auto-PEEP phenomenon, 88
Avascular necrosis, 433
AV nodal block, 53
Avulsion, of teeth, 303
Avulsion fracture, 420

B
Babesiosis, 183
Bacillus cereus gastroenteritis, 119
Back pain, 240–243, 241b, 241t, 243b
Bacteremia, in pediatric patients, 359–361
Bacterial conjunctivitis, 282
Bacterial gastroenteritis, 118–119
Bacterial meningitis, 161–163, 359
Bacterial pharyngitis, 347–348
Bacterial pneumonia, 351–352
Bacterial skin infections
 cutaneous abscesses, 269–270
 impetigo, 268–269, 269f
 scarlet fever, 268
Bacterial tracheitis, 349
Bacterial vaginitis, 326–327
Bacteriuria, 137
Bacteroides, 150
Bag-valve-mask ventilation, 10
Balanoposthitis, 147
Barlow syndrome, 59

Barotrauma, 88
Bartter syndrome, 186
Basilar artery migraine, 212
Basilic veins, 15
Battle sign, 207
Beck triad, 64
Beef tapeworm, 179
Bell's palsy, 226
Bend fracture, 420, 421f
Benign intracranial headache, 213–214
Benign paroxysmal positional vertigo, 221
Benign postural syncope, 52
Benzodiazepine overdose, 451–452
Bifascicular blocks, 49
Bilateral orchiopexy, 149
Bilateral rales, 90
Biliary colic, 130–131
Biochemical derangements from cancer, 396–400
Bite wounds, 441
Black widow spider, 486–487
Bladder injury, 411–412
Bleeding
 diverticula, 124–125
 esophageal, 113–115
 evaluation of, 379
 therapy for, 380–383
 vaginal. *See* Vaginal bleeding
Blepharitis, 278–279
Blood components, 380–381
Blood type, 380
Blue dot sign, 149
Blue toe syndrome, 77
Blunt trauma
 abdomen, 409
 chest, 406–408, 407b
Boerhaave syndrome, 112–113. *See also* Acute
 esophageal perforation
Bone biopsy, 178
Bone crisis, 391
Bone infections, 177–178
Bone scan, 178
Borrelia burgdorferi, 180
Botulism, 226
Bouchard nodes, 250
Boutonniere deformity, 427
Bowel obstruction, 122–123, 313
Bowel sounds, 109b, 128, 208
Boxer's fractures, 427–428
Bradyarrhythmias, resuscitation with, 22, 22f
Bradydysrhythmia, 53
Brain abscess, 163–164, 164t
Branch retinal artery occlusion, 276
Breach of duty, 492b
Breathing
 assessment of, 1–2, 9–10
 failure of, 11
 interventions for, 10–11
 in pediatric patients, 331
Breech, 325
Bronchial foreign bodies, 340
Bronchiolitis, in pediatric patients, 345–347
Bronchiolitis obliterans, 345
Bronchitis, chronic, 88
Bronchopneumonia, 179, 345
Bronchopulmonary dysplasia, 346
Bronchoscopy, 341
Bronchospasm, 233
Brown recluse spider, 487–488, 488f
Brown-Séquard syndrome, 404b
Bruises, 377, 419
Bruits, 109b
Bubo, 145
Buckle fracture, 420, 421f
Bulimia nervosa, 307–308
Bullae, 255t, 258
Bundle branch blocks, 48–49

Bupivacaine, 336
Burning pain, 107
Burns, 377, 416–418, 416b, 417f, 418b
Butterfly fracture line, 420, 420f
By-proxy neglect, 376

C
C1q esterase deficiency, 234
Caffeine, 213, 338
Calcaneal fractures, 432
Calcium channel antagonist overdose, 457–458
Calcium imbalance, 189–191
Calcium oxalate and phosphate stones, 137, 138b
Calcium pyrophosphate deposition disease (CPPD),
 245
Campylobacter gastroenteritis, 118
Campylobacter jejuni, 159
Candida, 111–112, 158, 160
Candida albicans, 136, 263, 326
Candidiasis, 263
Capillary refill, delayed, 413
Capnometry, 12
Caput medusae, 109b
Carbamates, 468–469
Carbonic anhydrase inhibitors, 274b, 276
Carbon monoxide, 416, 465–466, 482–483
Carboxyhemoglobin level, 465
Carbuncle, 269
Cardiac box, 406
Cardiac contusion, 407
Cardiac pump theory, 12
Cardiac remodeling, 38
Cardiac tamponade, 26, 39, 64–65
Cardiac troponins, 27, 28t, 34, 34t
Cardiogenic shock, 36–37, 58, 401
Cardiomyopathies
 dilated, 67–68, 68t
 hypertrophic, 53, 59–60, 68t, 68–70, 70f
 restrictive, 68t, 70–71
Cardiopulmonary arrest, 1
Cardiopulmonary bypass, 13
Cardiopulmonary resuscitation (CPR)
 cardiopulmonary bypass, 13
 DNR and, 1
 for hypothermia, 474
 noninvasive compression, 12–13
 open chest compression, 13
Cardiovascular syphilis, 167
Cardioversion, 20, 42, 45
Carotid artery, 217b, 218f, 294
Carotid hypersensitivity, 52
Carpal injuries, 428, 428f
Carpal tunnel syndrome, 428
Catarrhal enteritis, 179
Catecholamines, 204
Cavities. *See* Dental caries
Cecal volvulus, 124
Cellulitis, 176–177, 280–282, 280f, 281b
 of hand, 427
 Ludwig angina, 298–299
 orbital, 280f, 281–282, 281b
 periorbital, 280–281, 280f
 peritonsillar, 297–298
 staphylococcal, 177
 streptococcal, 177
Central chemoreceptors, 2
Central cord syndrome, 404b
Central nervous system (CNS)
 AIDS and, 158–159
 altered mental status and, 208–210, 208t, 209t,
 210b, 210f
 infections of
 brain abscess, 163–164, 164t
 encephalitis, 163
 meningitis, 161–163
 rabies, 164–165
 tetanus, 165–166, 166b

primary tumors of, 215–216
sepsis at, 153
thyroid storm and, 202
Central retinal artery occlusion (CRAO), 275–276, 275f, 276f
Central retinal vein occlusion (CRVO), 277, 277f
Central vertigo, 221–222, 222t
Cephalic tetanus, 166b
Cerebellar function, 210
Cerebellar hemorrhage, 221
Cerebellar infarction, 221
Cerebellar pontine angle tumors, 221
Cerebral artery, 217b, 218f
Cerebrovascular accident
anemia and, 392b, 394
heat and, 482
stroke, 216–220, 217b, 218f, 219f, 220b
transient ischemic attack, 220
Cerebrovascular insufficiency, 53
Cervical cancer, 329b
Cervical nerves, 238
Cervical polyps, 329b
Cervical spondylosis, 236–237, 240
Cervical vertebrae, 236
Cervicitis, 312, 327–328
Chagas disease, 180
Chancre, 167
Chancroid, 143t, 145
Charcoal hemoperfusion, 451
Charcot triad, 130
Chemical asphyxiants, 482, 483b
Chemical burns, of eyes, 287–288
Chemical-induced hypoglycemia, 196
Chemical restraint, 307
Chest, in pediatric patients, 333
Chest crisis, 391
Chest pain, 25–28, 28t
with pleural effusion, 97
with pulmonary embolism, 94
Chest tube placement, 408
Cheyne-Stokes respiration, 208
CHF. See Congestive heart failure
Chickenpox. See Varicella
Chilblain, 475–478
Child abuse, 376–378
Chip fracture, 420
Chlamydia, 168
Chlamydia pneumoniae, 99, 101
Chlamydia trachomatis, 136, 145–146, 149, 168, 327–328
Chloral hydrate, 336
Chlorhexidine, 436
Cholecystitis, 130–131
Cholelithiasis, 128, 391
Cholinergic toxidrome, 445b
Chronic arterial insufficiency, 76–77, 77t
Chronic blood loss anemias, 387
Chronic bronchitis, 88
Chronic hypertension, 321–323, 322b
Chronic kidney disease, 143
Chronic laryngitis, 173
Chronic obstructive pulmonary disease (COPD), 88–90, 89t
Chronic venous insufficiency, 83
Circulation
for acute respiratory failure, 85
assessment of, 1–2, 11
for hemoptysis, 93
interventions for, 12–16, 15t–18t, 19f
in pediatric patients, 331–332
Circumferential casts, 424b
Civil law, 491
CK. See Creatinine kinase
CK-MB, 27, 28t
Classic heat stroke, 480
Classic migraine, 211
Clavicle fractures, 430

Clonic seizures, 223
Clonidine toxicity, 459
Closed-fist injuries, 441
Clostridium, 150
Clostridium difficile, 119
Clostridium tetani, 165
Cluster headache, 213
CMV. See Cytomegalovirus
CMV Epstein-Barr virus leptospirosis, 127
CMV retinitis, 158, 159f, 160
CNS. See Central nervous system
Coagulation, cascade, 384f
Cocaine, 460–461
Cold agglutinin disease, 387–388
Cold agglutinin titer, 351
Cold autoimmune hemolysis, 387
Colitis, 179
Collagen synthesis, 435b
Colles fracture, 428
Colorado tick fever, 183
Colubrids, 484
Coma, nonketotic hyperosmolar, 198–199
Coma cocktail, 445–446
Comminuted fracture, 420
Common migraine, 212
Compartment syndromes, 433
Complete cord injuries, 404
Completed abortion, 317b
Complete fracture, 420, 421f
Complete heart block, 48
Complex migraine, 212
Complex partial seizures, 223
Compression fractures, 244, 420
Computed tomography (CT)
for nephrolithiasis, 139, 139f
for periorbital cellulitis, 280, 280f
for SAH, 214–215, 215f
Concussion, 402
Conduction, 471b
Condylomata acuminatum, 143t, 145–146
Congenital heart disease, 71
in pediatric patients, 354–357
Congenital valve deformity, 58, 61
Congestive cardiomyopathy. See Dilated cardiomyopathy
Congestive heart failure (CHF), 38–41, 40f
Conjunctivitis, 282–283
Connective tissue disease, 58
Consolidated Omnibus Budget Reconciliation Act/Emergency Medical Treatment and Active Labor Act, 495–496
Constrictive pericarditis, 65–66
Contact dermatitis, 261
Contact vaginitis, 327
Contamination of wound, 434
Convection, 471b
Conversion reactions, 309–310, 309b, 310t
COPD. See Chronic obstructive pulmonary disease
Core temperature, 473
Corneal abrasion, 284–285, 285f
Corneal laceration, 285
Corneal ulcers, 282–283, 283f
Coronary artery occlusion, 28–29
Cor pulmonale, 89, 391
Corticotropin stimulation test, 205
Corynebacterium diphtheriae, 170
Coryza syndrome, 173–174
Costochondritis, 251
Cotton wool spots, 158, 159f, 160
Coumadin therapy, 359
Coxiella burnetii, 182
CPPD. See Calcium pyrophosphate deposition disease
CPR. See Cardiopulmonary resuscitation
Crabs, 143t, 146
Cramping pain, 107
Cranial nerve assessment, 209, 209t
CRAO. See Central retinal artery occlusion

Creatinine kinase (CK), 27, 28t
Creatinine phosphokinase, 34, 34t
Cricothyrotomy, 9, 173
Criminal law, 491
Crohn disease, 120–121, 121b
Crossed straight leg raising, 242
Crotalids, 484
Crotamiton, 264
Croup syndrome. See Laryngotracheobronchitis
Crust, 255t
CRVO. See Central retinal vein occlusion
Cryoprecipitate transfusions, 155, 381, 386
Cryosurgery, for condylomata acuminatum, 146
Cryptococcal CNS infection, 158, 160
Cryptococcus, 161
Cryptococcus neoformans, 158, 245
Cryptosporidiosis, 119, 159
CT. See Computed tomography
Cullen sign, 109b
Cutaneous abscesses, 269–270
Cutaneous candidiasis, 263
Cutoff sign, 129
Cyanotic congenital heart disease, 354
Cycloplegics, 274–275, 286–288
Cystic fibrosis, 345
Cystine stones, 138b
Cystitis, 136–137, 137t
Cytomegalovirus (CMV), 111–112, 158–159, 283

D
Dacryocystitis, 279–280
Datura stramonium, 466
DDAVP. See 1-Deamino-8-d-arginine vasopressin
D-dimer testing, 82
1-Deamino-8-d-arginine vasopressin (DDAVP), 386
Debridement, 438, 486
Deep venous thrombosis (DVT), 79–82, 80t–81t
Defibrillation, 2, 13–14
Degenerative calcific aortic stenosis, 55
Degenerative disk disease, 240
Delirium, 306–307
Dementia, 306–307
Dental abscesses, 300–301
Dental anatomy, 300, 301f
Dental caries, 300
Dental trauma, 301–303, 302b, 302f
Depolarizing blockade, 9
Depression, 306–307
suicide and, 310–311, 311b
Dermal suturing, 440
Dermatologic lesions, 254–255, 255b
Dermatomyositis, 227–228
Dermatophytoses, 263
Desmopressin, 384, 386
Desquamation, 358
Dextrose, 197, 445
Diabetic ketoacidosis, 197–198
Diaphragmatic injury, 407–408
Diarrhea, 118, 119, 372
Diastolic murmur, 60
DIC. See Disseminated intravascular coagulation
Dicloxacillin, 269
Diffuse axonal injury, 402
Diffuse brain injuries, 402
Diffuse idiopathic skeletal hyperostosis, 236
Digitalis toxicity, 458–459
Digoxin, 44t
Dilated cardiomyopathy, 67–68, 68t
Diltiazem, 19, 21f, 43t
Diphtheria, 170–171, 348
pharyngeal, 170
Diphtheria antitoxin, 171
Diphyllobothrium latum, 179
Discitis, 236
Disk disease, 240

Index

Dislocations, 419, 423–424, 424b
  ankle, 432
  elbow, 429
  finger, 427
  glenohumeral, 430, 430f
  hip, 431
  knee, 432
  wrist, 428, 428f
Disorders of cardiac conduction, 48–49
Disseminated gonococcal arthritis, 244–249
Disseminated gonorrhea, 166–167
Disseminated intravascular coagulation (DIC),
  394–396, 395b, 396t
Distal DVT, 79
Distal humerus fracture, 429
Distal radius fractures, 428
Distended colon, 123
Diverticular disease, 123–125
Diverticulitis, 124–125
DNR. See Do not resuscitate
Do not resuscitate (DNR), 1
Dressler syndrome, 62
Drop attacks, 374
Drug-induced hemolytic anemia, 388
Drug-induced vertigo, 221
Duchenne muscular dystrophy, 227, 227t
Duodenal ulcers, 116–118, 117b
Duodenum, 408
Duroziez sign, 57
Duty to treat, 492b
DVT. See Deep venous thrombosis
Dysmenorrhea, 313–314
Dysphagia, 113
Dyspnea, exertional, 57
Dysrhythmias
  resuscitation with, 16–22, 20f–22f
  supraventricular. See Supraventricular
    dysrhythmias
  treatment of, 36
  ventricular, 47–48, 47f

E
Early appendicitis, 312
Ears
  altered mental status and, 207
  foreign body in, 290–291
  infections of, 288–290
  tympanic membrane rupture, 291–292
Ebstein anomaly of the tricuspid valve, 355
Ecchymosis, 207
Eclampsia, 321–323, 322b
Ectopic pregnancy
  clinical features of, 315
  differential diagnoses for, 315
  discussion of, 314–315
  disposition of, 317
  evaluation of, 315–316, 316f
  pelvic pain with, 312–313
  therapy for, 316–317
Ectopic supraventricular tachycardia, 46
EEG. See Electroencephalogram
Elapids, 484
Elbow injuries, 429
Electrical alternans, 64
Electrical pacing, 14
Electrocardiographic monitoring of circulation, 2
Electrocautery, 118, 146
Electrocution, resuscitation for, 22–23
Electrodesiccation, 146
Electroencephalogram (EEG), for seizures, 375
Ellis classification, 301–302, 302b, 302f
Emancipated minors, 492
Embolectomy, for pulmonary embolism, 97
Embolic strokes, 216
Emergency implied consent, 491
Emergent therapy, 37

EMLA. See Eutectic mixture of local anesthetics
Emotional neglect, 376
Emphysema, 88
Encephalitis, 163
Endocarditis
  infectious, 56, 60, 71–74, 72t, 74t
  rheumatic, 55
Endogenous anovulation, 329
Endogenous insulin excess, 196
Endometrial carcinoma, 329b
Endometriosis, 312, 314
Endoscopic variceal ligation, 114
Endoscopy, 113, 115–116, 118
Endotracheal intubation, 2, 11
Entamoeba histolytica, 159, 179
Enterobacter, 136, 152
Enterobius vermicularis, 178, 178f
Enterococcus, 151
Enteropathic arthritis, 250–253
Environmental seclusion, 307
Epididymal appendage torsion, 149
Epididymitis, 149–150, 168
Epidural hematomas, 402–403, 403f, 413
Epigastric pain, 107, 128
Epiglottitis, 171–173, 172f, 297, 343
  in pediatric patients, 348–350
Epilepsy, 222
Epinephrine, 22, 335–336, 437
Episioproctotomy, 325
Epistaxis, 293–295, 296f, 303, 386
Epithelialization, 435b
Epstein-Barr virus, 170, 283, 358
Erysipelas, 176
Erythema chronicum migrans, 181b
Erythema infectiosum, 267
Erythema multiforme, 256–258, 257f
Erythema nodosum, 262–263, 262f
Escharotomy, 418
Escherichia coli, 119, 136, 149–150, 245, 359
Escherichia coli 0157:H7, 119
Esophageal disorders, 27
  Boerhaave syndrome, 112–113
  esophageal bleeding, 113–115
  esophageal dysphagia, 113
  esophagitis, 111–112
  GERD, 111
Esophageal foreign bodies, 115–116, 115b
Esophageal varices, 114–115
Esophagitis, 111–112
  with AIDS, 158, 160
Esophagoscopy, 112
Esters, 437
Ethanol, 464, 464b
Ethylene glycol, 462–463, 463b, 464b
Eutectic mixture of local anesthetics (EMLA), 335
Euvolemic hyponatremia, 184
Evaporation, 471b
Exertional dyspnea, 57
Exertional heat stroke, 480
Exogenous anovulation, 329–330
Expiratory airflow obstruction, with COPD, 88
Extraocular motion, 272, 273t
Extrapancreatic neoplasms, 196
Extremities
  DVT of, 79–82, 80t–81t
  edema of, 109
  innervation of, 239t, 241t
  in pediatric patients, 333
Extrinsic asthma, 86
Eyes
  altered mental status and, 207
  angle closure glaucoma, 273–274, 274b
  anterior uveitis, 274–275
  examination of, 272
  infections of, 278–282, 280f, 281b
  trauma of, 284–288, 285f
  vision loss, 275–278, 275f, 276f, 277f

F
Factitious disorder, 309b
Factitious hypoglycemia, 196
Factor IX, 384–386
Factor VIII, 384–385
Fascicular blocks, 49
Fascioscapulohumeral muscular dystrophy, 227,
  227t
Fasting hypoglycemia, 196
Febrile nonhemolytic transfusion, 382
Febrile seizures, 373, 373b
Felon, 426
Femoral hernia, 133
Femoral shaft fractures, 431
Femoral vein, 16, 18t, 19f
Femur, injuries to, 431
Fetomaternal hemorrhage, 415
FFP. See Fresh frozen plasma
Fiberoptic intubation, 9
Fibrinous pericarditis, acute, 62
Finger test, 272
Fingertip
  amputations, 427, 442
  injuries, 442
Finger trauma, 427–428
First-degree AV block, 48
First-degree burn, 416
Fish tapeworm, 179
Fitz-Hugh–Curtis syndrome, 313, 329
Flail chest, 406
Flavoxate therapy, 141
Floppy valve syndrome, 59
Flumazenil, 446
Focal lesions, 402
Folate, 464
Follicular cysts, 313
Folliculitis, 269
Fomepizole, 463–464, 464b
Food poisoning, 118–119
Foot injuries, 432
Forearm injuries, 428–429
Foreign bodies
  corneal abrasion, 284
  in ears, 290–291
  gastrointestinal, 115–116, 115b
  intraocular, 285–286
  in nose, 293
  in pediatric patient, 339–342, 340b, 341f
  urethral, 140, 148
  in vaginitis, 326–327
  in wound preparation, 438
Fournier gangrene, 150
Fourth-degree burn, 416
Fractures
  ankle, 432
  with child abuse, 377
  clavicle, 430
  compression, 244, 420
  femur, 431
  finger, 427–428
  foot, 432
  of forearm, 428–429
  knee, 432
  lower leg, 432
  management of, 423–424, 424b
  mandibular, 303, 303f, 305
  maxillary, 303, 304f, 305b
  of nose, 295–297
  orbital, 286–287
  pelvis, 431
  renal, 410, 411f
  of ribs, 408
  of teeth, 301–302, 302b, 302f
  types of, 419–421, 420f, 421f
  upper arm, 429
Francisella tularensis, 183
Frank breech, 325

Frank-Starling mechanism, 38
Free wall rupture, 36
Fresh frozen plasma (FFP), 381
  for esophageal varices, 114
  for hemophilias, 385
  for sepsis, 155
Friction rub, 97
Frostbite, 475–478, 476b, 477b
Fulminant hepatic failure, 127
Functional hypoglycemia, 196
Fundi, 207, 272
Fungal meningitis, 161–163
Fungal skin infections, 263–265, 264f
Fungal vaginitis, 327
Furuncle, 269

G

G6PD deficiency. *See* Glucose-6-phosphate dehy-
  drogenase deficiency
Gag reflex, 3
Galeazzi fracture, 429
Gallbladder, 130–131
Gallstones, 128, 130
Gammaglobulin, 156
Gardnerella, 136
Gardnerella vaginalis, 326
Gastric decontamination procedures, 446
Gastric lavage, 446
Gastric ulcers, 116–118, 117b
Gastroenteritis
  of infectious origin, 118–120
  in pediatric patients, 361–363
Gastroesophageal reflux disease (GERD), 111
Gastrointestinal foreign bodies, 115–116, 115b
Gauze packing, 295, 296f
Generalized seizures, 223, 374
Generalized tetanus, 166b
Genital lesions, 143t
  chancroid, 145
  condylomata acuminatum, 145–146
  genital herpes, 144, 144f
  LGV, 143t, 145
  molluscum contagiosum, 146
  pediculosis pubis, 146
  primary syphilis, 143–144
Genital warts. *See* Condylomata acuminatum
Genitourinary trauma, 410–413, 411f, 412b
GERD. *See* Gastroesophageal reflux disease
German measles, 267
Gestational hypertension, 321–323, 322b
Giardiasis, 119, 159, 180
Glasgow Coma Scale, 208, 208t
Glaucoma, angle closure, 273–274, 274b
Glenohumeral dislocations, 430, 430f
Glomerulonephritis, 142
Glucagon, 456–457
Glucose
  in alcoholic ketoacidosis, 200
  for altered mental status, 207
  for nonketotic hyperosmolar coma, 199
Glucose-6-phosphate dehydrogenase (G6PD) defi-
  ciency, 387–389
Glucose levels
  in alcoholic ketoacidosis, 200
  in hypoglycemia, 196
  in nonketotic hyperosmolar coma, 199
Glycogen storage diseases, 227
Gonococcal cervicitis, 327–328
Gonorrhea, 166–167
Gout, 244–249
Graft-versus-host disease, 382
Graves disease, 201
Greenfield filters, for pulmonary embolism, 97
Greenstick fracture, 420, 421f
Grey-Turner sign, 109b, 129, 129f
Griseofulvin, 264–265

Group A β-hemolytic streptococci, 169–170, 176,
  268, 289, 297–298, 347
Group B streptococcus, 154
Guillain-Barré syndrome, 226
Gunshot wounds, 409
Gynecomastia, 109

H

Haemophilus ducreyi, 145
Haemophilus influenzae, 90, 99–100, 154, 245, 279,
  281, 289, 345, 348–349
  vaccination against, 156, 173
Hallucinogens, 462
Hamman sign, 112
Hampton hump, 95
Hand-foot-and-mouth syndrome, 268
Hand injuries, 425–428, 425b, 426f, 428f
Haustra, 123
Head
  altered mental status and, 207
  in pediatric patients, 332
  trauma of, 377, 402–404, 403f
Headache
  benign intracranial, 213–214
  cluster, 213
  hypertensive, 213
  migraine, 211–212
  post–lumbar puncture, 213, 213b
  subarachnoid hemorrhage, 214–215, 215f
  temporal arteritis, 214
  trigeminal neuralgia, 214
Head tilt/chin lift, 3
Heat cramps, 478–479
Heat exhaustion, 479–480
Heat-related illness, 478
Heat-related inhalation injuries, 482
Heat stroke, 480–481, 480b
Heat syncope, 478–479
Heberden nodes, 250
Helicobacter pylori, 116–117
Hematuria, 137, 139, 386, 395
Hemodialysis, 451, 463
Hemolysis, 382, 387
Hemophilias A and B, 384–386, 396t
Hemoptysis, 57–58, 91–93, 92b
Hemorrhagic strokes, 216, 220
Hemorrhoids, 125–126, 125b
Hemothorax, 406
Hepatic injuries, 409
Hepatitis, 127–128, 131
Hepatobiliary radionuclide scan, 131
Hepatosplenomegaly, 179
Herald patch, 260, 261f
Hereditary angioedema, 234
Hereditary spherocytosis, 387, 388, 389
Hernia, incarcerated, 133, 367–368, 367b
Herpangina, 348
Herpes, 169, 169f
  eye infection with, 283–284
  genital, 144, 144f, 143t
  hepatitis, 127
Herpes simplex virus (HSV), 169
  with AIDS, 156, 158–159
  in cervicitis, 327–328
  encephalitis and, 163
  esophagitis, 111–112
  genital herpes with, 144
Herpes zoster (shingles), 255–256, 256f
Hidradenitis suppurativa, 269
High-pressure injection injuries, 442
Hilar adenopathy, 262
Hip, injuries to, 431
Histamine, 230
Histamine-2 antagonists, for GERD, 111
Histamine receptor blockade, 233
Histoplasma capsulatum, 158

HIV infection, 156, 157b
Hookworm infection, 179
Hoover test, 242
Hordeola, 279
HSV. *See* Herpes simplex virus
HSV polymerase chain reaction, for encephalitis, 163
Human diploid cell vaccine, 165
Human papillomavirus, 160
Humerus fracture, 429
Hydatidiform mole, 318–319, 318f
Hydralazine, 322b
Hydrocarbons, 469
Hydrochlorothiazide therapy, 139
Hydrogen cyanide poisoning, 483
Hydrogen peroxide, 436
Hydrogen sulfide poisoning, 483–484
Hydroxocobalamin, 483–484
Hymenoptera, 233, 489–490, 489b
Hypercalcemia, 190–191, 396–400
Hyperkalemia, 187–189, 188f, 399
Hypermagnesemia, 191–192
Hypernatremia, 185–186
Hyperosmolar coma, nonketotic, 198–199
Hyperosmotic agents, 274b
Hyperphosphatemia, 399
Hypertension
  emergency, 50–51
  management of, 219
  overview of, 49–50
  in pregnancy, 321–323, 322b
  thoracic aortic dissection with, 74
  urgency, 49–50
Hypertensive headache, 213
Hyperthermia, 481–482
Hypertrophic cardiomyopathy, 53, 59, 68t, 68–70, 70f
Hyperuricemia, 399
Hyperventilation, 53–54, 208, 404
Hyperviscosity syndrome, 396–400
Hypervolemia, 382
Hypervolemic hyponatremia, 184
Hyphema, 286, 392b, 394
Hypocalcemia, 189–190
Hypochloremic alkalosis, 368
Hypochromic anemia, 388
Hypochromic diseases, 387, 387b
Hypoglycemia, 54, 196–197, 207, 445, 450
Hypokalemia, 186–187, 187f, 368, 451
Hypomagnesemia, 191
Hyponatremia, 184–185
Hypoperfusion strokes, 216
Hypoplastic left heart syndrome, 356
Hypotension, 88
Hypothermia
  clinical features of, 473
  differential diagnoses for, 473
  discussion of, 470–473, 471b, 472f, 473b
  disposition of, 475
  evaluation of, 473–474
  resuscitation for, 23–24, 474
  therapy for, 474–475
  with transfusion, 382
Hypothyroidism, 202–204
Hypoventilation, 1, 208
Hypovolemic shock, 401

I

ICH. *See* Intracerebral hemorrhage
Icteric phase, 127
Idiopathic hypoglycemia, 196
Idiopathic pericarditis, 62, 64
IgE. *See* Immunoglobulin E
Immersion foot, 475, 476f
Immune-mediated thrombocytopenia, 396, 399–400
Immunization. *See also* Vaccination
  for tetanus, 166
Immunoglobulin E (IgE), 230

Index

Immunologic complications from cancer, 396–400
Impetigo, 268–269, 269*f*
Incarcerated hernia, 133
  in pediatric patients, 367–368, 367*b*
Incisional hernia, 133
Incomplete abortion, 317*b*
Incomplete cord injuries, 404, 404*b*
Induced hypoglycemia, 196
Industrial chemicals, 467–469, 467*b*
Inebriation, 493, 495
Inevitable abortion, 317*b*
Infections
  bone, 177–178
  of CNS. *See* Central nervous system
  of ears, 288–290
  of eyes, 278–282, 280*f*, 281*b*
  of hand, 426–427
  parasitic, 178–180, 178*f*
  skin. *See* Skin infections
  with transfusion, 382
  upper respiratory tract. *See* Upper respiratory tract
    infections
  urinary tract, 136–138, 137*t*
  in wounds, 443
Infectious blepharitis, 278–279
Infectious endocarditis, 56, 60, 71–74, 72*t*, 74*t*
Infectious esophagitis, 111–112
Infectious mononucleosis, 170, 348
Inferior vena cava filters, for pulmonary
  embolism, 97
Inflammatory arthritis, 236, 240
Inflammatory bowel disease, 120–122, 121*b*
Inflammatory phase, 435*b*
Inflammatory polyarthritis, 249–252
Informed consent, 491–493
Inguinal hernia, 132–133
Inguinal syndrome, 145
Inhalation burns, 416
Inhalation injuries, 482–484, 483*b*
Innervation
  of lower extremity, 241*t*
  of upper extremity, 239*t*
Inotropic support, for cardiogenic shock, 37
Insect stings, 486, 489–490
In situ thrombosis, 78
Insulin
  in diabetic ketoacidosis, 197–198
  for hyperkalemia, 188
  for nonketotic hyperosmolar coma, 199
Insulin-induced hypoglycemia, 196
Insulinomas, 196
Intermuscular abscess, 126
Internal hordeola, 279
Intersphincteric abscess, 126
Intertrochanteric fractures, 431
Intervertebral disks, 236–237
  disease of, 240
  herniated, 243–244
Intestinal disorders
  bowel obstruction, 122–123
    in pediatric patients, 364–366, 365*f*
  diverticular disease, 123–125
  inflammatory bowel disease, 120–122, 121*b*
Intra-articular fracture, 420
Intracerebral hemorrhage (ICH), 215–216
Intracerebral vascular catastrophe, 54
Intracranial aneurysm, 214
Intracranial bleeding, 386
Intraocular foreign body, 285–286
Intraocular pressure, 272
Intrauterine devices, 329
Intravenous access, 14–16, 15*t*–18*t*, 19*f*
Intravenous drug abuse, 71–72, 72*t*
Intravenous fluids, for traumatic shock, 401
Intravenous immunoglobulin, 358
Intrinsic asthma, 86
Intrusion, of teeth, 302–303

Intubation
  endotracheal, 2, 11
  fiberoptic, 9
  lighted stylet, 9
  nasotracheal, 4, 5*t*
  orotracheal, 4, 4*t*
  rapid sequence, 4–9, 6*t*–7*t*, 9*t*
  retrograde wire, 9
Intussusception, 123
  in pediatric patients, 369–370
Inverted three sign, 129
Involuntary holds, 493, 495
Iridocyclitis, 274
Iris, 272
Iritis, 274
Iron deficiency anemia, 387*b*, 389–390
Irrigation, 438
Ischemic heart disease, 53
Ischemic strokes, 216, 217*b*, 219–220, 220*b*
Ischiorectal abscess, 126
Isopropyl alcohol, 464–465
Isospora, 159

J

Janeway lesions, 72
Jaundice, 109, 128, 130
Jaw thrust, 3
Jimsonweed, 466
Jock itch, 263
Joint crisis, 391
Joint stiffness, 433
Jugular vein, 15, 16*t*, 19*f*
Jugular venous distention, 60–61
Junctional arrhythmias, 46–47, 47*f*
Junctional rhythm, 46, 47*f*
Junctional tachycardia, 47

K

Kaposi sarcoma, 156, 158, 158*f*, 160
Katayama fever, 179
Kawasaki disease, 357–359
Keratoconjunctivitis, 283
Kerion, 264, 264*f*
Ketoacidosis, 198
  alcoholic, 199–200
  diabetic, 197–198
Ketonemia, 198
Kidney injuries, 410, 411*f*, 412
Kiesselbach plexus, 294
Klebsiella, 99–101, 136, 149, 151
Kleihauer-Betke test, 415
Knee injuries, 431–432
Koplik spots, 266, 267*f*
Kussmaul respirations, 197, 200
Kussmaul sign, 64

L

Labor. *See* Parturition
Labyrinthitis, 221
Lachman test, 431
Lactate dehydrogenase, 34, 34*t*
Lactic acid, 154
Lactic acidosis, 194, 200–201, 200*b*
Large-bore thoracostomy tube, for pneumothorax,
  105
Laryngeal foreign bodies, 340
Laryngeal mask airway (LMA), 3–4
Laryngitis, 173–174, 343
Laryngoscopy
  for epiglottitis, 172–173, 350
  for gastrointestinal foreign bodies, 115
  video-assisted, 9
Laryngotracheal injuries, 405
Laryngotracheobronchitis, in pediatric patients,
  342–345
Laser surgery, 146

Latrodectus mactans, 486–487
Le Fort fractures, 303, 304*f*, 305*b*
Left lower quadrant pain, 107
Leg. *See also* Extremities
  lower. *See* Lower leg injuries
  ulcers of, 391
Legionella, 99–100, 154
Leptospirosis, 358
Leriche syndrome, 76
Lesions
  dermatologic, 254–255, 255*b*
  focal, 402
  genital. *See* Genital lesions
  Janeway, 72
  vesicular, 255–256, 256*f*
  vesiculobullous, 256–259, 257*f*, 258*f*
Leukocyte esterase test, 137
LGV. *See* Lymphogranuloma venereum
Lidocaine, 5, 36, 43*t*, 48, 232, 335–336
Lighted stylet intubation, 9
Limb–girdle muscular dystrophy, 227, 227*t*
Lipid emulsion, 456–457
Listeria monocytogenes, 162
Lithium toxicity, 453
LMA. *See* Laryngeal mask airway
Local anesthesia, 436–437
Local tetanus, 166*b*
Lower extremity, innervation of, 241*t*
Lower leg injuries, 432
Loxosceles reclusa, 487–488, 488*f*
Ludwig angina, 298–299
Lumbar back pain. *See* Back pain
Lunate injuries, 428, 428*f*
Lund-Browder burn diagram, 416*b*
Luteal cysts, 313, 329
Lyme disease, 180–181, 181*b*
Lymphadenopathy, 144–146, 179, 268, 357
Lymphangitis, 177
Lymphogranuloma venereum (LGV), 143*t*, 145

M

Macules, 255*t*
Magnesium depletion, 186
Magnesium imbalance, 191–192
Magnesium replacement, 186, 191
Male urogenital problems
  of penis, 146–148, 147*f*, 148*b*
  of prostate, 151–152, 151*t*
  of scrotum, 150–151
  of testicles and epididymis, 148–150
Malignant effusions, 64, 396–397
Malignant hypertension, 50–51
Malignant hyperthermia, 481
Malingering, 309*b*
Malleolar fractures, 432
Mallet finger, 427
Mallory-Weiss tears, 115
Malpractice, 491, 492*b*
Malunion, 433
Mandibular fractures, 303, 303*f*, 305
Mania, 306–307
Manual defibrillator, 13–14
Marcus Gunn pupil, 275, 276*f*
Marrow function suppression, 396
Massive hemothorax, 406
Mastoidectomy, 290
Mastoiditis, 290
Maternal resuscitation, 323
Maxillary fractures, 303, 304*f*, 305*b*
McBurney point, 132
McRoberts maneuver, 325
Measles, 266, 267*f*
Mechanical complications from cancer, 397–400,
  398*f*
Mechanical positive-pressure ventilation, 11, 90
Mechanical ventilation, 87–88, 90–91, 155

Meckel diverticulum, in pediatric patients, 370–371
Meckel radionuclide scan, 371
Median veins, 15
Medical negligence, 491, 492*b*
Medicolegal considerations, 491
Megaloblastic anemia, 387–388, 390
Meibomian glands, 279
Melanotic stools, 371
Ménière disease, 221
Meningismus, 214
Meningitis, 161–163
  nonsuppurative, 179
  in pediatric patients, 334, 359–361
Meningococcus, 154
Meniscus injuries, 432
Menstrual cramps, 312
Mental illness, 493
Mesenteric ischemia, 134
Metabolic acidosis, 192*b*, 194–195, 195*b*
Metabolic alkalosis, 192*b*, 195
Metacarpal fractures, 427–428
Metatarsal fractures, 432
Methamphetamine, 460–461
Methanol, 463–464
MI. *See* Myocardial infarction
Microangiopathic hemolytic anemias, 387, 395
Microcrystalline disease, 252
Migraine, 211–212
Migratory polyoligoarthritis, 181*b*
Minor heat illness, 478–479
Miosis, 207
Miotics, 274*b*
Miscarriage, 317–319
Missed abortion, 317*b*
Mitral regurgitation, 58–59
Mitral stenosis, 57–58
Mitral valve disease, 57–60
Mitral valve prolapse, 27, 59–60
Mittelschmerz, 313
Mobitz type I block, 48
Mobitz type II block, 48
Molar pregnancy, 318–319, 318*f*
Moll glands, 279
Molluscum contagiosum, 143*t*, 146, 160
Monarticular arthritis, 166
  clinical features of, 246
  differential diagnoses for, 246–247
  discussion of, 244–246
  disposition of, 249
  evaluation of, 247–248, 248*t*
  therapy for, 248–249, 249*t*
Mononucleosis, infectious, 170, 348
Monteggia fracture–dislocation, 429
Moraxella catarrhalis, 90, 289
Multifocal atrial tachycardia, 42
Mumps orchitis, 150
Munchausen syndrome, 309*b*, 376
Mupirocin, 268
Mural thrombi, 77
Murmur, 357
Murphy sign, 130
Muscarinic sites, 467–468, 467*b*
Muscle disorders, 226–228, 227*f*
Muscle spasm, 236
Muscle strength assessment, 209, 209*t*
Muscular dystrophy, 227, 227*t*
Musculoskeletal disorders, 27
Mycobacterial pulmonary disease, 102–103, 103*b*
Mycobacterium avium-intracellulare, 102–103, 103*b*, 158
Mycobacterium tuberculosis, 99–100, 102–103, 103*b*, 158, 161
Mycoplasma, 152, 345, 350
Mycoplasma hominis, 328
Mycoplasma pneumoniae, 99–100, 351
Mydriasis, 207

Myelosuppression, 396
Myocardial biopsy, 67
Myocardial disease, primary. *See* Primary myocardial disease
Myocardial hypertrophy, 38
Myocardial infarction (MI)
  clinical features of, 33
  differential diagnoses of, 33
  discussion of, 32–33
  disposition of, 36
  evaluation of, 30*f*–31*f*, 33–35, 34*f*, 34*t*
  serum markers of, 27
  therapy for, 34–36, 35*t*
Myocardial ischemic disease
  angina, 28–32, 30*f*–31*f*, 31*t*
  cardiogenic shock, 36–37
  myocardial infarction, 32–37, 34*f*, 34*t*–35*t*
Myocardial oxygen demand, 28
Myocarditis, 66–67, 179
Myoclonic seizures, 223, 374–375
Myoglobin, 27, 28*t*, 34, 34*t*
Myopathies, 226–228, 227*f*
Myotonic muscular dystrophy, 227, 227*t*
Myringotomy, 290
Myxedema coma, 202–204

N
Naegleria, 163
Nail bed injuries, 442
Naloxone, 207, 445–446, 459–460
NAPQI, 447–449
Narrow-complex supraventricular tachycardia, 45–46
Nasal cannula, 10, 85
Nasal trumpet, 3
Nasogastric decompression, 365
Nasogastric lavage, 124
Nasogastric tube placement, 2, 123
Nasopharyngeal airway, 3
Nasopharynx, 294
Nasotracheal intubation, 4, 5*t*
Navicular fracture, 425*b*, 426*f*, 428
NCPE. *See* Noncardiogenic pulmonary edema
Near-drowning, resuscitation for, 23
Necator americanus, 179
Neck pain, 236–240, 236*b*, 239*t*
Neck stiffness, 237
Needle aspiration, 105–106, 298
Needle thoracostomy, for pneumothorax, 104
Neisseria gonorrhoeae, 136, 150, 166, 244–245, 327–328
Neisseria meningitidis, 334
Neonatal seizures, 374–375
Neonatal tetanus, 166*b*
Neoplasia, vaginal bleeding with, 329, 329*b*
Neovascularization, 435*b*
Nephrolithiasis, 138–140, 138*b*, 139*f*, 140*b*, 313
Neurogenic shock, 401, 404
Neuroleptic malignant syndrome (NMS), 228–229, 481
Neurologic injuries, 405
Neuromuscular blockade, 8–9, 9*t*
Neuropathies, peripheral, 225–226
Neurosyphilis, 167
Nicotinic sites, 467–468, 467*b*
Nightstick fractures, 429
Nikolsky sign, 174, 175*f*, 270
Nitrites, UTIs and, 137
Nitrous oxide, 336
NMS. *See* Neuroleptic malignant syndrome
Nodules, 255*t*
Noncardiogenic pulmonary edema (NCPE), 90–91, 91*f*, 382, 450
Nondepolarizing blockade, 8, 9*t*
Nondepolarizing neuromuscular junction blocking agents, 229

Nonesophageal foreign bodies, 116
Nongonococcal arthritis, 244–249
Nongonococcal cervicitis, 327–328
Noninflammatory polyarticular arthritis, 249, 252
Noninvasive compression, 12–13
Nonketotic hyperosmolar coma, 198–199
Nonoliguric, 141
Nonrebreather mask, 10
Nonsexually transmitted epididymitis, 149
Non-ST elevation MI, 30*f*, 33
Nonsteroidal anti-inflammatory drugs (NSAIDs)
  for back pain, 243
  for crystal-induced arthritis, 249
  for migraine, 212
  for osteoarthritis, 253
  for otitis media, 289
  for sickle cell anemia, 393
Nonstrangulatory sigmoid volvulus, 123
Nonsuppurative meningitis, 179
Nonunion, 433
Norwalk agent, 118
Nose
  altered mental status and, 207
  epistaxis, 293–295, 296*f*
  foreign body in, 293
  fractures of, 295–297
  sinusitis, 292–293
NSAIDs. *See* Nonsteroidal anti-inflammatory drugs
Nursemaids' elbow, 429

O
Oblique fracture line, 420, 420*f*
Obturator sign, 132
Occult bacteremia, 359
Ocular toxicity, 463
Oliguric, 141
Omnibus Budget Reconciliation Act, 496
Oncologic emergencies
  clinical features of, 397–398, 398*f*
  differential diagnosis for, 398
  discussion of, 396–397, 397*b*
  evaluation of, 398–399
  therapy for, 399–400
One-way catheter insertion, for pneumothorax, 105
OPA. *See* Oropharyngeal airway
Open chest compression, 13
Open fracture, 420
Open pneumothorax, 406
Opiate
  ingestion, 445
  overdose, 459–460
Opioid toxidrome, 445*b*
Optic neuritis, 278
Oral candidiasis, 263
Orbital cellulitis, 280*f*, 281–282, 281*b*
Orbital fractures, 286–287
Orchiopexy, 149
Orchitis, 150
Organic brain disorders, 306–307
Organomegaly, 109*b*, 208
Organophosphates, 467–468, 467*b*
Oropharyngeal airway (OPA), 3
Oropharyngeal dysphagia, 113
Oropharyngeal odynophagia, 112
Orotracheal intubation, 4, 4*t*
Orthopedic emergencies
  complications of, 433
  diagnosis of, 421–422
  management of, 423–424, 424*b*
  types of, 419–421, 420*f*, 421*f*
Osler nodes, 72
Ossicles, 291
Osteoarthritis, 240, 244, 249–250, 252–253
Osteomyelitis, 177–178, 236, 433

Otitis externa, 288–289
Otitis media, 289–290
   in pediatric patients, 352–354
Ovarian carcinoma, 329b
Ovarian cyst, 312–314, 329
Ovarian torsion, 313–314
Oxybutynin therapy, 141
Oxygen administration, 2, 10

P

Pacemaker, prophylactic placement of, 36
Packed red blood cells (PRBCs), 380–381
Paget disease, 236
Pain
   abdominal. See Abdominal pain
   with appendicitis, 131–132
   back. See Back pain
   burning, 107
   chest. See Chest pain
   with cholecystitis, 130
   control for, 442–443
   neck. See Neck pain
   in pediatric patient, 335–337
   pelvic, 312–314
   periumbilical, 134
Pain-induced syncope, 52
Palmar erythema, 109
Palpation, 109b, 422
Pancreatic injuries, 409
Pancreatitis, 128–130, 129f
Panic attacks, 308–309, 308t
Papillary muscle rupture, 36
Papillitis, 278
Papules, 255t
Papulosquamous eruptions, 259–260, 260f, 261f
Parainfluenza virus 3, 345
Parallel margin infiltration, 436
Parapharyngeal abscess, 299
Paraphimosis, 140, 147, 147f
Parasitic infections, 178–180, 178f
Parasitic skin infections
   pediculosis, 266
   scabies, 156, 265–266, 265f
Paronychia, 426
Parotitis, 150
Paroxysmal supraventricular tachycardia,
   resuscitation with, 19–20, 21f
Partial seizures, 223, 374
Parturition, complications of, 323–326
Pasteurella multocida, 171, 176
Patches, 255t
Pathologic fractures, 420
Pathologic postural syncope, 52
Patient confidentiality, 493, 494b
Patient transfer laws, 495–496
PCP. See Pneumocystis carinii pneumonia
Peak expiratory flow rate (PEFR)
   for asthma, 86
   for COPD, 89, 89t
Peau d'orange, 176
Pediatric patients
   approach to, 331–334, 332b
   bacteremia, meningitis, and sepsis in, 359–361
   child abuse, 376–378
   congenital heart disease, 354–357
   foreign bodies, 339–342, 340b, 341f
   gastrointestinal disorders in
      appendicitis, 372–373
      gastroenteritis, 361–363
      incarcerated hernia, 367–368, 367b
      intestinal obstruction, 364–366, 365f
      intussusception, 369–370
      Meckel diverticulum, 370–371
      pyloric stenosis, 368–369
      volvulus, 366–367
   Kawasaki disease, 357–359

otitis media, 352–354
pain in, 335–337
respiratory tract infections in
   bronchiolitis, 345–347
   epiglottitis, 348–350
   laryngotracheobronchitis, 342–345
   pharyngitis, 347–348
   pneumonia syndrome, 350–352
seizures in, 373–376, 373b
SIDS, 337–339, 338b
trauma, 413–414, 413b
Pedicle injury, 410, 411f
Pediculosis, 266
Pediculosis pubis, 143t, 146
PEFR. See Peak expiratory flow rate
Pelvic brim, 138
Pelvic inflammatory disease (PID), 166, 168,
   312–313, 328–329
Pelvic pain, 312–314
Pelvic trauma, 409–410
Pelvis
   injuries to, 431
   in pediatric patients, 333
Pemphigus vulgaris, 259
Penetrating injury
   abdominal, 409
   chest, 406–408, 407b
Penis
   injury to, 412
   problems of, 146–148, 147f, 147f, 148b
Pentad of Reynold, 130
PERC. See Pulmonary Embolism Rule Out Criteria
Percussion, 109b
Percutaneous suturing, 439–440, 440f
Percutaneous transluminal coronary angioplasty
   (PTCA), for myocardial infarction, 35
Perforated peptic ulcers, 26, 117
Perianal abscess, 126–127
Pericardial disease, 61–66, 62t, 63f
Pericardial effusion, 62t, 64
Pericardial friction rub, 63
Pericardial tamponade, 407–408
Pericardiocentesis, 64–65
Pericarditis, 27
   acute, 62–64, 62t, 63f
   constrictive, 65–66
Perilunate injuries, 428, 428f
Periodic paralysis, 227
Periodontal abscesses, 300–301
Periorbital cellulitis, 280–281, 280f
Peripheral artery disease, 76–79, 77t, 78f
Peripheral chemoreceptors, 2
Peripheral nerve block, 336
Peripheral neuropathies, 225–226
Peripheral pauciarticular arthritis, 250
Peripheral polyarthritis, 250
Peripheral polyarticular arthritis, 250
Peripheral vertigo, 221–222, 222t
Peristalsis, 109b
Peritoneal signs, 109b, 364
Peritonitis, 116
Peritonsillar abscess, 297–298, 297f, 343, 349
Peritonsillar cellulitis, 297–298
Periumbilical pain, 134
Perniosis, 475
Pertussis syndrome, 345
Petechiae, 176, 377
Phalanx fractures, 427, 432
Pharyngeal diphtheria, 170
Pharyngeal gonorrhea, 166, 170
Pharyngitis
   in pediatric patients, 347–348
   streptococcal, 169–170, 170b
Phimosis, 140, 146, 147f
Phlegmasia alba dolens, 80
Phlegmasia cerulea dolens, 80

Phosphate replacement, 187
   for diabetic ketoacidosis, 198
   for nonketotic hyperosmolar coma, 199
Phthiriasis, 143t, 146
Physical abuse, 376
Physical neglect, 376
Physical restraint, 307
Physostigmine salicylate, 466
PID. See Pelvic inflammatory disease
Pill esophagitis, 112
Pinworm infection, 178–179, 178f
Pit vipers, 484
Pityriasis rosea, 260, 261f
Pityrosporum ovale, 278
Placenta abruption, 319–321
Placental previa, 319–321
Plantar fasciitis, 251
Plaques, 255t
Platelet abnormalities, 390
Platelet infusion, 380–381
   for esophageal varices, 114
   protocol for, 381
   for sepsis, 155
Pleural effusion, 97–98, 98t
Pneumococcal vaccination, 156
Pneumocystis carinii, 99, 101
Pneumocystis carinii pneumonia (PCP), 156, 158,
   160–161, 351
Pneumonia, 26, 39, 99–102, 99t, 101t, 102t, 109
   in pediatric patients, 350–352
Pneumothorax, 26, 88, 104–106, 105b, 105f, 406, 408
Podagra, 246
Police holds, 495
Polyarthralgia, 252
Polyarticular arthritis
   clinical features of, 250–252
   differential diagnosis for, 252
   discussion of, 249–250
   disposition of, 253
   evaluation of, 248t, 252–253
   therapy for, 253
Polymorphic VT, resuscitation with, 21, 21f
Polymyositis, 227–228
Pork tapeworm, 179
Porphyrias, 387
Postcardiac injury pericarditis, 62
Posterior shoulder delivery, 325
Post–lumbar puncture headache, 213, 213b
Post-MI pericarditis, 62
Postmortem evaluation, 338, 338b
Postpartum hemorrhage, 325–326
Postpericardiotomy syndrome, 62
Postprandial hypoglycemia, 196
Postreduction immobilization, 424, 424b
Posttraumatic pericarditis, 62
Postural syncope, 52
Potassium hydroxide (KOH) slide preparation, 254,
   264
Potassium imbalance, 186–189, 187f, 188f
Potassium replacement, 186
   for diabetic ketoacidosis, 198
   for nonketotic hyperosmolar coma, 199
Povidone–iodine solutions, 435
Poxvirus, 146
Pralidoxime, 468
PRBCs. See Packed red blood cells
Prediabetic glucose intolerance, 196
Preeclampsia, 321–323, 322b
Preexcitation syndromes, 49
Pregnancy. See also Parturition
   ectopic. See Ectopic pregnancy
   hypertension in, 321–323, 322b
   molar, 318–319, 318f
   respiratory alkalosis with, 193
   resuscitation with, 24
   right upper quadrant pain in, 127
   sickle cell disease in, 394

thoracic aortic dissection with, 75
trauma in, 414–416, 415*b*
vaginal bleeding during
  first-trimester, 317–319, 317*b*, 318*f*
  second- and third-trimester, 319–321
Prehn's sign, 149–150
Premature junctional beats, 46
Premature labor, 324–325
Premature membrane rupture, 324
Premature ventricular contractions (PVCs), 47
Priapism, 148, 148*b*, 392*b*, 394
Primary hypothermia, 473
Primary myocardial disease
  cardiomyopathies, 67–71, 68*t*, 70*f*
  myocarditis, 66–67
Primary syphilis, 143–144, 143*t*, 167
Prinzmetal angina, 29
Proctitis, 168
Prodromal phase, 127
Prolapsed umbilical cord, 325
Prophylactic pacemaker placement, 36
Prostate
  enlargement of, 140
  problems of, 151–152, 151*t*
Prostatitis, 151
  acute, 151–152, 151*t*
  chronic, 152, 151*t*
  nonbacterial, 152, 151*t*
Prostatodynia, 152
Prosthetic valves, 71, 72*t*
Proteinuria, 154
Proteus, 136, 151–152
Prothrombin, 386
Protozoal gastroenteritis, 119
Proximal DVT, 80
Proximal humerus fracture, 429
Proximate cause, 492*b*
Pseudogout, 244–249
Pseudohyperkalemia, 188
Pseudohyponatremia, 184
Pseudomembranous enterocolitis, 119
Pseudomonas, 99–101, 136, 149, 151–152, 288
Pseudomonas aeruginosa, 156, 177, 245, 441
Psoas sign, 132
Psoriasis, 259–260, 260*f*
Psoriatic arthritis, 250–253
Psychogenic syncope, 54
Psychosis, 306–307
PTCA. *See* Percutaneous transluminal coronary
  angioplasty
Pubic lice, 143*t*, 146
Pulmonary atresia, 355
Pulmonary contusion, 407
Pulmonary edema
  clinical features of, 38–39
  differential diagnosis of, 39
  discussion of, 38–39
  disposition of, 41
  evaluation of, 39–40, 40*f*
  mitral regurgitation and, 58–59
  therapy for, 40–41
Pulmonary embolism, 26
  clinical features of, 94
  differential diagnoses for, 94
  disposition of, 97
  evaluation of, 94–96, 94*b*, 94*t*, 95*b*, 95*f*, 96*f*
  therapy for, 96–97
Pulmonary Embolism Rule Out Criteria (PERC),
  94, 95*b*
Pulmonary embolus, 39
Pulmonary fat embolus, 433
Pulmonary hypertension, 61
Pulmonary infarction, anemia and, 392*b*
Pulmonary laceration, 407
Pulmonic regurgitation, 61
Pulmonic stenosis, 61
Pulmonic valve disease, 61

Pulseless electrical activity (PEA)
  with pulmonary embolism, 94
  resuscitation with, 17–18, 20*f*
Pulsus paradoxus, 64
Puncture wounds, 441
Pupils
  altered mental status and, 207
  inspection of, 272
Pure red cell aplasia, 388–389
Purpura fulminans, 395
Pustular dermatitis syndrome, 166
Pustules, 255*t*
PVCs. *See* Premature ventricular contractions
Pyelonephritis, 136–138
Pyloric stenosis, in pediatric patients, 368–369
Pyridoxine, 225, 464*b*
Pyrimethamine, 160
Pyuria, 137, 149–150

Q

Q fever, 182
Quincke pulse, 57

R

Rabies, 164–165
Rabies immune globulin, 165
Raccoon's eyes, 207
Radial head subluxation, 429
Radial shaft fracture, 429
Radiation, 471*b*
Radiography
  for foreign bodies, 341, 341*f*
  for orthopedic emergencies, 422–423
  in pediatric patients, 333
Range-of-motion testing, 242, 422
Ranson criteria, 129–130
Rapid sequence intubation (RSI)
  guidelines for, 5, 6*t*
  indications and contraindications for, 4–5
  neuromuscular blockade for, 8–9, 9*t*
  overview of, 4
  pharmacologic adjuncts for, 5
  unawareness induction, 5–8, 6*t*–7*t*
Rash, 262, 262*f*, 266–268
RBCs. *See* Red blood cells
Reactive airway disease, 345
Recombinant Factor VII, for esophageal varices,
  114
Rectal prolapse, 179
Red blood cells (RBCs)
  for esophageal varices, 114
  formulations of, 380
  mechanical disruption of, 387
  for sepsis, 155
Red cell aplasia, 387
Reduction, 424
Reentrant supraventricular tachycardia, 45–46, 45*f*
Reflex (hypertonic) bladder, 141
Reflexes, 210, 210*b*
Refractory anaphylaxis, 233
Refusal, 493
Regional anesthesia, 436
Regional lymphadenopathy, 143
Reiter syndrome, 250–251, 253
Relapsing fever, 182
Renal calculi, 138*b*
Renal colic, 135
Renal failure
  AKI, 141–143, 142*t*
  chronic kidney disease, 143
  metabolic acidosis and, 194
Renal injuries, 410, 411*f*, 412
Renal pelvis, 138
Renal tubular acidosis, 186
Reperfusion arrhythmias, 35
Reperfusion injury, 35

Reperfusion therapy
  for cardiogenic shock, 37
  for myocardial infarction, 34–35
Reportable conditions, 493, 494*b*
Rescue breathing, 10
Respiration, 471*b*
Respiration effectors, 2
Respiratory acidosis, 192–193, 192*b*
Respiratory alkalosis, 192*b*, 193–194
Respiratory control center, 2
Respiratory syncytial virus, 345
Respiratory tract infections
  in pediatric patients
    bronchiolitis, 345–347
    epiglottitis, 348–350
    laryngotracheobronchitis, 342–345
    pharyngitis, 347–348
    pneumonia syndrome, 350–352
  upper. *See* Upper respiratory tract infections
Rest, immobilization, compression and cold packs,
  and elevation (RICE), 423
Restrictive cardiomyopathy, 68*t*, 70–71
Resuscitation
  airway, 3–9, 4*t*–7*t*, 9*t*
  breathing, 9–11
  circulation, 11–16, 15*t*–18*t*, 19*f*
  maternal, 323
  for near-drowning or submersion incident, 23
  with pregnancy, 24
  prognosis for, 1
  for SIDS, 338
  termination of, 1
Resuscitation catheters, 14–16, 15*t*–18*t*, 19*f*
Retinal detachment, 277–278
Retinal hemorrhages, 377
Retrobulbar neuritis, 278
Retrograde wire intubation, 9
Retropharyngeal abscess, 299–300, 343, 349
Reverse Monteggia fracture, 429
Rhabdomyolysis, 228
Rheumatic endocarditis, 55
Rheumatic fever, 71
Rheumatic heart disease, 56–58, 60
Rheumatoid arthritis, 250–253
Rheumatoid nodules, 251
Rh incompatibility hemolysis, 382
Rho(D) immune globulin, 415
Rhus dermatitis, 261–262
Rhythm disturbances. *See also* Dysrhythmias
  disorders of cardiac conduction, 48–49
  supraventricular dysrhythmias, 42–47, 43*t*–44*t*,
    45*f*, 47*f*
  ventricular dysrhythmias, 47–48, 47*f*
Rib fractures, 408
RICE. *See* Rest, immobilization, compression and
  cold packs, and elevation
Rickettsia rickettsii, 181, 350
Right lower quadrant pain, 107, 131–132
Right-sided heart strain, with pulmonary embolism, 95
Right upper quadrant pain, 107, 130
  in pregnancy, 127
Ringworm, 263
Rinne-Weber hearing tests, 291
Rocky Mountain spotted fever, 181–182, 358
Roentgenographic examination, 341
Roseola infantum, 267–268
Rotavirus, 118
Rovsing sign, 109*b*, 132, 372
Rubeola. *See* Measles
Rule of nines, 416*b*, 417*f*
Rule of palms, 416*b*
Rumack-Matthew nomogram, 448, 448*f*

S

SAD PERSONS suicide risk scale, 311, 311*b*
SAH. *See* Subarachnoid hemorrhage

Salicylate therapy, 358–359
Salicylate toxicity, 193, 449–451
Salmonella, 245
Salmonellosis, 118, 159, 177
Salpingitis, 315
Salter-Harris fractures, 421, 421f
Sarcoptes scabiei, 265
Scabies, 156, 265–266, 265f
Scalp wounds, 404, 413
Scaphoid fracture, 425b, 426f, 428
Scarlet fever, 268, 358
Schistosomiasis, 179
Schizophrenia, 306–307
Sclerotherapy, for peptic ulcer disease, 118
Scorpion stings, 488–489
Scrotum, problems of, 150–151
Seborrheic blepharitis, 278–279
Secondary bacteremia, 359
Secondary hypothermia, 473
Secondary syphilis, 167, 168f
Second-degree AV block, 48
Second-degree burn, 416
Seizures, 54, 222–225
  in pediatric patients, 373–376, 373b
  treatment of, 404
Sengstaken-Blakemore, 114
Sensory examination, 210, 210f
Sepsis, 153–156, 154b, 156t, 157t
  in pediatric patients, 359–361
Septic abortion, 317b
Septic arthritis, 244–249, 427
Septic shock, Boerhaave syndrome and, 112
Sequestration crisis, 391
Serratia marcescens, 177
Sexual abuse, 376
Sexually transmitted diseases
  AIDS. *See* AIDS
  chlamydia, 168
  gonorrhea, 166–167
  herpes, 169, 169f
  syphilis, 167, 168f
  trichomoniasis, 168–169
Sexually transmitted epididymitis, 149
Shattered fracture, 420
Shattered kidney, 410, 411f
Shigellosis, 119, 159
Shingles. *See* Herpes zoster
Shoulder
  dystocia, 325
  injuries to, 429–430, 430b, 430f
  presentation of, 325
SIADH. *See* Syndrome of inappropriate antidiuretic hormone
Sickle cell anemia
  clinical features of, 391, 392b
  differential diagnosis for, 391–392
  discussion of, 390–391
  evaluation of, 392–393
  therapy for, 393–394
Sickle lung disease, 391
Sick sinus syndrome, 53
SIDS. *See* Sudden infant death syndrome
Sigmoidoscopy, 124
Simple alveolar fractures, 303
Simple partial seizures, 223
Simple pneumothorax, 104–106, 105f, 406
Sinus arrhythmia, 42
Sinus bradycardia, 46
Sinusitis, 292–293
Sinus tachycardia, 42
  with pulmonary embolism, 95
Six Ps, 78
Skin
  AIDS and, 156, 158, 158f
  cleansing of, 435–436
  lesions of, 254–255, 255b. *See also specific disorders*
  sepsis at, 153

SSSS, 174–175, 175f, 270–271, 271t
  TEN, 270, 271t
Skin biopsy, 255
Skin infections
  bacterial, 268–270, 269f
  fungal, 263–265, 264f
  parasitic, 156, 265–266, 265f
SLE. *See* Systemic lupus erythematosus
Sleeping sickness, 180
Slipped capital femoral epiphysis, 431
Small artery disease, 217
Small-bore thoracostomy tube, for pneumothorax, 105
Small bowel obstruction, 123
Smith fracture, 428
Smoke-related inhalation injuries, 482, 483b
Smoking
  abdominal pain and, 108
  COPD and, 88–89
  GERD and, 111
  wounds and, 434
Snakebites, venomous, 484–486
Snellen eye chart, 272
Sodium imbalance, 184–186
Sodium reduction, 185
Sodium replacement, 185
Sphenopalatine artery, 294
Spider bites, 486–488
Spina bifida, 240
Spinal cord compression, 141, 238, 241, 397b, 398–400
Spinal injuries, 404–405, 404b, 413
Spinal shock, 404
Spinal stenosis, 240, 244
Spiral fracture line, 420, 420f
Spleen, 409
Splenomegaly, 390
Splinting, 423, 424b
Spondylarthritides, 251, 253
Spondylolisthesis, 240, 244
Spondylolysis, 240, 244
Spontaneous hypoglycemia, 196
Spontaneous pneumothorax, 104–106, 105f
Sprain, 419, 423
  ankle, 432
  finger, 427
  knee, 432
SSSS. *See* Staphylococcal scalded skin syndrome
Stable angina, 26, 29–31
Stab wounds, 409
Staphylococcal cellulitis, 177
Staphylococcal food poisoning, 119
Staphylococcal scalded skin syndrome (SSSS), 174–175, 175f, 270–271, 271t
Staphylococcus, 426
Staphylococcus aureus, 99, 119, 156, 177, 245, 268–269, 278–279
Staphylococcus epidermidis, 278
Staples, 440
Status epilepticus, 223–224, 374, 376
ST elevation MI, 30f–31f, 33
Stevens-Johnson syndrome, 258–259, 258f
Stokes-Adams syndrome, 53
Straight leg raising, 242
Strain, 419
Strangulated hernia, 133
Streptococcal cellulitis, 177
Streptococcal pharyngitis, 169–170, 170b
Streptococcal toxic shock–like syndrome, 176
Streptococcus, 269, 426
Streptococcus pneumoniae, 90, 99–101, 154, 289, 359
Streptococcus pyogenes, 176
Stress fractures, 420
Stridor, 343
String-of-pearls sign, 123
Stroke
  clinical features of, 217, 217b, 218f
  discussion of, 216

evaluation of, 217–219, 217b, 218f, 219f
  therapy for, 219–220, 220b
Strongyloides stercoralis, 179
Struvite stones, 138b
Subarachnoid hemorrhage (SAH), 214–215, 215f, 402, 403f
Subchorionic hemorrhage, 319–321
Subclavian steal, 53
Subclavian vein, 15–16, 17t, 19f
Subdiaphragmatic abscesses, 26
Subdural hematomas, 377, 402, 403f, 413
Subluxation, of teeth, 302–303
Submersion incident, resuscitation for, 23
Subtrochanteric fractures, 431
Sudden infant death syndrome (SIDS), 337–339, 338b
Suicide, depression and, 310–311, 311b
Superficial hordeola, 279
Superficial thrombophlebitis, 82–83
Superior vena cava syndrome, 397, 397b, 398f, 399–400
Supplemental oxygen, 10
Supralevator abscess, 126
Supraventricular dysrhythmias
  atrial fibrillation, 42, 45
  atrial flutter, 42, 43t–44t, 45f
  junctional arrhythmias, 46–47, 47f
  multifocal atrial tachycardia, 42
  sinus arrhythmia, 42
  sinus bradycardia, 46
  sinus tachycardia, 42
  supraventricular tachycardia, 45–46, 45f
  wandering atrial pacemaker, 42
Supraventricular tachycardia, 45–46, 45f
Sutures, 439–440, 440f
Swallowing, assessment of, 3
Swelling, 423
Swyer-James syndrome. *See* Unilateral hyperlucent lung syndrome
Sympathomimetic toxidrome, 445b
Symptomatic anemia, 391
Syncope, 52–55
Syndrome of inappropriate antidiuretic hormone (SIADH), 396–400
Syphilis, 167, 168f
  with AIDS, 156
  primary, 143–144, 167
  secondary, 167, 168f
  tertiary, 167
Systemic inflammatory response syndrome criteria, 153, 154b
Systemic lupus erythematosus (SLE), 250–252
Systemic vascular resistance, 470
Systolic click–murmur syndrome, 59
Systolic murmur, 69

T
T₃. *See* Triiodothyronine
T₄. *See* Thyroxine
Tachycardias
  junctional, 47
  multifocal atrial, 42
  paroxysmal supraventricular, 19–20, 21f
  pediatric, 413
  sinus, 42
  supraventricular, 45–46, 45f
  ventricular, 20–21, 21f
  ventricular (wide-complex), 47–48, 47f
  wide-complex supraventricular, 45
Tachydysrhythmia, 53
Tachypnea, 10
  with asthma, 86
  with NCPE, 90
  pediatric, 413
  with pulmonary embolism, 94
Taenia saginata, 179
Taenia solium, 179

Tapes, 441
Tapeworm infections, 179
Teeth
  abscesses, 300–301
  anatomy of, 300, 301f
  avulsion, 303
  cavities of, 300
  fractures of, 301–302, 302b, 302f
  subluxation or intrusion of, 302–303
Temporal arteritis, 214
TEN. *See* Toxic epidermal necrolysis
Tendinitis, 236
Tendon injuries, of hand, 427
Tenosynovitis, 426–427
Tension pneumothorax, 26, 104–106, 105b, 105f, 406, 408
Terbinafine, 263–265
Tertiary syphilis, 167
Testicular appendage torsion, 149
Testicular injury, 412
Testicular masses, 150
Testicular torsion, 148–150
Tetanospasmin, 165
Tetanus, 165–166, 166b
  immunization to, 434
Tetanus immune globulin, 166
Tetanus toxoid, 166
Tetralogy of Fallot, 355, 357
Thalassemias, 387
Thiamine, 197, 200, 207, 225, 445, 464b
Thiopental, 5, 6t–7t, 7
Third-degree AV block, 48
Third-degree burn, 416
Thoracentesis, for pleural effusion, 98, 98t
Thoracic and lumbar back pain. *See* Back pain
Thoracic aortic dissection, 74–76, 76f
Thoracic outlet syndrome, 236
Thoracic pump theory, 12
Thoracic trauma, 406–408, 407b
Threadworm infection, 179
Threatened abortion, 317b
Throat
  altered mental status and, 207
  Ludwig angina, 298–299
  parapharyngeal abscess, 299
  peritonsillar cellulitis and abscess, 297–298, 297f
  retropharyngeal abscess, 299–300
Thrombocytopenia, immune-mediated, 396
Thrombocytosis, 390
Thrombolysis, for myocardial infarction, 35, 35t
Thrombotic strokes, 216
Thrush, 263
Thyroid function tests, 202–203
Thyroid-stimulating hormone (TSH), 202
Thyroid storm, 201–202
Thyroxine (T₄), 202, 204
TIA. *See* Transient ischemic attack
Tibia–femur dislocations, 432
Tibial plateau fractures, 432
Tibial shaft fractures, 432
Tick-borne disease
  babesiosis, 183
  Colorado tick fever, 183
  Lyme disease, 180–181, 181b
  Q fever, 182
  relapsing fever, 182
  Rocky Mountain spotted fever, 181–182
  tick paralysis, 182
  tularemia, 183
Tinea, 263–265, 264f
Tissue plasminogen activator, 220, 220b
Tocolysis, 325
Tonic–clonic seizures, 223, 374
Tonic seizures, 223
Toothache, 301
Tophi, 245
Torsades de pointes, 47. *See also* Polymorphic VT

Torticollis, 236
Torus fracture, 420, 421f
Total anomalous pulmonary venous return, 355–356
Toxic epidermal necrolysis (TEN), 174, 270, 271t
Toxic megacolon, 122
Toxicodendron dermatitis, 261–262
Toxicologic emergencies
  acetaminophen toxicity, 447–449, 448b, 448f
  β-adrenergic antagonist overdose, 455–457
  alcohols, 462–465, 463b, 464b
  anticholinergics, 466–467
  antipsychotic overdose, 454–455
  approach to, 444–447, 444b, 445b
  benzodiazepine overdose, 451–452
  calcium channel antagonist overdose, 457–458
  carbon monoxide, 465–466
  clonidine toxicity, 459
  digitalis toxicity, 458–459
  drugs of abuse, 459–462
  industrial chemicals, 467–469, 467b
  lithium toxicity, 453
  salicylate toxicity, 449–451
  tricyclic antidepressant overdose, 453–454
Toxicology screens, 446–447
Toxic shock syndrome (TSS), 174–175, 358
Toxidromes, 445, 445b
Toxoplasmosis, with AIDS, 158, 160
Tracheal foreign bodies, 340
Tracheitis, 343, 349
Tracheobronchial injuries, 407
Tracheostomy, for epiglottitis, 173
Tranexamic acid, 386
Transcutaneous pacing, 14, 22
Transesophageal echocardiography, for thoracic aortic dissection, 75
Transfusion
  blood components for, 380–381
  complications with, 382–383
  protocols for, 381–382
  for sepsis, 155
  for sickle cell anemia, 393–394
  for traumatic shock, 401–402
Transient arthritis, 358
Transient hypertension, 49
Transient ischemic attack (TIA), 220
Transposition of the great vessels, 355
Transtracheal jet insufflation, 9
Transvenous intrahepatic portosystemic shunt, 114
Transvenous pacing, 14
Transverse fracture line, 420, 420f
Transverse lie, 325
Trauma
  abdominal, 408–409, 408b, 409f
  approach to, 401, 402f
  of eyes, 284–288, 285f
  genitourinary, 410–413, 411f, 412b
  of hand, 427–428
  to head, 377, 402–404, 403f
  to neck, 405–406, 405f
  pediatric, 413–414, 413b
  pelvic, 409–410
  in pregnancy, 414–416, 415b
  to teeth, 301–303, 302b, 302f
  thoracic, 406–408, 407b
  vaginal bleeding with, 329
Traumatic arthritis, 433
Traumatic pneumothorax, 104–106, 105f
Traumatic shock, 401–402, 402b
Traveler's diarrhea, 119
Trench foot, 475–478, 476f
Treponema pallidum, 143, 161, 167
Triamcinolone acetonide, 260
Trichinellosis, 179
Trichomonas vaginalis, 136, 326
Trichomoniasis, 168–169, 326–327
Trichuris trichiura, 179
Tricuspid insufficiency, 60–61

Tricuspid regurgitation, 60–61
Tricuspid stenosis, 60
Tricuspid valve, Ebstein anomaly of the, 355
Tricuspid valve disease, 60–61
Tricyclic antidepressant overdose, 453–454
Trigeminal neuralgia, 214
Triiodothyronine (T₃), 202, 204
Triquetrum injuries, 428, 428f
Trismus, 297, 305
Truncus arteriosus, 356
Trypanosomiasis, 180
TSH. *See* Thyroid-stimulating hormone
TSS. *See* Toxic shock syndrome
Tubal adhesions, 315
Tuberculosis, 102–103, 103b
Tuberculous meningitis, 161–163
Tubo-ovarian abscess, 329
Tularemia, 183
Tumor lysis syndrome, 396–397, 399–400
Tumors. *See also* Oncologic emergencies
  of CNS, 215–216
  complications of, 397b
Tympanic membrane rupture, 291–292
Tympanometry, 353
Tympanostomy tube placement, 354
Typhoidal tularemia, 183
Typical pneumonia, 99
Tzanck slide preparation, 254
Tzanck smear, 144

U

Ulcerative colitis, 122
Ulceroglandular tularemia, 183
Ulcers, 258
Ultrasound
  for ectopic pregnancy, 316, 316f
  for intestinal obstruction, 365, 365f
  of molar pregnancy, 318, 318f
Ultraviolet light therapy, 260
Umbilical hernia, 133
Unawareness induction, 5–8, 6t–7t
Uncomplicated hypertension, 49
Unilateral hyperlucent lung syndrome, 345
Unstable angina, 29, 31–32
Upper arm injuries, 429
Upper extremity, innervation of, 239t
Upper respiratory tract infections
  diphtheria, 170–171
  epiglottitis, 171–173, 172f
  laryngitis, 173–174
  streptococcal pharyngitis, 169–170, 170b
Ureaplasma, 152
Urecholine therapy, 141
Uremia, 64
Uremic pericarditis, 62
Ureter injury, 411
Ureteropelvic junction, 138
Ureterovesical junction, 138
Urethra injury, 412–413, 412b
Urethral foreign bodies, 140, 148
Urethral strictures, 140
Urethritis, 136, 149, 166, 168
Uric acid stones, 138b, 139
Urinary alkalinization, 451
Urinary retention, 140–141
Urinary tract, sepsis at, 153
Urinary tract infections (UTIs), 136–138, 137t, 149, 312
Urticaria, 233–235
Urticarial vasculitis, 234
Urticaria pigmentosa, 234
Uterine dehiscence and rupture, 319–321
Uterine fibroids, 312
Uterine leiomyomas, 329b
Uterine rupture, 415
UTIs. *See* Urinary tract infections

Index

V

Vaccination
against *H. influenzae*, 156, 173
human diploid cell, 165
pneumococcal, 156
Vagal maneuvers, 20
Vaginal bleeding
abnormal, 329–330, 329*b*
during pregnancy
first-trimester, 317–319, 317*b*, 318*f*
second- and third-trimester, 319–321
Vaginitis, 136, 168–169, 312, 326–327
Valvulae conniventes, 123
Valvular disease
aortic, 55–57
mitral, 57–60
pulmonic, 61
tricuspid, 60–61
Vaporization, 343
Varicella (chickenpox), 255
Varices, esophageal, 114–115
Varicose veins, 82
Vascular disease
peripheral artery disease, 76–79, 77*t*, 78*f*
thoracic aortic dissection, 74–76, 76*f*
venous disease, 79–83, 80*t*–81*t*
Vascular disorders
abdominal aortic aneurysm, 134–135
mesenteric ischemia, 134
Vasoactive drugs, 52
Vaso-occlusive pain crisis, 391
Vasovagal syncope, 52
Venography, for DVT, 81
Venomous snakebites, 484–486
Venous disease, 79–83, 80*t*–81*t*
Venous insufficiency, chronic, 83
Venous valvular competence, 79
Ventilatory control, 2
Ventilatory support, 2, 10–11. *See also* Mechanical
ventilation
for acute respiratory failure, 85
Ventricular dysrhythmias, 47–48, 47*f*

Ventricular fibrillation (VF), 48
resuscitation with, 16–17, 20*f*
Ventricular tachycardia (VT), resuscitation with,
20–21, 21*f*
Ventricular (wide-complex) tachycardia, 47, 47*f*
Venturi mask, 10
Vertebrobasilar insufficiency, 221
Vertebrobasilar system, 217*b*, 219*f*
Vertigo, 221–222, 222*t*
Vesicles, 255*t*, 258
Vesicular lesions, 255–256, 256*f*
Vesiculobullous lesions
erythema multiforme, 256–258, 257*f*
pemphigus vulgaris, 259
Stevens-Johnson syndrome, 258–259, 258*f*
Vestibular neuritis, 221
VF. *See* Ventricular fibrillation
Vibrio parahaemolyticus gastroenteritis, 119
Vibrio vulnificus, 176
Video-assisted laryngoscopy, 9
Viral cervicitis, 327–328
Viral conjunctivitis, 282
Viral exanthems
erythema infectiosum, 267
German measles, 267
hand-foot-and-mouth syndrome, 268
measles, 266, 267*f*
roseola infantum, 267–268
Viral gastroenteritis, 118
Viral meningitis, 162–163
Viral pharyngitis, 347–348
Viral pneumonia, 351–352
Virchow triad, 79
Vision loss
branch retinal artery occlusion, 276
CRAO, 275–276, 275*f*, 276*f*
CRVO, 277, 277*f*
optic neuritis, 278
retinal detachment, 277–278
Volume expansion, 37
Volvulus, in pediatric patients, 366–367
von Willebrand disease, 383–384, 384*f*, 396*t*

V/Q scan, for pulmonary embolism, 96
VT. *See* Ventricular tachycardia

W

Wallenberg syndrome, 217, 219*f*
Wandering atrial pacemaker, 42
Warm autoimmune hemolysis, 387
Wash-out syndrome, 461
"Water-hammer" pulse, 57
Well criteria, 81–82, 81*t*, 94
Wenckebach block, 48
Wernicke-Korsakoff syndrome, 197, 445
Westermark sign, 95
Whiplash, 237
Whipworm infection, 179
Whistle-tip suction catheter, 291
Whole-bowel irrigation, 446
Wide-complex supraventricular tachycardia, 45
Wolff-Parkinson-White (WPW) syndrome, 49
Wood maneuver, 325
Wood's light examination, 254, 264
Wounds
care of, 435–438, 436*b*, 438*f*
closure of, 439–441, 439*t*, 440*f*
contraction of, 435*t*
evaluation of, 434–435
follow-up care of, 442–443, 443*b*, 443*t*
gunshot and stab, 409
healing stages, 435*t*
scalp, 404, 413
types of, 441–442
WPW syndrome. *See* Wolff-Parkinson-White
syndrome
Wrist injuries, 425–428, 425*b*, 426*f*, 428*f*

X

Xanthine stones, 138*b*, 139

Z

Zavanelli maneuver, 325
Zeis glands, 279
Zipper entrapment, 148

CD062022

Index